D0756745

The
CANNABIS
HEALTH
INDEX

Also by Uwe Blesching:

Spicy Healing: A Global Guide to Growing and Using Spices for Food and Medicine

Cuba's Carnival: Origins of the Biggest Party on Earth

How the Old Man Learned to Smile

The

CANNABIS
HEALTH
INDEX

Combining the Science
of Medical Marijuana
with Mindfulness
Techniques to Heal
100 Chronic Symptoms
and Diseases

Uwe Blesching, PhD

North Atlantic Books
Berkeley, California

Copyright © 2013, 2015 by Uwe Blesching. All rights reserved. No portion of this book, except for brief review, may be reproduced, stored in a retrieval system, or transmitted in any form or by any means—electronic, mechanical, photocopying, recording, or otherwise—without the written permission of the publisher. For information contact North Atlantic Books.

Published by
North Atlantic Books
Berkeley, California

Cover photo © underworld/shutterstock.com
Cover design by Howie Severson
Interior design by Brad Greene

Printed in the United States of America

The Cannabis Health Index: Combining the Science of Medical Marijuana with Mindfulness Techniques to Heal 100 Chronic Symptoms and Diseases is sponsored and published by the Society for the Study of Native Arts and Sciences (dba North Atlantic Books), an educational nonprofit based in Berkeley, California, that collaborates with partners to develop cross-cultural perspectives, nurture holistic views of art, science, the humanities, and healing, and seed personal and global transformation by publishing work on the relationship of body, spirit, and nature.

North Atlantic Books' publications are available through most bookstores. For further information, visit our website at www.northatlanticbooks.com or call 800-733-3000.

MEDICAL DISCLAIMER: The following information is intended for general information purposes only. Individuals should always see their health care provider before administering any suggestions made in this book. Any application of the material set forth in the following pages is at the reader's discretion and is his or her sole responsibility.

DISCLAIMER: The following information is intended for general information purposes only. The publisher does not advocate illegal activities but does believe in the right of individuals to have free access to information and ideas. Any application of the material set forth in the following pages is at the reader's discretion and is his or her sole responsibility.

Library of Congress Cataloging-in-Publication Data

Blesching, Uwe, 1958-
    The cannabis health index : combining the science of medical marijuana with mindfulness techniques to heal 100 chronic symptoms and diseases / Uwe Blesching, PhD.
        pages cm
    First published: Berkeley, Calif. : Logos Publishing House, [2013].
    ISBN 978-1-58394-962-7 (pbk.) — ISBN 978-1-58394-963-4 (ebook)
    1. Cannabis—Therapeutic use. 2. Marijuana—Therapeutic use. 3. Medicine, Psychosomatic. 4. Mind and body. I. Title.
    RM666.C266B54 2015
    615.7827—dc23
                                                                        2014043656

3 4 5 6 UNITED 19 18 17
Printed on recycled paper
North Atlantic Books is committed to the protection of our environment.
We partner with FSC-certified printers using soy-based inks and
print on recycled paper whenever possible.

CONTENTS

Chapter III

How to Use The Cannabis Health Index (CHI)

Chapter IV

Diseases and Symptoms A–Z

Chapter V

Integrating Mind-Body Medicine for Deeper Healing 473

PREFACE

Allow me to tell you the story of how, when I was a mobile intensive-care paramedic in San Francisco, I witnessed the murder of a patient and how my partner and I used magic to bring him back to life.

It was late, a few hours past midnight, and the storefront lights on Chestnut Street were dim. The streets were empty except for some late-night clubbers looking for a taxi. We had been working a string of highly stressful emergencies nonstop for twenty-three hours with no sleep and little time to eat. We were burned out in attitude and exhausted in body when we got a call for an unconscious person lying on the sidewalk.

Lights and sirens on, our ambulance was briefly airborne as we flew over the top of the steep hill on Franklin. We came down hard and sped on until we found the person lying face down on the sidewalk in front of an elegant store selling evening gowns. He was oozing bodily fluids from every orifice.

We did a quick, head-to-toe assessment: no signs of blood or broken bones, blood test for sugar within normal limits, no sign of recent injection. The patient's pupils were dilated, so we could rule out narcotics overdose. I got the gurney and aligned it next to his limp 220-pound body. Lifting him was difficult and strenuous. Once he was in the ambulance, I placed an EKG monitor on his chest and fitted an oxygen mask over his face. He was breathing okay; pulse oximeter was a bit low but not too bad; his cardiac rhythm was normal.

My partner, as he was trying to adjust the gurney's safety belts, slipped. He tried to break his fall by bracing himself against the gurney and his hand ended up in the wet, warm puddle that had pooled between the patient's legs.

"Just die," he said, following up this fatigue-induced directive with an expletive.

I looked at the monitor at that very moment. The patient's normal heart rhythm instantly flat-lined. My partner and I looked at each other. All of our exhaustion and bad attitude was washed away by an immediate flood of adrenalin. We initiated CPR, and I placed a tube in the patient's lungs while my partner hooked up an intravenous line.

I injected the first ampule of epinephrine into his system. No response. He was still flat-lining.

Without making the conscious connection to what had happened a few minutes earlier, I yelled, "Come on! Stay with us!"

Nothing happened.

"Come back!" I shouted again, but this time I followed the command with a colorful expletive. To my surprise and instant relief, his heart started to beat again. His breathing returned spontaneously and his oxygen saturation improved dramatically.

The rest of the transport to the emergency room was uneventful. Later we learned that our passenger had overdosed on GHB (a euphoria-inducing substance known to most people as the "date rape drug"). The patient was kept at the hospital for a day and released the next morning with no complications.

I, however, was put on a fast track to studying anything I could find about mind-body medicine and that elusive bridge between them. Little did I know that the scientific evidence would lead me directly to the recent discovery of the body's own endocannabinoid system.

INTRODUCTION: YOU'RE SICK!

You're sick with a chronic condition. In a world of cause and effect, the exact cause of most chronic illnesses escapes modern medicine. To make things worse, cures are few and far between. In many cases, the best you can hope for is to be managed by pharmaceuticals . . . in other words, by the mighty corporate world.

Should you manage to make it to the doctor's office, what may make you even sicker is to find out the hard way that only about 15% of medical interventions are actually based on solid scientific evidence.[1] Even if the actual evidence were double that estimate, it would still seem like a walk somewhere between a wish and a prayer.

How can that be? For instance, when Vioxx entered the market it was approved (i.e., tested for) an immune deficiency disease called rheumatoid arthritis. However, once it was on the market, doctors quickly began prescribing it to patients with various conditions, a common practice called "off-label use." By the time the medical community caught up with the deadly reality, Vioxx had killed an estimated 55,000 to 500,000 patients by causing heart attacks and strokes. The company settled the resulting class-action lawsuit for a little less than US$5 billion. Sounds tough, but they still made about ten billion in revenue over the life of the drug.

Consider this: the Food and Drug Administration (FDA) actually has very little power and in fact does not approve drugs or devices but only the marketing of them. Before the FDA approves the marketing of a drug, the pharmaceutical company has to prove that it is more or less safe and that it is more effective than a placebo. Once the company has done so (usually at significant expense), the drug or device enters the market.

Many of us make the mistake of assuming that because of the successes of some specialized fields within medicine—such as emergency medicine or reconstructive plastic surgery, which are predominantly evidence-based—that all of medicine, especially those branches that treat chronic degenerative illness, follows the same ideals. Not true, as cases like the Vioxx scandal clearly show.

So what is one to do? Well, don't fret—change is in the air. Concerned doctors and patients' advocates alike have been pushing for a different approach to medical decision-making such as that of the Cochrane Collaboration and Library. Currently, Cochrane consist of thousands of health care practitioners, researchers, and advocates from more than 120 nations with the purpose of providing and promoting evidence-informed health decisions by producing high-quality, relevant, accessible systematic reviews and other research evidence.

Here's their definition: "Evidence-based medicine is the conscientious, explicit, and judicious use of current best evidence in making decisions about the care of individual patients. The practice of evidence-based medicine means integrating individual clinical expertise with the best available external clinical evidence from systematic research."[2]

To date, demand for evidence-driven health care has prompted the U.S. Department of Health to fund 13 evidence-based practice centers located throughout the country, such as the Mayo Clinic, Duke University, and Johns Hopkins, for example.[3]

Over the past twenty years the available scientific literature on medical cannabis has grown to more than 15,000 entries at the National Library of Health. But a systematic evidence-based model of the plant's safe and targeted use has largely been lacking—until now.

The Cannabis Health Index (CHI) is an evidence-based compilation and review of the available literature relevant to more than 100 different chronic diseases or stubborn symptoms. The CHI model takes into consideration the practical value of each study design (such as studies conducted in the laboratory on one hand, and double-blind, placebo-controlled human trials on the other) as well as the key findings. Is cannabis a viable treatment for your chronic condition, your stubborn symptom, or do studies say it doesn't work? The Cannabis Health Index rates on a scale ranging from possible to probable to actual and gives therapeutic evidence for a particular illness or symptom. In other words, the CHI rating system shows current degrees of confidence at a quick glance.

Equipped with evidence-based research results at your fingertips, the task of making more informed decisions about medical cannabis becomes practical and doable.

The Cannabis Health Index features an additional innovation that many readers may find helpful. The book combines and correlates evidence-based research results and specific techniques from mind-body medicine for your consideration. In other words, physical scientific evidence is presented alongside well-studied theories of psychological and emotional involvement in disease states.

The Cannabis Health Index features a free app and companion monthly eMagazine that support, supplement, and update the book. The CHI app puts evidence-based medicine for over 100 diseases at your fingertips. It provides the same rating system as the book, making it easy to determine at a glance what the current scientific consensus says about how cannabis may work for a specific condition. *CHI Magazine* explores how the endocannabinoid system works as a bridge between the body and the mind. Monthly editions examine new research and offer innovative articles on topics such as mind-body medicine, cannabinoid-based medicine, and emotional intelligence.

As many patients have discovered, whenever we engage in the process of exploring and learning about evidence-based medicine and include a mind-body approach, we are empowered to make more informed decisions. Better decisions mean we have access to more options and possibilities for regaining our health and fully healing.

Cannabis Health Index

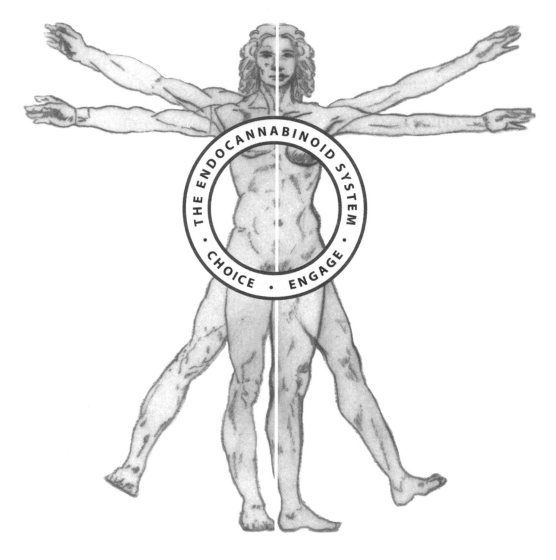

Using the **CHI** for health and healing

Chapter I

The Evidence-Based Science of Medical Cannabis

The Endocannabinoid System (A Brief Introduction)

All mammals have an endocannabinoid system (ECS). The ECS is involved in many important functions, including initiating a host of physiological and psychological changes needed to adjust to ever-changing internal and external environments. This is true from the very beginning of life, when ECS signaling determines if a fertilized egg will implant in the uterine wall or not. Throughout our life the ECS produces nurturing responses to injuries and inflammations. It is involved in protective mechanisms against numerous cancers, neurological diseases, and nerve damage, and it may mitigate changes associated with aging.

The scientific identification of the endocannabinoid system in 1990 is a relatively recent development that stemmed from research into the cannabis plant, for which it is named.[1] Since then, about ten new studies have been published every month examining the impact of the ECS, its range, and its complexity.[2] Presumably this is a reflection of the excitement and hope that the early results have generated in the medical research community and among physicians, patients, and caregivers.

The ECS is a biological regulatory mechanism that operates much like a lock and key. Understanding the ECS is a critical task if we are to more effectively manage diseases, especially chronic, debilitating diseases for which there is no orthodox cure. For instance, if properly activated, the ECS is capable of suppressing numerous cancers and may be protective against Alzheimer's disease.

In addition to its preventive and protective mechanisms, the ECS balances and strengthens our nervous and immune systems, initiates pain control, and calms inflammation. The ECS initiates neurogenesis[3] (the production of new nerve cells), which is essential to recovery from brain damage, and crucial to protecting nerve cells and enhancing memory function. The ECS increases our ability to try out new perspectives and experiences. When we try new things, we literally change our brain functions for the better in a process called neuroplasticity. Evidence suggests that the ECS may be involved in generating subtle but therapeutic shifts in the ways we perceive the world, relate to our internal landscape, think and feel about ourselves, and interact with each other.

The role of the ECS in neurogenesis, neuroplasticity, learning, and opening us to new experiences demonstrates connections between our frame of mind and the development of illness or expansion of health and well-being. For example, a frame of mind that frequently leads to guilt or shame produces specific negative changes that impact the body's ability to defend against pathogens.[4] On the other hand, many cannabis-using patients notice the positive health effects of open-mindedness, creativity, humor, laughter, bliss, acceptance, tolerance, gratitude, and forgiveness despite an often-difficult healing process.

These shifts in frame of mind can be induced by endocannabinoids (cannabinoids produced by the body itself) or by cannabinoids extracted from plants or synthesized in a laboratory. Either way, the ECS can be activated to help us move beyond limiting ways of being and behaving based on past experiences. The ECS can be activated to support movement toward whatever can produce enhanced health and vitality *now*.

Cannabinoids and Their Receptors

Large numbers of cannabinoid receptors are embedded in specific cell membranes throughout the human body. These receptors can be activated in three ways: by release of the body's own cannabinoids (for example, anandamide), through the introduction of plant-based cannabinoids such as cannabis, or through manufactured cannabinoids such as Dronabinol.

The two most common types of cannabinoid receptors are the CB1 and the CB2 receptors. Scientists suspect there are three more endocannabinoid receptors whose locations and functions will be more fully understood after more research. For the time being, these other receptors are referred to as non-CB1 and non-CB2.

Cannabinoid Receptor Chart A

Endocannabinoid receptors influence, modulate or regulate the function of each of the cells, tissues, glands, organs and systems in which they are contained.

CB1 RECEPTORS ARE LOCATED IN THE CELLS OF THE:

CB1 AND CB2 RECEPTORS ARE LOCATED IN THE CELLS OF THE:

Brain/CNS/Spinal cord (CB1)
Cortical regions (CB1): (neocortex, pyriform cortex, hippocampus , amygdala)
Cerebellum (CB1)
Brainstem (CB1)
Basal ganglia (CB1): globus pallidus, substantia nigra pars, reticulata
Olfactory bulb (CB1)
Thalamus (CB1)
Hypothalamus (Endocrine-brain link CB1)
Pituitary (CB1)

Thyroid (endocrine gland (CB1)

Upper airways (of mammals CB1)

Liver (CB1): Kupffer cells (macrophage immune cells), Hepatocytes (liver cell), Hepatic stellate cells (fat storage cell)

Adrenals (endocrine gland CB1)

Ovaries (gonads and endocrine gland CB1)

Uterus (myometrium CB1)

Testes (gonads and endocrine gland CB1): Leydig cells; Sperm cells

Prostate (CB1): Epithelial and smooth muscle cells

Eye (CB1 and CB2): Retinal pigment epithelial/RPE cells

Heart : CB1 and CB2)

Stomach (CB1 and CB2)

Pancreas (CB1 and CB2)

Digestive tract (CB1 and CB2)

Bone (CB1 and CB2)

Affinity of major cannabinoids on CB receptors:
Anandamide binds relatively equally with CB1 and CB2
THC binds relatively equally with CB1 and CB2

For key study references for CB receptor site location see endnotes 22 through 34.

Rather than creating a long list of organs, cells, and systems that contain cannabinoid receptors and the diseases they influence, I have generated the following charts to show 1) the specific cannabinoid receptors discovered to date and 2) a list of chronic diseases for which cannabinoid therapy has shown promise. (See Cannabis Health Index Chart on page 513).

If cannabinoid receptors function as a lock, cannabinoids are the key. Scientific knowledge of cannabis and its most potent constituents is expanding exponentially, reflective of the far-reaching implications for human health and medicine. Cannabis has repeatedly demonstrated profound therapeutic efficacy for multiple conditions, many of which you will find in the index. A search in the U.S. National Library of Medicine using the single keyword "cannabinoids" currently yields more than 15,000 studies.[5]

Worldwide, millions of patients rely on cannabis or cannabinoid prescriptions to maintain health and well-being and mitigate the assault of chronic degenerative illness or the terrible adverse effects of allopathic treatments such as chemotherapy. Hundreds of medical and scientific organizations support the use of medical marijuana including Kaiser Permanente, the California Medical Association, and the American Nurses Association. Even the conservative American Medical Association now supports research on cannabis for medicinal use.

This support from the medical community is hardly surprising considering the level of frustration felt by a large number of physicians and health care providers who lack adequate and safe treatment options for the many chronic degenerative diseases listed in these pages.

One of the plant's many astounding capabilities is that it simultaneously relaxes and stimulates the autonomic nervous system. Cannabinoids induce these changes by enhancing and balancing individual cellular function as well as that of the whole organism. This occurs in the mind as well as elsewhere in the body. Marijuana's constituents enhance left-brain and right-brain functioning, inducing an expanded state of consciousness that embraces logic and intuition, individuality and oneness, thought and feeling.

To date, more than 111 cannabis-based cannabinoids have been isolated, and researchers are beginning to look at other plant constituents such as terpenoids as important co-factors in inducing therapeutic effects.[6]

Cannabinoid Receptor Chart B

Endocannabinoid receptors influence, modulate or regulate the function of each of the cells, tissues, glands, organs and systems in which they are contained.

CB2 RECEPTORS ARE LOCATED IN THE CELLS OF THE:

NON-CB1 AND NON-CB2 ARE LOCATED IN CELLS OF THE:

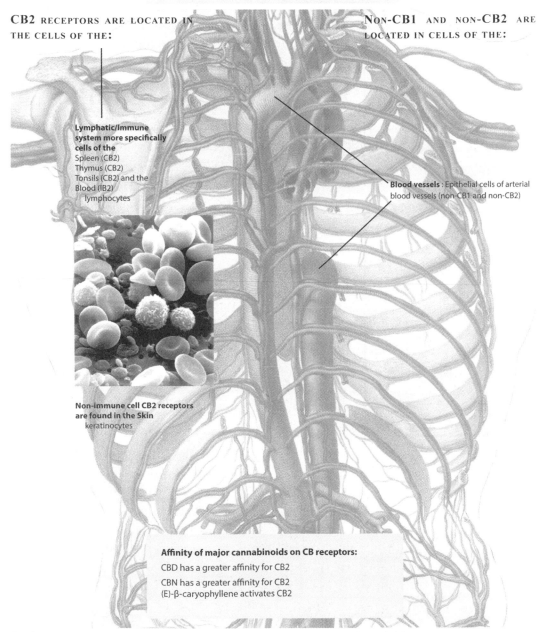

Lymphatic/Immune system more specifically cells of the
Spleen (CB2)
Thymus (CB2)
Tonsils (CB2) and the
Blood (IB2)
    lymphocytes

Blood vessels : Epithelial cells of arterial blood vessels (non-CB1 and non-CB2)

Non-immune cell CB2 receptors are found in the Skin
    keratinocytes

Affinity of major cannabinoids on CB receptors:

CBD has a greater affinity for CB2

CBN has a greater affinity for CB2
(E)-β-caryophyllene activates CB2

For key study references for CB receptor site location see endnotes 22 through 34.

Four Prime Cannabinoids (AEA, THC, CBD, and (E)-BCP)

Anandamide—AEA (produced by the body)

The discovery of the "Bliss Molecule" anandamide[7] in the 1990s was a major scientific breakthrough that led to a better understanding of the interaction between cannabinoids and the endocannabinoid system of the human body. Like all other cannabinoids, anandamide is a "key" molecule. It fits relatively equally into both CB1 and CB2 receptors ("locks").[8] Once the connection is made, the lock opens and a signal is generated. At that point, numerous physiological as well as mental and emotional changes take place. In general, anandamide initiates simultaneously a host of changes in both the central nervous system (CNS), consisting of brain and spinal cord (primarily via CB1) and the immune system (primarily via CB2), as well as the autonomic nervous system (ANS) with its two subdivisions of parasympathetic (downer effect, feed and breed, rest and digest) and sympathetic (upper effect, fight or flight or freeze). More specifically, anandamide enhances pleasure,[9] may be involved in mitigating episodes of acute schizophrenia,[10] destroys numerous types of cancers,[11] and soothes coughs.[12]

Five Distinct Endocannabinoids (produced by the human body) have been Identified:

Anandamide (N-arachidonoylethanolamide) (AEA)

2-arachidonoyl glycerol (2-AG)

2-arachidonoyl-glyceryl-ether (Noladin ether)

O-arachidonoyl-ethanolamine (Virodhamine)

N-arachidonoyl-dopamine (NADA)

Tetrahydrocannabinol—THC (sourced in cannabis)

Under a microscope, tetrahydrocannabinol (THC) looks like a sticky liquid crystal when warm and a glass-like solid when cool. It is the primary mind-altering constituent of marijuana, responsible for generating complex changes that occur physically as well as mentally and emotionally.

The chemical structure of THC was discovered in 1964 by two Israeli scientists, Raphael Mechoulam and Yechiel Gaoni.[13] It is without a doubt the most studied cannabis constituent. However, despite this vast knowledge base, this unique molecule keeps surprising scientists as new information comes to light about its immense influence on human physiology and psychology.

Like anandamide, THC binds relatively equally to both CB1 and CB2 receptors[14] and thus initiates simultaneously a host of changes in the CNS (primarily via CB1), the immune system (primarily via CB2), and the ANS. It is interesting to note that changes in our frame of mind (e.g., fear vs. relaxation) can similarly affect our nervous and immune systems.

Whenever applicable, the therapeutic impact of THC is examined in the discussion of specific diseases in this book. Rather than repeat information included elsewhere, I'd like to mention a highly significant discovery relevant to the number-one killer in the United States: heart disease.

THC may protect the heart from damage and may mitigate damage from an infarction (heart attack). Recent discoveries have isolated several mechanisms by which THC demonstrates heart-protective abilities. While these latest insights are still in their beginning stages, it is likely that the way we will treat acute and chronic heart disease in the future will change as a result: THC reduced heart attack size in mice;[15] THC may protect heart cells against damage from hypoxia by induction of nitric oxide, in a sense THC preparing heart cells to better withstand hypoxia (poor perfusion of heart cells and a direct cause of heart attacks);[16] THC is neuroprotective via CB1;[17] THC causes bronchodilation (enlargement of the airways leading to increased air supply—a potent therapeutic element in heart disease);[18] THC causes weight gain and an increase in walking distance in chronic obstructive pulmonary disease (COPD).[19]

Synthetic drugs containing THC include Sativex, Dronabinol, Marinol, and Nabilone. These pharmaceuticals are approved by the FDA and are used to treat a large number of conditions, some of which include AIDS-related anorexia/cachexia, nausea and vomiting secondary to chemotherapy cancer treatments, neurological disorders, inflammatory conditions, and PTSD.

With the exception of Sativex, which is essentially a plant-derived tincture, pharmaceuticals that contain THC do not contain any of the other biologically active components of cannabis that may play an important therapeutic role in the human body.

Plant-based THC content varies by cannabis strain and depending upon whether it is fresh or dried (and if dried, its age), and whether it is grown indoors or outdoors. Some strains may be especially potent in

THC while others may contain only trace amounts. Fresh cannabis contains THC in the form of THC-carboxylic-acid, which is considered only minutely psychoactive. Once dried, however, the chemical composition of THC-acid changes, and it becomes decarboxylated through heat (as it dries or when it is burned). Once devoid of its carboxyl group, THC becomes psychoactive. Talk to your local medical dispensary for information on the THC profiles of current strains.

THC content decreases over time and is affected by UV light, heat, and exposure to moisture. Indoor cultivation follows a three-month cycle, while outdoor cultivation follows an annual or biannual cycle. Indoor crops tend to contain a markedly higher THC content than outdoor crops.

Cannabidiol—CBD (sourced in cannabis)

Sourced in cannabis, cannabidiol (CBD) is a non-psychoactive cannabinoid. CBD has a greater affinity for CB2 receptors than CB1 receptors,[20] but much of its therapeutic influence stems from its ability to suppress the enzyme (fatty acid amide hydrolase or FAAH) that breaks down anandamide, thus keeping "the Bliss Molecule" active at higher concentrations and for a longer duration. At the same time, CBD tames the psychoactive influence of THC, allowing patients to focus on THC's other therapeutic powers at higher concentrations.

While the full complexity of how CBD interacts with the body's endocannabinoid system is yet to be revealed, numerous studies have shown that CBD affects diseases of both the mind and the body, particularly neurological diseases, inflammatory illness, and cancer.

More specifically, CBD is considered a very promising agent with the highest prospect for therapeutic use in the treatment of neurodegenerative illness.[21] An oil-based solution of CBD has been documented as effective for pediatric patients suffering from epileptic seizures who failed to respond to traditional pharmaceutical anti-seizure medications.[22] CBD may also be useful in preventing nerve damage associated with alcohol poisoning.[23]

In addition to providing neuroprotection, CBD appears to calm autonomic responses to stress (such as rapid heart rates) by engaging receptors that select serotonin to achieve a calming effect.[24] Cannabidiol's therapeutic potential in psychological disorders is based on its antipsychotic,[25] anxiolytic, and antidepressant effects.[26] CBD is able to reduce symptoms of acute paranoid schizophrenia as well as the pharmaceutical drug Amisulpride which (unlike CBD) has significant adverse side effects.[27]

CBD has been shown to have a clear and measurable therapeutic impact on inflammatory and anti-inflammatory regulation mechanisms[28] such as in inflammatory bowel disease,[29] arthritis,[30] periodontitis,[31] and atherosclerosis.[32]

As regards cancer, CBD is able to produce significant anti-tumor activity both in vitro and in vivo.[33] Further, CBD has been shown to selectively produce oxidative stress in cancer cells, thus producing apoptosis (cancer cell suicide) without impacting normal cells.[34]

(E)-β-Caryophyllene (primarily sourced in spice plants)

An international group of researchers from Switzerland, Germany, Italy, and the U.S. (2008, 2012) reported that certain plants, most notably spice-producing plants, contain a functional non-psychoactive CB2 agonist called (E)-β-caryophyllene or (E)-BCP. This molecule is considered by some researchers to be a food-based cannabinoid. And, while some chemists may be more inclined to stick with more traditional nomenclature and consider the molecule a terpene or terpenoids, this distinction has little if no practical value to the many patients who may benefit from its use. Scientists suggest that activation of CB2 receptors via this newly discovered dietary plant-based cannabinoid might present a new and additional therapeutic strategy in the treatment of a multitude of diseases associated with inflammation and oxidative stress, both underlying factors in a host of different pathologies.[35] Additional research has shown that (E)-β-caryophyllene may also protect against microbes, pain, and cancer.[36]

This food-based cannabinoid is fully accepted by the U.S. government with the FDA's seal of approval, and key (E)-β-caryophyllene-containing organic spices are relatively easy to obtain. Spices that contain (E)-β-caryophyllene include black and white Ashanti (West African) peppers, Indian bay-leaf, alligator pepper, basil, cinnamon, rosemary, caraway, black pepper, Mexican oregano, and clove.

Black and White "Ashanti Peppers" *(Piper guineense):* The (E)-β-caryophyllene content contained in test samples of Black Ashanti pepper was 58% and in White Ashanti pepper 52%.[37] In comparison, the (E)-β-caryophyllene content in a sample of *Cannabis sativa* ranges from 12 to 35%.[38]

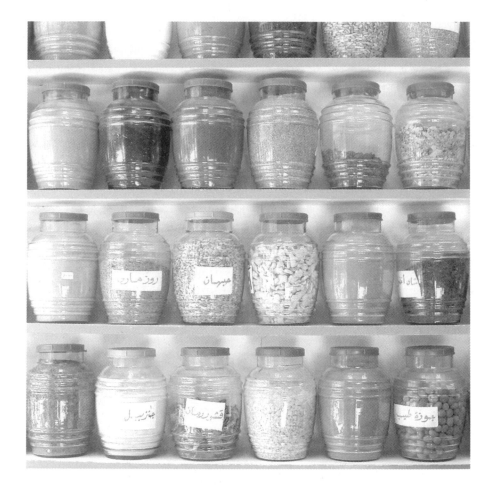

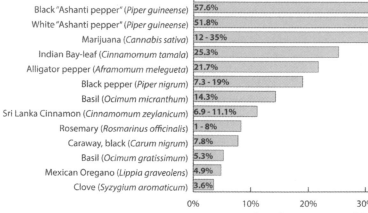
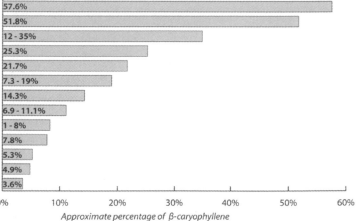

Black "Ashanti pepper" (*Piper guineense*)	57.6%
White "Ashanti pepper" (*Piper guineense*)	51.8%
Marijuana (*Cannabis sativa*)	12 - 35%
Indian Bay-leaf (*Cinnamomum tamala*)	25.3%
Alligator pepper (*Aframomum melegueta*)	21.7%
Black pepper (*Piper nigrum*)	7.3 - 19%
Basil (*Ocimum micranthum*)	14.3%
Sri Lanka Cinnamon (*Cinnamomum zeylanicum*)	6.9 - 11.1%
Rosemary (*Rosmarinus officinalis*)	1 - 8%
Caraway, black (*Carum nigrum*)	7.8%
Basil (*Ocimum gratissimum*)	5.3%
Mexican Oregano (*Lippia graveolens*)	4.9%
Clove (*Syzygium aromaticum*)	3.6%

0%   10%   20%   30%   40%   50%   60%

Approximate percentage of β-caryophyllene

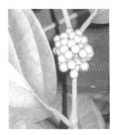

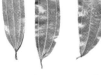

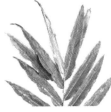

Black "Ashanti Pepper" *Indian Bay-Leaf* *Aligator Pepper*

These peppers also have antibacterial properties against *E. coli* and *Staphylococcus aureus.*

Indian Bay-Leaf *(Cinnamomum tamala):* The (E)-β-caryophyllene content of a tested sample was 25%.[39] In addition, Indian Bay-Leaf, a prominent herb in Ayurvedic traditions, exhibits proven antioxidant and antidiabetic properties.[40]

Grains of Paradise *(Aframomum melegueta):* The (E)-β-caryophyllene content measured in this spice was 22%.[41] Additional medicinal uses and properties supported by scientific studies include the promotion of wound healing by cell membrane support.[42] It is also an antioxidant,[43] anti-inflammatory,[44] analgesic,[45] molluscicidal (destroys snails),[46] anti-diarrheal agent,[47] antimicrobial agent,[48] and may enhance sexual interest and function.[49]

Black Pepper *(Piper nigrum):* Samples of black pepper yielded an (E)-β-caryophyllene content ranging between 7% and 19%.[50] Scientific studies have documented additional medicinal benefits including antibacterial properties,[51] use as a protective agent against colon cancer,[52] and antioxidant activity.[53]

African Basil *(Ocimum micranthum):* This type of basil typically contains a (E)-β-caryophyllene content of 14%.[54] There are many varieties of basil with similar constituents. However, not all species have been fully explored. The medicinal uses and properties of *Ocimum basilicum,* a form of basil commonly used worldwide, include antimicrobial (giardia) properties, it may assist in dyspepsia and high blood pressure (diuretic), it is potentially effective against cholera-induced diarrhea, has antiviral activity against herpes virus I and II, adenoviruses, hepatitis B virus, and the RNA

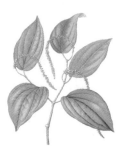

Black Pepper

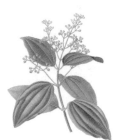

Sri Lanka Cinnamon

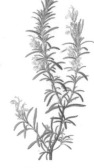

Rosemary

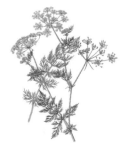

Caraway, black

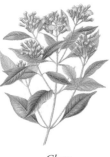

Basil

Clove

viruses (coxsackievirus B1 and enterovirus 71), is an antibacterial for mid-dle-ear infections, and has anti-inflammatory properties.[55]

Sri Lanka Cinnamon *(Cinnamomum zeylanicum):* A tested sample of Sri Lanka (Ceylon) cinnamon contained 7–11% (E)-β-caryophyllene.[56] Other medicinal uses and properties supported by scientific studies include improved fat and sugar metabolism, a possible treatment for high blood pressure, antioxidant properties, broad-spectrum antibiotic properties, and the ability to cure mite infestation in animals.[57]

Rosemary *(Rosmarinus officinalis):* Approximately 1% and 8% of (E)-β-caryophyllene was contained in two different samples of rosemary.[58] Medicinal uses and properties supported by scientific studies include use of rosemary as an antimicrobial (bacteria, fungi), to treat dyspepsia (digestive complaints), to promote circulation, as a radio protective, to possibly prevent skin cancer tumors and other kinds of tumors, as an anti-inflammatory, and in the prevention and treatment of diabetic, cardiovascular, and other neurodegenerative diseases.[59]

Caraway, black *(Carum nigrum)*: Levels of (E)-β-caryophyllene in a sample of black caraway were measured at 8%.[60] Essential oil of *Carum nigrum* has demonstrated potent antioxidant, antibacterial, and antifungal properties.[61]

Basil *(Ocimum gratissimum)*: (E)-β-Caryophyllene content in a sample of this type of basil was measured at 5%.[62] See also African Basil, above. Basil has shown protective gastrointestinal abilities[63] and antibacterial properties against *E. coli* and *Staphylococcus aureus*.[64]

Mexican Oregano *(Lippia graveolens)*: The (E)-β-caryophyllene content in a sample of Mexican oregano was measured at 5%.[65] This herb, commonly used in Mexican traditional healing, has demonstrated abilities to inhibit acyclovir-resistant herpes virus in the laboratory.[66]

Clove *(Syzygium aromaticum)*: A sample of clove contained almost 4% (E)-β-caryophyllene.[67] Studies have shown the essential oil of clove to work as an analgesic, anti-inflammatory, antioxidant, antimicrobial, antifungal, antiviral (*Herpes simplex* I & II and hepatitis C), antibacterial (including several of the multi-drug-resistant *Staphylococcus epidermidis*), anticancer, cancer protective (skin and lung), antidiabetic, and insect repellant. It contains aphrodisiac properties. A cream from clove works as an effective treatment for chronic anal fissures.[68]

Cannabis

Numerous good books have been written on the history of cannabis and its place among the people and cultures of the world, so I will keep this section brief and relevant to healing. There are hundreds of varieties of cannabis with similar appearance and characteristics. With the exception of Antarctica, the species grows on every continent.

For our purposes two basic distinctions are of importance. First, the name "hemp" is used to indicate extremely low or non-psychoactive cannabis species. And, while hemp plants are a good source of nutrition (e.g., essential fatty acids), the medicinal quality of hempseed oil is limited to some mild anti-inflammatory properties. Hemp is a legal crop in numerous countries, utilized for food, drink, fiber, oil, paper, building materials, erosion control, fuel, biodegradable plastics, and a multitude of other uses.

Second, medicinal cannabis consists of two basic species, *Cannabis sativa* and *Cannabis indica*. Both are psychoactive and both contain the cannabinoids required to engage the endocannabinoid system for specific therapeutic purposes. These two strains look different and contain different ratios of the primary cannabinoids, which is relevant when selecting a strain for specific therapeutic purposes.

Indica plants tend to be short and stalky, with wider leaves than sativas, which usually grow longer, higher, and display a finer leaf structure. More important, however, indicas and sativas produce different THC:CBD/CBN ratios. These ratios are important, because the ratio determines the degree to which the balancing properties of the whole plant's constituents are additive or cancel each other out.

Sativa vs. Indica

Sativa: Higher THC to Lower CBD/CBN Ratio	Indica: Lower THC to Higher CBD/CBN Ratio
Generally stimulating, energizing, uplifting	Generally sedating, relaxing, grounding
Generally more mental/emotional	Generally more physical
Usually more extrovert	Usually more introvert
Best for daytime use	Better after work is done, bedtime
Increases alertness	Sleeping aid
Consider with depression	Consider with anxiety
Pain relief, muscle relaxant	Pain relief, muscle relaxant
THC binds both CB1 and CB2 receptors	CBD has a greater affinity for CB2

Many cannabis-using patients use the plant not only as medicine but as a means to seek a deeper and longer-lasting healing. The cannabis-induced "high" is employed to explore one's frame of mind associated with illness and disease, reach a deeper understanding, gently accept oneself, and initiate nurturing changes that support health and healing and desired levels of energy.

A carefully balanced and finely tuned body and mind can more easily surpass ordinary states of consciousness and open doors to spiritual dimensions of reality. Ascetics of India and modern urban shamans alike consider this dance of expanding consciousness between plant and human a literal infusion of spirit. The ingestion, topical application, or inhalation of marijuana is employed as a tool to learn and explore, and to seek knowledge, insights, and spiritual revelations about the self in an ever-expanding and mysterious universe. And it is precisely this infusion of spirit with its vibrancy, aliveness, and enthusiasm that ultimately allows for a renewed sense of health and well-being.

Cannabis Lore and Legend

In one sense, the cannabis-using patient reaching for deeper healing is not dissimilar to those who use the plant to access realms that are beyond the comprehension and imagination of ordinary consciousness. Those who use the plant as a spiritual practice echo a tradition that dates back to ancient times. In India and Nepal, some of the wandering yogis and *sadhus* (ascetics who have dedicated their life to exploring the ineffable presence of God) use cannabis as a means to this end. To Rastafarians in Jamaica, "the herb is the key to new understanding of the self, the universe, and God. It is the vehicle to cosmic consciousness."[69] Ancient Scythians used cannabis to produce trance states, divination,[70] delight, and joy.[71] According to the Bible,[72] God instructs Moses to make holy anointing oil containing keneh bosem (cannabis)[73] to ". . . anoint Aaron and his sons, sanctifying them as priests to Me." The Egyptian Ebers papyrus, which documents medical practices dating from 3400 BC,[74] describes the use of cannabis ground in honey as a remedy for vaginal illness.[75]

Among the numerous fun, informative, and interesting stories and legends surrounding cannabis, this is my favorite one:

> Once upon a time, long, long ago, legend has it that "Warrior Gods" from the star system Orion (the hunter), traveling in their "divine ships" through the vastness of space, had discovered the third planet from the sun. Apparently fascinated with the sheer abundance and variety of life on this watery world, they made it a playground for "scientific" experimentations. They carelessly cloned beasts with the primitive humans of that time, just to see what would happen. And, while the agonizing pains and labored breaths produced by experiments gone terribly wrong echoed up into the endless firmament, they were neither lost nor left unanswered.

Histories recorded the elemental cries of Cyclops, Sphinxes, Centaurs, Medusas, and many other creatures long turned to stone. They are remembered in countless sculptures, in the annals of the world's mythologies, and to this day on the magic screens—the movie theatres of "modern-day" man and woman.

Near neighbors of the universe such as those from the blue-star constellations of the Seven Sisters (Pleiades) and Alpha Canis Majoris (which contains Sirius, the night sky's brightest star) noticed these horrible things and would not allow them to go on. They took steps to intervene. Since war and confrontation was not their way, they instead engaged in a grand and creative adventure. It started by taking away the source of the energy the "Warrior Gods" needed to conduct their experiments.

Furthermore, it was decided that these neighboring cultures would actively participate in a co-creation that blended their own DNA with that of these earlier humans. The "Blue Star Adventurers" brought love to the table of chaos and creation and engaged the permission and collaboration of the early humans' spirit and soul alike.

As a result of this collaborative spiritual and genetic adventure, humanity rapidly transcended with extraordinary new abilities such as perceiving the color blue. Other examples are said to be: the ability to consciously select gene expression; an expansion of the visual spectrum; the awareness of creating one's life experience deliberately; the ability to know when someone is telling the truth; the ability to heal oneself or another; communication with other realms; or new and creative means to inspire solutions to all kind of problems.

Having been faced with the loss of their energy source and a "new" humanity with potential abilities similar to that of the "Gods," the "Warrior Gods" themselves were effectively robbed of their advantages to continue horrific and loveless activities on Earth. And from their dominator point of view, this co-creative activity between the Blue Star Alliance and humanity was a betrayal of the highest order.

The "snake" had dared to give the "carnal apple of knowledge" to their "toy" creatures. And, one form of the apple was said to be cannabis. When taken at the proper therapeutic dose, especially during times of chronic stress and stubborn disease, the cannabis experience is said to function to remind us of our stellar inheritance, those abilities that are now part and parcel of our human-stellar nature.

In that sense cannabis is a plant imbued with a resonance that can catalyze and bring to consciousness what is already within. Once remembered, we are invited to further transcend by utilizing our capacity for growth and healing without the help of the catalyst.

According to this legend, the cannabis experience can be a reflection of the vast human capacity for self-healing.

1. The ability to consciously select gene expression is explored in Chapter II, "The Art and Science of Mind-Body Medicine."
2. Expansion of the visual spectrum can ensue with extraordinary states of consciousness born from meditation, mindfulness, or a shamanic practice (for example), which can bring revealing vision and healing insight.
3. The awareness of creating one's life experience deliberately contributes new depth of freedom and responsibility.
4. The ability to know when someone is telling the truth, also called intuition, is a skill that can be developed and honed.
5. The ability to heal oneself or another can arise when we enter a state of deep relaxation that supports and balances our capacity for self-healing; we can understand what makes us vulnerable to illness and disease and make healthier choices.
6. Communication with other realms in visionary, dream-like states can be employed for meaning and healing.
7. New and creative means to inspire solutions to all kind of problems are readily available when we learn to let go of control and domination and instead embrace a non-defensive, vulnerable, and curious mind.

Is Cannabis a Cure-All?

Even though cannabis has more proven therapeutic applications than any other plant in the world, working with cannabis is by no means a panacea. However, an informed and responsible use of cannabis that engages mind-body medicine opens a door to a new and potent synergy that can take our healing journey to new depths, far beyond temporary relief or mere cessation of symptoms. We might discover places of profound understanding, combined with a deep sense of empathy. Perhaps it will show up as a newly found freedom, rooted in responsibility without blame. The journey might reveal a love emerging from an ancient hatred, or the lifting of a humiliating shame that was crushing our spirit. Or we may surprise ourselves by the emergence of a tender intimacy that transcends the lingering sensation of worthlessness like dew in the morning fog.

Is Cannabis Safe?

As with any medicine that affects the mind and the body, cannabis evokes numerous concerns and questions worthy of examination. Chief among them are: What can I expect from using cannabis? What is the potential for adverse effects? How do I reduce the risk of adverse effects? Does the use of marijuana lead to addiction? How does the use of the plant affect the development of adolescents, or the developing fetus in pregnant women? Concerns about fertility are raised. The smoking of plant material and its effect on the lungs is another commonly expressed concern. What about the plant's impact on the heart, or the development of cancer? Some studies have suggested that marijuana may be implicated as a co-factor in developing schizophrenia, or cause traffic accidents from irresponsible use. Could smoking pot encourage use of other illegal and/or dangerous "recreational" drugs (an idea known as the Gateway Theory)? Lastly, is it possible to overdose on cannabis?

Without going into the social, historical, and political aspects of cannabis, I will attempt to briefly address these reasonable health concerns in descending order. I used to judge a drug by the harmful impact it had on the people I treated as a paramedic and the frequency with which people needed to call 911 due to drug use. The number-one drug responsible for generating 911 emergency calls is nicotine contained in tobacco cigarettes, due to the lasting and serious damage that smoking causes, followed closely by alcohol abuse. Next come heroin, stimulants (cocaine, crack, methamphetamine, diet pills), and PCP.

On the other side of the spectrum are occasional calls to 911 related to use of psychogenic substances such as LSD, ecstasy, and psilocybin. During my twenty years working in emergency services, I can barely recall an incident in which someone called 911 for cannabis use alone. However, many studies show large numbers of cannabis-related visits to the ER. Upon closer examination, it is clear that the majority of such visits were due to cannabis used in combination with other drugs, or incidences of people experiencing anxiety. Government statistics seem to echo my experience.

According to several U.S. government sources, there were zero deaths due to the exclusive use of cannabis in the periods studied, which range from January 1997 through June 2005.[76] (Deaths in which cannabis was one of several drugs used are not counted here.) In contrast, recent CDC (Centers for Disease Control) estimates suggest that, on average, tobacco (particularly cigarette smoking) claimed 110,750 lives per year from 2000 to 2004.[77] The average number of alcohol-related fatalities was estimated at 75,766 in 2001.[78]

WHAT CAN I EXPECT (MENTALLY/EMOTIONALLY) FROM USING CANNABIS?

Commonly noted effects of cannabis include, at once, an energizing euphoria and grounding relaxation, intensification of sensory experiences, an occasionally infectious laughter and talkativeness, and "feeling stoned."

However, as we will see in Chapter II and its supplementary appendix, we can get even more out of the cannabis experience when we gain a basic understanding of what is possible in a supportive environment and by setting a conscious and caring intention. In doing so we may expect to stay more deeply in the present moment, cultivate an inner silence, and allow a deeper relaxation to flood the areas of the body that are normally tight, tense, and achy. We may now, perhaps for the first time, allow emotions to surface that before were considered intolerable. We may now find it easier to suspend whatever stands in the way and allow our innate capacity for self-healing (always ready to engage) to flow unencumbered and freely to realize the healing we are all capable of.

WHAT ARE POTENTIAL ADVERSE EFFECTS (PHYSICAL, MENTAL, EMOTIONAL)?

Adverse effects may include increased appetite, reduced attention span, red sclera (reddening of the normally white part of the eyes), dry mouth, and decreased cognitive and motor skills. Other side effects, more common when ingested or when used at higher than the subjective therapeutic dose, include ataxia (unsteady gait), aphasia (inability to speak clearly), unusual perceptions of all senses including hallucinations, anxiety (though this can be addressed by reassurance), slight increase in heart rate, subtle shifts in blood pressure depending on the position of the body, and panic (moderated by reassurance) upon first-ever use.

HOW DO I REDUCE THE RISK OF ADVERSE EFFECTS?

To reduce the risk of adverse effects it is imperative to start by taking a small and measured amount and then slowly increasing the dosage by the same amount until the desired effect is achieved. This process is called "finding your subjective therapeutic window."

WHAT IS A SUBJECTIVE THERAPEUTIC WINDOW AND HOW DO I ESTABLISH IT?

OR

HOW DO WE TURN CANNABIS MEDICINE INTO A PRECISE MEDICINE?

Evidence has shown that the vast majority of adverse effects are directly related to using cannabis in excess of the subjective therapeutic window. In other words, taking too little can be sub-optimal, while too much can actually increase the very symptoms you are attempting to treat. For instance, it is an age-old tradition in various healing practices to use cannabis to reduce anxiety and return to a state of relaxation and general calm. However, if too much cannabis is used too rapidly, the feeling of apprehension and anxiety may actually multiply.

Establishing one's own therapeutic window is governed by three things: the body's present endocannabinoid state (relative balance or deficiency), the cannabinoid profile in the medicine to be taken, and the form in which it is consumed.

If you're a patient who deals with neurological disorders or mental/emotional problems, you are most likely lacking CB1 activation. On the other hand, if you're immune-compromised or experience chronic inflammation, you're most likely CB2-deficient. In these cases you would want to choose a strain with a higher THC:CBD ratio or a lower THC:CBD ratio, respectively, because each would modulate your specific deficiency accordingly.

Important Safety Tip: Inhaling vapors produces near-instant results, while ingesting plant materials may not show effects until hours later, especially when taken on a full stomach.

When inhaling cannabis smoke or vapors, take one short to medium inhalation and wait 5 to 10 minutes. See how you feel. Did this dose achieve your desired effect? If not, inhale another vapor of about the same length. Wait again for 5 to 10 minutes. Don't be impatient—the line between an effective dose that really meets your needs and an adverse effect is indeed very thin. Continue this process until you have found the sweet spot and stop. Do not inhale more. More is not better.

Also, stop if you're experiencing unwanted effects. In the case of adverse effects you might want to wait a full day and start again at a lower dosage (shorter inhalation).

If, however, you were happy with the results—let's say it took two medium-size inhalations to feel the desired therapeutic effect—then use two inhalations for relief of symptoms in the future. This is your subjective therapeutic window or optimal dose with this delivery mechanism and cannabis batch.

When it comes to ingesting cannabis-containing medicine such as cookies, oils, and tinctures, it is advisable to use an exact and measured amount, preferably on an empty stomach, and wait at least one hour (in case of a full stomach, wait two hours) before increasing the dose by the same amount. Repeat this process until you achieve the desired effect. Do not be impatient.

If you are happy with the results, remember the amount it took to achieve the effect. They next time you need to use this medicine and in accordance with the recommendations of your health care provider, repeat the total amount of drops (or cookies) minus about 20% (to allow for changes due to time and rate of digestion) as your starting dose.

Many patients have made the mistake while eating cannabis of saying to themselves, "I'm not feeling anything," and then continuing to eat until it's too late and adverse effects occur. In case of ingesting too much cannabis, the effect may last many hours and can be intense and very unpleasant.

So, start slow, be as precise as you can be, be patient, and remember what it took to achieve the desired result, and you will know the secret to the optimal therapeutic dose that is right for you.

DOES THE USE OF MARIJUANA LEAD TO ADDICTION?

In the context of addiction, both opponents and proponents of medical marijuana have numerous studies to support their arguments. However, one distinction is usually agreed upon. If dependency occurs, it is an addiction in psychological terms rather than in the physical realm, as is the case with many other substances such as tobacco, alcohol, and heroin. The large numbers of people enrolled in drug treatment centers is often cited to substantiate claims that the plant is psychologically addictive. This overlooks the reality that many court judges do not believe marijuana users should go to jail, but as they are bound to uphold present laws, they are left with no other option but to mandate drug treatment instead of jail or prison time.

Compared to pharmaceuticals, some of which have a more significant addiction potential, cannabis carries a considerably reduced risk of adverse side effects (including death). An FDA (federal Food and Drug Administration) report compared marijuana to seventeen common FDA-approved pharmaceutical drugs used to treat similar symptoms and conditions. The findings make a compelling argument for medical marijuana. Between 1997 and 2005, no deaths were attributed to the exclusive use of cannabis, while the FDA recorded 10,008 deaths due to the seventeen FDA-approved pharmaceutical drugs in the study.[79]

If you are concerned about developing a dependence on cannabis, you may reduce this potential risk by infusing mindfulness into your process of healing and/or using raw preparations of cannabis, which have little or no psychoactive effect.

> Walter had sexual performance anxiety. The use of cannabis reduced his anxiety and otherwise enhanced his sensual experience. Rather than becoming dependent on the use of the plant each time he wished to engage in sexual activity, he used the cannabis-induced state of mind to explore the deeper causes for his anxiety and took corrective action, which eventually cured his anxiety and eliminated his need for cannabis.

HOW DOES USE OF THE PLANT AFFECT THE DEVELOPMENT OF ADOLESCENTS, ISSUES OF FERTILITY, OR THE DEVELOPING FETUS IN PREGNANT WOMEN?

When it comes to fertility, to the developing fetus, or to the still physically developing adolescent, the use of any mind-body-altering substance is cause for concern. As before, various studies are cited as evidence by those on both sides of this issue. No long-term studies examining the exclusive use of cannabis on fertility, the fetus, and adolescents have been conducted. Instead, people enrolled in most studies were exposed to other substances, thus complicating the overall picture.

However, a study conducted at Duke University[80] which collected subjective observational data from New Zealand residents over a period of about 38 years[81] concluded that while cannabis use by adults has no effect on intelligence, "cannabis dependency" in adolescents (defined by the authors as continued use despite major health, social and/or legal problems related to its use) may contribute to reduced IQ test scores later in life. The study has limitations: data were described subjectively, the study had a small sample size (17% or 153 people fit the authors' dependency definition), and only some factors that may alter IQ were considered in the analysis. Still, no other study to date has examined the impact of adolescent use of cannabis on intelligence measured over time. Until more is known, it is advisable to assume a possible correlation.

WHAT ARE THE EFFECTS OF INHALING BURNED PLANT MATERIAL ON THE LUNGS?

Whenever plant matter is burned, smoke is released, and with it potentially harmful particles. However, the largest population-based case-controlled study ever conducted of cannabis-only use yielded somewhat counter-intuitive results. For the 2,252 people observed in a Los Angeles, California, study, smoking (only) cannabis was found to be mildly lung-protective and was not associated with an increased risk of lung cancer.[82]

Cannabis oil produces therapeutic effects in patients with chronic obstructive pulmonary disease (a serious lung disorder) and asthma. (See also the section on Lung Diseases in Chapter IV.) To minimize any potential risk of negative consequences to one's lungs, some people use vaporizers to inhale cannabis rather than smoking cannabis wrapped in paper. Use of a vaporizer eliminates the inhalation of carbon compounds from burned paper. An infused oil or alcohol-based tincture can also be used to address symptoms related to lung diseases.

WHAT IS THE PLANT'S IMPACT ON THE HEART?

Endocannabinoid receptors are present in the heart and thus are involved in regulating heart function. THC can increase one's heart rate, but not to a dangerous extent. Furthermore, numerous studies have shown that THC, CBD, and CBN have potentially potent cardio-protective properties. (See the section on Cardiovascular Disease/Heart Disease in Chapter IV.)

WHAT IS THE PLANT'S IMPACT ON THE DEVELOPMENT OF CANCER?

In the context of cancer, the constituents of cannabis have demonstrated remarkable abilities to produce apoptosis (cancer cell death) in a great variety of cancer manifestations. (See the section on Cancer in Chapter IV.)

MARIJUANA AND SCHIZOPHRENIA?

Observational studies have concluded that consuming cannabis as an adolescent may increase one's risk of developing schizophrenia later in life. While cannabis is not itself a causal factor for schizophrenia, in some instances it may be a co-factor. Based on the current evidence, it would be prudent for adolescents or young adults with a known family history of psychosis or schizophrenia to stay away from cannabis or any other mind-altering substance, especially speed-based drugs such as cocaine or methamphetamines. (See the section on Mental Disorders/Schizophrenia in Chapter IV.)

CANNABIS A "GATEWAY DRUG"?

The controversial gateway theory suggests that adolescents who experiment with cannabis are more likely to subsequently try, and become addicted to, other illicit drugs. While the gateway theory has never attempted to address therapeutic uses of legally obtained medicine, the suggestion that even short-term cannabis use could lead to addiction to other drugs still lingers in many people's minds. In fact, a recent study of more than 4,000 cannabis smokers concluded that cannabis use leads to a decrease in the use of alcohol, tobacco, and hard drugs.[83]

CAN CANNABIS KILL YOU?

A laboratory study conducted in 1973 reported the median lethal dose of oral THC in rats as 800–1900 mg/kg, depending on the sex and genetic strain of the animal.[84] If body weight is used as the sole criteria, this study suggests that 200 grams of herb per kilogram of body weight is required to approach a lethal dose in humans. Accordingly, a person weighing 70 kg or 154 lbs would need to consume 14 kg of herb to approach a fatal dose. A 2004 study was much more conservative, stating "628 kg of cannabis would have to be smoked in 15 min. to induce a lethal effect."[85]

"Unlike many of the drugs we prescribe every day, marijuana has never been proven to cause a fatal overdose."

— Joycelyn Elders, MD, former U.S. Surgeon General

WHAT ABOUT CONTAMINANTS?

Another area of concern for some is the possibility that external toxins or biological pathogens could be present on the cannabis plant, particularly pesticides or aspergillus fungus. The presence of pesticides on any consumed plant material may increase the body's toxic load and can contribute in numerous and unpredictable ways to ill health, but this risk can easily be eliminated by purchasing or growing organic cannabis. Aspergillus is a mold that grows on many agricultural products throughout the world and is a common contaminant of bread, potatoes, and peanuts. Because cannabis is not regulated, growers do not routinely test for aspergillus nor report concentration amounts as is required for, say, peanut growers. Patients with an already depressed immune system could be particularly vulnerable to any negative effects of aspergillus fungus-contaminated cannabis. Use caution to determine the presence of the fungus on any plant product before consumption. Many cannabis patients believe that heating cannabis at temperatures of 300°F (-149°C) for a period of 5 minutes will kill the pathogen, but I have not been able to find any studies to verify this suggestion. However, one study suggested that aspergillus fungus was not present in any samples of ten medicinal herbs dried and stored with a water activity of less than 0.81 in temperature ranges of 25 +/- 2°C (77 +/- 3.6°F),[86] highlighting the importance of proper drying practices.

In summary, the bottom line is that extensive evidence indicates that cannabis is neither dangerous nor harmless. Consideration of its medicinal use should include a risk versus benefit analysis, focused on the specific therapeutic needs and health challenges of the individual in question. This book is written and organized in order to facilitate exactly that.

Forms of Cannabis

Cannabis is used medicinally in many forms. Most often, patients utilize dried buds, flowers, and leaves of the cannabis plant. To minimize inhalation of burned carbon products, many patients prefer the use of a vaporizer to heat the plant material to a precise temperature that will evaporate the cannabinoids just below the burning point of the plant matter.

Cannabis can be cooked into other foods such as a cookie, brownie, or savory dishes. Cannabis is usually added to recipes in the form of an herbed butter, infused oils, or tinctures. A dropper may be used to measure medicine precisely and thereby stay within an established optimum therapeutic window.

Fresh cannabis leaf is consumed by many self-growing patients as a salad mixed with other greens. Fresh raw leaves can also be juiced; this is often diluted with other vegetable juices to disguise its bitter taste. Fresh cannabis contains CBD and THC in their acid forms. As THC is not psychoactive in this form, fresh raw cannabis is ideal for patients advised to consume large quantities of CBD for its numerous therapeutic and preventative purposes. While studies are underway to determine the therapeutic value of raw cannabis, to date only physician case studies and patient testimonials are available.

Kief and hashish are the collected resin of mature and ripe cannabis flower buds. Separation and collection of the resin is usually accomplished by using a sieve or ice water. Kief is the name given to resin crystals in their loose form, while hashish is merely heated and pressed kief.

Alcohol or glycerin may be used as a medium to dissolve plant material and produce a tincture useful in oral or topical preparations. This is often called "green dragon." Tinctures extracted using alcohol, glycerin, or oil form the basis of various medicinal creams, balms, and lotions. Alternatively, hemp oil, almond oil, or coconut oil (preferably of the virgin, organic variety) may be mixed with cannabis as an additive to create topical skin creams and food products.

Solvents such as hexane, butane, or isopropyl alcohol may be employed to dissolve the ingredients of cannabis. While this method produces the highest concentration of cannabinoids, it is also dangerous due to the flammability of the solvents. Explosions have led to serious injuries and deaths. Also, solvent residue may linger in the concentrate and add a toxic material to the medicine.

Pharmaceutical Prescription Cannabinoids:

Dronabinol

Nabilone

Sativex

Rimonabant (no longer available)

Synthetic Cannabinoids Primarily Used in Research

CB1 agonists:

CP 55,940 (is equally strong at CB1 and CB2 receptors)

HU 210 (primarily CB1)

HU 239 (ajulemic acid)

a potential CB1 agonist:

WIN55,212-2 (binds with both but stronger at CB1)

CB1 antagonists:

SR 141716A (Rimonabant)

AM 251

CB2 agonists:

AM 1241

CP 50556-1

CP 55,940

JWH-015

JWH-133

JWH-300

JWH-359

JWH-361

GW-405,833 (primarily CB2)

WIN55,212-2

CB2 antagonists:

SR144528 (blocks both but much stronger at CB2)

AM 630

Modes of Administration

Cannabis may be eaten raw, cooked into other foods, drunk as juice, inhaled after vaporization, smoked in a pipe, wrapped in paper and smoked, or rubbed into the skin. It is not safe to drive or operate heavy machinery after taking any psychoactive form of cannabis.

When you receive a prescription from your doctor for medical marijuana, your doctor will probably recommend a preferred method for taking your medicine. Medical marijuana dispensaries typically have literature available and staff prepared to teach new patients how to correctly use medical marijuana as prescribed. Your local pharmacist can also discuss derivatives of cannabinoids in pill or liquid form with you if you are unsure how to follow your doctor's instructions.

Inhalation of cannabinoids via vaporization quickly reaches the bloodstream, and effects are often experienced in minutes or even seconds. However, effects are of a shorter duration than other modes of administration.

If eaten, it may take 45 minutes to an hour and a half for cannabis to be absorbed through the gastrointestinal tract. The effects of consumed cannabis thus tend to be delayed, last much longer, and are noticeably different compared to the effects of inhalation. Some patients who want to deliver cannabinoids to the lower half of the intestinal tract use suction-bulbs filled with cannabis-infused oils inserted into the rectum similar to a suppository.

Any favorite recipes can be fortified with cannabis-infused oil, or an alcohol-based tincture that supports your specific needs. Add the oil or tincture after the cooking process is completed, and at the right dose specific to your therapeutic window.

Infused oils or tinctures often come in dropper bottles, which allow for precise dosing. As always, start slowly with a few drops, and wait at least one hour to feel the effect. Then slowly increase the dosage by a couple of drops, repeating the process until you have achieved the desired therapeutic effect. Many patients start with 3 or 4 drops and work from there. The oil or tinctures can easily be made at home or bought at most dispensaries. Since most products are not standardized, you may need to repeat the process each time you make or purchase a new bottle.

Topical creams are used to deliver medicine to specific and isolated problem areas. Absorption rates may be similar to that of ingestion but tend to be less systematic and more local.

Summary

- The endocannabinoid system is a bridge between the body and mind.
- Bodies make their own cannabinoids to regulate, regain, or maintain a healthy body and mind.
- Cannabinoid sources: our body, cannabis, certain plants, and man-made.
- The endocannabinoid system is involved in healing 100(+) chronic symptoms and stubborn diseases.
- Cannabinoids are essential to life, health, and well-being.
- Cannabis is neither dangerous nor harmless.

Chapter II

The Art and Science of Mind-Body Medicine

A Brief Introduction to Mind-Body Medicine

In the following multiple-choice questions, which answer is closest to what you believe?

1. Disease/symptom (_____) happens to me for NO reason. ☐
2. Disease/symptom (_____) happens to me for a reason. ☐
3. Disease/symptom (_____) is part of who I am. ☐
4. Disease/symptom (_____) is something I allow. ☐

The answers to these questions are not right or wrong, but they are important to the healing environment they engender. When we believe that something happens to us for no reason, we limit our options. We are often left with a frustrated medical profession that has no cure for most of the chronic diseases or stubborn symptoms listed herein and is limited to managing ever-shifting expressions of the chronic condition.

If, however, we believe that an illness happens to us for a reason, if it is part of how we think of ourselves, or if it is something we have a say in, we create many options. This book is, in part, an invitation for the reader to consider studies, approaches, and perspectives that offer numerous opportunities and approaches in the domain of conscious intervention.

Mind-Body Medicine is relevant to physicians and patients alike because it operates on research results that suggest that whenever we include the mind in the healing process we allow any healing methodology of our choice to be more effective. Patients and physicians alike become empowered. Patients enhance their capacity for self-healing, and as a result physicians tend to be more effective.

While modern medicine and current scientific consensus have long accepted symptoms and diseases such as rheumatoid arthritis, chronic pain (such as pain affecting the neck, wrist, and elbow), insomnia, irritable bowel syndrome, and fibromyalgia as having a mind-body component, Helen Flanders Dunbar, MD,[1] and psychoanalyst Franz Alexander, MD,[2] founders of modern psychosomatic medicine, posited a hundred years ago and sixty years ago, respectively, that emotions influence all illness.

Dunbar writes: "We know now that many physiological processes which are of significance for health of the individual can be controlled by way of emotion. In this knowledge we have the key to many problems in the prevention and treatment of illness, yet we have scarcely begun to use what we know."[3] Alexander states: "It is well established that emotional influences can stimulate or inhibit the function of any organ."[4] In that sense, both Alexander and Dunbar draw attention to the importance of identifying and targeting specific emotions on equal footing with identifying and targeting specific biological parts or systems affected by the disease.

Alexander Summarized the Following Factors that Play a Role (in different proportions) in the Development of Illness:

1. Hereditary constitution
2. Birth trauma
3. Nature of infant care (weaning habits, toilet training, sleeping arrangements, etc.)
4. Accidental physical traumatic experiences of infancy and childhood
5. Accidental emotional traumatic experiences of infancy and childhood
6. Emotional climate of family and specific personality traits of parents and siblings
7. Late physical injuries
8. Later emotional experiences in intimate and occupational relations
9. Organic diseases of infancy which increase the vulnerability of certain organs

Currently we have four basic approaches that attempt to integrate mind-body medicine in very different ways; following are very brief descriptions.

In **psychiatry,** the problem is diagnosed by the psychiatrist (who is viewed as the expert). The patient is given mostly a mind/mood-altering pharmaceutical treatment with little or no focus on underlying influences. It's not that the psychiatrist does not believe in underlying causes—the expediency is primarily for practical reasons. The waiting room is most always full and the waiting list is long (unless you are in private practice and your client list is wealthy). So, to help as many patients as possible, it is much faster to just fill out a prescription.

Psychology offers the patient support from a psychologist, therapist, or intern (therapist apprentice). The therapist is most often viewed as the expert. An initial interview is conducted, a problem area is identified (including underlying causes), and the therapist will suggest and employ a given technique to work with the client together to produce the desired changes.

Transpersonal psychology is an Eastern-influenced psycho-spiritual approach where the patient embarks on a therapeutic journey that emphasizes self-responsibility for problem discovery, origins, and self-guided treatments such as mindfulness and/or a spiritual practice (for instance). If a therapist is employed s/he acts mostly as a catalyst for the patient on their way to uncovering their own truth about what ails them and how to deal with it to bring about the desired health and healing.

As a fourth area of practice, **a shamanic** approach may be taken in which the person engages the assistance of a plant ally such as cannabis (to stay with the focus of this book) to find and make conscious that which is in the way of healing and to explore ways of replacing it with what supports health and well-being.

And while there are many more options and fields between these basic divisions that can be chosen and utilized for help and assistance, for our purpose in this book, these shall suffice. Similarly, the historical and contemporary practical applications of mind-body medicine cover a huge spectrum. They can be found in the various alternative medical traditions such as Traditional Chinese Medicine, Naturopathic medicine, and Osteopathic medicine, to name but a few. For the reader interested in the broader context of psychosomatics (another term for mind-body medicine) it is easy to find relevant material in print or on the internet.

At this point, however, I want to briefly mention the work of two researchers and authors: pharmacologist Candace Pert, PhD, and developmental cell biologist Bruce Lipton, PhD, because of the relevance of their findings to much of what we will be exploring in this chapter.

In his book *The Biology of Belief,* Lipton suggests that each of the trillion cells working in concert to provide balance and well-being in the human body have self-receptors in their membrane.[5] It is these receptors that know the difference between a virus or bacteria and the body's own structures.[6] A mismatch in self-receptors can trigger a severe immune response, such as the dreaded rejection of a transplanted organ, which is needed to sustain life.

It is these cellular self-receptors that demonstrate that our mind is omnipresent in a trillion cellular membranes, all connected with each other and operating in concert. This may explain how the impact of nonphysical influences, such as suppressed emotions, can induce signals throughout the body at a cellular level that generate the transcription of disease-producing proteins instead of those involved in the production of health.

Pert echoes Lipton's findings in more depth and detail in her book *Molecules of Emotions: The Science Behind Body-Mind Medicine.*[7] One of her key findings shows that intelligence is present in each cell of the body, and that the dance between emotions and molecules is indeed a two-way street. Pert's discoveries of a two-way communication between the environment (physical or nonphysical) and the production of either health-supporting or disease-producing molecules are further supported by research conducted in the field of epigenetics.

Epigenetics is a new and still-evolving term,[8] generally used to describe the study of environmental signals (epigenators) such as temperature, nutrition, or emotions that initiate specific change in genetic expressions via a direct pathway into the cellular nucleus, without changing the DNA sequence. Once the signal is received, an intra-cellular epigenetic initiator determines the precise location in the nucleus for the pathway, and an epigenetic maintainer sustains the change through succeeding generations. In other words, an environmental signal (physical or nonphysical) begins a two-way communication with the human body at a cellular level that produces a switch that either turns a gene on or off. This switch can be inherited by future generations.

For instance, studies on mice have shown that emotional material from traumatic experiences produces immediate changes in the biology of the animals, and that these changes can be passed on to the next generation of offspring.[9] A review of relevant studies including on humans similarly demonstrated that horrific emotions experienced during the Holocaust produced physiological changes in the coating of the victims' chromosomes (thread-like strands of total DNA found in the nucleus of each cell) that are passed on to the next generation, leaving the offspring more vulnerable to developing anxiety disorders such as phobia or PTSD.[10]

Since our mental and emotional architecture is part of the environment that sends constant signals to every cell in our body, and vice versa, the implications for mind-body medicine are significant. Epigenetics may provide a basis for better understanding the results of clinical trials indicating that chronically suppressed or repressed emotions exacerbate a variety of medical conditions such as hypertension,[11] cardiovascular disease,[12] and breast cancer,[13] and thus eventually reduce life expectancy.[14]

Now, after having reported on the vast and significant potential of health benefits using mind-body medicine, it is also important to look at the rare but potential downside. Observations from long-term mindfulness practitioners, psychotherapists, meditation teachers, and shamanic practitioners alike suggest that a very small percentage of people using mind-body medicine modalities such as mindfulness, meditation practices, or emotional release work may experience disturbances.[15]

The disturbance may express itself through confusion, feeling lost, a psychotic episode, the end of a relationship, or difficulty concentrating while working, for instance. In the Christian spiritual traditions this type of disturbance brought on by a practice such as prayer or visionary awareness is referred to as "the dark night of the soul" and reflects a spiritual crisis on a person's way to union with God. In the world of meditation this type of disturbance may be spoken of as "enlightenment's evil twin" and often related to irreversible insights such as staring into "emptiness" or experiencing "no-self." Stanislav Grof, MD, who conducted research into extraordinary states of consciousness using LSD and later holotropic breath work, called these events "unresolved ego-deaths."

The U.S. National Institutes of Health addresses the potential problem with meditation by publishing the following partial text on their website:

> Meditation is considered to be safe for healthy people. There have been rare reports that meditation could cause or worsen symptoms in people who have certain psychiatric problems, but this question has not been fully researched. Individuals with existing mental or physical health conditions should speak with their health care providers prior to starting a meditative practice and make their meditation instructor aware of their condition.[16]

A proper setting, a safe environment, and a good match between method or facilitator and student can minimize the risk of adverse effects. If you work with a teacher, guide, physican, or therapist, make sure they are trustworthy, use evidence-based and/or time-proven methods, have the capacity to track your process, and can provide you with the best support possible. And while a supportive and experienced teacher, therapist, or peer (group) can make a positive difference, consider that you are the most important member on your growth and healing team. During time of crisis employ forgiveness (for whatever part you may have played in it) and give yourself as much compassion, kindness, and love as possible.

Molecules, Emotions, and Conscious Interventions—Complex Connections in the Endocannabinoid System

Consider this: Every cell of the human body is in constant communication with other cells. The way signals are communicated is either by chemical or non-physical signals. Molecules are physical (chemical) signals, and sunlight or emotions are examples of non-physical signals. With speeds similar to that of sound, both types of signals "fly" back and forth, through the vast expanse of our nervous system, on a constant basis. For instance, adrenalin (epinephrine), a hormone and a neurotransmitter, is associated with the emotional counterparts of fear (fight or flight or freeze responses). When we encounter (or simply imagine) a fearful situation we instantly send an emotional signal to the adrenal glands (on top of the kidneys), which in turn instructs cellular DNA to code for proteins that combine into adrenalin in rapid succession. Adrenalin enters the bloodstream and increases the body's heart rate and blood pressure, and diverts blood supply from the gastrointestinal tract to the large muscle groups, getting you ready for fight or flight. After all, there is a tiger in front of you. And what are you going to do?

> *"We know now that many physiological processes which are of significance for health of the individual can be controlled by way of emotion."*

—Flanders Dunbar, MD, MedScD, PhD

Acute fear can tell you to step away from that cliff and in that sense is a great motivator that has your body's survival in mind. However, with chronic fears that just won't go away, stress molecules such as adrenalin and cortisol are produced on a continuous basis and in higher amounts, which in turn can have numerous real and serious ill-effects such as making the body more vulnerable to infections and increasing your risk of developing a host of potentially life-threatening diseases including heart disease and hypertension.

Here is the good news: reducing stress hormones is in the domain of conscious intervention. To stay with the example of adrenalin and cortisol and by extension the emotions of fear and anxiety, consider the ten options on page 49. Some of the suggestions may not resonate with you at all, while you may find others especially useful. The idea is that we have options to consciously influence our internal chemistry, not by denying our emotional realities, which only functions to suppress them, but by reducing our fears and anxieties in constructive ways so we can be done with them and their debilitating impact on body and mind.

As you will see in the following pages, understanding the two-directional nature of our emotions and the body's associated physical reactions provides us with the potentially powerful opportunity for self-healing. We can, in fact, begin to release emotions associated with unhealthy molecules and instead foster emotional signals that support our ability to heal and thrive.

At this point, it is important to remember that constricting emotions and stress are not themselves harmful to our health provided they are expressed and let go of appropriately.

Generally speaking, all appropriately expressed emotions are healthy. Anger, while normally seen as a negative emotion, can certainly be destructive, but it can also bring about positive change. The constricting emotion of fear can paralyze a life, but it can save one from falling off the edge of a cliff. Hopelessness can kill or give birth to determination. Worthlessness can imprison or produce compassion. Blame can fuel violence toward others, and it can demonstrate what matters.

Conversely, the expansive and positive emotion of love can be a true wonder to behold and experience, but it can also be used to control or smother another. Hope can sustain life in difficult times or maintain a negative influence. Trust can propel a positive reality, while inappropriate trust can destroy it.

However, there are three types of emotions that by definition have only a negative impact, namely guilt, harbored anger, and martyrdom. (See "Exploring Unhealthy Emotional Habits" in the Appendix.)

The up-side of stress comes into play when we love what we do. When we are engaged in work that is meaningful and important to us, stress turns into a positive by propelling motivation, growth, and evolution. Healthy stress produces a molecular balance in which our mechanism for processing stress is fortified and quite able to handle most everything we experience biologically as well as psychologically.

Molecules and Emotions—A Two-Way Street

Have a look at this partial list of endogenous molecules (made by the human body) and their known or suspected emotional counterparts. Consider the possibility that by generating specific emotional content you are also changing the very chemistry of your body, either fully or partly modulated via the endocannabinoid system. In doing so we can consciously direct and support the self-healing abilities of our body.

Also, remember that the evidence-based patterns represented in this section are a sampling of a much larger body of scientific studies and do not represent a comprehensive review. They do serve, however, to demonstrate the intricately linked mind-body connection and its influence on our health and well-being.

The Biology of Emotions (Summary)

Molecules primarily associated with expansive emotions:

Acetylcholine: I remember

Anandamide: I am at ease

Endogenous opioids: It feels so good when the pain stops

Gamma-aminobutyric acid (GABA): I am melting

Oxytocin: I feel for you

Serotonin: I am happy

Molecules primarily associated with constricting emotions:

Epinephrine: I am afraid

Dopamine: I am motivated

Norepinephrine: I am attentive!

Cortisol: I am stressed

Glutamate: I am excited

Vasopressin: I am aggressive

The Biology of Emotions
Building and Balancing Chi

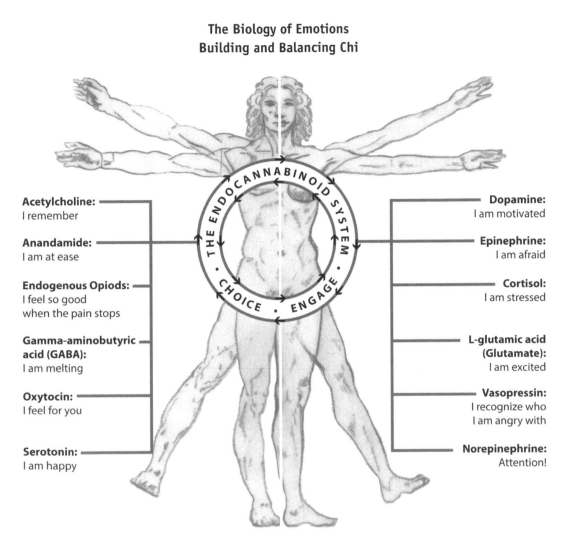

Acetylcholine:
I remember

Anandamide:
I am at ease

Endogenous Opiods:
I feel so good
when the pain stops

**Gamma-aminobutyric
acid (GABA):**
I am melting

Oxytocin:
I feel for you

Serotonin:
I am happy

THE ENDOCANNABINOID SYSTEM
· CHOICE · ENGAGE ·

Dopamine:
I am motivated

Epinephrine:
I am afraid

Cortisol:
I am stressed

**L-glutamic acid
(Glutamate):**
I am excited

Vasopressin:
I recognize who
I am angry with

Norepinephrine:
Attention!

Molecules Primarily Associated with Expansive Emotions
ACETYLCHOLINE

- Produced by neurons throughout the body
- Neurons contain CB1

Acetylcholine is a naturally occurring neurotransmitter of the autonomic nervous system and the only neurotransmitter of the voluntary nervous system. Depending on location, the molecule produces different effects. For instance, acetylcholine produces contraction of skeletal muscles while it inhibits contraction of the muscles of the heart.

Animal studies show that a low to medium dose of THC can increase acetylcholine in the brain (while a high dose of THC may lower it, an effect not confirmed in human trials).[1]

Emotional Keywords: I remember (learning, memory, plasticity, arousal, attention, reward)

Potential Ill-Effects: Reduced acetylcholine levels are associated with insomnia, impaired creativity, and dementia in Alzheimer's patients. Too much acetylcholine may contribute to anxiety, restlessness, or heightened levels of fear.

Potential Health Benefits:
Increased sense of creativity, ability to enjoy life's pleasures and passions.
Enhanced ability for learning and remembering.
May help you sleep.
May reduce risk of dementia.

To Boost or Balance Your Acetylcholine Availability:
- learn and use a new word(s) every day
- meditate to enhance focus and concentration
- improve your memory (crossword puzzles, riddles, etc.)
- recall a rare emotion in detail until you feel it
- think of a feeling you never had and imagine what it feels like
- consider CB1 activating cannabinoids

ANANDAMIDE
- Produced in human cell membranes
- Human cell membranes contain CB1 and CB2

Anandamide is an endogenous (made by the human body) cannabinoid and neurotransmitter very similar to THC (from the cannabis plant). THC binds at the same receptor sites (CB1 and CB2) as anandamide and at the proper therapeutic dose produces very similar effects.

Emotional Keywords: I am at ease (bliss, relaxation, social)

Potential Ill-Effects: Not known

Potential Health Benefits:
Anandamide may reduce hypertension, depression, fear, and anxiety as well as contribute to social play behavior.[1] The molecule may also

be relevant in the treatment of psychiatric disorders characterized by impairments in social behavior such as autism.

The presence of corticosteroids stimulates the body's production of anandamide, which may account for the way in which anandamide influences the neuropathic and antidepressant effects of exercise.[2]

Both THC and the synthetic cannabinoid CP 55,940 reduce pain by inducing the release of the endogenous opioid dynorphin A and dynorphin B, respectively. Anandamide similarly reduces pain but by a potentially novel mechanism not very well understood.[3]

Anandamide inhibits the movement of cancer cells and may prevent metastasis without negative effects to the patient's immune system.[4]

To Boost or Balance Your Anandamide Availability:

- Exercise such as high-intensity endurance running significantly increased anandamide and "runner's high."[5]
- Meaningful social interactions may increase anandamide levels naturally.
- Anandamide inhibits norepinephrine.[6]
- Meditation practices may increase anandamide levels naturally.
- Consider a balanced CB1:CB2 activating cannabinoids.

How to meditate: About thirty years ago I was interested in learning about Buddhist philosophy and healing practices, and I went straight to the source. I traveled to Northern Thailand, to a town called Chiang Mai. I visited a temple called Wat Tapotaram. While there I noticed a Thai family bring in a severely disturbed woman who was hearing voices "telling her to do terrible things." A young monk was brought to talk to her. About an hour later she had visibly changed and appeared at peace and was taken home. I learned that this young monk was well known to be able to help the psychologically disturbed, or as the villagers called them, the "possessed."

I wanted to learn more about how he was able to assist the patient and her family to allow such a significant change in such a short period of time. Believing in learning by doing, I ordained as a monk. I lived at Wat Tapotaram, where the old Abbott taught me the following simple technique called Samatha (Tranquility), which develops single-point concentration as a way to calm the mind.

Samatha (Tranquility Meditation): Kneeling on a meditation bench (I could never sit cross-legged for long), I listened intently as he taught me to focus my attention on my abdomen (about an inch or so above my navel), i.e., to place my mind's attention there. (The focus point should lie on the vertical midline of the body.)

As I breathe in, my abdomen expands until it peaks or pauses; as I breathe out, it contracts until I reach the bottom of the exhale or pause again. He said, "This never changes as long as you live." As the abdomen expands, pauses, contracts, and pauses, follow the motion from beginning to end with your mind's eye. Just be with your breath throughout these four phases. That's all there is to it.

If you get distracted or your mind starts to wander, bring it gently back to that focus point on your belly. After I had some time to practice I began to notice changes in my ability to maintain equanimity, and I experienced a deeper sense of peace and overall calm.

A month or so later the Abbott introduced another technique to me called Vipassana. This technique is designed to understand and develop insights into self that lead to transformation and healing. Mindfulness practices are employed to contemplate the constructs of the mind (sensation, thoughts, and feelings) and how they contribute to one's health and healing or the lack thereof.

Vipassana is taught in many countries including the U.S. (for example, by Jack Kornfield, Ruth Denison, Sharon Salzberg, Joseph Goldstein). It has been adopted by numerous psychotherapists, neuroscientists, and clinicians alike as a means to further therapy, achieve stress reduction, and deepen personal and spiritual growth as a pathway to health. Vipassana is taught in various prisons in Asia and the U.S. to remarkable effect in reducing violence and establishing compassion among inmates.

Jon Kabat-Zinn, Professor Emeritus of Medicine at MIT, developed a technique based in part on Vipassana called "mindfulness-based stress reduction," which has been studied extensively for its positive impact on numerous diseases such as hypertension, anxiety, depression, and fibromyalgia.

If you don't like to sit but would like to practice meditation, you can look at moving meditations such as simple Walking Meditation, Tai Chi, or Qi Gong.

ENDOGENOUS OPIOIDS (PAIN-BLOCKING MOLECULES MADE BY THE HUMAN BODY)

- Produced by central nervous system (CNS) and pituitary
- CNS and pituitary contain CB1

Five groups of endogenous opioids have been discovered: beta-endorphins, enkephalins, dynorphins, endomorphins, and nociception.[1] Endogenous opioids bind with opiate receptors and reduce stress and pain perceptions; they are also involved in the formation of emotions, interpersonal relationships, and hunger, among other feelings and physical states.

Emotional Keywords: It feels so good when the pain stops

Potential Ill-Effects: None known

Potential Health Benefits:

In addition to modulating pain, endorphins can produce feelings of euphoria and elation.

Both THC and the synthetic cannabinoid CP 55,940 reduce pain by inducing the release of the endogenous opioids dynorphin A and dynorphin B, respectively.[2]

To Boost or Balance Your Endorphin Availability:

- Strenuous exercise
- A pleasurable massage
- A deeply relaxing acupuncture session
- Sex
- Inducing deep relaxation response via cannabis or relaxation technique of choice
- Consider CB1 activating cannabinoids

GAMMA-AMINOBUTYRIC ACID (GABA)

- Made in brain cells from glutamate
- Brain cells contain CB1

GABA (the brain's own Valium) is an amino acid that acts as an inhibitory neurotransmitter and thus functions as the body's "downer." It regulates excitability of nerve cells and muscle tone. GABA also influences speech and language by putting a pause between our words.

A pilot study conducted at the University of Boston demonstrated a mind-body link via measuring a significant increase in brain GABA after subjects practiced yoga.[1]

When GABA and glutamate balance each other, relaxation and excitement balance each other and vice versa. Find your emotional balance.

Emotional Keywords: I am melting (relaxed, calm, slowed down)

Potential Ill-Effects: Low levels of GABA are related to irritability, anxiety, panic attacks, lack of empathy, aggression, attention deficit hyperactivity disorder (ADHD), antisocial behavior, depression, craving for carbohydrates, and adrenal fatigue.

Potential Health Benefits:

GABA inhibits fear signaling in the amygdala.[2]

May reduce sleep problems, anxiety, and depression.

The dual capacity of the endocannabinoid system to simultaneously balance upper (via cortical glutamate) and downer effects (via GABA) may present a new approach to treating ADHD.[3]

To Boost or Balance Your GABA Availability:

- Yoga (asana) sessions increased brain GABA level by 27%.[4]
- Chronic stress reduces GABA. Reduce toxic stress with the method of your choice.
- Consider the calming effects of CB1 activating cannabinoids.

OXYTOCIN

- Produced in hypothalamus and stored in pituitary
- Hypothalamus and pituitary contain CB1

Oxytocin is a hormone produced by both genders. In orthodox medicine it is used to stop post-partum bleeding and to induce labor.

Emotional Keywords: I feel for you (empathy, generosity, trust, and reduced fear)

Potential Ill-Effects: Lack of oxytocin (or imbalance) has been associated with the development of autism, low libido, eating disorders, social anxiety disorders, schizophrenia, and depression.

Potential Health Benefits: You may already know that a mutual hug is fun, free, and feels good. But you may not know that recent scientific discoveries have shown that hugs[1] (warm relationships[2] but also sex and orgasms[3]) create oxytocin and by extension measurable health benefits, helping you not just improve the quality of your life but also stimulate and empower your innate capacity for self-healing.

Oxytocin is commonly referred to as the "cuddle molecule." It is involved in the development of bonding, closeness, tenderness, and intimacy. It increases trust[4] and generosity.[5] Additionally, it initiates the release of endorphins with their own deep relaxation and emotional benefits. And while the scientific community acknowledges that understanding the "cuddle hormone" is just beginning, here is a list of physical benefits we already know about.

Oxytocin reduces high blood pressure and protects the heart in women.[6]

Oxytocin reduces cravings such as your sweet tooth and thus can have an impact in preventing diabetes, excess weight gain, and drug use.[7]

The cuddle hormone enhances the healing of wounds, making hugs an important benefit in any recovery.[8]

Oxytocin reduces the sensation of pain, making hugs an important adjunct analgesic.[9]

Intimacy reduces inflammation and oxidative stress by increasing endorphin levels and ridding the body of pro-inflammatory hormones, which translates into better immunity and faster recovery.[10] (Most chronic degenerative illnesses involve inflammation and oxidative stressors.)

Oxytocin released by hugs reduces anxiety and fear and enhances the development of trust.[11]

The "cuddle hormone" may also be implicated in getting an erection, suggesting that male virility may be related to developing good relationships.[12]

Remember, "vitamin O" has a short half-life and last only for a few seconds in the bloodstream, which suggests that to maximize the potential health benefits of oxytocin we need to keep our focus on generating these qualities.

Oxytocin and the Endocannabinoid System: Recent studies suggest that the endocannabinoid system is involved in the production and release of oxytocin.[13] Anandamide has been discovered to modulate oxytocin levels,[14] and the CB1 receptor plays a key role in the ability of oxytocin to reduce pain.[15]

How to Make "Vitamin O"

- Hugs
- Warm relationships
- Sex and orgasm
- Closeness
- Tenderness
- Intimacy
- Trust
- Generosity
- Consider CB1 activating cannabinoids

Self-Love (A "Tell All" Technique)

Close your eyes, enter a state of relaxation, and begin by touching your feet. Make physical contact with them and, as you feel them, convince them that you love them. Explain why. Thank them for getting you around the beautiful world all by themselves, for allowing you to go places and have adventures. Love them for the work they do so well. Move to the ankles: love them for the support, strength, and flexibility they bring to your steps, jumps, and bounce. Your calves for the power of motion they bring to each step you take. The support and solidity your shin bones provide day in and day out, without you ever having to even think about it. Your knees for their flexibility, endurance, and range of motion they provide. Your strong thighs whose powerful muscles and bones carry your weight so easily. Your pelvic girdle, your biggest joint (no pun intended), between your upper and lower halves that allows for motion in all directions. Your buttocks that allow you to sit and contemplate the world, to work long hours, and to grind to the rhythm of your bass. It also contains your genitals that offer sensuality and pleasure, as well as your anus, which releases what is no longer needed. Your abdomen with all the organs that digest, assimilate, and eliminate in a process so essential for your life and well being. Your chest, with the ribs that protect your heart, and the lungs that deliver fresh oxygen and nutrients to every cell of your body. Your arms and hands that allow you to reach and touch whatever your heart desires. Your neck and spinal cord, that spring that supports you with strength and flexibility. Your face rich with sensory treasures and home to your taste, smell, sound, and sight. Your skin and hair sensitive to the slightest touch of wind, letting you know where you end and the outside world begins.

Let each of your body's parts know you love them and you will have found an avenue that leads to self love. After practicing this technique, see and feel how your day may unfold differently. I still surprise myself at how much better my day goes when I do this.

SEROTONIN

- Made primarily in the digestive tract
- Gut contains primarily CB2

Serotonin is a neurotransmitter especially abundant in the gastrointestinal tract (assisting appetite regulation and bowel movement). To a lesser degree it is found in the central nervous system (affecting mood, sleep, memory) and in blood cells called platelets that are responsible for clotting; thus serotonin is involved in wound healing.

Research has shown a direct correlation between mood and serotonin. Positive mood = increased serotonin while negative mood = reduced serotonin.[1] Positronic brain imaging has shown that healthy people who underwent positive or negative mood induction produced more serotonin when happy and less when sad.[2]

The endocannabinoid-induced modulation of stress-related disorders such as anxieties or depression appears to be mediated, at least in part, through the regulation of the serotoninergic system.[3]

Emotional Keywords: I am happy (relaxed, sensual, happy, safe, positive, flexible, easy-going)

Potential Ill-Effects: Low levels of serotonin are linked to difficulty finishing things, poor impulse control, irritability, depression, and anxiety disorders. Too much serotonin (e.g., resulting from serotonin reuptake inhibitors/SSRIs) can cause excessive nerve cell activity and serotonin reuptake syndrome, with potential deadly consequences.

Potential Health Benefits:
Increased sense of well-being, sensuality, and happiness.
May protect against depression and anxieties.

To Boost or Balance Your Serotonin Availability:
- Reduce toxic stress (chronic stress reduces serotonin)
- Be Happy! Merely remembering happy situations and memories gives you a boost. Also, happiness tends to occur naturally when you meet your basic human needs for safety, security, pleasure, and belonging.

- Get a massage to boost your happiness and your serotonin.
- Consider CB2 activating cannabinoids
- Exercise increases serotonin production and release.
- Balanced exposure to sunlight increases vitamin D, which is involved in promoting serotonin production.

Molecules Primarily Associated with Constricting Emotions
CATECHOLAMINE FAMILY (EPINEPHRINE, DOPAMINE, AND NOREPINEPHRINE)

EPINEPHRINE

- Produced primarily by the adrenal glands
- Adrenals contain CB1

Epinephrine, also known as adrenalin, is a hormone and neurotransmitter associated with fight, flight, or freeze responses as well as the long-term memory of intense events. It is produced in the adrenal glands, which are located on top of each kidney. Physiologically arousing epinephrine increases heart rate and raises blood pressure (by constricting the smooth muscles of the arteries), but at the same time it relaxes the smooth muscles of the airways (all in anticipation of a fight or flight stimulus).

Psychologically the hormone is clearly associated with fear. Consider one of numerous experiments with similar results. Healthy students were injected with epinephrine and then watched film clips that induce emotions such as fear. Those injected with the hormone responded with greater fear and intensity than the control group, whose members received a non-reactive saline injection.[1]

Emotional Keywords: I am scared

Potential Ill-Effects: Too much epinephrine (adrenalin) causes adrenal fatigue, rapid heartbeat and palpitations, high blood pressure, anxiety, weight loss, sweating, and cold extremities. The good news is that adrenalin has a half-life of about 5 minutes in the bloodstream, which means that once the chronic stressor (e.g., fear) is removed, so is epinephrine.

Potential Health Benefits: Epinephrine can save your life by enabling you to quickly respond to a real threat.

10 Proven Strategies to Reduce Stress Hormones by Ending the War with Fear and Anxiety

1. Accept Your Fear and Make It Bigger

One way to diminish fear's stranglehold is to embrace it. In fact, try this technique: Retreat to a quiet place, get comfortable, close your eyes, and breathe a few deep breaths.

Notice where in your body you experience fear.

What does it look like (shape and color); do you notice a sound, smell, or taste of fear?

Say, "Greetings fear, I welcome you to this moment."

Now, allow fear to grow bigger. Let it become as big as it wants to be.

Notice your fear-based thoughts and feelings and welcome those as well.

Try to get a sense of the boundaries, dimensions, and the edges of fear. What is its shape? Is it sharp-edged or like an amorphous blob?

Thank fear for its intention (whatever that may be).

Now, release fear back whence it came. Sense it depart.

Flood your senses with compassion, love, and gratitude.

You may try filling yourself with white light.

Allow the light to flood every single cell in your body.

How do you feel now?

2. Create a Plan B (this technique is best done in writing)

Identify your fear and let it tell you its story (each fear has a story).

Ask yourself the following questions and write out the answers, in detail, like you were writing in a journal.

What if I fail? (create a plan B, break it down into small steps that you can do)

What happens if I do nothing?

What happens if I succeed?

This simple writing idea will often let you give dimensions to your fear and allow you to realize that fear does not have to be overwhelming, never-ending, or all-powerful.

3. Tsunami Technique—Reclaiming Your Imagination

Close your eyes and use any relaxation method you like. When you have entered the safety of your meditative space, imagine yourself in the middle of your worst-case scenario. Your nightmare is here and everything is falling apart. See and feel in detail what it would be like to be lost in the tsunami of your fear realized. Now, STOP. Lift out of the wave of destruction and let it collapse below you. Above you imagine a reality in which you succeed and your best-case scenario unfolds instead of your worst. Lift into it and see and feel the details of this version of reality. Come out of meditation and notice how you feel.

4. Flip the Switch from Fear to Wonder

You may not be able to control the circumstances of your fear, but you do have control about how you are going to respond to it. Instead of responding with fear, consider wonder instead. What can be learned from this situation? What does fear tell you about yourself, about others, or the values you hold dear? Perhaps it is informing you that trust is earned and should only be given to those who are worthy of it. Perhaps it is showing you your motivation, creativity, the power of your imagination, and what it is you truly love.

5. Surrender

There is a fine line between fear and exhilaration. I talked to a skydiver who described it this way: "I feel intense fear all the way up in the airplane. But, when the door opens and I climb outside there is the moment when I let go. And in that moment all that fear turns instantly into pure, orgasmic exhilaration." Now, granted skydiving is a risky activity. But consider something that for you is exciting and scary at the same time. For instance, "I like to have intimacy but just the thought of it terrifies me." What do you have to let go of to turn the switch? What would have to happen for you to surrender and consider intimacy fun, safe, and exciting?

6. Breathe

Fear has a specific breath pattern of rapid inhalations and exhalations with short pauses in between. Accelerated heart rate, increases in blood pressure, and fear go hand in hand. By changing the way we breathe, we can change the way we feel. Taking successful control of your breathing (the only one of the three that is subject to conscious intervention) will lower heart rate and blood pressure and by extension reduce your fear.

Breathe in deeply and hold your breath at the height of inhalation.

Count to five (slowly).

Breathe out, deeply.

Hold your breath at the bottom of your exhalation.

Count to five (slowly).

Repeat for at least five cycles.

7. Analyze Your Fear

Determine if your fear is keeping you from real danger or if it is just a fabrication of a fear-fueled imagination. For instance, are you standing at the edge of a cliff and your fear is asking you to step back to safety, or is your fear telling you that love is for fools because your first date as a teenager didn't go so well?

8. Slow Down

Studies have shown that when we are afraid we limit our choices and close down to many otherwise possible responses. Fear, like most of the constricting emotions (such as anxiety, anger, defensiveness), flourishes with the speed of thought and speech. In other words, the more dangerous tigers you imagine, the more your mind will try to protect you by rapidly trying to find a safe place to hide. We think fast and we speak fast. However, a person in constant fear always imagines more tigers. So, slow down your thinking. It is your imagination; it does not belong to fear. Take it back and go slow motion in your mind's eye or ear. Slow down your speech. In conversation speak one or two sentences, then take a break and breathe, relax, and listen to the response. Repeat.

9. Work with Cannabis (Consider strains with slightly higher THC: CBD ratio to favor CB1 activation)

Cannabis is broadly recognized for its capacity to diminish chronic negative affect (fear, anxieties, anger) and replace it with a gentle attitude, an easy smile, and more optimistic outlook, all of which have proven to support out natural self-healing abilities.

When working with cannabis it is important to remember the idea of the therapeutic window. Your subjective therapeutic window is established by bottom and top threshold. Using too little (below your therapeutic threshold) is sub-optimal and ineffective. Using too much (above your therapeutic threshold) may worsen the very symptoms you are trying to alleviate. For instance, if you are working to reduce your anxiety then taking in excess of your top threshold can make your anxieties worse. (You might want to review the section "Is Cannabis Safe: What is a subjective therapeutic window?" in Chapter I.)

10. Heart Rhythm Coherence (HeartMath Technique)

A study conducted by the Santa Cruz County Children's Mental Health Agency in California used this HeartMath Technique on seriously emotionally disturbed youths and found that it could help the kids feel calmer during times of stress.[2]

Step 1. Focus your attention on your heart (the center of your chest).

Step 2. Feel your breath coming in and out of your heart area (breathe deeply but normally).

Step 3. As you continue to focus on your heart and your heart-centered breathing, choose to experience a positive feeling. (The study participants were instructed to create a library of positive feelings, thoughts, and memories on which they could focus at any given moment.)

DOPAMINE

- Made primarily by adrenal glands
- Adrenal glands contain CB1

Dopamine, a hormone and neurotransmitter that is primarily produced by the body in the adrenal glands located on top of each kidney, is associated with emotional and behavioral motivation (positive and negative)[1] such as reward, emotional memory, and arousal (e.g., pleasure, love, money, food, and sex). In a way the molecule is saying, "Pay attention, this is worth remembering." The more intense, unpredictable, or novel the experience, the greater the reward and associated dopamine release. Dopamine is also involved in the processing of emotions, making this molecule makes especially relevant to patients with PTSD or autism.[2]

Dopamine modulates neurons in the substancia nigra (a portion of the mid-brain) via dopamine receptors and CB1.[3] The loss of dopamine-producing nerve cells in this portion of the brain is associated with numerous mental and neurological disorders such as schizophrenia, ADHD, and Parkinson's.

Emotional Keywords: I am motivated (arousal, emotional processing, and memory)

Potential Ill-Effects: Lack of dopamine is associated with fatigue, failure to finish tasks, low libido, and burdensome emotional memory. Too much dopamine (e.g., pharmaceuticals such as L-dopa drugs, or drugs such as methamphetamine) is associated with psychosis and/or aggression.

Potential Health Benefits:

Increased motivation, productivity, sensuality and libido; sufficient dopamine reduces risk of developing Parkinson's disease.

Abnormal dopamine transmission in the striatum (the part of the forebrain that modulates the endocannabinoid system) plays a pivotal role in ADHD. Researchers point to CB1 receptors as novel molecular players in ADHD, and suggest that therapeutic strategies aimed at engaging the ECS might prove effective in this disorder.[4]

To Boost or Balance Low Dopamine Availability:

- Listen to music that accesses and moves deep emotions.[5]
- Learn to play music (play an instrument).
- The natural amino acid tyrosine is a precursor to dopamine.

- Meditation induced changes of consciousness.[6]
- Consider CB1 activating cannabinoids.
- Explore Extended Attention Span Training (EAST), a technique developed by NASA, and its offshoot called Self Mastery and Regulation Training (SMART), a biofeedback-based video game.

NOREPINEPHRINE

- Produced primarily by the adrenal glands
- Adrenal glands contain CB1

Norepinephrine, another hormone and neurotransmitter, functions physiologically in a similar way to epinephrine (fight and flight), and it is also produced in the adrenal glands. Psychologically norepinephrine is associated with focused and sustained concentration.

GABA, THC, and anandamide inhibit norepinephrine levels.[1]

Emotional Keywords: Attention! (excitement, alertness, urgency, concentration, focus, and motivation)

Potential Ill-Effects: On the mental-emotional plane, excess norepinephrine can increase anxiety and restlessness, and heighten levels of fear. Physical effects may include rapid heart rate and elevated blood pressure. Lack of the hormone is common in Alzheimer's patients and may play a contributing role.

Potential Health Benefits:

Norepinephrine can speed a heart beating too slowly or increase the force of contraction, thus improving circulation of oxygen and nutrients. It can tighten the smooth muscles in the arteries and raise blood pressure in hypotensive patients such as those suffering from forms of shock (i.e., hypovolemic, septic).

Psychologically the hormone produces excitement, alertness, urgency, concentration, focus, and motivation. It reduces symptoms of ADHD or ADD.

Modulating Norepinephrine

- Reduce toxic stress with the relaxation method of your choice.
- Consider the calming effects of cannabinoids.
- Increase your anandamide availability (see Anandamide, above).
- Consider CB1 activating cannabinoids.

CORTISOL

- Made primarily by the adrenal glands
- Adrenal glands contain CB1

Cortisol is a steroidal hormone that is released into the bloodstream when we experience stress. Cortisol, like epinephrine and norepinephrine, is produced by the adrenal glands, situated on top of the kidneys.

The presence of corticosteroids stimulates the body's production of anandamide, which may account for the way in which anandamide influences the antidepressant effects of exercise.[1]

An experiment conducted at the University of California suggests a connection between the emotions of shame and guilt and the psychological constructs of self-worth and self-esteem.

People burdened with shame and those with low self-esteem and a low sense of self-worth exhibited increased levels of cortisol when compared to a random control group.[2]

Emotional Keywords: I am stressed (fear, anxiety, restlessness, shame, guilt, low self-esteem, low self-worth)

Potential Ill-Effects: Sustained and increased levels of cortisol are highly self-destructive (weaken the immune system, weaken bones, skin, muscles, tendons, and other connective tissue, thereby increasing vulnerability to infections and injuries).

Potential Health Benefits: Cortisol is a steroid-based hormone that, similarly to epinephrine, helps to produce energy to escape dangerous situations and is beneficial in the acute (initial) phase of an injury.

To Reduce or Balance Your Cortisol:

- See Epinephrine, above ("10 Proven Strategies to Reduce Stress Hormones").
- Reduce feelings of shame and guilt; rediscover your self-worth and build self-esteem.
- Consider CB1 activating cannabinoids.

Giving Shame Back Technique
(a meditative process, not a real-life action)

1. In the safety of your meditative space, relax and breathe.
2. Set the intention of finding and releasing shame (feelings of "there is something seriously wrong with me").

3. Scan your body for where you sense shame, and allow your body to show you (it remembers).

4. Allow yourself to get into the feeling of shame and explore what is there (you may find a memory, or a set of memories, or a perpetrator or not).

5. Either way feel the ugliness, the hurt, the violation…(and the debilitating meaning of it).

6. Now grab hold of it (i.e., if you sense it as a tarry goo, pull it off and out of you and throw it at its source—the perpetrator). If you can't sense or it is too scary to deal with a perpetrator (that's okay), throw the shame in whatever form you sense it into a hole in the ground. Earth can handle shame and transform it into fertilizer just fine.

7. The perpetrator will take it and leave your meditation and take their shame with them (after all, it is your meditation, you are in charge, and it is their shame to process, not yours).

8. Now, flood the area previously occupied by shame with light (color of your choice) to flush out any remaining residue. Remember that the autonomic nervous system does not know the difference between a real or an imagined event. Once you end shame by returning it from whence it came, you can be free of the mental construct that constantly produces shame-based cortisol.

9. Alternate process/ending: If you believe in a celestial architect (by whatever name) you can ask them to take the shame away (they know what to do with it) and flush your body and mind with the light of their choice.

GLUTAMATE

- Most likely produced by mitochondria and released by brain cells (astroglia)
- Astroglia contain CB1 and possibly CB2

L-glutamic acid is the most abundant excitatory neurotransmitter, but it only exists in low concentrations. Glutamate is glutamic acid to which a mineral ion (salt) has been attached (e.g., sodium glutamate or potassium glutamate, etc.). L-glutamic acid made by the human body is healthy. All L-glutamic acid made outside contains unhealthy impurities and at high concentrations (e.g., MSG or 99% pure labels). Glutamine, an amino acid, is a precursor to glutamate. Gluten and synthetic glutamate are unrelated except in that they both may contribute to neurological illnesses.

Emotional Keywords: I am excited (the body's "upper")

Potential Ill-Effects: Too much glutamate is a major contributing factor in anxiety disorders, insomnia, neurological illnesses such as autism, Parkinson's, MS, seizures, and increased risk of strokes. Too much glutamate can overly increase acetylcholine, which can further increase anxiety, restlessness, and fear. Excitotoxicity is defined as excessive stimulation of nerve cells (e.g., by too much glutamate, or too concentrated an amount), causing inflammation, damage, or death to cells of the nervous system. Inflammation increases glutamate over-excitation and neurotoxicity.

Potential Health Benefits:

Activation of CB1 stimulates the release of glutamate, thus modulating synaptic transmission and plasticity.[1] The dual capacity of the ECS to balance upper (cortical glutamate) and downer effects (GABA) at the same time may present a new approach to treating ADHD.[2]

Chronic stress and acute stress associated with severe emotional trauma can reduce natural endocannabinoid production as well as reduce receptor-site sensitivity, thus removing an important biological mechanism to end anxieties. The body utilizes the endocannabinoid system to reduce stress responses and anxieties by reducing glutamte.[3]

Modulating Glutamate:

- Reduce or cease using foods that contain glutamate.
- Reduce fear, worry, and stress with any technique of your choice (see Epinephrine).
- Consider CB1-activating cannabinoids.

VASOPRESSIN

- Produced by hypothalamus and stored and released by pituitary
- Both contain CB1

The hormone vasopressin functions physiologically primarily to hold on to water and thus is important in maintaining hydration and the utilization of molecular sugars and salts. Vasopressin also constricts blood vessels, which makes it relevant to blood pressure regulation.

On the mental-emotional plane, the hormone is associated with aggression and defensive and territorial behavior (especially in males). Vasopressin is also involved in social recognition of facial expressions (i.e., happy and angry), which serve as important cues in developing intimacy in humans.[1]

In an experiment a group of men and women were exposed to a significant stressor. Blood level and emotions were assessed immediately after the stressful event. Results showed that men (but not women) had more vasopressin in their blood and reported increased anger in response. Hence the correlation of anger and vasopressin in males.[2]

Another study focused on 12 heterosexual couples in which the male partner suffered from PTSD, with the symptoms of difficulties with emotional intimacies. When patients received vasopressin they were able to antidote the effects of PTSD by making emotional connections.[3] Thus vasopressin was associated with social cognition.

Recent studies suggest that the endocannabinoid system is involved in the production and release of vasopressin.[4]

Both vasopressin and oxytocin modulate the portion of the brain responsible for social and emotional interaction and thus may be relevant to other-regarding behavior such as empathy, compassion, and kindness (altruism).[5]

Emotional Keywords: Move over, I see you (aggression, defensive and territorial behavior especially in males, social recognition of facial expressions such as happy and angry)

Potential Ill-Effects: Low levels of vasopressin contribute to polyuria (excess urination), excess thirst, and hypernatremia (excess salt retention). Too much vasopressin can cause hyponatremia (lack of sodium concentrations in blood).

Potential Health Benefits: Vasopressin may act in the brain to induce assertiveness and is involved in social (re)cognition.

Modulating Vasopressin:

- Reduce fear, worry, and anger-related stress states with any technique of your choice.
- Consider developing empathy and compassion by paying attention to subtle cues such as facial expression, tone of voice, or body language, for example.
- Employ open, non-defensive, and vulnerable inquiries or any other method of developing intimacy skills.
- See the section on oxytocin (above), since it is very likely that both hormones are produced and utilized to achieve similar outcomes.
- Consider CB1 activating cannabinoids.

NOTE: For more mindfulness techniques related to healing, please see Chapter V: Integrating Mind-Body Medicine for Deeper Healing.

Chapter III

How to Use The Cannabis Health Index

What Is a CHI Score?

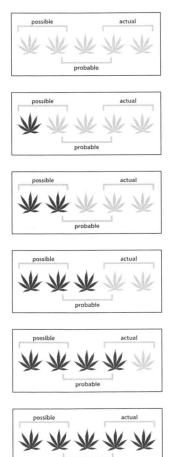

Simply put, the CHI score is an evidence-based rating system that shows degrees of confidence in cannabis as an effective treatment for a specific condition.

More specifically, the CHI score is a rating system that takes into account both the type of research study (which impacts the reliability of a study's conclusions) and the study's findings, which may be positively associated with medical use of cannabis (that is, the study reports that cannabis is a viable treatment) or negatively associated with it (the study says it doesn't work).

Each experiment is scored based on type of study (between 1 and 5—see chart below), and then this number is multiplied by +1 if the study concluded that cannabis was effective, or multiplied by -1 if the study concluded that cannabis was ineffective. Studies with inconclusive or mixed results may be included in the text for your reference, but they do not contribute to the overall disease CHI score.

Finally, all the scores for individual studies included in the analysis of a disease are added together to create an overall disease CHI score. (An overall high disease score means that many studies have been conducted for this particular illness or that the studies conducted were of high caliber.) The overall CHI score is then divided by the total number of studies in each section ranging between 0 and 5 (or to a maximum of five leaf symbols), and this number is the CHI number that can be used to approximate degree of confidence about the current state of scientific inquiry for any particular disease listed.

While the CHI may not provide you with all the information that you need, the CHI can be an indispensable tool at your fingertips. Nevertheless, you may still want to discuss these studies with your health care practitioner. The CHI makes that possible, particularly if you have concerns about the effectiveness and/or safety of other methods available to you.

For ease of use and improved availability, the CHI is also available as an app on the website www.cannabishealthindex.com.

Importance of the Type of Research Study

Not all study types and designs, and their respective findings, translate equally well into practically useful insights. The scientific method informs and guides basic research and experiments. Different types of research studies attempt to test hypotheses—for example, that cannabis is an effective treatment for multiple sclerosis. Within medical research, double-blind, placebo-controlled, and clinical human trials provide the strongest evidence (that is, are deemed most likely to determine the truth). Next in line are controlled human trials. Studies that review and compare available published research are also highly respected, strong pieces of evidence. Less convincing, in order, are human case studies and case studies of individual clinical experiences, animal experiments, and laboratory studies. In this book, values are assigned to reviewed research studies that reflect the intrinsic strength of evidence associated with each type of study. The following chart gives the value assigned to each category at a glance.

How Should I Use the CHI Score in General?

This book concentrates on diseases and conditions for which cannabis shows promise, so it should be no surprise that you will rarely see negative CHI scores. However, you may see negative as well as positive scores for individual studies if various studies reached different conclusions. Published studies were primarily extracted from MEDLINE, the U.S. National Library of Medicine's bibliographic database. Inclusion criteria

Possible CHI Scores

Study Designs	Evidence-based Rating of Possible CHI Scores
Double-blind, placebo-controlled, clinical human trials and double-blind, placebo-controlled, clinical, crossover human trials	+/–5
Clinical human trials and cohort studies	+/–4
Reviews (of relevant literature and studies) and human case studies	+/–3
Animal studies	+/–2
Laboratory studies	+/–1

focused on the influence of the endocannabinoid system, cannabis and/ or cannabinoids on symptoms and diseases listed (A–Z) in the *Cannabis Health Index*.

Please note that a high total score reflects the amount of available published research to a much larger extent than it reflects the degree of efficacy of cannabis to treat the particular disease. The disease CHI score is a simple sum of all the individual study scores for that disease, so higher overall CHI numbers indicate that a large amount of research has been conducted for that disease.

How Should I Use the CHI Score for a Particular Study?

When comparing CHI values for one disease versus another, it is important to realize that the values are relative to the available academic literature. A lower value does not necessarily mean that cannabis is a less effective treatment. On the other hand, a higher CHI value does indicate not just a greater knowledge base but also a higher degree of scientific certainty that medical marijuana is beneficial for treating a specific disease (or disease group).

A CHI score of 3.5 to 5 for a particular study means that there is solid, **actual** evidence that cannabis may be a useful treatment. If it is relevant to your health issues, you may wish to share this citation with your doctor for his or her review.

A score of 1.5 to 3.4 for a particular study means that while more research needs to be done, it is **probable** that cannabis could be a useful treatment. While this is not conclusive evidence, you may still want to discuss these studies with your doctor, particularly if you have concerns about the effectiveness and/or safety of other methods available to you.

A score of 0 to 1.5 suggests that it is **possible** that cannabis is therapeutic or that study results were nonexistent, mixed, or inconclusive.

Evidence-Based Strain- and Form-Specific Considerations

Sativas and indicas as well as their respective dominant hybrids present with a different cannabinoid profile. Sativas and sativa-dominant strains present with a higher THC to CBD ratio when compared to indicas or indica-dominant strains. THC binds with both CB1 and CB2 receptors, while CBD has a greater affinity for CB2.

In general, if you require focused CB1 activation, you may want to select a strain with a higher THC to CBD ratio, namely sativas or sativa-dominant hybrids. On the other hand, if you are trying to enhance CB2 activation, select an indica or indica-dominant strain with a lower THC to CBD ratio, thus favoring CB2 expression.

Most cannabis dispensaries will have a laboratory-tested cannabinoid profile available for each of the strains they carry.

To fine-tune therapeutic effects, in addition to carefully selecting the ideal strain of cannabis with the most appropriate ratios, also consider the "method of administration," meaning how you take your medicine. There are several options.

In fresh and raw cannabis leaf, CBD and THC cannabinoids exist as CBD-acid and THC-acid, both of which are non-psychoactive in the raw state. Once the plant cannabinoids become heated, dried, or stored, decarboxylation takes place, changing the molecular structure and its resultant properties. While CBD remains non-psychoactive after decarboxylation, THC-acid becomes THC, the main psychoactive molecule in cannabis, which limits the maximum potential dose accordingly.

William L. Courtney, MD, a physician who has been working with dietary raw cannabis, considers fresh and raw cannabis leaf an especially rich form of CBD, further increasing CBD influence potential. Courtney suggests that unheated large cannabis leaf or leaf juice can be tolerated at doses 60 times higher than when cannabis is heated. The juice tastes bitter and can be diluted with another vegetable juice at a ratio of 1:10. Mix one part cannabis juice with nine parts vegetable juice to mask the taste. Ten to twenty large fan leaves juiced daily is a commonly recommended dose.

Additionally, research is beginning to show that raw plant THC-acid has unique and potent therapeutic properties of its own and does not make users "high." Dutch scientists' research suggests that raw THC-acid inhibits tumor necrosis factor alpha (TNF-α) levels,[1] which have become associated with the promotion of inflammation and the overall regulation of specific immune responses.

Raw, fresh cannabis leaf medicine allows patients to benefit from the potent therapeutic properties of cannabis without altering their state of consciousness. Thus they remain able to safely operate heavy machinery, drive to and from work, and make delicate decisions.

The Setting

Find a place where you can sit or lie comfortably, without interruptions, for 2 to 4 hours. Consider a day or an evening where you are not called upon to do something or drive after your experience. Give yourself a day to nurture, explore, and heal. You can work in silence (turn off the telephone) or play music that is conducive to go within. If you use music it helps to use a list of songs that you have not heard before (you can choose a list based on genre).

The Intention

Intention is not wishful thinking, which tends to be broad, nebulous, and abstract in comparison. Integrating mind-body medicine benefits from setting a conscious intention. Placebo,[2] nocebo,[3] and quantum research[4] suggest that focused, clear, and direct intention supported by an unwavering commitment can activate and support the body's capacity for self-healing.

You may want to begin by deciding: "I want to heal" or "I want to heal, even if I don't know how" or "I want to discover what is blocking my healing." Or, you may want to ask a specific question relevant to your specific symptoms. You can use the section "Powerful Questions" (associated with diseases A–Z) as a way to find one that resonates with you, or you may want to just read them over and see if they stimulate the question(s) that is right for you. Remember, the innate part within that is looking for healing has been trying to get your attention for a while. It will respond.

The Exploration

Enter a deeply relaxed state by using the appropriately dosed amount of cannabis or any meditative practice of your choice. Allow yourself to focus on the tension, sensations, or feelings of your symptom or disease that you are working to heal. In particular, try to focus on how you feel about what your illness is preventing you from doing.

Think of these feelings as the needle of a compass that points to underlying issues that require your attention. Often, at this point of the process, patients report the emergence of a memory or a related scenario. Sometimes several memories or scenarios emerge and, not unlike layers of an onion, they produce tears or reveal an emotional connection or similarity, and thus a theme that may be important to notice on your journey to health and well-being.

Being with What Surfaces

Like many others who have used this method for deep healing, you may become (more) aware of some internal resistance to getting better, which could be any behavior that propels your attention outward, such as paying attention to noise elsewhere, wanting to talk to someone, or wanting to move around. Signs that relevant material is emerging may include feeling uncomfortable, distracting pains, or falling asleep. Try to stay focused within. Notice your sensations, desires, and impulses; be curious and try to discover what lies beneath. Under the influence of cannabis or through engaging a spirit of gentle mindfulness, you may find, to your surprise, that you are fully able and willing to forgive yourself for any resistance present. This is an excellent start.

You may discover that merely being with whatever emotions or resistances surface, no matter how unpleasant or difficult it at first seems, is the beginning of true, deep healing. Once you have discharged blocked emotional energy, you will be able to identify the beliefs, attitudes, and choices that are contributing to your ill health and which are in need of replacement.

Powerful Questions (Self-Guide to Deeper Healing)

People are like fingerprints or snowflakes in that we are all unique. Human beings each have their own set of questions to explore, including those raised by the crisis of a mild, acute, or debilitating illness. However, there are common threads that may weave through the internal architecture of a manifest disease. The questions used in the "Mind-Body Medicine" part of each disease discussion attempt to address these common threads. You could ponder them during meditation, or engage the plant's help to examine them together.

The exploration of these questions, or your own versions of them, makes it possible to look through your unique veil of misery and pain to discover what lies beyond. The learning that can take place on the fulcrum between life and death, between body and mind, between doing and being, can play an integral part in health and healing.

In general, or if the current state of mind-body medicine offers no guidance for a particular illness, you can employ this set of six questions to gain insight and direction about how best to proceed.

1. What are the symptoms keeping you from doing?
2. How do you feel about that?
3. Where do these feelings take you?
4. What scenarios or memories are associated with these feelings?
5. What is the meaning (messages, unhealthy beliefs/attitudes, etc.) you have given to that scenario?
6. Can the answers to these questions direct your focus to support your capacity for self-healing?

Suggested Blessings

Some people like to engage the spiritual, by whatever name or form they may hold dear. One way to engage something larger than ourselves is to ask for a blessing to seed new, healthier thoughts and feelings as part of our daily health routines. This section of each disease discussion suggests sample blessings to spur your own imagination.

Suggested Affirmations

Thoughts and words affect the immune system. We can be imprisoned by our own words and thoughts, or we can use them to set us free. For those people who like to work with carefully and consciously chosen words to support their health and healing, this section suggests affirmations directly related to the possible internal architecture of each illness described.

Anecdotes

Although this book emphasizes scientific findings and evidence-based methods, some readers may have difficulty relating to mind-body healing without personal accounts to put these findings in context. Where personal accounts have been included, the names and context of the cases have been altered. Healing journeys are often complex and multi-layered. Due to space constraints, the examples chosen are necessarily simplified, focusing on only one, or at best a handful, of key elements in a person's experience of using cannabis and/or consciousness to foster their health and healing.

Let Food Be Thy Medicine/Take Notice

The efficacy of ancient healing practice using spices as medicine has been confirmed by the recent scientific discoveries related to (E)-β-caryophyllene —a common food-based cannabinoid fully accepted by the Food and Drug Administration (FDA). The (E)-β-caryophyllene contained in specific exotic spices activates the endocannabinoid system via CB2, which makes these spices a potentially novel form of treatment available to everyone. These food-based cannabinoids can activate CB2 receptors for therapeutic purposes. Used in conjunction with cannabis, a synergy of beneficial effects may result.

The "Take Notice" section of this book may also report on other natural therapeutic possibilities such as mindfulness techniques related to the particular illness being discussed.

Spice Power

The (E)-β-caryophyllene contained in certain spices activates the endocannabinoid system via CB2, which makes these spices an accessible form of treatment.

It is well known that ingesting cannabis enhances taste and smell and stimulates the appetite. It is less well known that your spice rack, a treasure chest of wondrous culinary delights, is also an inexpensive natural pharmacy. Research has shown that (E)-β-caryophyllene protects against microbes, inflammation, oxidative stress, pain, and cancer.[5]

In addition to listing relevant CB2-activating (E)-β-caryophyllene-containing spice plants, this section focuses on knowing how to select and use medicinal spices, whether you do so alone or in combination with an appropriate strain of cannabis for your unique healing journey.

While the spice, herbal, and nutritional information in this publication is primarily based on Western herbal philosophies, you can choose how and how much to include them as building blocks in your overall therapeutic regimen.

The spices and plant products listed here are based mainly on the prior research I conducted on the medicinal benefits of spice, published in the book *Spicy Healing—A Global Guide to Growing and Using Spices for Food and Medicine.* Many more spices with therapeutic potential are available than are discussed in this text, which is focused on cannabinoids.

It's important to realize that while scientific studies are available to highlight certain therapeutic potentials, and while the time-proven use of spice for health and healing speaks of its general efficacy and safety, the use of spices should not be construed as a silver bullet that will cure all ailments. Spices can, however, be helpful for bringing an awareness or mindfulness to how we prepare and enjoy food, and they encourage us to make food choices based on the impact on our health.

Those using Ayurvedic prescriptions based on the three *doshas* (body types) or working with Five Element considerations can further fine-tune the potential effectiveness of food and recipe choices with the information provided here. Suggested spices can easily be added or subtracted from most meals.

Summary

So, in summary, and for ease of use, each disease or symptom listed in this index is organized in the same fashion and presented in the same pattern, though not every section appears for each disease:

Description of Disease (from an orthodox perspective)

Cannabis and the Disease (evidence-based research results)

Cannabis Study Summary (chart)

Cannabis Strain- and Form-Specific Considerations (based on the given information)

Exploring Mind-Body Medicine for each disease/symptom listed

Powerful Questions

Suggested Blessings

Suggested Affirmations

Anecdotes

Let Food Be Thy Medicine/Take Notice

Ideally this book will be a useful tool for you, or perhaps for your friends, clients and/or loved ones on the journey toward greater health and deeper awareness of the power of mind-body healing. We can exercise the power to create and promote our health in the midst of these explorations. In doing so, we can dissolve issues, release whatever needs releasing, gain new perspectives, try new beliefs and the new set of feelings they induce, make healthier choices, and walk our own unique path to better health and healing. Some manage to do it instantly, as in spontaneous remission, while others embark on a more gradual, slower journey.

Where we go from here is up to us.

Chapter IV

Diseases and Symptoms A–Z

Aging /Anti-Aging

Evidence-Based Confidence Level and Therapeutic Potential

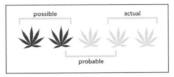

Total Number of Studies Reviewed: 1

Combined CHI Value: 2

Scientists do not yet have a thorough understanding of the physiological mechanism of aging. Various theories have been proposed to explain the loss of cellular integrity that we recognize as aging (wrinkles, age spots, or decline in physical and mental function). Such theories largely focus on the cumulative effects of exposure to radiation, toxins, or pathogens contributing to mutation in cellular DNA over time.

Specifically, the following are believed to be causal agents in the process of aging: accumulation of toxins, the long-term effect of ionizing radiation, changes in hormone profiles, damage from exposure to free radicals (oxidative stressors), exposure to parasites, fungi, bacteria, viruses, or other pathogens, shortening of the end strings of DNA (called telomeres, which occurs with each cell division and in the presence of environmental toxins), and the accumulation of senescent (older) cells.

Anti-Aging

Animal studies have shown that longevity is achievable through external means such as modest caloric restriction. These decades-old findings were confirmed by a recent study in which scientists proposed a potential mechanism underlying the inverse relationship between calories and longevity. Researchers observed that a reduction of cellular sugar (glucose) caused an increase in free radicals. While we ordinarily think of free radicals as damaging, in this case cells responded rapidly to the reduction of glucose by producing an enzyme (catalase). This enzyme breaks down the radical before it causes any damage. Researchers theorized that it is this enhanced mechanism in response to the presence of free radicals that explains the longer lifespan of test animals fed less food (but not so much less as to be malnourished).[1] It would appear that repetitive, low-stress exposure to free radicals might have anti-aging effects. If this theory is correct, the use of high doses of antioxidants to "fight" aging may be counterproductive.

Other life-extension research has focused on the potential of specific nutritional supplements. Alpha lipoic acid, in conjunction with acetyl-L-carnitine, has demonstrated protective abilities from perceived effects of aging in animal studies.[2] Similarly, a recent Mayo Clinic study found that typical signs of aging were not observed in mice whose senescent cells were eliminated.[3] (Senescent cells tend to aggregate in aging tissue and cause chronic low-grade inflammation.) However, it is important to note that these results have not been confirmed with human subjects.

In the year 2009 the Nobel Prize in Physiology or Medicine was awarded to three scientists (Elisabeth Blackburn, Carol Greider, and Jack Szostack) who discovered how the aging or degradation of cellular chromosomes is limited by telomeres and the enzyme telomerase.

In a nutshell, when telomeres are shortened, cells age. Conversely, when telomerase is abundant, telomere length is sustained and cellular aging arrested. This singular discovery has infused a lot of excitement into the various treatment communities. For example, since cancer cells are immortal because of high telomerase activity, products are currently being tested to reduce the enzyme in cancerous tissue. In healthy tissue, however, high telomerase activity protects the cell from aging. Based on these observations, drug companies and nutritional industries have launched efforts to introduce pharmaceutical drugs (e.g., GRN163L by Geron) and nutritional formulations (e.g., Product B by Isagenix) that are designed to decrease or increase telomerase activity in the human body with the goal of suppressing cancer and extending life, respectively.

Cannabis and Aging

Scientists from Columbus University in Ohio discovered that the synthetic cannabinoid WIN55,212-2 (WIN-2) can enhance cognition and have an anti-inflammatory effect in older rats.[4] This effect found in animals has not yet been confirmed in humans.

Study Summary

Drugs	Type of Study	Key Results	CHI
WIN55,212-2	Animal study	Potential anti-inflammatory and cognitive-enhancing effect in aged rats.[4]	2

Total CHI Value 2

Strain- and Form-Specific Considerations

The synthetic cannabinoid WIN55,212-2 binds more securely ("with higher affinity") to CB2 receptors than CB1 receptors,[5] which suggests that the CB2 receptor may be more important for the desirable anti-inflammatory and cognitive-enhancing effects seen in older rats in the Columbus study.

Similarly, non-psychoactive cannabidiol (CBD) has a greater affinity for CB2 receptors. Indicas and indica-dominant hybrids generally present with a lower THC:CBD ratio when compared to sativa-based strains, thus favoring CB2 signaling.

Raw, fresh cannabis leaf or juice contains CBD and THC in the form of THC-acid and CBD-acid, which can be consumed in larger quantities, since THC in that state is considered non-psychoactive.

Mind-Body Medicine and Aging

Aging clichés have become clichés by repetition. Each alone, but especially together, reveals much of society's negative programming and individual negative beliefs about aging. "You cannot teach an old dog new tricks" implies that we cannot learn when we are older. "Dirty old man" insinuates that it is unnatural for an older man to be sexually active. An "old wives' tale" dismisses the wisdom of older women. "If the devil can't come himself, he will send an old woman" suggests that an older woman cannot be trusted.

Opposing those negative clichés is a sense of wonder about the experiences beneath the signs of age, along with a curiosity about the potential value and wisdom brought on by experience, knowledge, conscientiousness, and emotional stability. Positive aging beliefs include "It is never too late to learn," "Age bestows wisdom," "It's never too late to have a happy childhood," and "Death is the ultimate healer of any physical ailment."

The secrets of longevity will be difficult to discover for those of us who look at aging as failure. Those who believe that old age is ugly will miss the opportunity to discover new depths of beauty that cannot be found in the polished exterior of the "body perfect" but in ever-deeper dimensions of consciousness. If we think aging is the enemy, we will miss out on befriending life and will forego the adventure that comes with lasting friendships.

While its significance varies among cultures, aging is regarded by most modern societies as something to be feared and avoided. Corporations exploit and reinforce societal ideals of beauty and youth in order to increase demand for their products, elevating the mythical "body perfect" in the process. If accepted blindly, these unrealistic archetypes supplant the complex flavors and fabrics of a deeper and richer experience that could otherwise be there, and one that only age, the very thing we are taught to fear, can bestow.

The field of medical psychosomatics is concerned with the impact of social, psychological, and behavioral factors on bodily processes and quality of life. Psychosomatic research has expanded knowledge of the specific physiological components of aging. "Positive affect seems to protect individuals against physical declines in old age."[6] "Longevity was associated with being conscientious, emotionally stable, and active."[7] "Positive emotional content reported in early-life autobiographies was strongly associated with longevity six decades later."[8]

A study conducted at the University of California–Davis (2011) demonstrated that intensive meditation training not only decreased psychological stress and improved overall well-being but also significantly increased the enzyme telomerase, a known predictor of cellular longevity that is achieved by repairing and rebuilding of telomeres (end points of cellular chromosomes).[9]

Combining the perspectives of different medical disciplines makes it possible to better understand various elements of aging and even to shift our attitude toward aging. This new perspective focuses on deeper and broader experiences of life itself. Insights from medical, nutritional, and food sciences can be integrated with knowledge of how our belief systems, thoughts, feelings, choices, decisions, and attitudes impact our health and quality of life.

Now instead of looking at aging as failure, we can see that with each experience—each day, each year that passes—we have an opportunity to learn more, to love more, and explore more of the interactive dance that is our awareness of the world.

We can now see the beauty of experience that only age can bestow. Instead of functioning merely as a body, we can become more aware of previously unexplored dimensions of consciousness.

The more we release repressed or suppressed emotions, the better we understand our tendencies to focus on the negative or previous experience of feeling lousy. By understanding how frequent fear or any other chronically constricting emotion hinders our healing process, we may more easily identify how our frame of mind, consciously or otherwise, interferes with our health. The more we challenge faulty beliefs that support disease at the core of each illness, the better able we are to reverse the damage. The more access we gain to our subconscious mind, and the more we explore the sliver of the unconscious at the edge of mindfulness, the more multidimensional we can become.

Change may come slowly and incrementally, almost invisibly, but every action to bring more consciousness to the healing process enhances our essential capacity for wisdom. Wisdom comes from the cumulative experience of conscious living, not simply the passage of time.

Powerful Questions

Think of eight to ten words or phrases that mean "getting older."
Are you eagerly looking forward to your own "old age"? Why or why not?
What does it mean to be old?
What negative beliefs do you have about aging?
Can you replace these negative beliefs with more positive beliefs?
What does it mean to be an elder?
How do I want to return to the source of all life: as an infant or as a wise person?

Suggested Blessings

May I learn the wonders of the world.

May I love in ways I have never loved before.

Suggested Affirmations

I allow my wonder, my love, and my wisdom to show my true age.

My age has been changing since the day I was born; every day I get better at embracing continual change.

Aging takes a lot of courage, so the task can only be given to those with a lot of life experience.

Take Notice: Age Spots

Cannabis-using patients have reported that a daily drop of cannabis-infused hemp or coconut oil applied to moles and age spots has resulted in the reappearance of normal tissue in time periods ranging between three weeks and three months. Here is an example from one of my own moles.

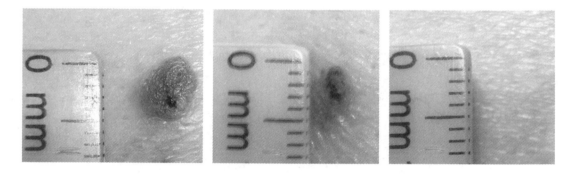

Let Food Be Thy Medicine

(E)-β-Caryophyllene or (E)-BCP is a FDA-approved dietary plant-cannabinoid that activates CB2 receptor sites and initiates potent anti-inflammatory actions and protection from oxidative stress,[10] both potential underlying factors in aging. Spice plants known to contain significant amounts of (E)-BCP in descending order include: Black "Ashanti Pepper" *(Piper guineense),* White "Ashanti Pepper" *(Piper guineense),* Indian Bay-Leaf *(Cinnamomum tamala),* Alligator Pepper *(Aframomum melegueta),* Basil *(Ocimum micranthum),* Sri Lanka Cinnamon *(Cinnamomum zeylanicum),*

Rosemary *(Rosmarinus officinalis)*, Black Caraway *(Carum nigrum)*, Black Pepper *(Piper nigrum)*, Basil *(Ocimum gratissimum)*, Mexican Oregano *(Lippia graveolens)*, and Clove *(Syzygium aromaticum)*.

Anorexia and Cachexia

Evidence-Based Confidence Level and Therapeutic Potential

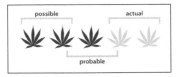

Total Number of Studies Reviewed: 11
Combined CHI Value: 28

Anorexia nervosa is a lack of interest in or a refusal to eat sufficient food and nutrients to maintain a healthy body weight due to psychological reasons. Anorexia is distinct from bulimia nervosa, which is defined as binge eating followed by purging or laxative abuse. Cachexia, also called wasting syndrome, refers to a loss of body mass that cannot be replaced through nutrition. It presents as generalized weakness, overall poor health, malnutrition, and emaciation. Cachexia is usually a secondary condition in chronic destructive diseases such as end-stage cancer, AIDS, terminal tuberculosis, multiple sclerosis, or chronic obstructive pulmonary diseases such as emphysema.

Patients with progressive or late-stage cancer who experience weight loss due to limited appetite, nausea, and increased weakness are suffering from cancer-related anorexia-cachexia. AIDS-related anorexia is defined as a lack or loss of appetite leading to weight loss of fat and muscle tissues due to appetite-depressing disease progressions.

Cannabis and Anorexia

Cannabis has been mentioned as an effective plant remedy to stimulate appetite and weight gain in almost every culture and medical tradition. Building on this traditional knowledge, many scientific studies have evaluated the evidence base for various uses of cannabis in allopathic medicine. It has been discovered that cannabinoids play a part in modulating the desire to eat. Most studies have focused on cannabis and anorexia in the context of cancer, AIDS, and Alzheimer's disease. In general, study results indicate that cannabinoids are effective in reducing anorexia in AIDS and Alzheimer's patients.

Results for cancer patients with anorexia were more mixed. Cancer anorexia studies reported that cannabis is relatively safe, but usage under the individual study protocols produced some positive and some neutral reports of efficacy. For example, in a 2006 Swiss study, 164 cancer patients were divided into three groups and given a six-week course of cannabis extract, oral THC, or a placebo to evaluate differences in cancer-related anorexia-cachexia syndrome. The results of this randomized, double-blind, placebo-controlled clinical trial showed no difference in appetite or quality of life with cannabis, THC, or placebo. No reports of toxicity were noted.[1]

An animal-based experiment conducted in Madrid and published in 2002 provided scientists with the initial evidence that peripheral endocannabinoid (CB1) receptors play a complex role in the regulation of eating.[2] In a 2007 study conducted in St. Louis, Missouri, 29 senior long-term care patients suffering from weight loss were treated with oral doses of Dronabinol. Over a period of twelve weeks, study participants gained an average of almost 8 pounds.[3]

Based on earlier studies that established that endocannabinoid CB1 receptors are related to eating behavior, scientists in New York examined the possibility of reducing appetite by influencing CB1 receptors. Results showed that reducing CB1 expression does in fact produce a reduction of appetite. Thus CB1 blockers may warrant further exploration as a possible novel weight-loss product.[4]

Cannabis and Cachexia

One hundred and seventeen people living with HIV/AIDS and suffering from loss of both appetite and weight were enrolled in a three- to twelve-month trial based in Orlando, Florida, and given regular oral doses of Dronabinol. Researchers reported that the majority of study participants' appetites quickly improved and weight loss was reduced.[5]

A researcher from the University of Liverpool in England summarized the scientific basis for treating cachexia with cannabinoids this way: ". . .

considerable research has examined endocannabinoid involvement in appetite, eating behavior, and body weight regulation. It is now confirmed that endocannabinoids, acting at brain CB1 cannabinoid receptors, stimulate appetite and ingestive behaviours. [...] Moreover, there is strong evidence of an endocannabinoid role in energy metabolism and fuel storage."[6]

Inspired by scientific evidence that oral cannabinoid-containing medications reduce chemotherapy-induced nausea as well as AIDS wasting syndrome, researchers hypothesized that cannabinoids might also mitigate the severe side effects of antiviral therapy used to treat hepatitis C. In a study conducted in Ottawa, Canada, in 2009, researchers found that 64% of patients undergoing interferon-ribavirin therapy experienced improvements in their symptoms when also administered cannabinoids.[7]

Cannabis and AIDS-Related Anorexia-Cachexia

A Tulsa, Oklahoma, study followed 139 patients with AIDS, half of whom received Dronabinol as treatment. Patients rated their appetite, mood, and nausea three times a week. The group receiving Dronabinol reported increases in appetite (38% vs. 8% for placebo), improvement in mood (10% vs. -2% for placebo), and decreased nausea (20% vs. 7% for placebo). Body weight was stable in those patients receiving Dronabinol, while recipients receiving a placebo had a mean loss of 8.8 pounds (or 4 kg). The authors of the study concluded: "Dronabinol was found to be safe and effective for anorexia associated with weight loss in patients with AIDS." Further, these excellent results were achieved without significant adverse effects. Researchers Beal et al. reported that "side effects were mostly mild to moderate in severity (euphoria, dizziness, thinking abnormalities)."[8]

Cannabis and Cancer-Related Anorexia-Cachexia

Cancer anorexia studies generally report that cannabinoids are relatively safe and produce both positive and neutral effects.

Scientists in Toronto, Canada, collected data from 82 cancer patients who received Nabilone for 53 days for cancer-related pain and other symptoms. Their study results, published in 2006, indicate a potential therapeutic benefit in cancer-related anorexia with improvement seen in pain levels, nausea, depression, anxiety, insomnia, and night sweats.[9]

A study in Cleveland, Ohio, evaluated the impact of tetrahydrocannabinol (THC) on cancer patients with anorexia. The patients were given 2.5 mg of THC orally, three times per day, one hour after a meal for four weeks. Of the 18 patients who completed the course, 13 reported an increase in appetite. The study authors concluded: "THC is an effective appetite stimulant in patients with advanced cancer. It is well tolerated at low doses."[10]

A study of Dronabinol used to treat patients with symptomatic HIV infections and/or cancer was conducted in Somerville, New Jersey. Researchers found that ". . . Dronabinol caused weight gain in seven of ten patients with symptomatic HIV infection. In both HIV and cancer patients, Dronabinol improved appetite at a dose which was well tolerated for chronic administration."[11]

Strain-Specific Considerations

Cannabis constituents are well-known for their ability to induce appetite, reduce nausea and vomiting, and gently lift the energy of body and mind, thereby addressing both physiological and psychological system needs. Cannabinoids, acting at brain CB1 cannabinoid receptors (especially anandamide and THC), stimulate appetite and ingestive behaviors. Most anorexia/cachexia research has been done on patients with Alzheimer's disease, AIDS, and cancer. Study results have shown that the cannabinoid THC increases appetite, reduces nausea, and increases weight gain.

Cannabis-using anorexia and/or cachexia patients often prefer sativa strains of cannabis with higher concentrations of tetrahydrocannabinol (THC) relative to cannabidiol (CBD) and cannabinol (CBN). Or, patients may seek isolated synthetic THC medication that is available by prescription. However, patients' individual needs and preferences vary.

Mind-Body Medicine and Anorexia/Cachexia

Researchers in North Carolina studied 753 female patients diagnosed with anorexia nervosa (AN) to discover possible underlying causes. Results showed that exposure to abuse resulting in post-traumatic stress disorder

Study Summary

Drugs	Type of Study	Published Year, Place, and Key Results	CHI
Oral cannabinoid-containing medications	Human trial conducted on patients with hepatitis C	2008—University of Ottawa, Canada: May stabilize weight loss during interferon-ribavirin therapy in chronic hepatitis C patients.[7]	3
Dronabinol	Human trial on 29 senior long-term care patients suffering from weight loss	2007—Saint Louis University, St. Louis, Missouri, USA: Average weight gain of 8 lbs. in long-term care patients.[3]	3
Dronabinol (isomer of THC)	117 people living with HIV/AIDS	2007—Orlando Immunology Center Orlando, Florida: Improved appetite, weight gain, and reduction of nausea.[5]	3
Cannabis extract containing 2.5 mg THC and 1 mg CBD, or THC 2.5 mg, or placebo twice daily for 6 weeks	164 cancer patients	2006—Oncology and Palliative Medicine, Cantonal Hospital, St. Gallen, Switzerland: No difference in appetite or quality of life between cannabis, THC, and placebo. No reports of toxicity.[1]	0
Nabilone	82 cancer patients	2006—William Osler Health Center, Toronto, Canada: Reduction in pain, nausea, depression, anxiety, insomnia, and night sweats. Drowsiness, tiredness, appetite, and well-being remained the same but decreased in control group.[9]	3
Studied the effects of reducing CB1 expression	Animal study (mice)	2005—Columbia University, New York: Endocannabinoid (CB1) receptors are involved in appetite.[4]	2
Endocannabinoid acting at brain CB1 cannabinoid receptors studied	Analysis	2005—University of Liverpool, United Kingdom: CB1 endocannabinoid receptors stimulate appetite and ingestive behaviors. Moreover, there is strong evidence of an endocannabinoid role in energy metabolism and fuel storage.[6]	1
Anandamide and other cannabinoid agonists	Animal study (rats)	2002—University Complutense of Madrid, Spain: Endocannabinoid (CB1) system modulates feeding.[2]	2
2.5 mg of Dronabinol twice daily, or placebo	139 people living with AIDS	1995—St. John's Hospital, Tulsa, Oklahoma: Increased appetite, mood, and weight gains with reduction of nausea.[8]	5
THC 2.5 mg three times daily	18 cancer patients	1994— Palliative Care Program, Cleveland Clinic Foundation Ohio, Cleveland, Ohio: 13 patients reported an improvement in appetite.[10]	3
Dronabinol	HIV and cancer patients	1991—UNIMED, Inc., Somerville, New Jersey: Dronabinol improved appetite in both cancer and HIV patients.[11]	3

Total CHI Value 28

(PTSD) was a significant co-factor (13.7%) in developing AN. One hundred and three women who met the *DSM-IV* criteria for PTSD had suffered mostly sexual abuse during childhood or as an adult.[12]

To learn more about possible personality traits or temperaments of people suffering from AN, Australian scientists examined a prior study that followed 1,002 same-sex female twins in which one twin had AN but the other did not. Results showed that those with AN are prone to an elevated need for order, reward dependence, an elevated concern over mistakes, very high personal standards, and constant doubt about their actions (perfectionism).[13]

Researchers from Munich, Germany, and San Diego, California, discovered that AN patients, perhaps similarly to autistics, are not able to normally recognize and respond to different facial emotional expressions. The authors write: "Differences in brain dynamics might contribute to difficulties in the correct recognition of facially-expressed emotions, deficits in social functioning, and in turn the maintenance of eating disorders."[14]

A person suffering from AN without an underlying physical pathology may deny any suggestion that s/he is underweight because of an overwhelming false perception of the self as overweight. Here, belief has significant health consequences. Extreme self-loathing may also result in the rejection of any nurturing influences. Intense guilt, with its demand for punishment, has a similar effect.

Lack of appetite, as well as nausea/vomiting after eating even small amounts, may be related to fear or dread of an emotion or experience.

Factors that can aid and speed recovery include healing prior traumatic events and abuse, allowing shame to be lifted by something larger than ourselves, and returning shame to the source from whence it came without harming anyone (a process done in meditation, with a therapist, or consider the "giving shame back" technique on page 54).

Powerful Questions

Can I find a way to embrace my emotional experience (not my disease)?

If I were to let myself sink into the heart of fear, what would I find there?

How can I make any feeling a safe experience for me?

If weakness is the result of constant self-judgment, what is the source of my strength?

Can I accept and forgive myself for getting in the habit of self-judgment and negative self-talk?

Do I fully understand that human perfection is, by definition, unachievable?

Can I accept and forgive myself for the mistakes I've made?

How might I discover any false beliefs, conscious or unconscious, that influence my unhealthy behavior?

See also sections on Bacterial and Viral Infections–HIV/AIDS and Cancer.

Suggested Blessings

May you realize that it is safe to feel anything.

May you discover the source of your fear, and perhaps replace it with the seeds of love.

Suggested Affirmations

I accept myself just as I am.

I find appropriate ways to experience and release all my feelings without hurting anyone.

I can learn to nurture myself gently, a little more each day.

Let Food Be Thy Medicine

Cannabis-infused oils or tinctures can easily be added to your favorite recipes to suit your specific dietary requirements.

Anise ✿ Basil ✿ Cardamom ✿ Cinnamon ✿ Fennel ✿ Garlic Ginger Rosemary ✿ Turmeric

Anise: Scientists have tested Brazilian *curanderos'* age-old herbal medicinal practice of using anise to cure digestive difficulties resulting from gas or overeating, cramps, and nervous stomach. A University of São Paulo study confirmed the use of anise as an antispasmodic agent.[15]

Basil: A tea made of basil relieves symptoms of abdominal discomfort due to gas. As a diuretic, it treats high blood pressure.[16]

Cardamom: Cardamom is approved by the German Commission E (a government program to evaluate the safety and efficacy of herbal medicine) for the treatment of dyspeptic complaints (digestive difficulty).[17] These findings echo the time-proven Unani and Ayurvedic application of cardamom as a treatment in certain gastrointestinal diseases.

Cinnamon: In Cuba, a cinnamon infusion (tea) is prescribed to stimulate appetite and the immune system in patients with tendencies toward bacterial and fungal infections.[18] The German Commission E approved cinnamon for the treatment of "loss of appetite, dyspeptic complaints such as mild spasms of the gastrointestinal tract, bloating, flatulence."[19]

Fennel: Veterinary scientists from Afyon, Turkey, confirmed some of fennel's time-proven applications such as its beneficial use as a treatment for certain digestive problems.[20] Another study from Turkey concluded that the essential oil of fennel protected rats from chemically induced liver damage,[21] lending further credibility to fennel's reputation as a useful agent for gastrointestinal disorders.

Garlic: Garlic is one of the world's most versatile herbs and may help in cases of anorexia or cachexia by acting as an overall tonic, and by preventing and treating infections caused by bacteria, fungi, viruses, and parasites, according to studies in Cuba, where it is used extensively for health and wellness.[22]

Ginger: Ginger supports natural appetite by functioning as an anti-emetic (morning sickness, sea sickness, post-surgery sickness), analgesic, anti-inflammatory, antioxidant, antibacterial *(Helicobacter pylori)* stomach ulcer preventative, and hepatoprotective agent (protects the liver).[23]

Rosemary: An infusion of rosemary leaves is used in Cuba to treat liver and gallbladder complaints, and it is also used to reduce spasms due to gas and flatulence.[24] The German Commission E approved rosemary for "internal dyspeptic complaints."

Turmeric: Almost considered a wonder drug with a broad therapeutic potential, turmeric has been the subject of numerous studies conducted on the plant's constituents and its efficacy for gut health.[25] The German Commission E approved turmeric in the treatment of digestive difficulties with a dose range of 1.5–3 grams daily.[26]

Bacterial and Viral Infections (in general)

Evidence-Based Confidence Level and Therapeutic Potential

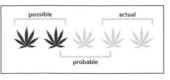

Total Number of Viral and Bacterial Studies Reviewed: 15

Combined CHI Value: 31

The scientific method has determined that the diseases listed in the left column of the table below are caused by viruses. Antibiotics are useless in fighting a viral disease but may work to eliminate bacterial infections such as those listed below.

Viral Infections

Chicken pox

Colds (parainfluenza virus)

Conjunctivitis (pink eye)

Croup (parainfluenza virus)

Dengue fever

Ebola

Epstein-Barr (a herpes virus)

Encephalitis

Flu (influenza virus)

Hepatitis A,B,C (inflammation of the liver)

Human papilloma virus (HPV)

Herpes simplex virus (HSV 1&2)

Kaposi's sarcoma (herpes virus 8)

Measles (rubella virus)

Meningitis (inflammation of the lining of the brain and spinal cord)

Mumps virus

Myocarditis (inflammation of the heart muscle)

Polio virus

Rabies virus

Reye syndrome (influenza virus)

Rubella virus

Shingles (*Herpes zoster* virus)

Smallpox virus

Yellow fever virus

Bacterial Infections

Anthrax

Chlamydia

Cholera

Conjunctivitis (can also be viral)

Escherichia coli (aka E. *coli*)

Diphtheria

Dysentery

Gonorrhea

Helicobacter pylori (stomach ulcers)

Legionnaire's disease

Leptospirosis

Viral Infections	Bacterial Infections
Streptococcus	Leprosy
Syphilis	Meningitis (bacterial)
Tuberculosis	Pneumonia
Typhoid	Rocky Mountain spotted fever
Urinary tract infections (UTI)	Salmonella
Yersinia pestis (bubonic and pneumonic plague)	Staphylococcus

How Do Scientists Determine the Cause of a Disease?

The answer, in part, is what scientists call Koch's Postulates. In the late 1800s, a virologist named Robert Koch created a set of criteria helpful for identifying a causal relationship between a microbe and a disease. His four primary criteria are not absolute truths, though they continue to inform scientific inquiry today. The criteria are:

> The microorganism must be found in abundance in all organisms suffering from the disease, but should not be found in healthy organisms.
>
> The microorganism must be isolated from a diseased organism and grown in pure culture.
>
> The cultured microorganism should cause disease when introduced into a healthy organism.
>
> The microorganism must be re-isolated from the inoculated, diseased experimental host and identified as being identical to the original specific causative agent.

Bacterial Infections
Gonorrhea

No Evidence-Based Confidence Level and Therapeutic Potential available

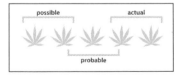

Gonorrhea is caused by gonococcus or *Neisseria gonorrhea* bacteria. It is usually sexually transmitted, though an infected mother can transmit the disease to an infant during birth. Gonorrhea symptoms in infants are mostly limited to infections of the eyes. In adults, gonorrhea affects the

mucous membranes of the genitals, reproductive organs, the anus, or the throat. It is estimated that about 1 in 10 infected males and 5 in 10 infected females show no or very mild physical symptoms of the disease. Early symptoms of the disease usually occur within the first week after exposure but may present up to 30 days after infection.

Early symptoms in women are usually milder than in males, and include burning or painful sensation when urinating, unusual vaginal discharge (sometimes with an odor), and spotting or bleeding between menstrual cycles. If the disease remains undetected and untreated in females, gonorrhea may progress over time and manifest years later as pelvic inflammatory disease, abscesses along the affected mucous membranes, damage to the reproductive organs, and an increased risk for ectopic pregnancies and infertility.

Early symptoms in males include penile discharge (white, yellowish) and painful, burning urination. If allowed to progress, gonorrhea may move deeper into the tissue of the genitals and affect the male reproductive organs, causing inflammation of the epididymis and testicles, with associated pain and swelling of the groin and scrotum. Untreated gonorrhea can cause infertility in men as well as women.

Both sexes may experience rectal or throat infections of gonorrhea. While rectal infection may produce less severe symptoms, rectal discharge, anal itching, and pain during bowel movements may be present. Throat infections may also be asymptomatic, or they may cause sore throat, swollen tonsils, and discharge at the site of the infected tissue.

Fever and chills, as well as joint aches, may be present from the onset of infection or only after the initial symptoms have passed. In the latter stages of the disease, gonorrheal arthritis may develop, causing pain in the wrist, knee, and ankle joints.

A urine test or a swab sample from the affected mucous membranes, examined under a microscope, can determine if gonorrhea is present. Both orthodox and holistic doctors recognize that if one sexually transmitted disease is present, others may be also, so testing for other sexually transmitted diseases is usually recommended. When gonorrhea is suspected, chlamydia and HIV screens are also routinely conducted.

Orthodox medical treatment uses antibiotics exclusively to eliminate the bacteria. While penicillin was initially advertised as able to cure gonorrhea in four hours, today it and most other antibiotics are generally ineffective. The bacteria have become resistant and easily survive most antibiotic treatments. For that reason, treatment guidelines of the U.S. Centers for Disease Control recommend cephalosporin antibiotics to treat all gonococcal infections.[1] Gonorrhea may soon become a "superbug" infection, resistant to all known antibiotics. As a consequence, there is global interest in the search for new and effective remedies for gonorrhea.

Cannabis and Gonorrhea

Five major cannabinoids (THC, CBD, CBG, CBC, and CBN) have been discovered to be potent against bacteria, including multi-drug-resistant bacteria, most notably methicillin-resistant *Staphylococcus aureus* (MRSA).[2] However, the precise mechanism of their antiseptic effect is still under study. While cannabinoids have been effective in treating MRSA in laboratory settings, no studies are available examining the potential antibacterial impact of cannabinoids on the gonorrhea bacterium.

However, Arabic and Indian Ayurvedic physicians have long applied the diuretic, sedative, and anti-inflammatory properties of cannabis to treat cystitis and gonorrhea.[3] Prior to the discovery of penicillin, cannabidiolic acids were commonly prescribed for bacterial infections such as gonorrhea. An 1892 treatment guideline describes the use of cannabis to treat gonorrhea: "it lessens the discharge, inflammation, burning pains, and restlessness, and allays chordee (downward curvature of the penis)."[4] Cannabis was apparently applied as a tincture, extract, or tannate (a salt made from cannabidiolic acids). As late as 1935, a cannabis preparation was sold in the U.S. in the form of pills to be dissolved in clean water and injected into the urethra using a pipette.[5] A Japanese team of scientists recently discovered (2008) that CBD-acid selectively inhibits COX-2, an enzyme responsible for inflammation and pain in general.[6]

Strain- and Form-Specific Considerations

The major cannabinoids, THC, CBD, CBG, CBC, and CBN, are present in both sativa and indica, the primary strains of cannabis. Non-psychoactive CBD-acid is present in relatively high concentrations in raw, fresh cannabis flower, leaf, and juice. CBD activates CB2 receptors in immune cells and may play a part in modulating immune responses. It is important to remember that to date no studies are available examining the potential antibacterial impact of cannabinoids on the gonorrhea bacterium.

Mind-Body Medicine and Gonorrhea

Sexually transmitted disease (STD) is not exclusively a physiological problem. The field of mind-body medicine examines mental and emotional factors that can make individuals vulnerable to disease, unable to recognize disease, unwilling to request treatment, or even predisposed to spreading disease. A lack of social responsibility may be associated with a lack of self-care or empathy for others. Unhealthy body image or post-traumatic stress disorder following sexual assault can lead people to disassociate during sex or ignore entire regions of their body.

While understanding how STDs are mechanically transmitted is important, it is also relevant to consider conscious and unconscious mental and emotional factors that impact the genesis, transmission, progression, and outcome of disease. Individuals often do not know that they are infected with a STD, or even how or when they were exposed to it. But sometimes individuals know that they are infected and continue to have unprotected sex anyway, spreading the disease to others. A drug addict with an STD may trade sex for drugs, oblivious to the damage this causes to herself and others when her next "fix" is her only priority. An assault victim may refuse to get treatment for an STD, insisting that the pain in his genitals is less onerous than a doctor's physical exam and the admission that he was unable to defend himself. A distorted self-concept based on unresolved childhood shame may induce an adult to validate their (perceived) "worthlessness" by repeatedly taking excessive risks in the sexual arena.

Guilt, fear, and shame figure prominently in the emotional context of STDs. Our sexuality and the meanings and value that we attach to it are very complex, and significantly influenced by religious, cultural, family, and personal circumstances. It should come as no surprise then that conflicts between these perspectives and our own, or conflicting desires within us, can lead to "cognitive dissonance" or discomfort and stress. Stress, especially chronic stress, gives rise to an internal environment in which the body becomes vulnerable to disease. Many pathogens involved in STDs are found in a dormant state within the body under normal circumstances, and they are given an opportunity to activate when the body is under stress and therefore vulnerable.

"There is light and there is shadow on the mountain of Aphrodite from whence life came."[7] The light is the pleasure, the intimacy, the fun, the beauty, and the embrace of primal creative energy. In the shadow we find the guilt, the shame, the blame, and the controls and judgments bringing pain to the self or others. It is estimated that more than half of all people will have a sexually transmitted disease at some point during their lifetime.[8]

The remainder are able to stay healthy. Our beliefs about ourselves, beliefs about our bodies, beliefs about the validity of our choices, and beliefs about our prospects for happiness all interact with the physical functioning of our bodies (and any diseases and discomforts we face). Our thoughts impact our emotions; our emotions impact our actions; our actions impact our health; our health impacts our thoughts, and so on. The pursuit of excellent health may be the same path that allows us to calm our fears and increase our access to and experience of love.

Mental and emotional constructs that may make us more vulnerable to STDs such as gonorrhea include: sexual guilt demands for purification through punishment, sex without care, sex without love, sex without intimacy, emotional manipulations or taking payoffs that come with sexual guilt such as the lack of principles related to sex, entitlements around sex, righteous angers around sex, suppressed emotions around sex (e.g., fears, anxieties, angers, shame, self-pity).

Mental and emotional constructs that may make us less vulnerable to STDs such as gonorrhea: Develop healthy principles around sex and abide by them on a consistent basis. Discover and replace all beliefs that initiate guilt, fear, or shame around sex. Find a way to release guilt, fear, anger, and shame around sex without hurting yourself or others. Consider adding care and love to balance lust and desire.

Powerful Questions

Do you consider sex natural and "good," or something dirty and wrong?

Do you know what constitutes safe sex?

Have you thought through what level of risk is acceptable to you?

Do you engage in unsafe sex?

Do you use alcohol or other drugs to give you "permission" to be sexual?

Do you use alcohol or other drugs to give you "permission" to take risks you otherwise would not?

What sexual situations scare you?

When you experience sexual difficulties, how do you react?

How do you deal with difficult emotions (for example, anger or shame) accompanied by arousal?

Do you struggle with "unacceptable" sexual desires or thoughts?

When have you felt guilty about your sexual conduct?

When have you felt ashamed by your own behavior?

When have you felt ashamed of your body's appearance or response to sexual attention?

Are there sexual acts you think should be punished? Who would be served by such punishment?

Do you harbor shame or guilt about having a STD?

Does fear of contracting STDs prevent you from experiencing a fully satisfying sex life?

Are you willing to explore your sexual desires?

Are you willing to explore the sexual desires of your partner(s)?

Can you find a way to own and release your fears, resentments, guilt, and shame appropriately?

Do you find guilt a useful and welcome signal that your desires and values are in conflict? Or are you sickened and paralyzed by chronic guilt?

How can you set sexual boundaries to protect yourself and others?

How can you increase the love and intimacy in your life?

Suggested Blessing

May you realize that your genitals are essentially good, healthy, natural, beautiful, and this organ is a necessity for all of life.

Suggested Affirmation

I am an adult and I celebrate my sexuality freely and with harm to none.

Let Food Be Thy Medicine

Coconut ∽ Spices containing (E)-β-Caryophyllene

Coconut: In a laboratory study in Iceland, researchers discovered that medium-chain fatty acids, especially capric acid ($C_{10}H_{20}O_2$), worked effectively in killing all strains of *Neisseria gonorrhea*.[9] Another laboratory study from the island determined how well medium-chain fatty acids destroy or inhibit the growth of other groups of bacteria. Both lauric acid and capric acid showed strong antibacterial abilities.[10] Again, researchers demonstrated another aspect of lauric and capric acids' broad antimicrobial properties in the laboratory—this time against a fungus associated with yeast infections.[11] Lauric acid and capric acid were also found to effectively inactivate chlamydia in the laboratory. This suggests that these two fatty acids, found in relatively high concentrations in coconut milk and coconut oil, may play a role in the prevention of this particular bacterial infection as well.[12]

(E)-β-Caryophyllene: (E)-β-caryophyllene or (E)-BCP is a fully FDA-approved dietary cannabinoid that activates CB2 receptor sites and initiates potent anti-inflammatory actions and protection from oxidative stress, both commonly associated factors in pathogen-based inflammations. Spice plants known to contain significant amounts of (E)-BCP include (in descending order) Black "Ashanti Pepper" *(Piper guineense)*, White "Ashanti Pepper" *(Piper guineense)*, Indian Bay-Leaf *(Cinnamomum tamala)*, Alligator Pepper *(Aframomum melegueta)*, Basil *(Ocimum micranthum)*, Sri Lanka Cinnamon *(Cinnamomum zeylanicum)*, Rosemary *(Rosmarinus officinalis)*, Black Caraway *(Carum nigrum)*, Black Pepper *(Piper nigrum)*, Basil *(Ocimum gratissimum)*, Mexican Oregano *(Lippia graveolens)*, and Clove *(Syzygium aromaticum)*.

Methicillin-Resistant *Staphylococcus aureus* (MRSA)

Evidence-Based Confidence Level and Therapeutic Potential

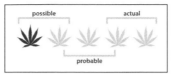

Total Number of Studies Reviewed: 1

CHI Value: 1

Certain strains of staphylococcus, an otherwise common bacterium, have developed a resistance to the usual antibiotic pharmaceuticals, which is the reason they are also referred to as "superbugs" or Multi-drug-Resistant *Staphylococcus aureus* (MRSA). People with weakened immune systems, chronic open wounds, surgical implants, and exposure to the bacteria are its most likely victims. The bacteria are spread via close skin-to-skin contact, contaminated items and surfaces, crowded living conditions, and poor hygiene.

Many of the MRSA infections are acquired in hospitals, nursing homes, and prisons. Hospitals isolate infected patients and disinfect medical tools and the environment to reduce the risk of public health hazards. If an infection occurs, treatments with standard antibiotics are ineffective, making this microbe a potentially deadly agent. Infections are usually limited to the skin, where they commonly form abscesses, but in severe cases can affect internal organs, leading to sepsis and death.

If a strong suspicion exists that MRSA may be involved, a specific test is performed to determine the exact strains present. The test may take several days to complete, and given that in some cases disease progression is very rapid (2–3 days after first sign of topical symptoms), presumptive treatments are strongly recommended by the allopathic community. However, the problem is discerning which of the few remaining antibiotics, if any, are still able to kill the bacteria. Clinical trials are currently underway to develop updated guidelines on treatment options.

Cannabis and MRSA

Various cannabinoids have antibacterial properties, but the mechanism through which the plant constituents are able to destroy even antibiotic-resistant bacteria remains elusive. An international group of scientists conducted a laboratory experiment where researchers examined five major cannabinoids (cannabidiol, cannabichromene, cannabigerol, Δ9-tetrahydrocannabinol, and cannabinol) and their effectiveness against MSRA. Results showed potent activity against a variety of methicillin-resistant *Staphylococcus aureus* (MRSA) strains of current clinical relevance.[1]

Study Summary

Drugs	Type of Study	Published Year, Place, and Key Results	CHI
CBD, CBC, CBG, THC, and CBN	Laboratory	2008—Multi-center international study: All five major cannabinoids showed potent activity against a variety of MRSA strains.[1]	1

Total CHI Value 1

Strain-Specific Considerations

Both indica and sativa flowers contain these five major cannabinoids (cannabidiol, cannabichromene, cannabigerol, Δ9-tetrahydrocannabinol, and cannabinol). Possible synergistic effects of using complete cannabinoid profiles against MRSA have not yet been tested.

Mind-Body Medicine and MRSA

While MRSA has been known to affect the bloodstream, lungs, and urinary tract, its primary target is the skin, possibly suggesting an underlying vulnerability connected to image and identity. The rapid destructiveness of MRSA suggests an extreme defenselessness against something that is literally eating the patient.

See also Skin Diseases and Cancer/Skin Cancer.

Powerful Questions

What is eating me?
Where, or with whom, do I feel completely defenseless?

Suggested Blessing

May I find ways to release the helplessness, no matter what its source.

Suggested Affirmations

I allow all that eats at me from the inside to dissipate like dew on a warm
summer morning breeze.

I can transcend any punishment with forgiveness.

Let Food Be Thy Medicine

Garlic: A laboratory study in London, England, determined that allicin, a
major antibacterial component of garlic, is a very effective defense against
MRSA.[2] This result was confirmed by another study conducted on mice
infected with MRSA, which concluded that the garlic extract, consisting
of diallyl sulphide and diallyl disulphide, possessed multiple protective
functions against MRSA infection.[3] Reports from case studies conducted
by Dr. Cutler, a member of the research team, have shown that topical and
internal use of allicin (provided by Allicin International) has cured patients
infected with MRSA.

Take Notice

Essential Oils ∾ Maggot Debridement Therapy

Essential Oils: Using topical applications, highly volatile essential oils
and extracts have been studied in an attempt to find ways to mitigate
MRSA. Researchers discovered that grapefruit seed extract (Citricidal)
together with geranium oil showed the greatest antibacterial effects against
MRSA, while a combination of geranium and tea tree oil was most active
against the Oxford strain (methicillin-sensitive *S. aureus*).[4] Another study
discovered that the multiple constituents of the essential oils of peppermint, spearmint, and Japanese mint exhibited properties that inhibited
the growth of several different kinds of disease-causing bacteria, including
MRSA.[5] Essential tea tree oil was discovered to be very effective in vitro
(laboratory) against MRSA.[6] Other studies confirm similar results of essential oils used to treat MRSA, including lavender, lemongrass, cinnamon,
melissa, and mountain savory (*Satureja cuneifolia* Ten.), a common fragrant
plant frequently used as a spice and herbal tea in Turkey.

Warning: Essential oils are usually used externally. As with all essential oils,
do not rub on mouth, nose, or near the eyes, especially those of infants

or children. Gagging and throat spasms may occur. Be extra careful when pregnant; any systemic allergic reaction may affect the fetus. You may want to use a small amount and test on a small skin area, then wait a few hours to see if an allergic reaction occurs. Discontinue use if reddening, swelling, or pain on site occurs. If you want to try again, dilute it with some other non-essential carrier oil first.

Maggot Debridement Therapy: Sterile maggot debridement therapy has proven an effective way to clean infected skin wounds, abscesses, ulcers, infected tissue, and necrotic or gangrenous tissue.[7] Besides cleaning the infected area, maggots also disinfect the wounded tissue and stimulate wound healing. While the antibacterial effect of maggot therapy is not systemic, MRSA is effectively killed in the topical area of application.

Viral Infections

Evidence-Based Confidence Level and Therapeutic Potential

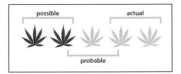

Total Number of Viral Studies Reviewed: 14
CHI Value: 30

Virus is a Latin word that means "slime" or "juice." Modern medicine has identified hundreds of different viruses. Some are completely harmless, while others can cause specific diseases in the plant, animal, and human kingdoms. Viruses are extremely small and omnipresent. The biggest virus is about the same size as the tiniest bacterium. In comparison to the smallest of all bacteria, the average virus is, relatively speaking, the size of a grain of sand next to a skyscraper.

A dormant (sleeping/inactive) virus is described as a simple organism that basically consists of DNA, RNA (a chemical blueprint of itself), and a protective protein (protein is usually a mixture of several elements, like carbon, oxygen, nitrogen, sulfur, and phosphorus). It seems to want but one thing, and that is to make more of itself. Based on a yet-to-be-discovered signal, the virus "wakes up" and begins to develop when it comes across a vulnerable host cell.

The virus either attaches itself to the host cell or enters the host cell. Once attached or inside, it tells the cell to stop doing what it has been doing, namely maintaining your well-being, health, and healing, and instead to produce the elements the virus needs to make more of itself. In the case of many viruses, when a copy has been made, it bursts out of the host cell, destroying the host cell in the process. When this occurs a million times over, viruses make people sick or even sometimes kill them.

However, the immune system, the police department of the body, is extremely smart, and if healthy and strong it is more than capable of fighting viruses. For example, many viruses are inactivated or destroyed by a body temperature slightly more than normal. Thus, fever is an effective immune-system defense to a viral invasion.

The immune system also produces antibodies and sensitized cells (virus-fighting police) that are made specifically to destroy a specific virus. These police circulate throughout the body long after the virus has been destroyed, keeping the body safe and protected. If the same virus reenters the body (for example, the chicken pox virus), the person will not get sick with chicken pox a second time. One is usually immune for life.

Mind-Body Medicine and Viral Infections

A review and analysis of psychosomatic studies published since 1939 shows that negative emotions, hostility, and stressful experiences directly influence pro-inflammatory cytokine production, which is associated with slower healing and acceleration of age-related illness.[1]

In every epidemic, there are people who do not get ill. While it is clear that pathogens such as viruses play a part in the contraction of disease, pathogens are not the sole cause of disease. Mental-emotional states directly affect the immune system. Mental-emotional states may induce a susceptibility or vulnerability to disease, and they are also capable of initiating a formidable defense and rapid immune response. They thus play a critical role in determining whether or not an individual will get sick.

Infectious agents are more likely to result in disease whenever negative affect is present, because negative emotional and mental states are resource-intensive and deplete the reserves that protect immunity. So we are at greater risk of disease whenever we experience chronic lack of support, insecurity, mistrust, fear, mental or emotional defenselessness, defensiveness, victimization, powerlessness, or a violation of personal boundaries. Conversely, a balanced and powerful immunity results from the experience of emotional support, safety, security, trust, love, intimacy, functional coping mechanisms, confidence, and belief in one's inner strength and abilities.

Suggested Blessings

May you begin the process of expanding already-present strengths and abilities.

May you also find new depths of gratitude, love, and trust in yourself and those who are truly trustworthy.

Suggested Affirmations

I trust that I will find a way to deal with whatever life brings my way. Thus I can relax, release all excess stress, fears, and anxieties.

Let Food Be Thy Medicine

Acacia ❧ Basil ❧ Cardamom ❧ Clove ❧ Coconut ❧ Turmeric ❧ Spices containing (E)-β-Caryophyllene

Acacia: A study from Mumbai, India, presented at the Eighth International Congress on Drug Therapy in HIV Infection in 2006, indicated that the aqueous extract of acacia pods is effective in vitro against the viral enzyme reverse transcriptase.[2]

Basil: Basil has been used in Traditional Chinese Medicine for thousands of years. Now researchers from the island nation of Taiwan have taken a closer look at the possible antiviral properties of basil extract and several of basil's specific compounds against DNA viruses, herpes virus, adenoviruses, hepatitis B virus, and the RNA viruses (coxsackievirus B1 and enterovirus 71). The results showed that: "... crude aqueous and ethanolic extracts of basil *(Ocimum basilicum)* and selected purified components, namely apigenin, linalool, and ursolic acid, exhibit a broad spectrum of antiviral activity. Of these compounds, ursolic acid showed the strongest activity against HSV-1... whereas apigenin showed the highest activity against HSV-2...."[3]

Cardamom: At the University of Cincinnati College of Medicine, scientists looked at cineole, a major constituent of cardamom, in the context of treating vaginal herpes infections in mice; it was determined that sufficient evidence exists to warrant more research on this compound as a potentially promising natural treatment modality.[4]

Clove: In a series of experiments, virologists from the Toyama Medical and Pharmaceutical University in Sugitani, Japan, determined that eugenine, a compound purified from the extracts of clove, inhibits viral DNA synthesis in several strains of herpes (I & II), including acyclovir-phosphonoacetic acid-resistant HSV-I.[5]

A Tunisian study reported in the National Library of Medicine determined that essential oil of clove extract has antiviral (*Herpes simplex*—HSV and hepatitis C) and antibacterial properties (including efficacy against several of the multi-drug-resistant *Staphylococcus epidermidis*).[6]

Coconut: The authors of a study from Staten Island, New York, state: "Lipids can inactivate enveloped viruses, bacteria, fungi, and protozoa." By adding medium-chain fatty acids (MCFA) to HIV-infected blood products, the researchers learned that they could reduce the virus concentration by a very large number. Further, the scientists expect that MCFA "... may potentially be used as a combination of spermicidal and virucidal agents."[7]

A crude extract of *Cocos nucifera L.* husk fiber demonstrated inhibitory activity against acyclovir-resistant *Herpes simplex* virus type I (HSV-I-ACVr).[8]

Turmeric: Researchers tested the hypothesis that curcumin, the main active constituent in turmeric, would block viral infection and gene expression of HSV-I by inhibiting promoters of herpes gene expression. Results showed that curcumin significantly decreased HSV-I infectivity and IE gene expression.[9]

(E)-β-Caryophyllene: (E)-β-Caryophyllene or (E)-BCP is a fully FDA-approved dietary cannabinoid that activates CB2 receptor sites and initiates potent anti-inflammatory actions and protection from oxidative stress, both commonly associated factors in pathogen-based inflammations.

Spice plants known to contain significant amounts of (E)-BCP include (in descending order) Black "Ashanti Pepper" *(Piper guineense),* White "Ashanti Pepper" *(Piper guineense),* Indian Bay-Leaf *(Cinnamomum tamala),* Alligator Pepper *(Aframomum melegueta),* Basil *(Ocimum micranthum),* Sri Lanka Cinnamon *(Cinnamomum zeylanicum),* Rosemary *(Rosmarinus officinalis),* Black Caraway *(Carum nigrum),* Black Pepper *(Piper nigrum),* Basil *(Ocimum gratissimum),* Mexican Oregano *(Lippia graveolens),* and Clove *(Syzygium aromaticum).*

Colds and Flu

No Evidence-Based Confidence Level and Therapeutic Potential available

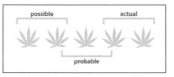

According to orthodox medicine, all common colds as well as all types of flu are caused by viral infections. There are hundreds of known and ever-mutating cold and flu viruses. However, during every flu outbreak in history there have been many people who did not get sick even when sufficiently exposed, so one must consider susceptibility as being a major contributing factor to whether a person falls sick or not. While the allopathic model is aware that people with lower immunity are more vulnerable to becoming sick, it has concentrated research primarily on microbes rather than susceptibility. The allopathic model has no cure for either colds or flu.

Many signs and symptoms of colds and flu tend to represent themselves in a similar fashion. A cold usually affects only the nose and throat and is associated with a low-grade fever. Flu may have the same symptoms, but they are usually more sudden, severe, and include a cough, higher fevers, muscle aches and pain, headaches, and fatigue. While most colds and flu are self-correcting, it is prudent to get help from a licensed health care practitioner when the following symptoms are present: loss of consciousness, disorientation, seizures, vomiting, or diarrhea with an inability to regain fluids, fevers over 102° F (39° C), a bloody cough or stool, sustained fever over several days, or inability to walk.

According to the World Health Organization, flu epidemics occur every year during fall and winter in temperate regions (regions without extreme heat or cold). "Worldwide, these annual epidemics result in about three to five million cases of severe illness, and about 250,000 to 500,000 deaths."[1] Most deaths associated with influenza in industrialized countries occur among people age 65 or older. In some tropical countries, influenza viruses circulate throughout the year, with one or two peaks during rainy seasons.

Other diseases that may look like a cold or flu but require different treatment approaches include asthma, pneumonia, bronchitis, sinusitis, allergies, strep throat, tuberculosis, emphysema, and chronic obstructive pulmonary disease (COPD).

Common Allopathic Treatment

Decongestants are a group of medications from a long list of vasoconstrictors, from A-Actifed through Z-Zephrex. Decongestants constrict blood vessels and are intended mainly to reduce the swelling of mucous membranes in the nose. Common side effects may include rebound congestion (the cold actually takes longer to heal), restlessness, dizziness, insomnia, elevated blood pressure, and an increased heart rate.

Antihistamines (for example Allegra, Benadryl, Claritin, and Seldane) are ineffective treatments for colds. A prominent medical text puts it plainly: "despite early claims and persistent popular belief, histamine-blocking drugs (antihistamines) are without value in combating the common cold."[2] Common side effects such as blurred vision, dry mouth, dry eyes, constipation, confusion, or sexual dysfunction are related to the anticholinergic properties of antihistamines, which block the effects of acetylcholine. Acetylcholine is a substance involved in the function of the parasympathetic nervous system. A suppression of the parasympathetic nervous system produces an increase in heart rate and less production of digestive juices, tears, sweat, and saliva.

Cough suppressants containing opiates (for example, codeine) reduce the reflex to cough up undesirable materials. They are, in most cases, counterproductive to what the body needs to do to rid itself of mucus, phlegm, and the materials encased in them. The most common side effects of cough suppressants are constipation, dizziness, sedation, nausea, and vomiting.

Opiates may be habit-forming and can produce respiratory depression ranging from mild hypoxia to respiratory arrest.

Expectorants (such as Robitussin) are drugs that are supposed to assist in the loosening, thinning, and bringing up of phlegm. However, a sufficient amount of water may be a better expectorant, and it avoids all the possible side effects of consuming expectorants: allergic reaction, dizziness, nausea, vomiting, abdominal discomforts, headache and/or a rash.

In 1997, U.S. poison control centers were contacted a total of 110,870 times about cases involving pharmacological cold and cough preparations; 22,073 patients had to be treated in a health care facility, and 14 people died.[3]

Prescription antiviral medication such as amantadine, rimantadine, oseltamivir (Tamiflu), and zanamivir are approved in the U.S. for the treatment of flu. Each has a set of potential side effects.[4] The CDC lists the side effects of amantadine and rimantadine as nervousness, anxiety, difficulty concentrating, lightheadedness, and gastrointestinal side effects like nausea and loss of appetite. Among some persons with long-term illnesses, more serious side effects can occur, such as delirium, hallucinations, agitation, and seizures. For zanamivir, the CDC lists side effects such as decreased respiratory function and bronchospasm, diarrhea, nausea, sinusitis, nasal infections, bronchitis, cough, headache, and dizziness. Finally, the side effects of oseltamivir (Tamiflu) include nausea, vomiting, and psychotic self-destructive behavior.

Antipyretic (fever-reducing) medications such as acetaminophen (Tylenol and many others) are commonly used to battle a cold or flu. This pharmaceutical medication is broken down in the liver and can cause liver damage and death. Acetaminophen overuse causes about 56,000 emergency room visits and 26,000 hospitalizations yearly, with approximately 500 of these cases ending in death.[5] Aspirin is another pharmacological medication commonly used to reduce fever and pain. Side effects include internal bleeding and liver damage, as just two examples. People under twenty years old should not take or be given aspirin products in conjunction with fever because aspirin is linked to Reye's syndrome, a potentially fatal condition.

Antibiotics are still commonly prescribed to treat the common cold or flu. Since, according to the allopathic model, both the cold and the flu are caused by viruses, and antibiotics only kill bacteria, there is no way antibiotics can help cure these diseases or speed up natural healing. Physicians usually justify prescribing antibiotics for cold and flu as a means to prevent bacterial infections such as pneumonia. However, among the many side effects of antibiotics is making a person more susceptible to a dangerous bacterial super-infection, such as pneumonia, which nowadays is often resistant to the antibiotic the person is taking. The Public Citizen's Health Research Group reports that "in 1983, more than 51% of the more than three million patients who saw doctors for treatment of the common cold were given an unnecessary prescription for an antibiotic."[6]

Allopathic doctors also prescribe steroidal inhaler and/or systemic steroids. Potential side effects include growth interference in children, weight gain, high blood pressure, stomach ulcers, pancreatitis and hyperglycemia, osteoporosis, and muscular weakness.

Flu vaccines are made from last year's viral strain. By the time a vaccine hits the shelves, the virus blamed for this year's "outbreak" is a different mutated kind, rendering the promise of immunity questionable. Furthermore, long-term studies on the potential effects of flu vaccines and their various ingredients have not been conducted, and their safety cannot be clearly determined as of yet. The decision to be vaccinated or not is yours, and yours alone. If you decide to receive a vaccination, look for any unusual signs or symptoms such as a high fever and/or changes in behavior. Signs of a serious allergic or anaphylactic reaction include shortness of breath, hives, paleness, weakness, a fast heartbeat, low blood pressure, dizziness and/or swelling of the throat. Other conditions to watch for are seizures—more common in the presence of a high fever, and especially in children under the age of three.

You can report cases of vaccine side effects to your doctor, nurse practitioner, nurse, or public health department and file a Vaccine Adverse Event Reporting System (VAERS) form, or call VAERS at 1-800-822-7967.[7]

Cannabis and Colds/Flu

While not a remedy for colds or flu per se, cannabinoids may be useful in alleviating the cough and fever often associated with colds and flu. (See Cough on page 105.)

Mind-Body Medicine and Colds/Flu

The Grace and Graham study focused on vasomotor rhinitis (stuffy or runny nose not caused by allergies or infection), and the psychosomatic similarities warrant inclusion of their findings in this section on colds. The researchers examined the psychosomatic underpinning of 12 patients with stuffy and runny nose diagnosed as rhinitis and discovered that symptoms occurred when a patient was faced with a life situation they wished would just go away, or they wished someone else would take responsibility for it and make it disappear, or felt avoidance would be the best course for them. Typical statements were: "I wanted them to go away." "I didn't want anything to do with it." "I wanted to blot it all out; I wanted to build a wall between me and him." "I wanted to hole up for the winter." "I wanted to go to bed and pull the sheets over my head." Grace and Graham concluded that: "The reaction of the respiratory mucous membrane to a noxious agent is to exclude it by swelling of the membrane with consequent narrowing of the passageway, and to dilute it and wash it out by hypersecretion."[8]

Another experiment used 334 healthy volunteers between 18 and 54 years who were assessed for their tendency to experience positive as well as negative emotions. Each was exposed to cold viruses and monitored in quarantine for the development of the symptoms of a common cold. Those who had tendencies to experience positive emotions had a significantly greater resistance to developing a cold.[9]

In cases of colds and flu, the body may become a metaphorical stage on which to act out various themes of dis-ease. This "lack of ease" may be the consequence of limiting beliefs such as "The glass is half empty rather than half full," "I don't want anything to change!", "I'll probably get sick because it's the cold season," or it may result from simply feeling overwhelmed. Likewise, when the fulfillment of a dream becomes a burden, we are ill at ease. ("I wanted this job, but in dealing with the daily grind I have forgotten how great it is to have a job." Or "I always wanted children, but all this nursing, teaching, and driving means I am constantly exhausted.") During difficult times, it is easy to simply forget to feel grateful. Then here comes fall and winter, and they offer an easy solution—"catch a cold." Now I can cough and sneeze my way into a break from it all.

The environment changes, daylight changes, and the air takes on a different feel in each season. Life is change. However, in the minds of many, change is not considered a friend and is often greeted with great dislike. In such cases, even a simple change in our routines may lead to irritation, anxiety, and attempts to wrestle with and dominate reality. Drained and overwhelmed by attempts to control the inevitable, one may want to curl up in bed, attempting to avoid dealing with change altogether.

The annual anxiety about getting sick during the "cold and flu season" may also contribute to lowered immunity to cold and flu viruses that otherwise would be easily handled by our immune system. Here, catching cold actually means release from the clutches of anxiety of getting sick. To many, the actual cold is preferable to constant anxiety.

It is interesting to note that those people who stay healthy undermine the collective belief in a cold and flu season. In fact, looking at the numbers, those who stay healthy are in the majority. In the U.S., it is estimated that about 1 in 4 will catch a cold, but 3 out of 4 will not. The estimates for flu are similar: 1 out of 10 Americans will catch a flu, but 9 out of 10 will stay healthy.

Powerful Questions

Have any of my fulfilled dreams become a burden?
Has the tedium of my daily routine eroded my gratitude?
Where is my glass "half empty" rather than half full?
Where am I feeling overwhelmed?
In what situations or circumstances am I averse to change?
Am I giving my power away to the cold season?

Suggested Blessings

May you slow down and stand still for a while.
Allow yourself to downshift your mind, take a deep breath, and relax.

Suggested Affirmations

I always find something to feel grateful for.
I maintain my living dreams with care and gratitude in mind.
I can ask for help.

I release the pressure of my to-do list by prioritizing.

I release my need to battle change.

I can relax in the face of change.

There is beauty in change.

I trust myself to find an appropriate way to handle change.

Let Food Be Thy Medicine

Anise ∽ Coconut ∽ Fennel ∽ Garlic ∽ Myrrh ∽ Oregano

Anise: Cuban physicians use the fruit (fresh or dried) of anise as an expectorant. It is used to treat coughs and sore throats as well as general low immunity.[10]

Scientists from Mashhad, Iran, discovered a possible mechanism that may explain why many traditional healers have been using anise extracts and oils in the treatment of certain respiratory ailments. Anise extracts and essential oils possess bronchodilatory (opens the upper airways) qualities derived from possible antihistamine-like properties.[11]

Coconut: The authors of a study from Staten Island, New York, state: "Lipids can inactivate enveloped viruses, bacteria, fungi, and protozoa." The scientists expect that medium-chain fatty acids (which are abundant in coconut) "may potentially be used as virucidal agents."[12]

Fennel: Fennel seeds and oil are approved by the German Commission E for the treatment of "catarrh of the upper respiratory tract."[13]

Garlic: In Cuba a syrup made from garlic is utilized to treat colds, coughs, and flu.[14]

Myrrh: Approved by the German Commission E for the topical treatment of mucous-membrane inflammation such as in sore throat during episodes of cold or cough.[15]

Oregano: Scientists from the University of Medicine in Varna, Bulgaria, discovered that tea of oregano may be effective in treating certain respiratory illness.[16]

Cough
Evidence-Based Confidence Level and Therapeutic Potential

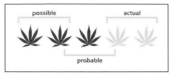

Total Number of Studies Reviewed: 4

Combined CHI Value: 11

While human physiology allows us to cough consciously, most coughs are sudden and involuntary reflexes designed to clear the upper airways of mucus, phlegm, microbes, irritants, or foreign bodies. Differentiations of coughs include onset, duration, and dry, productive, chronic, or tic coughs (psychogenic). The most common cause for a sudden-onset cough is a virus-based infection. Antibiotics are useless in these cases, as are anti-histamines. While most coughs will simply take their course and are by nature self-limiting, certain complications or conditions may warrant treat-ment. A cough remedy may be helpful if symptoms include severe pain, cough-induced insomnia, fainting, vomiting, incontinence, hernias, or tissue damage of the rib cage.

No cure exists within the orthodox model of medicine. For the past two hundred years of modern medicine, opiates have been its most effective anti-tussive. However, adverse effects are common, as is the possibility of addiction or abuse.

Cannabis and Cough

The anti-inflammatory, antispasmotic, and bronchodilating properties of cannabis all may play a part in the therapeutic impact of the herb as an anti-tussive.

As early as 1976 scientists experimenting on anesthetized cats had discov-ered that THC (but not CBD or CBN) had cough-suppressing capacities similar to that of codeine-PO4.[1]

An analysis conducted in 2006 by the University of California in con-junction with the U.S. federal government indicated that the immediate impact of smoking cannabis is bronchodilation. The abstract filed with the U.S. Patent and Trademark Office states: "The invention discloses the existence of cannabinoid receptors in the airways, which are functionally linked to inhibition of cough. Locally-acting cannabinoid agents can be administered to the airways of a subject to ameliorate cough, without causing the psychoactive effects characteristic of systemically administered cannabinoids. In addition, locally or systemically administered cannabinoid inactivation inhibitors can also be used to ameliorate cough. The present invention also defines conditions under which cannabinoid agents can be administered to produce anti-tussive effects devoid of bronchial constriction." The patent application also states that: "The Government may have certain rights in this invention."[2]

While the abstract is concerned that the long-term use of the plant might contribute to respiratory symptoms such as coughing, the review acknowledged that these symptoms might also be caused by other factors, such as tobacco. This possibility is highlighted by the discoveries made in a Vancouver study (2009): "Smoking both tobacco and marijuana synergistically increased the risk of respiratory symptoms and COPD (chronic obstructive pulmonary disease). Smoking only marijuana was not associated with an increased risk of respiratory symptoms or COPD."[3]

Studies have shown that THC opens the upper airways and ameliorates coughing. However, smoke of any kind may cause cough, spasm, reduced lung function and/or disease over long periods of time. Intravenous THC is anti-tussive in animal experiments but has not been tested in humans. Vaporizers that heat cannabis to 350°F do not burn the plant material or produce smoke, yet released THC and other cannabinoids may mitigate the irritation of smoke. The efficacy of taking cannabis-infused oils by mouth has yet to be studied. However, oromucosal sprays have been invented (UC Berkeley, U.S. Government 2006) and can be purchased in various forms at some dispensaries. The government patent states: "The present invention unexpectedly achieves the . . . desired anti-tussive effects without the dysphoric side effects and habit-forming properties characteristic of centrally acting cannabimimetic or opiate drugs."[4] The researchers believe their invention works via CB1 receptors.

Additionally, a systemic review (2007) of available studies conducted by researchers from numerous institutions discovered that short-term exposure to cannabis produces bronchodilation.[5]

Study Summary

Drugs	Type of Study	Published Year, Place, and Key Results	CHI
Tobacco, cannabis	Survey of 878 people over 40 with a history of tobacco and/or marijuana smoking	2009—Vancouver, British Columbia, Canada: Participants who reported smoking only tobacco, but not those who reported smoking only marijuana, experienced more frequent respiratory symptoms.[3]	3
Smoked cannabis	Meta-analysis including 34 studies	2007—Multi-institutional research team, West Haven Veterans Affairs Medical Center (Connecticut), Yale University School of Medicine (Connecticut), Case Western University School of Medicine (Ohio): Short-term use produces bronchodilation. Long-term use effects are inconclusive.[5]	3
Cannabinoids (incl. anandamide, THC)	Meta-analysis	2006—UC Berkeley, U.S. government: Locally acting cannabinoid agents can be administered to the airways of a subject to ameliorate cough.[2]	3
THC intravenously	Animal study (cats)	1976—Wallace Laboratories, Cranbury, New Jersey: THC is anti-tussive.[1]	2

Total CHI Value 11

Strain-Specific Considerations

Anandamide and THC bind with CB1 and CB2 receptors relatively equally. Sativa and sativa-prominent hybrids tend to present with a higher THC:CBD profile, thus providing a relatively balanced activation while favoring CB1.

Mind-Body Medicine and Cough

Coughing is a survival mechanism that by nature is self-correcting and a means to draw one's attention. Other people nearby, especially those who care, will pay attention to a person with a sudden cough. The natural question is "Are you okay?"

However, coughing is also a means to keep people at a distance, communicating the danger of infection: "Stay away." In a sense, coughing may represent a push–pull, as if to say, "Notice me, but do not come too close."

Powerful Questions

What is stuck in my throat that needs to be expressed?
Who do I want to pay attention to me?
Who would I like to keep at a distance?

Why do I need to be noticed?
Who is not listening to me?
Where do I feel I have not been heard?
What is not communicated until I shout it out?

Suggested Blessings

May you find a way to express yourself with ease and fun, so as to draw
only positive attention and care.
May our flowers soothe, relax, and open you to the knowledge that you
are loved and the certainty that your message has been heard.

Suggested Affirmations

People listen to me.
I always find the most appropriate way to bring my point across.
I express myself with ease and fun and harm no one.

Let Food Be Thy Medicine

See the section on supporting herbs under Viral Infections/Colds and Flu.

Encephalitis

Evidence-Based Confidence Level and Therapeutic Potential

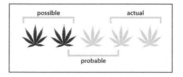

Total Number of Studies Reviewed: 1

CHI Value: 2

Encephalitis is an acute inflammation of the brain most commonly caused
by a virus (e.g., live virus vaccination, herpes, West Nile, or equine encephalitis), although it may also be produced by bacteria (e.g., syphilis, bacterial meningitis, Lyme disease), parasites (e.g., malaria), or an over-reactive
immune response to an inflammation or secondary infection (e.g., measles,
mumps, or rubella).

Symptoms may include headaches, blurred vision, fever, confusion, generalized weakness, seizures, stiff neck, and projectile vomiting. Diagnosis is done by physical examination, history, blood, urine or mucosa tests, spinal tap (to examine cerebrospinal fluid), electroencephalogram (EEG), brain biopsy, and a possible imaging of brain structure by magnetic resonance (MRI) or an x-ray CT scan.

Depending on underlying cause, treatment may include antiviral agents such as acyclovir (only in cases of herpes), other antimicrobial pharmaceuticals, anti-inflammatory drugs to reduce swelling and inflammation, analgesics (for pain), anti-emetics (for vomiting), and supportive care as needed (e.g., intravenous fluids, seizure medications, ventilation).

Cannabis and Encephalitis

A study conducted on rodents by researchers at the University of Manitoba, Winnipeg, Canada, (2013) discovered that CB2 signaling was a mechanism of controlling CNS (central nervous system) inflammation during viral encephalitis.[1]

Study Summary

Drugs	Type of Study	Published Year, Place, and Key Results	CHI
Synthetic CB2 agonist, HU308 (5 mg/kg ip once daily)	Animal study (rats)	2013—Department of Medicine (Neurology), University of Manitoba, and Department of Medical Microbiology, University of Manitoba, Winnipeg, MB, Canada: HU308 effect on CB2-mitigated inflammation during viral encephalitis by limiting viral infection and by reducing microglia activation.[1]	2

Total CHI Value 2

Strain-Specific Recommendations

The Manitoba study suggests mitigation of inflammation via CB2. To enhance CB2 activation, select an indica or indica-dominant strain with a lower THC to CBD ratio.

Mind-Body Medicine and Encephalitis

Depending on underlying cause or key symptoms, consult the sections of this book on bacterial and viral infection, inflammation, pain, or vomiting.

Powerful Questions

What are these symptoms keeping you from doing?

How do you feel about that?

Where do these feelings take you?

What scenarios or memories are associated with these feelings?

What is the meaning (messages, unhealthy beliefs/attitudes, etc.) you have given to that scenario?

Can the answers to these questions direct your focus to support your capacity for self-healing?

Hepatitis

Evidence-Based Confidence Level and Therapeutic Potential

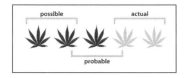

Number of Studies Reviewed: 3

Combined CHI Value: 8

The liver is a vital and large organ located in the upper right side of the abdomen. It is the largest gland of the body and plays a major part in a complex set of life-maintaining bodily functions. The liver excretes bile stored in the gallbladder, which is used for digestion. It is a major bodily filter, ridding the body of toxic substances whether natural or chemical. It breaks down hormones and hemoglobin, and stores iron and other substances along with vitamins A, D, and B_{12}. Liver cells participate in the production of glycogen, which functions as a rapid energy reserve and aids in maintaining blood volumes and clotting ability. There is no substitute for the liver. If the liver fails and is not replaced by a suitable donated liver, death results.

Hepatitis is inflammation of the liver and can be characterized as acute or chronic. Acute hepatitis usually lasts no more than a couple of months. Chronic hepatitis can be a lifelong debilitating disease. Most commonly, the liver becomes inflamed as a result of the hepatic viruses A, B, C, D, or E, which are a major health problem worldwide. Viral hepatitis is contagious, while non-viral forms of hepatitis are not. However, toxins, alcohol, and many pharmacological medications such as acetaminophen and ibuprofen can also produce hepatitis. Other viruses (such as those causing yellow fever or bacterial infections like leptospirosis) can affect the liver and cause inflammation. Hepatitis can also occur after ingesting poisonous mushrooms, or result from an autoimmune disease in which the body's own immune system attacks the liver.

Signs and symptoms vary from one person to another and include increased generalized weakness, decreased energy levels, loss of appetite, nausea, vomiting, diarrhea, clay-colored bowel movements, pain in the joints or muscles, and headaches. Symptoms may progress to include the presence of dark urine, the yellowing of the sclera (white of the eyes), or jaundice (yellowing of the skin). Tenderness or pain in the region of the liver and enlarged spleen, and lymph nodes may also be present. The general disease development of hepatitis is two-fold. The patient may go through an acute phase, then recover and gain lifelong immunity (in the case of hepatitis A). Or, the illness may progress into a chronic debilitating form, leading to cirrhosis (scarring of the liver), liver cancer and/or premature death.

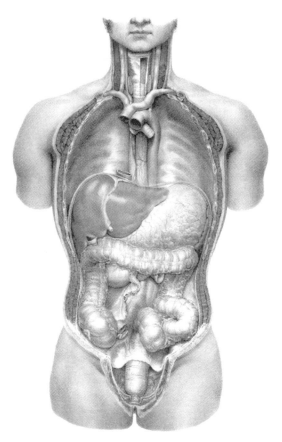

Until very recently, no treatment existed within orthodox medicine to cure hepatitis C. Treatment focused on supporting the body through different stages of the illness. Some of the most common pharmaceutical medications used in the management of hepatitis were immune globulin, interferon, and ribavirin, each with a set of potentially severe adverse effects. Sometimes liver transplants could sustain life. However, a new line of drugs just arrived (I'm writing this in 2015) which has achieved a relatively high cure rate (up to 90%) for hepatitis C (at least genotype 1). The cost for a course of a 12-week treatment of Harvoni, Sovaldi, or Olysio in specific combination can easily surpass six figures.

Overview of Hepatitis A, B, C

Type	Transmission Route	Diagnosis by	Orthodox Treatment	Severity
Hepatitis A virus (HAV)	Infected fecal-oral route	Hepatitis A-specific blood test	No cure; once recovered, person has lifelong immunity	Most people recover
Hepatitis B virus (HBV)	Contact with infected bodily fluids	Hepatitis B-specific blood test	No cure	Most people recover, but for some people it can become chronic
Hepatitis C virus (HCV)	Contact with infected blood	Hepatitis C-specific blood test	A new line of drugs is having a promising success rate with the new treatments	Most likely to become chronic, or may be cured

Cannabis and Hepatitis

Cannabinoids have demonstrated the ability to minimize the frequent adverse side effects of the most common pharmaceutical treatment regimen (which uses interferon and ribavirin), thus facilitating compliance with the full dose and length of the recommended treatment. A Columbia University study (2008) demonstrated that cannabinoids are themselves able to inhibit the virus.[1]

Study Summary

Drugs	Type of Study	Published Year, Place, and Key Results	CHI
THC, anandamide	Animal study (murine)	2008—Multi-institutional research team, Columbia University, New York: THC and anandamide and a lack of FAAH, an enzyme that breaks down anandamide, all can inhibit hepatitis.[1]	2
THC and Nabilone	21 patients with hepatitis C undergoing interferon and ribavirin therapy	2008—University of Ottawa, Canada: Oral THC and Nabilone reduce nausea, vomiting, improve appetite.[2]	3
Cannabis	71 recovering substance users with Hep. C	2006—Department of Medicine, University of California San Francisco: Cannabis users were able to maintain adherence to the challenging medication regimen.[3]	3

Total CHI Value 8

Strain-Specific Considerations

The primary cannabinoids tested in the context of hepatitis, or as an adjunct treatment to pharmaceutical treatment of hepatitis, were THC, anandamide, Nabilone, and whole-plant cannabis. THC and anandamide bind relatively equally to CB1 and CB2 receptors. Nabilone is a synthetic cannabinoid similar to THC; and whole-plant cannabis, depending on strain, binds to CB1 and CB2 receptors but at different ratios.

Sativas and sativa-dominant strains tend to have a higher THC:CBD ratio.

Mind-Body Medicine and Hepatitis

The liver functions as a major filter and is capable of ridding the body of physical toxins. When the liver tissue is infected and inflamed, its ability to break down toxins is diminished. As the toxic load increases, liver function continues to be impaired, ultimately producing the peculiar signs and symptoms of hepatitis.

This particular detoxification function of the liver may be mirrored in the mental-emotional realm by the accumulation of the toxins represented by unexpressed or harbored angers, resentment, and rage, and also by long-standing and unresolved fears, angst, sorrows, and anxieties.

Some patients completely recover and even gain lifelong immunity, while others struggle with the chronic forms of hepatitis for long periods or even the rest of their lives. This fork in the road suggests that some transcend underlying issues more rapidly than others.

Powerful Questions

Do I have long-standing feelings that are clogging me up and remain unprocessed?

Is a heavy load of negative feelings making me toxic?

Which emotions that I regularly experience might lead to toxic build-up?

Suggested Blessings

May you find, feel, and release all emotions hidden in the recesses of your mind.

May you uproot the beliefs from which they sprang.

May you succeed in seeding new and healing beliefs and attitudes.

Suggested Affirmations

I embrace all my feelings with appropriate intensity and harm no one.
I can find the belief(s) which produced chronic anger or fear, and replace
it/them with belief(s) that generate long-lasting love and well-being.

Let Food Be Thy Medicine

Basil ∾ Clove ∾ Saffron

Basil: Basil has been used in Traditional Chinese Medicine for thousands of
years. Now researchers from the island nation of Taiwan have taken a closer
look at the possible antiviral properties of basil extract. They found that
extracts of basil *(Ocimum basilicum)* exhibit a broad spectrum of antiviral
activity, including combatting hepatitis B.[4]

Clove: A Tunisian study determined that essential oil of clove extract has
antiviral effects against hepatitis C.[5]

Saffron: *Crocus sativus L.* or saffron may possess anticancer activity and
activity against hepatitis.[6]

Herpes

Evidence-Based Confidence Level and Therapeutic Potential

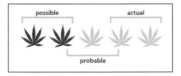

Total Number of Studies Reviewed: 3

CHI Value: 5

Herpes simplex is a common virus that belongs to the same family as
the chicken pox virus. There are currently eight known herpes viruses.
According to orthodox medicine, all herpes viruses can exist in the
body without any outward sign or symptom until a period of depressed
immunity suddenly results in an outbreak. Oral herpes (cold sores or
fever blisters) called HSV-I usually appears above the waist, in contrast
to genital herpes (HSV-II). While HSV I and II are relatively benign

physically, they often take a profound toll on the patient's emotional well-being.

No orthodox cure exists. A common allopathic treatment to "manage" herpes is Zovirax (acyclovir). Side effects may include nausea and/or vomiting, diarrhea, dizziness, anorexia, fatigue, swelling of the skin, skin rashes, leg pains, sore throat, and paresthesia (feeling of numbness). A month's supply for the maximum recommended dose costs about $870 (in 2015).

Cannabis and Herpes

A 2010 study conducted on humans in Münster, Germany,[1] confirmed that topical cannabinoids significantly reduce nerve pain after a flare-up of the herpes virus. Laboratory experiments from Tampa, Florida (2004),[2] and Johnson City, Tennessee (1980),[3] showed that THC has the ability to interfere with replication of the herpes virus even in instances related to the genesis of cancer.

Study Summary

Drugs	Type of Study	Published Year, Place, and Key Results	CHI
Cannabinoid-containing cream	Human	2010—Münster, Germany: Majority of patients experienced pain reduction by more than 80%.[1]	3
THC	Laboratory	2004—University of South Florida (Tampa, USA): THC specifically targets viral and/or cellular mechanisms required for replication.[2]	1
THC	Laboratory	1980—Johnson City, Tennessee: Herpes simplex I and II failed to replicate when introduced to dishes containing human cell cultures treated with THC.[3]	1

Total CHI Value 5

Strain-Specific Considerations

THC binds with CB1 and CB2 receptors relatively equally. Sativas and sativa-dominant hybrids have a higher THC:CBD ratio.

Mind-Body Medicine and Herpes

A study published by the American Psychosomatic Society acknowledges prior reports of precipitating emotional or psychic trauma as a component in herpes breakouts. In particular, the study focused on a patient with repeated outbreaks of HSV-I who was "... able to consciously associate a relationship between the outbreak of the skin lesions and the existence of repressed hostility."[4]

Guilt, with its demand for punishment and purification through suffering, is not benign. Guilt is damaging to oneself and to others. People who believe it is not acceptable to feel angry may be conscious only of guilt. However, since feeling angry is part of the human experience, where is the anger going to go? In the case of herpes, the unexpressed anger may shift into the physical realm. Herpes sores on the lips may represent guilt associated with affection, expressing affection, or one's inability to tell the truth, while herpes sores on the genitals may represent guilt associated with sexual activity and pleasures.

Herpes sores on the lips are punishing, forcing distance and halting kisses, a physical display of affection and intimacy whose loss impacts both members of a couple. Herpes sores on the genitals are also punishing, denying oneself and the other the experience of sexual fun, pleasure, and intimacy. In both cases, the complex function of a herpes breakout can be summarized by the practical impact it has on the patient's physical experience. It prevents sexual intimacy and displays of affection, it satisfies a need for purification through suffering, and it may assist the patient to express anger s/he believes it is not okay to feel.

People who are able to prevent or abort an outbreak acknowledge and appropriately express their emotions, fostering a deeper intimacy with themselves and others. Those who have achieved a cure have been able to change the beliefs that initially made suppression of "unacceptable" feelings seem necessary. As a result, they no longer need to suppress anger, suppress what is true for them, or suppress their sexual needs and sexual pleasure.

Powerful Questions (HSV-I)

Do I feel un-kissable, and if so, why?

What is my truth? Have I left my truth unspoken?

Why do I not want to kiss my intimate partner?

Why do I want to deny my affection?

Aggravating Factors (HSV-I)

Guilt/anger around affection and kissing; pressure to be affectionate; repressed anger/hostility

Healing Factors (HSV-I)

Appropriately express anger; appropriately express personal hostile experiences; establish principles around the expression of affection

Suggested Blessings (HSV-I)

May you see the anger hiding behind your guilt.

May you use your anger like a compass to guide you to the beliefs that need changing so that healing can begin.

Suggested Affirmations (HSV-I)

It is okay to feel angry.

I can find beneficial ways to own and express my anger so that I can trust others more and become closer to them.

I can identify and change limiting beliefs that tell me it is not okay to be angry.

I can appropriately express what is true for me, no matter how difficult this feels.

I can say what I need to say without hurting anyone.

Powerful Questions (HSV-II)

Am I angry about sex or my sexual pleasure?

Does it feel acceptable (seem reasonable) to be angry about these things?

Am I angry at my sexual partner?

Does it feel okay to be angry at my sexual partner?

Why do I want to take sex out of my relationship right now?

Who do I want to punish by not being able to have sex right now?

How can I honor my anger or guilt about sex without letting it ruin my sex life?

Can I show love and intimacy in non-sexual ways?

Aggravating Factors (HSV-II)

Guilt/anger around sex or the genitals; guilt around perceived sexual performance pressure; repressed anger; hostility about/surrounding sex.

Healing Factors (HSV-II)

Appropriately express anger related to sexuality and sexual performance; establish principles around the expression of sexuality; speak appropriately about negative sexual experiences and angers related to sex; identify the beliefs underlying suppressed emotions and replace them with beliefs that produce expansive, loving sexual experiences.

Suggested Blessings (HSV-II)

May you see the anger hiding behind your guilt.

May you use your anger like a compass to guide you to the beliefs that need changing so that healing can begin.

Suggested Affirmation (HSV-II)

Sex is natural and sex is fun, and it's done best with harm to no one.

Let Food Be Thy Medicine

Basil ∽ Cardamom ∽ Clove ∽ Coconut ∽ Turmeric

Basil: Researchers from the island nation of Taiwan have taken a closer look at the possible antiviral properties of basil extract. Extracts of basil *(Ocimum basilicum)* exhibit a broad spectrum of antiviral activity, including defending against herpes.[5]

Cardamom: At the University of Cincinnati College of Medicine, scientists looked at cineole, a major constituent of cardamom, in the context of treating vaginal herpes infections in mice. They determined that sufficient evidence exists to warrant more research using this promising natural treatment modality.[6]

Clove: In a series of experiments, virologists from the Toyama Medical and Pharmaceutical University in Sugitani, Japan, determined that eugenine, a compound purified from the extracts of clove, inhibits viral DNA synthesis in several strains of herpes (I & II), including acyclovir–phosphonoacetic acid-resistant HSV-I.[7]

A Tunisian study determined that essential oil of clove extract has antiviral properties against herpes.[8]

Coconut: A crude extract of *Cocos nucifera L.* husk fiber inhibits acyclovir-resistant *Herpes simplex* virus type I (HSV-I-ACVr).[9]

Turmeric: Researchers tested the hypothesis that curcumin, the main active constituent in turmeric, would block viral infection and gene expression of HSV-I by inhibiting promoters of herpes gene expression. Results showed that curcumin does significantly decrease HSV-I infectivity and gene expression.[10]

HIV/AIDS

Evidence-Based Confidence Level and Therapeutic Potential

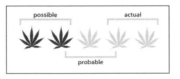

Total Number of Studies Reviewed: 1

CHI Value: 3

Mainstream orthodox medicine considers acquired immune deficiency syndrome (AIDS) to be a disease of the immune system that is caused by a human immunodeficiency virus (HIV) transmitted through sexual or blood contact.

Within a weakened immune system, infectious agents such as parasites, fungi, bacteria, or viruses encounter little resistance from our natural defenses. Regardless of where in the body the infection spreads, the response is fever, sweat, chills, and any other defenses still available. The body's natural filters (including lymph nodes, liver, and kidneys) can become overwhelmed by the invaders, which further increases symptoms of weakness, low energy, and weight loss.

This destructive process can develop into AIDS-related anorexia, cachexia, or wasting syndrome. Common opportunistic infections include lung infections by fungi (pneumocystis) or bacteria (pneumonia, tuberculosis), gastrointestinal infections such as candidiasis (thrush), infection of the nervous system and the brain by cryptococcal meningitis (fungus), progressive multifocal leukoencephalopathy (virus), or toxoplasmosis (parasite), which can lead to neuropathies (nerve pain) and dementia. Opportunistic diseases may also take the form of cancer (non-Hodgkin's lymphoma) or affect organs (hepatitis) or the skin (herpes).

Early signs and symptoms may include fatigue, weight loss, shortness of breath especially during mild exertion, dry coughs, swollen lymph nodes, recurring fevers and chills, frequent episodes of diarrhea, memory loss, blemishes (pink, brown, purple, red) of the mucous membranes and/or the skin, candidiasis, frequent colds, or pneumonia. Late-stage symptoms include higher fevers and chills lasting weeks, chronic diarrhea, and continuous weight loss that may develop into wasting, neuropathies, nausea, and vomiting. Pneumonia may progress into tuberculosis or pneumocystis. Memory loss may gradually evolve into an altered mental state and AIDS dementia.

No AIDS diagnostic test exists, but depending on what country a person lives in, diagnosis is done by symptoms alone, by testing for HIV, or by a combination of these methods. None of the tests are 100% accurate. Oral tests are available but produce numerous false positives, often indicating HIV infection when none exists. Blood tests include the ELISA and Western blot tests. ELISA tests may yield false positives due to a variety of common pathogens and the body's antibodies against them. In the U.S. ELISA positive results must be confirmed by a Western blot test.

The orthodox medical establishment has no cure for AIDS. Current treatment consists of pharmaceutical antiviral agents belonging to two classes, namely protease inhibitors and reverse transcriptase inhibitors.

Since the 1980s, an AIDS reappraisal movement has emerged that questions many of the orthodox positions. In particular, doubts have been raised about unsubstantiated AIDS epidemic predictions, changing surveillance definitions, unreliable AIDS tests, inconsistent diagnostic methods of AIDS, inconsistent African versus U.S./EU AIDS presentations, unsafe AIDS pharmaceuticals, curability, the HIV–AIDS hypothesis itself, AIDS and Koch's postulates, the fact that AIDS behaves unlike a contagious disease, and the lack of focus on other possible causative or contributing elements in the development of AIDS.

Cannabis and HIV/AIDS

Inspired by courageous early AIDS victims and their caretakers who discovered that cannabis reduces symptoms of AIDS and ameliorates the significant adverse effects of AIDS pharmaceuticals, scientists decided to take a closer look at cannabis in reference to AIDS. Today a growing body of scientific evidence elucidates how and why specific cannabinoids benefit patients with AIDS.

In one of the largest of any such studies ever conducted, scientists from Boston collected data from 775 patients living with HIV/AIDS who were suffering from six common symptoms (anxiety, depression, fatigue, diarrhea, nausea, and peripheral neuropathy). Participants came from Kenya, South Africa, Puerto Rico, and ten different U.S. locations. Results showed that while the differences were relatively small, cannabis was more effective than standard prescription and over-the-counter (OTC) medications for treating five of the six symptoms studied: anxiety, depression, diarrhea, fatigue, and neuropathy. Cannabis was slightly less effective than standard prescriptions and OTC medications for treatment of nausea.[1]

Study Summary

Drugs	Type of Study	Published Year, Place, and Key Results	CHI
Cannabis	775 patients living with HIV/AIDS	2009—MGH Institute of Health Professions, School of Nursing, Boston, Massachusetts: Cannabis is considered effective in treating anxiety and depression, diarrhea, fatigue, and neuropathy.[1]	3

Total CHI Value 3

Strain-Specific Considerations

HIV/AIDS patients use both basic strains of cannabis, often choosing a specific strain in response to the severity and presence of their unique symptoms.

Mind-Body Medicine and HIV/AIDS

When the "AIDS epidemic" was identified in the late '70s and early '80s, entire groups of people who dared to, or had to, live differently became visible. Social and moral rejection, marginalization, and judgment (often rooted in religious beliefs) rained down on the groups who experienced

AIDS first: gays, prostitutes, IV-drug users, and Haitians stricken with the ill-effects of abject poverty. Some voices in the religious community went so far as to call AIDS "God's punishment for breaking His rules." To many, gays were considered unnatural, prostitutes immoral, and IV-drug users worthless, while contemplating sick, poor, Third World minorities made people feel uncomfortable, anxious, or guilty.

AIDS was, in many ways, associated with a state of being a victim—a victim of ever-present social rejection, and vulnerable to a multitude of ever-present pathogens. Some people with HIV or AIDS may have taken these judgments into their bodies where issues surrounding love, hate, rage, punishment, vulnerability, defenselessness, or defensiveness become a deeply personal challenge.

This challenge was echoed by the dire early predictions of physicians and public health experts who fanned the fires of fear, warning of a new "plague" brought about by these marginalized groups. As a result, many patients with AIDS say that, through AIDS, they "found out who really loved them"—or not.

In summary, aggravating factors for HIV/AIDS may include: defensiveness, defenselessness, a love=sex mindset, self-destructive guilt, anger, rage, self-hatred, self-punishment, testing who loves me, and self-loathing.

Consider working with personal power instead of defensiveness; appropriate defenses instead of defenselessness; love as more than sex; constructive release of guilt, anger, hate, and rage; self-forgiveness instead of self-punishment; instead of testing who loves you, find elegant ways of loving and being loved; release self-hatred and loathing, and replace these with self-love and acceptance.

Suggested Blessings

May you realize that you are worth loving.

May you learn to raise the love you have to higher forms and expressions.

May you find constructive ways to release hate and rage.

May you choose self-acceptance instead of self-punishment.

May you release defensiveness and realize the powers that reside inside.

May you transcend your defenselessness into a new ability to cope.

Suggested Affirmations

I love myself just as I am. I accept myself just as I am.

I can raise my love to a higher octave. Sometimes just letting myself be with hate and rage is a release.

I am powerful, I am creative, and I am able to respond to insult appropriately without harming anyone.

I can respond constructively to judgments, and obtain immunity and protection.

Let Food Be Thy Medicine

Acacia ∾ Coconut

Acacia: A study from Mumbai, India, presented at the Eighth International Congress on Drug Therapy in HIV Infection in 2006, indicated that the aqueous extract of acacia pods was effective in vitro against the viral enzyme reverse transcriptase.[2]

Coconut: The authors of this study from Staten Island, New York, write: "Lipids can inactivate enveloped viruses, bacteria, fungi, and protozoa." By adding medium-chain fatty acids (MCFA) to HIV-infected blood products, researchers learned that they could reduce virus load. Furthermore, the scientists expect that MCFA ". . . may potentially be used as combination spermicidal and virucidal agents."[3]

Cancer (in general)

Evidence-Based Confidence Level and Therapeutic Potential for Cancer in General

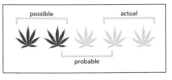

Total Number of Cancer Studies Reviewed: 50

Combined CHI Value: 100

Every year, cancer takes credit for 13% of all deaths worldwide; and, according to the orthodox model of medicine, 30% of all cancers are attributed to known and avoidable risk factors.[1] Cancer-inducing materials, called carcinogens, exist almost everywhere, and the list of known carcinogens grows as new information becomes available. A few of those hiding in plain view include tobacco smoke, industrial poisons in the environment, numerous household products (laundry soap with trisodium nitrilotriacetate), bath and beauty products (containing formaldehyde), pet products (certain flea collars), certain foods (hot dogs with nitrates), and modern medical procedures emitting ionizing radiation (mammograms, CAT scans, and any other x-ray devices).[2]

Certain types of infectious agents may also contribute to a cancer's development. For example, hepatitis B, an infection of the liver, is caused by a virus that may lead to liver cancer; human papillomavirus (HPV) may lead to cervical cancer; human herpes virus (HHV-8)—aka Kaposi's sarcoma-associated herpes virus (KSHV)—may produce skin cancer lesions; *Helicobacter pylori* may facilitate stomach cancer; and a parasite named *Schistosoma mansoni,* affecting the urinary tract, may initiate bladder cancer.

Within the orthodox model of medicine, cancer (malignant neoplasm) starts with the corruption of genetic material (a mutation) inside a normally healthy cell. Evidence suggests that cellular cancer may occur quite frequently in everybody, but that normally the body's own proper immune defenses can cure these threats. However, when the body's overall health is weakened, the growth of mutations may overwhelm the capacity of the body to cure them, and cancer can take over.

Scientists hypothesize that cellular corruption begins with exposure to a carcinogen (cancer-producing toxin). The now-corrupted cell begins to divide, but instead of generating healthy new cells, it begins producing new cancerous cells. Most cancer cells produce tumors but can also destroy adjacent tissue (metastasize) or affect the blood in cases of leukemia. Symptoms vary greatly, depending on where the cancer is located and how far it has progressed. Orthodox treatment is usually limited to chemotherapy, surgery and/or radiation.

Cannabis and Cancer

As early as 1974, the U.S. government knew of cannabis's effectiveness against certain types of cancer. While the publication of this particular study became a victim of the war on drugs, an article about the study published by the *Washington Post* survived. The story, written by Victor

Cohn, was entitled "Cancer Curb Is Studied: Doctors Eye Drug Found in Marijuana." Cohn reported that "the active chemical agent in marijuana curbs the growth of three kinds of cancer (lung cancer, breast cancer, and viral-induced leukemia) in mice, and may also suppress the immunity reaction that causes rejection of organ transplants, a Medical College of Virginia team has discovered."[3]

Since then the scientific evidence of cannabinoids' ability to counteract certain types of cancer has grown in quantity and detail. Major scientific journals continue to report in great detail about the trial results conducted by an international community of medical researchers and scientists examining the complex effects that cannabinoids have in preventing and treating specific cancer formations.

Furthermore, studies also lay claim to cannabinoids' abilities to mitigate common side effects of chemotherapeutic agents such as cisplatin.[4]

The scientific evidence of therapeutic effects of cannabinoids for patients with specific cancers begins after this introductory section, with the sections arranged alphabetically.

Strain- and Form-Specific Considerations

The review conducted in this section examined the results of 50 studies relevant to the use of cannabinoids and the endocannabinoid system in the context of the prevention and treatment of 15 types of cancer. A high overall CHI value of 100 suggests with relative confidence that cannabinoids may prevent, inhibit, and destroy cancer cells, as well as exhibit strong therapeutic influences to mitigate nausea, vomiting, pain, night sweats, and improve quality of life.

Research also shows that CB1- and CB2-mediated therapeutic influences may vary depending on the patient's type of cancer or symptoms. In some cases, therapeutic impact occurred via CB1; at other times, via CB2. In all other cases, it was the synergistic effects induced by activation of both CB1 and CB2 receptor sites that was therapeutic.

Sativa and sativa-heavy strains tend to present with a higher THC:CBD/CBN ratio, while indicas or indica-heavy hybrids tend to contain a lower THC:CBD/CBN ratio. While both strains will activate CB1 and CB2, in comparison, indicas or indica-heavy hybrids tend to activate more CB2 receptors than do sativas.

Raw, fresh leaf plant matter, such as cannabis juice, for example, has a significantly higher CBD content in the form of CBD-acid with a greater affinity to activate CB2.

Mind-Body Medicine and Cancer

Psychotherapists followed 1,353 people over a period of 10 years. The researchers discovered that in nine out of ten cases, cancer could be predicted in part on the basis of "an overly rational, anti-emotional attitude."[5] The longest study to date, conducted at Johns Hopkins, focused on 972 physicians who were followed over a period of 30 years. Results showed that those physicians characterized as "loners," and who were likely to suppress their emotions, were 16 times more likely to develop cancer than their more emotionally expressive peers.[6]

Psychotherapist Lawrence LeShan has worked with cancer patients for the past 50 years. Based on his extensive and numerous successful experiences with patients, including end-stage cancer patients, he published his findings in research papers and books highlighting a common denominator shared by those patients who went into and maintained remission: authenticity, or having learned to "sing their own song in life."[7] In other words, those patients who went into remission had learned to assertively communicate their needs and honestly express their emotions, even those hitherto considered taboo.

A study conducted at the Veterans Administration Hospital in Houston, Texas, revealed a possible correlation between an individual's body-image and the location of cancer development,[8] thus indicating that psychological constructs such as how we see ourselves may play a part in how and where cancer develops.

J. C. Holland, MD, wrote: "Over the last quarter of the past century, psycho-oncology became a subspecialty of oncology with its own body of knowledge contributing to cancer care. In the new millennium, a significant base of literature, training programs, and a broad research agenda have evolved with applications at all points on the cancer continuum: behavioral research in changing lifestyle and habits to reduce cancer risk; study of behaviors and attitudes to ensure early detection; study of psychological issues related to genetic risk and testing; symptom control (anxiety, depression, delirium, pain, and fatigue) during active treatment; management of psychological sequelae in cancer survivors; and management of the psychological aspects of palliative and end-of-life care. Links between psychological and physiological domains of relevance to cancer risk and survival are being actively explored through psychoneuroimmunology. Research in these areas will occupy the research agenda for the first quarter of the new century."[9]

Today, more than 200 different types of physical cancer classifications exist. And, while the mental/emotional architecture of a particular cancer may be unique to an individual, research suggests some common denominators: negative affect, hostility (overt and covert), lack of emotional authenticity, hopelessness, hopeless anger, and suppressed and repressed emotions foremost among them.

Often, people vulnerable to cancer share low self-esteem early in life. Overly critical authority figures, severe punishments, too much responsibility, a lack of praise or positive feedback, passive role models—these all can prevent the development of healthy self-esteem. These individuals then seek others' approval to counter their own insecurity. And, while there is nothing wrong with seeking the approval of others, it is not a substitute for self-esteem.

Cancer patients with low self-esteem may attempt to control anything that threatens the social hierarchy they believe in. So they live by the rules. They never rock the boat, do not like to say no, and are nice to everyone around them in order to win their group's appreciation. By the same token, they can be very judgmental of anybody whose values diverge from "normal" within their own social group.

Human emotions against anybody in "the group/family"—emotions such as hatred, hurt, shame, worthlessness, rage, or despairing hopelessness—must be hidden at all costs from the self and others. However, where are these feelings to go? Just because we deny them does not mean they don't exist. In cancer these "intolerable emotions," especially hopeless anger, demand to be acknowledged even if it kills us. Interestingly, researchers examining potential psychosomatic causes of breast cancer write: "In some of our patients, we had the feeling that the cancer was being utilized as a form of passive suicide."[10]

Cancer emerges as a living mirror of someone who has the need to demonstrate that s/he is perfect, static, unchanging, and permanent—all qualities that do not exist in life. The first physical symptoms appear. A visit to the physician produces the dreaded diagnosis. The crisis begins to erupt and grow.

Cancer dominates its environment and stubbornly imposes its will on everything in its path. It's almost as if cancer wants to be God-like, wants to be everywhere, to have power over everything. Cancer cells are theoretically immortal and can be cultured forever. However, cancer is also dumb, as it does not realize that the ultimate destruction of the body leads to its own demise as well.

While the patient previously refused to express thoughts or feelings deemed unacceptable, her body now erupts with these suppressed aspects in a last attempt to find a home for them. The body has no other option. It has harbored these ghosts for too long. To the body, it's either evict them or die. But where can these shadow aspects go?

Now the conscious mind has a unique opportunity to take them into its fold. To own the formerly unacceptable is a step toward authenticity and wholeness that provides support for possible healing.

Constructively used, cancer can serve as a way to integrate not only the shadow self but also the formerly denied depths of love, intimacy, and passion that were previously feared and similarly hidden away. This produces a real and solid foundation of self-realization where patients fully approve of all aspects of themselves. This can naturally grow into a more solid sense of self-esteem (love I earn from myself), self-respect (comes from feeling all of my feelings), and self-worth (appreciation of my already immortal spiritual nature).

In summary, aggravation factors include an overly rational, anti-emotional attitude; suppressed or repressed anger/hopelessness[11] (hopeless anger); tendencies for negative affect; seeking approval from other(s); valuing absolute judgments; self-loathing (repression, or the denial of the existence of anything we hate about ourselves, e.g., self-importance); refusal to change; little or no self-respect (respect comes from feeling all our feelings); lack of authenticity.

In contrast, healing factors may include the appropriate release of anger; hopeless anger replaced by will, determination, and vision; replacing tendencies for negative affect with those of positive affect; developing self-esteem; valuing discernment over judgment; self-acceptance (especially what we hate about ourselves, e.g., self-importance); finding positive ways of changing; developing self-respect (feeling and releasing all our feelings); developing authenticity.

Powerful Questions

Why am I not allowed to fail?

Why is it not okay to make a mistake?

What will happen to me if I stop judging people who have different beliefs?

Why do I have to be perfect?

Why do I have to avoid conflict within my group?

Why do I feel like a nobody on the inside?

Why do I have to project a perfect image to my group?

Why can't I help somebody without making it my problem?

How can I accept a feeling I absolutely hate to feel?

Is it okay for me to feel self-important?

Is it okay for me to feel aggressive, angry, or enraged at members of my group?

Can I, at least sometimes, put my needs above those of another?

Is it okay for me to be manipulative?

How can I stand up for myself?

What are my needs?

How can I meet my own needs?

How can I give myself the praise I've never gotten before?

What are good ways for me to feel angry?

How can I own and release my aggression?

What happened to my will to live?

Is my desire to live stronger than that of my cancer?

How can I increase my desire to live?

Can I get angry at my cancer?

What do I want to be angry about?

Can I laugh at myself for wanting to be angry?

How can I release the anger I want?

Suggested Blessings

May you realize that every feeling retrieved and embraced from the hidden recesses of your mind can serve to reduce the power of cancer.

May you become more conscious of your desire for growth and wholeness.

May your journey to the source of all life be the glorious return of a wise
wo/man who has become one with the light and with the shadows of
your own authentic life.

May you grow in the understanding that the universe offers a lot more
to explore than life and death.

May you release all worry and concern about what the world wants of
you, and instead be concerned with what brings you aliveness and
enthusiasm.

Suggested Affirmations

I am learning the most important word in the universe for me—NO!

There is nothing in my shadow that is not part of the human experience.

I can stand up for myself.

I can meet my own needs.

Sometimes my needs are more important than others.

It is okay to be angry.

I fully embrace my shadow without hurting anyone.

Let Food Be Thy Medicine

**Acacia ∾ Basil ∾ Bush Tea ∾ Caraway ∾ Cardamom ∾ Cayenne
Clove ∾ Cacao ∾ Garlic ∾ Ginger ∾ Myrrh ∾ Nigella ∾ Oregano
Rosemary ∾ Turmeric**

Acacia: An animal study from India found anti-tumor properties in acacia,
suggesting possible cancer-preventative abilities.[12]

Basil: Basil thwarted chemical attempts to produce stomach cancer in
rodents.[13]

Bush Tea: Laboratory studies found that bush tea (rooibos or red tea) possesses DNA-protective and antimutagenic properties.[14] The South African
researchers who found that topical application of bush tea inhibits skin
tumor formation also confirmed antimutagenic properties of rooibos.[15]

Caraway: Animal research conducted in India suggests that dietary caraway (at a dose of 60 mg/kg) can control lipid peroxidation and antioxidant

homeostasis, thereby preventing the development of chemically induced colon cancer lesions.[16] Japanese researchers echoed those results, asserting that a specific compound from caraway called Ogt-O6-methylguanine-DNA methyltransferase might be responsible for the antimutagenic activity.[17]

Cardamom: Aqueous suspensions of cardamom provide protective effects on experimentally induced colon carcinogenesis.[18]

Cayenne: After studying cayenne and prostate cancer in the laboratory and in patients, scientists from Madrid, Spain, concluded that capsaicin in cayenne "is a promising anti-tumor agent in hormone-refractory prostate cancer, which shows resistance to many chemotherapeutic agents."[19] Injecting capsaicin directly into a tumor resulted in the retardation not just of the injected tumor but also of other similar tumors nearby.[20]

Clove: One study from Kolkata, India, looked at the properties of aqueous solution of clove and found it to produce apoptosis of lung cancer cells in mice; it also had other possible cancer-protective properties.[21] Another Indian study determined that aqueous solution of clove might also have protective properties against skin papillomas (skin tumors).[22]

Cacao: Researchers at Georgetown University Medical Center in Washington, DC, examined a cacao-derived compound called pentameric procyanidin (pentamer) and discovered that it arrested human breast cancer cells in the laboratory.[23]

Garlic: Using a rodent model, scientists from Hong Kong reported for the first time the high level of success obtained with garlic in inhibiting primary tumor formation of the prostate and reducing secondary tumor formation. Another study revealed that garlic possesses potent anti-metastasis properties (metastasis is the spread of cancer to other than the primary site), which these scientists believed might also apply to other types of cancer.[24] Population-based case studies conducted in Gdansk, Poland, indicated that a relatively high garlic intake reduces the risk of developing certain cancers. It seems that certain compounds contained in garlic prevent and protect against cancer in vivo and in vitro. Researchers attributed the anticancer effect of garlic to its organosulfuric compounds.[25] Diallyl disulfide, a well-known component of garlic, demonstrated repeated ability to induce apoptosis (destruction) of many different cancer cells.[26]

Ginger: Researchers proved that ginger, a spice commonly used in Korean traditional medicine and cuisine, contains the ability to protect and strengthen the heart and liver and to function as an anti-inflammatory agent. Scientists are exploring ginger as a potential inhibitor of breast cancer cell growth.[27]

Myrrh: Based on traditional practice and evidence-based discoveries, a researcher from the National Institutes of Health in Bethesda, Maryland, reported that myrrh's significant antiseptic, anesthetic, and anti-tumor properties most likely stem from a specific alkene called furanosesquiterpene, present in essential oil of myrrh.[28] Scientists from the University of Texas discovered that naturally occurring steroids (guggulsterone) from a closely related species called *Commiphora mukul* could produce apoptosis, including destruction of the cells of leukemia, head and neck carcinoma, multiple myeloma, lung carcinoma, melanoma, breast carcinoma, and ovarian carcinoma. Guggulsterone also inhibited the proliferation of drug-resistant cancer cells (e.g., gleevac-resistant leukemia, dexamethasone-resistant multiple myeloma, and doxorubicin-resistant breast cancer cells).[29]

Nigella: Scientists at the Henry Ford Hospital in Detroit, Michigan, noted that a body of international reports, mostly from the Middle East and Asia, proved that nigella possesses an antineoplastic effect (it fights abnormal growth in cells of benign or cancerous tumors) in both the laboratory and actual patients. They isolated a component of nigella called thymoquinone and tested it in a rodent model. They discovered that the nigella-based compound produced apoptosis without notable side effects. These scientists also concluded that thymoquinone might help prevent prostate cancer.[30] A study from Béni-Mellal, Morocco, showed that injecting nigella essential oil into tumor sites significantly reduced solid tumor development, inhibited metastasis, and improved the overall survival of the test mice.[31] In a study from the University of Mississippi Medical Center, scientists explored time-proven treatment techniques from the Middle East. They examined the possible therapeutic effects of catechin, found in green tea, and thymoquinone, a major compound from black seed *(Nigella sativa),* on specific colon cancer cells. They compared the effectiveness of both natural products to the current chemotherapeutic drug of choice, 5-fluorouracil, for the treatment of colon cancer cells. Scientists determined that both the green tea catechin and the thymoquinone from nigella "have demonstrated incredible chemotherapeutic responses, thus suggesting that both may have similar chemotherapeutic effects as their pharmacological counterpart 5-fluorouracil, which unlike catechin and thymoquinone has known serious side effects, including cardiac toxicity."[32]

Oregano: Chemists at the University of Central Florida isolated several compounds from oregano. Studies showed that aristolochic acid I and II possessed cancer-fighting abilities, specifically against leukemia.[33]

Rosemary: Scientists from the island nation of Taiwan conducted a series of experiments using a super-critical fluid extraction technique and identified several biologically active constituents of rosemary that can be considered herbal anti-inflammatory and anti-tumor agents.[34]

Turmeric: Research during the past five decades, time-proven records from alternative medical traditions, and numerous case studies point toward turmeric's potential to prevent and treat certain forms of cancer. Turmeric has the ability to diminish the creation, production, and spread of a wide variety of tumor cells.[35]

Take Notice: Radiation Protection

Bush Tea ∾ Cacao ∾ Garlic ∾ Nigella ∾ Nutmeg ∾ Rosemary (E)-β-Caryophyllene

Bush Tea: Laboratory studies found that bush tea (rooibos or red tea) contains DNA-protective and antimutagenic properties.[36] The South African researchers who determined that topical application of bush tea inhibits skin tumor formation also confirmed the antimutagenic properties of rooibos.[37]

Cacao: Researchers from Tokyo, Japan, discovered that cacao bean extract, among other compounds, has protective properties against wrinkles caused by excessive UV-light exposure.[38]

Garlic: In a study from New Delhi, Indian scientists discovered that giving garlic extract to rodents reduced gamma ray-induced damage to their chromosomes in only five days. The animals were given doses of 125, 250, and 500 mg of garlic extract per kilogram of body weight.[39]

Nigella: Doctors use ionizing radiation to treat many human cancer patients. However, the radiation does not discriminate between cancer cells and healthy cells, and thus can result in massive tissue damage. A study from Turkey using rodents found that *Nigella sativa* oil ingestion (1ml/kg body weight) and injections of glutathione might minimize radiation damage to healthy tissue. The study reported: "These results clearly show that NS and GSH treatment significantly antagonize the effects of radiation. Therefore, NS and GSH may be a beneficial agent in protection against ionizing radiation-related tissue injury."[40]

Nutmeg: University of Rajasthan (India) scientists evaluated nutmeg's potential to protect mice from the damaging effects of gamma radiation. Gamma radiation resembles x-ray emissions, the major difference being the source. Both are ionizing radiations that penetrate the skin, possibly producing changes in the DNA of each cell. These permutations can result in a variety of cancers and congenital conditions, which may be passed to future generations.[41]

Rosemary: In a controlled study from the University of Rajasthan, researchers concluded that rosemary can protect laboratory animals from the damage of ionizing radiation.[42]

(E)-β-Caryophyllene: (E)-β-Caryophyllene or (E)-BCP is a FDA-approved dietary cannabinoid that activates CB2 receptor sites and initiates potent anti-inflammatory actions and protection from oxidative stress,[43] both commonly associated with cancer and ill-effects of exposure to ionizing radiation. Spice plants known to contain significant amounts of (E)-BCP include (in descending order): Black "Ashanti Pepper" *(Piper guineense)*, White "Ashanti Pepper" *(Piper guineense)*, Indian Bay-Leaf *(Cinnamomum tamala)*, Alligator Pepper *(Aframomum melegueta)*, Basil *(Ocimum micranthum)*, Sri Lanka Cinnamon *(Cinnamomum zeylanicum)*, Rosemary *(Rosmarinus officinalis)*, Black Caraway *(Carum nigrum)*, Black Pepper *(Piper nigrum)*, Basil *(Ocimum gratissimum)*, Mexican Oregano *(Lippia graveolens)*, and Clove *(Syzygium aromaticum)*.

Bone Cancer

Evidence-Based Confidence Level and Therapeutic Potential

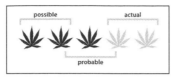

Total Number of Studies Reviewed: 3

CHI Value: 8

This type of cancer is relatively rare. The cancer cells proliferate within the bones' tissues, eventually forming tumors. Orthodox medicine differentiates between bone cancers that originate in the bone, calling these primary, and secondary cancers that develop in the bone tissue after spreading from another place (metastasizing).

Tumors may develop slowly over time, making their presence known through gradually increasing discomfort, visible deformities, and pain. The tumor often exerts pressure from the inside, which, combined with loss of bone density and strength, may produce fractures of the bones or make them much more vulnerable to breakage.

Orthodox medical treatments are limited to chemotherapy, radiation, and surgeries (amputations).

Cannabis and Bone Cancer

Patients with bone cancer are often stricken with severe pain. Opiates, while perhaps reducing the pain initially, have been recently associated with further bone destruction, thus contributing to more pain over time. A Tucson, Arizona, study in 2010 treated animals with bone cancer using peripheral synthetic cannabinoids (AM1241) to determine whether the treatment had any therapeutic potential. Results suggested that daily use (over seven days) of AM1241 significantly reduced both spontaneous and evoked bone cancer pain. Further, the authors of the study discovered that sustained use of AM1241 significantly reduced bone loss and decreased the incidence of cancer-induced bone fractures. Thus, the CB2 cannabinoid AM1241 achieved reductions in pain, bone cancer-induced fractures, and bone loss without the detrimental effects of opiates in animals with bone cancer.[1]

Similarly, researchers from Minnesota (2008) wanted to learn more about the role and effect of endocannabinoids on pain associated with bone cancer. Higher levels of anandamide reduced pain, while lower levels increased pain. The results of this rodent study prompted the authors to write: "the data provide evidence that manipulation of peripheral endocannabinoid signaling is a promising strategy for the management of bone cancer pain."[2]

Lastly, British scientists (2008) conducted a review of the existing literature of cannabinoids and bone disorders, which supported the notion that "cannabinoid receptor ligands show a great promise in the treatment of bone diseases associated with accelerated osteoclastic bone resorption, including osteoporosis, rheumatoid arthritis, and bone metastasis."[3]

Study Summary

Drugs	Type of Study	Published Year, Place, and Key Results	CHI
AM1241	Animal study (murine)	2010—University of Arizona: Reduction in bone cancer pain, bone cancer-induced fractures, and bone loss without the detrimental effects of opiates.[1]	2
Anandamide (AEA)	Animal study (mice)	2008—University of Minnesota: Higher levels of anandamide reduced pain.[2]	2
Endocannabinoid system	Review	2008—University of Edinburgh: Cannabinoid receptors show a great promise in the treatment bone metastasis.[3]	4

Total CHI Value 8

Strain-Specific Considerations

The animal study from Tucson, Arizona, employed the CB2-stimulating synthetic cannabinoid AM1241. Similarly, CBD has a greater affinity for CB2 receptors than for CB1. Indica strains have relatively less THC and relatively more CBD/CBN, thus favoring CB2 signaling.

Mind-Body Medicine and Bone Cancer

The human body contains 206 bones.[4] The skeleton protects vital organs and produces a rigid support system that enables the attached flexible counter system of muscles to exert force, allowing the body to contract and expand, thereby producing movement and enabling physical tasks.

Interestingly, a bone's hollowness provides its strength and light weight. The hard outer material is made from collagen and minerals, while the inside is filled with soft and spongy yellow and red bone marrow. Red marrow produces blood cells, and yellow marrow stores fat cells as energy reserves.

Thus, the outer shell of bones can be thought of as representing protection and support, while the inner parts correlate with blood (family, tribe, joy of life) and energy reserves (passion, intensity). Consider this line of thought. Bone cancer ultimately causes the complete reversal of protection and support when these natural functions are replaced by attack and destruction.

Unexpressed and long-standing resentment or guilt about having to uphold the rules, laws, and regulations of the family or tribe may become the force that ultimately destroys the patient's own protection and support.

Often the internal architecture of guilt is a self-imposed mechanism to force adherence to the perceived rules that "should" be complied with. Fractures result from built-up pressure exerted by the growing resentments and accumulated guilt for railing against outside authority, the fathers, the rulers, the gods, and their "shoulds" and "shouldn'ts." At this point, patients are unable to move about and are limited in their ability to complete daily tasks.

Powerful Questions

What will you do if I express my hatred for the rules?

What will happen if I let myself rail against my adopted authority?

Will I still be protected, supported, and loved if I do not follow the outside rules?

Can I become my own authority?

Suggested Blessings

May you become your own authority, with your own ideals, principles, and the character to enforce them.

May you discover your authentic passions.

May you accept yourself as good and true and beautiful.

Suggested Affirmations

Based on my authentic passion, I choose my own ideals.

I make my own rules as to how to get closer to my ideals.

I am the only enforcer of my rules.

I employ forgiveness, joy, love, and intimacy.

I can express all my feelings about authority without hurting anyone.

Brain Cancer
Evidence-Based Confidence Level and Therapeutic Potential

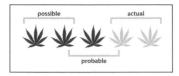

Total Number of Studies Reviewed: 9

CHI Value: 26

The location and size of cancerous brain tumors largely determine survivability and the various signs and symptoms likely to develop. As tumors grow, impairment increases. As a result, the whole body as well as the mind may be impacted. Generally speaking, the lower in the brain structure the tumor is, the poorer the survival outcome. This is because the brain's lower portions control most vital functions such as breathing and heart rate.

Signs and symptoms cover a relatively wide range and can include altered levels of consciousness ranging from mild confusion to epileptic seizures, from odd behavior to full-blown stroke-like handicaps. Additional commonly reported symptoms include headache, visual impairments, and nausea with vomiting.

Orthodox medicine does not know what causes brain cancer. It can neither prevent nor cure it. Its methods of diagnosis include a careful patient history and physical examination, electroencephalography (EEG) measuring the electrical activity of the brain, an extensive eye examination, and the use of imaging techniques such as MRI or CT scans.[1] However, within this model of medicine a definite diagnosis can only be arrived at by using a needle biopsy (a risky procedure of sticking a needle into the affected part of the brain), open brain surgery, or an autopsy. Management consists of the usual three: chemotherapy, radiation, and surgery. Brain cancer progression and treatment may leave the patient with severe impairment, similar to a stroke victim. The five-year survival rate for the most common brain tumors (glioblastomas, astrocytomas, and meningiomas) is 2%, 30%, and 70%, respectively.[2]

Cannabis and Brain Cancer

Starting in 2001, an international research team began looking at cannabinoids and brain cancer. The team demonstrated that local injections of the synthetic cannabinoid JWH-133 (a potent CB2 receptor agonist) into mice with brain cancer cells considerably reduced the size of malignant tumors.[3] By 2003, two Italian studies expanded our understanding of brain cancer and cannabinoids by suggesting that the non-psychoactive CBD was able to produce a significant anti-brain tumor activity, both in vitro and in vivo,[4] and that CBD selectively produced oxidative stress in brain cancer cells, thus producing apoptosis, leaving normal cells unaffected.[5]

A 2004 Spanish experiment produced another perspective as to why cannabinoids may present a new therapy for patients suffering from brain cancer. Results showed that cannabinoids effectively inhibited a chemical signal needed for the brain tumor to build its blood supply, an essential element for its survival and proliferation. The Spanish researchers considered the blockade of this signal to be one of the most promising anti-tumor approaches currently available, and the work proposed "a novel pharmacological target for cannabinoid-based therapies."[6]

To discover whether THC could be injected safely into humans, scientists from Madrid (2006) enlisted the cooperation of nine patients with brain cancers that had failed to respond to the standard treatments of either surgery or radiation. The researchers concluded that THC could be safely injected into human brain tumors without causing any overt psychoactive effects.[7]

In 2008, a team of researchers from Israel discovered another way in which cannabinoids may mitigate brain cancer. In this study E2F1 and Cyclin A, two proteins that promote cell cycle progression, were downregulated and later able to arrest glioblastoma multiforme (brain cancer cells) under the influence of THC.[8]

Two additional Spanish studies conducted on mice and humans with recurring glioblastoma multiforme brain cancers suggest two more mechanisms by which cannabinoids may counteract cancer. Tissue inhibitors of metalloproteinases (TIMPs) play critical roles in the acquisition of migrating tumor cells and their invasive capacities. TIMP-1 up-regulation is associated with high malignancy and negative prognosis of numerous cancers. Similarly, as matrix metalloproteinase (MMP)-2 up-regulation is associated with high progression and poor prognosis of gliomas (brain cancer), scientists discovered that TIMP-1 down-regulation and MMP down-regulation may be hallmarks of cannabinoid-induced inhibition of glioma progression.[9]

In a more recently published San Francisco study (2010) on brain cancer and cannabinoids, researchers showed in part that two cannabinoids, THC and CBD, acted synergistically to inhibit brain cancer cell growth by inducing reactive oxygen species to produce apoptosis.[10]

Strain- and Form-Specific Considerations

Both THC and CBD have been found to be potent inhibitors of cancer cell development and to produce apoptosis (cancer cell death). Each works independently in this regard; still greater effect may be produced synergistically when THC and CBD are applied together.

Both basic strains (sativa and indica) deliver the full range of plant cannabinoids. Most patients consider their mental and emotional preferences before determining if a more relaxing or uplifting effect is needed. Indicas are considered generally more relaxing, sedating, or grounding while sativas are more energizing or uplifting. Patients wishing to employ a non-psychoactive form of plant material may take raw juice made from fresh cannabis leaves.

Mind-Body Medicine and Brain Cancer

The brain commonly represents the physical structure associated with the mind; we often use the words "mind" and "brain" interchangeably. Both are considered the seat of consciousness.

Cancer in the brain affects the mind and the whole body, forcing changes of great magnitude. Formerly independent people may become unable to communicate normally, walk, or even complete simple tasks without help. Brain cancer severely disrupts the status quo of free will, consciousness, and the authority to govern actions of the body.

Another consideration centers on the brain's naturally soft and moist environment, consisting of a folded mass of grey matter that thrives on constant changes delivered by the senses. Rigid adherence to mental constructs

Study Summary

Drugs	Type of Study	Published Year, Place, and Key Results	CHI
CBD and THC	Animal study (rodent)	2010—California Pacific Medical Center Research Institute, San Francisco: Both cannabinoids acted synergistically to inhibit cancer cell growth by inducing reactive oxygen species to produce apoptosis.[10]	2
THC and JWH-133 injected into the tumors	Animal study and two human patients with recurrent glioblastoma multiforme (grade IV astrocytoma)	2008—Complutense University, Madrid, Spain: TIMP-1 down-regulation may be a hallmark of cannabinoid-induced inhibition of glioma progression.[9]	2+3
THC and JWH-133	Animal study and two human patients with recurrent glioblastoma multiforme	2008—Complutense University, Madrid, Spain: MMP-2 down-regulation constitutes a new hallmark of cannabinoid anti-tumoral activity.[9]	2+3
THC	Laboratory study	2008—Multi-institutional research team, Israel: THC is shown to significantly affect viability of glioblastoma multiforme (GBM) by down-regulation of E2F1 and Cyclin.[8]	1
Intracranial injections of THC into the tumor site	Nine end-stage brain cancer patients with recurrent glioblastoma multiforme	2006—Complutense University, Madrid, Spain: Cannabinoid delivery was safe.[7]	3
THC, WIN55,212-2 and anandamide	Laboratory, animal (mice) and human tests	2004—Complutense University, Madrid, Spain: Reduced VEGF gene expression, depressed VEGF pathways, decreased production of VEGF, and decreased the activation of VEGF receptors in the brain cancer cells. Corresponding reductions in tumor size in mice.[6]	2+3
Cannabidiol (CBD) at 0.5 mg	Laboratory and animal tests (mice)	2003—Multi-institutional research team: Apoptosis of U87 and U373 human glioma cell lines in the laboratory and significant growth inhibition of U87 implanted in mice.[4]	2
Cannabidiol	Laboratory	2003—University of Milan, Italy: CBD selectively produces oxidative stress in brain cancer cells, thus producing apoptosis, but not in normal cells.[5]	1
JWH-133 (local injection into tumor 50 µg/day)	Animal tests (mice)	2001—International and multi-institutional research team: Induced a considerable regression in size of the malignant tumors.[3]	2

Total CHI Value 26

fueled by fears of change or an unwillingness to change may cause rigidity in a naturally soft and ever-changing organ.

The mind/brain interprets the continuously incoming sensual data it receives and delivers a response. This is the realm of choices, decisions, thoughts, feelings, attitudes, and beliefs. Cancer in this realm may be reflective of conflicting beliefs, and thereby conflicting thoughts and feelings, making the mind and by association the brain an internal battlefield. The strain of this internal battle against change drains energy, increasing the body's vulnerability.

Change is thrust upon the patient. The body thus becomes the stage to act out the stubborn patterns that may have kept the patient from accepting and working in a healthy way with the inevitable nature of life, which is change.

It is important to remember that in the context of healing, a particular belief (system) is never right or wrong but is measured by its ability to support the health of an individual and the healing process of the patient.

Suggested Blessings

May you make it easy for yourself to trust the process of life.

May you choose authentic beliefs, birthed by your free will and your conscious care.

Suggested Affirmations

Change is within me and all around me, and I embrace change freely and easily.

It is easy to change my mind.

It is easy to replace a belief.

It is easy to make a new choice.

I am the author of my life, and I can write a whole new chapter whenever I am ready.

Breast Cancer
Evidence-Based Confidence Level and Therapeutic Potential

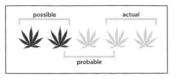

Total Number of Studies Reviewed: 6

CHI Value: 11

By 2004, reported global estimates of breast cancer deaths exceeded 500,000 victims.[1] The vast majority were women. This type of cancer most commonly originates in the milk ducts from a corrupted breast cell(s), which left unchecked can invade surrounding breast tissue with devastating results.

While often benign in origin, a dreaded lump in the breast can develop into a cancerous growth. Chronically swollen lymph nodes around the breast or in the armpit may be signs of cancer. Other symptoms include single nipple discharge, pain in the area, inverted nipple, discoloration, heat, redness, and swelling of the affected tissue, or a change in breast tissue texture. Orthodox treatment is usually limited to surgery, pharmaceuticals (chemotherapy), or radiation.

Although a multitude of possible known factors contribute to the genesis of cancers (see the introduction to this Cancer section), one controllable risk factor for breast cancer is high levels of estrogen. In fact, the development of breast cancer remains a serious effect of hormone replacement therapy. Body fat is another source of high levels of estrogen. Women's fat cells store excess estrogen after menopause.

Exposure to ionizing radiation is another known risk factor.[2] Mammograms, CAT (or CT) scans, and any other x-rays produce ionizing radiation. Dr. Gofman, Professor Emeritus from UC Berkeley, demonstrated that past exposure to ionizing radiation—primarily medical x-rays—is responsible for about 75% of breast cancer cases in the United States. He also reported some good news. Since the radiation dosage given today in hospitals and doctors' offices can be significantly reduced without interfering with a single useful procedure, numerous future cases of breast cancer can be prevented.[3]

Women who breast-feed longer tend to form greater protection against breast cancer.[4]

Cannabis and Breast Cancer

In 1998, a team of researchers from Naples, Italy, discovered that the endogenous cannabinoid anandamide blocks human breast cancer cell growth in vitro.[5] By 2000, researchers discovered a potential mechanism by which anandamide might inhibit breast cancer cell growth. Cannabinoids suppressed certain growth factors and prolactin receptors, which leads to an inhibition of certain types of breast cancer cell lines.[6]

By 2006, another Italian team had formulated more interesting insights. Researchers compared the specific anti-tumor properties of five individual cannabinoids to an extract of whole cannabis. Of the five individual cannabinoids (cannabidiol, cannabigerol, cannabichromene, cannabidiol acid, THC acid, and cannabis extract), cannabidiol emerged as the most potent anti-breast cancer substance, on par with the cannabidiol-rich whole plant extract. The authors wrote: "our experiments indicate that the cannabidiol effect is due to its capability of inducing apoptosis via [...] elevation of intracellular Ca2+ and reactive oxygen species."[7]

In the same year, a team of Spanish scientists found that cannabinoids are involved in the process of breast cell proliferation, differentiation, and survival. The authors of this study suggested several specific mechanisms, one of which proved "that Δ9-tetrahydrocannabinol (THC), through activation of CB2 cannabinoid receptors, reduces human breast cancer cell proliferation by blocking the progression of the cell cycle, and by inducing apoptosis."[8] The Spanish researchers concluded: "Taken together, these data might set the basis for a cannabinoid therapy for the management of breast cancer."

In 2007, a team from San Francisco examined cannabinoids in the context of cases involving a rapid spread of aggressive breast-cancer cells. To date, oncologists have a very limited set of options, each with its own toxic or dangerous adverse effects. In this experiment, scientists wrote about a key finding: "Here, we report that cannabidiol (CBD), a cannabinoid with a low-toxicity profile, could down-regulate gene (Id-1) expression in aggressive human breast cancer cells. [...] In conclusion, CBD represents the first nontoxic exogenous agent that can significantly decrease Id-1 expression in metastatic breast cancer cells leading to the down-regulation of tumor aggressiveness."[9]

Perhaps the most exciting research comes from Spain, where scientists discovered for the first time that cannabinoids therapeutically influence a genetic component involved in breast cancer progression. The authors wrote: "In summary, this is the first report showing not only that cannabinoids regulate a protein called transcription factor jun-D, which in humans is encoded in a JUND gene but, more generally, that jun-D activation reduces the proliferation of cancer cells, which points to a new target to inhibit breast cancer progression."[10]

Study Summary

Drugs	Type of Study	Published Year, Place, and Key Results	CHI
THC	Laboratory and animal study (mice)	2008—Complutense University, Madrid, Spain: Discovery of a mechanism by which THC reduces proliferation of human breast cancer cells.[10]	1+2
CBD	Laboratory and animal study (mice)	2007—California Pacific Medical Center, San Francisco, USA: CBD represents the first nontoxic agent that can significantly decrease breast cancer aggressiveness.[9]	1+2
THC	Laboratory	2006—Multi-institutional research team, Madrid, Spain: THC reduces human breast cancer cell proliferation.[8]	1
Cannabidiol, cannabigerol, cannabichromene, cannabidiol acid, and THC acid vs. whole-plant extract	Animal study (mice)	2006—Multi-institutional research team, Italy: Cannabidiol was the most potent anti-breast cancer substance, on par with the cannabidiol-rich whole-plant extract.[7]	2
Anandamide	Laboratory	2000—Multi-institutional research team, Naples, Italy: Inhibiting prolactin-responsive human breast cancer cells was achieved by down-regulating of the long form of the prolactin receptors.[6]	1
Anandamide	Laboratory	1998—Multi-institutional research team Naples, Italy: Anandamide blocks human breast cancer cell growth.[5]	1

Total CHI Value 11

Strain-Specific Considerations

Pre-clinical animal trials demonstrated that anandamide, the body's own endocannabinoid, and numerous plant cannabinoids such as THC but especially CBD have the ability to limit breast cancer cell proliferation and produce apoptosis (death of cancer cells). Current research results also suggest that therapeutic mechanisms begin at CB2 receptor sites.

Indica strains or indica-heavy hybrids tend to have a higher CBD profile. A CBD profile of more than 3–4% is considered potent.

Mind-Body Medicine and Breast Cancer

As early as the 1950s, physicians examined possible correlations between the psyche and cancer. Researchers enrolled 40 breast cancer patients in a study to evaluate the prevalence of common behavioral characteristics. Results exposed unresolved conflicts with their mothers. These included: competition and guilt; sexual inhibition; inhibited motherhood; masochistic character structures; denial; self-sacrifice; an inability to discharge or deal appropriately with anger, aggressiveness, or hostility; and a tendency to hide these emotions behind a façade of pleasantness.[11]

More recently, London scientists examining a possible link between emotional expressions and breast cancer discovered that "... IgA levels[12] were found to be significantly higher in patients who habitually suppressed anger than in those who were able to express anger."[13]

Another study, from the University of Arizona, similarly confirmed that acceptance of emotions and emotional processing decreased overall mortality from breast cancer. Furthermore, research results showed that close relationships that included confiding and dependable support were protective against breast cancer progression.[14] In addition, psychiatrists trying to understand the impact of emotional states on patients' personalities prior to the clinical manifestation of breast cancer suggested that a depressive reaction decreased host immunity, especially disturbances in the personal, sex, and maternal drive.[15]

Contrary to these above-mentioned study results, a large-scale research project from Australia found no significant correlation between anger management or negative affect and risk of breast cancer (and only weak links between anger management and prostate, lung, and colorectal cancer).[16]

For mothers and infants, breasts are a source of love, pleasure, life, and nourishment. Breastfeeding after giving birth releases oxytocin, a hormone that induces uterine contractions and thereby stops post-partum bleeding (a great benefit to the health and survival of the mother).[17] Oxytocin also relaxes the mother and increases her feelings of love for and bonding with the child. Breast milk provides all the food, immune protection, and nourishment the infant needs. Breastfeeding also supplies the mother with a host of health benefits. It is interesting to note that mothers who breastfeed lower their risk for developing breast cancer and a host of other diseases.[18]

Breasts also represent nurturing and the pleasure of nurturing in general. In a healthy situation, offering the breasts to another human being brings pleasure to the child or the lover, as well as the woman herself. Taking pleasure in a woman's breast can be a beautiful part of the human experience. The breast tissue, especially the areolas and nipples, is very sensitive, and sucking produces intensely pleasurable experiences for the happy infant, the aroused lover, and the woman alike. However, sometimes there is trouble in paradise.

Feeling arousal in the nipples during sex is considered normal, but arousal during breastfeeding is often discomforting. To women who consider motherhood holy and sex dirty, this sensation does not fit into the mental construct of what life should be like. Here we have a source of possible guilt and conflicting emotions involving the breasts. Many of these feelings can never be communicated, and may even have to be hidden from her. But where can they go?

Most kids take mom's love for granted. "A face only a mother could love." "No matter what I do mother loves me." It is assumed that her love is unconditional. But what about the many times when a mother doesn't feel that way? She is a human being, capable of feeling emotions not normally associated with the impossible and idealized version of motherhood: arousal, anger, rage, self-importance, and envy or jealousy of those in her care, be they child, husband, mother, father, or God. Yet she is a mother now, or a wife, or a loving daughter, or a God-fearing woman, and she likes to see herself and others as being only loving. Her soft bosoms, which should provide loving, nurturing hugs, may become a repository for all those distasteful and unwanted emotional experiences that are part of anybody's life.

When it comes to sex, the breasts are everywhere. No other organ induces such primary urges in males as the mammary glands of women. No other organ is as used and abused in social power plays by entire industries, as well as by both genders. Unexpressed hurt, anger, and silent rage born of this use and abuse may find the breast a perfect stage and repository to force attention on the core issues, thus presenting a serious demand for change.

While the intense focus on the importance of breasts is virtually everywhere, it is also reflected in medical statistics. In 2008, more than 300,000 women in the U.S. received voluntary cosmetic breast augmentations,[19] while in 2010, another 200,000 women were diagnosed with dreaded breast cancer.[20] Inside this soft place of pleasure, love, nurturing, and nourishment now looms an aggressive, hurtful threat, not just to the perceived front of womanhood but also to life itself.

Women who give and give might feel that their breasts exist solely for the pleasure of others. In such cases, women may forget to take pleasure in their own breasts, and by extension in the capacities they represent. Here, these capacities for life, love, pleasure, and nourishment are not applied to herself. Over time, a woman may feel chronically stressed by this costly one-way giving and lack of replenishment. She might even blame her lot in life (her gender) for the stress that she feels.

Her stress can soon form into feeling unappreciated, fueling a righteous control of those in her care. When left unchecked, this disintegrating process may even turn love or her loving bosoms into a form of smothering. It is as if her pattern of suppressing anything not in line with her ideal of what a good mother, woman, daughter, or member of her church should be superimposes itself onto those who behave differently than she thinks they should. She can become disrespectful, hard, and invasive, using righteous indignation as justification for dominating others into behaving according to her values and beliefs. She may treat others as she treats herself.

In summary aggravating factors for breast cancer may include suppressed anger; depressive reaction; decreased immunity; unresolved conflicts with one's mother, such as competition and guilt, sexual inhibition, inhibited motherhood; masochistic character structures; denial; self-sacrifice; an inability to discharge or deal appropriately with anger, aggressiveness, or hostility; and the desire to hide behind a façade of pleasantness.

Healing factors may include acceptance of emotions, willingness to process emotions, and the presence of close relationships, particularly those which include confiding and dependable support.

Powerful Questions

What does it mean to me to be a woman?
Is it okay for me to enjoy my breasts as a celebration of my sensuality?
How do I feel about wearing clothes that reveal my cleavage?
How do I feel about women who prominently display their breasts?
How do I feel about women who have larger or smaller breasts than mine?
What beliefs underlie those feelings?
Do these beliefs and the feelings they engender serve me well?

What does it mean to be a mother?
Is it okay for a mother to be aroused?
Is it okay to be aroused by breastfeeding my child?

What does it mean to be a daughter?
What does it mean to be a good daughter?

What does it mean to be a lover/wife?
What does it mean to be a good wife?

Do I have to "put out" to be a good wife?
What does it mean to be a God-fearing woman?
Is motherhood/martyrdom where I must suffer for the noble cause?
If I did not have breasts, how would I define being a woman?

Does nurturing necessarily entail sacrifice?
What do I get from nurturing others?
What does nurturing mean to me?
Do I make time to nurture myself?
How do I feel if I make time to nurture myself?
Can I trust myself to find my authentic self?
Can I support others in their attempt to become their ideal selves?

Suggested Blessings

May you find your own authentic means to be a woman.

May our flowers assist you in realizing that a woman who nurtures can also be nurtured.

May you find a way to lighten your heart by feeling and releasing all that is hidden, with ease and fun, and harm to none.

Suggested Affirmations

I am free to be me. I will discover and live my own definition of womanhood.

I respect my needs.

I care for myself because I matter.

I accept myself as I am, and I extend the same courtesy to others.

I seek to develop trust instead of control.

Let Food Be Thy Medicine

Anise ∾ Cacao ∾ Ginger ∾ Myrrh

Anise: Greek herbalists have long used anise and fennel to promote menstruation, increase breast milk production, facilitate birth, and enhance libido. Scientists at the University of Athens have taken a closer look at anise in the context of finding a safe alternative to estrogen replacement therapies to prevent osteoporosis. Anise exhibited estrogen receptor modulator-like properties that produce bone-cell formation without causing breast and cervical cancer cells to proliferate.[21]

Cacao: Researchers at the Georgetown University Medical Center in Washington, DC, examined a cacao-derived compound called pentameric procyanidin (pentamer) and discovered that it arrested human breast cancer cells.[22]

Ginger: Researchers from Seoul proved that ginger, a spice commonly used in Korean traditional medicine and cuisine, has the ability to protect and strengthen the heart and liver and to function as an anti-inflammatory agent. Scientists are exploring ginger as an inhibitor of breast cancer cells.[23]

Myrrh: Based on traditional practice and evidence-based discoveries, one author reported that myrrh's significant antiseptic, anesthetic, and anti-tumor properties most likely stem from a specific alkene called furanosesquiterpene, which is present in essential oil of myrrh.[24] Scientists from the University of Texas discovered that naturally occurring steroids (guggulsterone) from a closely related species called *Commiphora mukul* could produce apoptosis (destruction of cancer cells) "including leukemia, head and neck carcinoma, multiple myeloma, lung carcinoma, melanoma, breast carcinoma, and ovarian carcinoma. Guggulsterone also inhibited the proliferation of drug-resistant cancer cells (e.g., gleevac-resistant leukemia, dexamethasone-resistant multiple myeloma, and doxorubicin-resistant breast cancer cells)."[25]

Cancer Caused By Cannabis?
Evidence-Based Confidence Level and Therapeutic Potential

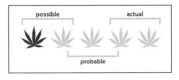

Total Number of Studies Reviewed: 6

CHI Value: -7

Plant and animal products, such as those used in smoking or barbequing, are known to produce carcinogenic substances. Smoking tobacco has been clearly implicated in the genesis of lung cancer. Inhaling any smoke (burned carbon and other toxic pollutants) is not healthy. This is especially true for highly concentrated toxic smoke or long-term exposure.

However, studies examining whether cannabis smoke leads to lung cancer have been confounded by test subjects who also smoked tobacco. No study examined risk of lung cancer when cannabis was ingested. No study examined the possible risk of lung cancer associated with smoking cannabis using various vaporizers (which produce no or very little smoke). And most studies reviewed were case studies or contained only a small sample of subjects.

A large-scale population study (2006) conducted on more than 2,000 residents of Los Angeles County yields perhaps the most reliable current scientific indicator. It concluded that "the association of these cancers with marijuana, even long-term or heavy use, is not strong and may be below practically detectable limits."[5]

When the five negative study results included below are contrasted against the 59 positive studies that suggest cannabis may be therapeutic and protective against cancer, the evidence-based scale tips in favor of cannabis, especially when smoke inhalation is avoided.

Study Summary

Drugs	Type of Study	Published Year, Place, and Key Results	CHI
Cannabis smoke	Human case study (interview based) with 187 patients and 148 men without the disease	2011—National Institutes of Health, Department of Health and Human Services, Rockville, Maryland, USA: Results suggested that cannabis might be associated with one of two types of testicular cancer.[1]	-3
Cannabis smoke	Laboratory	2009—University of Leicester, United Kingdom: Cannabis smoke can damage DNA.[2]	-1
Cannabis with tobacco smoke	Conducted in Morocco with 430 human patients with lung cancer and 778 healthy individuals	2008—International Agency for Research on Cancer, Lyon, France: Cannabis smoking may be a risk factor for lung cancer. However, residual confounding by tobacco smoking or other potential confounders may explain part of the increased risk.[3]	-3
Cannabis with tobacco smoke	79 patients with lung cancer and 324 people without	2008—Medical Research Institute of New Zealand, Wellington: Long-term cannabis smoking increases the risk of lung cancer in young adults.[4]	-3
Cannabis smoke	2,252 human subjects surveyed	2006—International Agency for Research on Cancer, Lyon, France; University of Michigan; Yeshiva University; UCLA; University of California; LA School of Public Health; University of Southern California: The association of these cancers with marijuana, even long-term or heavy use, is not strong and may be below practically detectable limits.[5]	3
Cannabis smoke	Meta-analysis of 14 case studies and 2 cohort studies	2005—International Agency for Research on Cancer, Lyon, France: In general, increased risk of lung cancer was not observed. However, the review found a potential increased risk of other cancers.[6]	0

Total CHI Value -7

Cancer-Induced Night Sweats
Evidence-Based Confidence Level and Therapeutic Potential

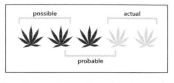

Number of Studies Reviewed: 1

CHI Value: 3

Night sweats, relatively common in end-stage cancer patients, are partly responsible for disrupted sleep patterns. This factor directly and indirectly further reduces the patient's overall quality of life. The orthodox medical system believes that the sympathetic nervous system controls sweating via the hypothalamus. This almond-sized, centrally located portion of the brain releases hormones to control numerous autonomic functions, such as temperature, circadian cycles, sleep, hunger, and thirst. Environmental signals such as light, stress, smell, or pheromones can activate the hypothalamus. It responds quickly to these indicators and other changes in heart rate, respiratory rate, blood, hormonal profile, and the presence of pathogens.

Perspiration also functions as a balancing mechanism by releasing excess water, dumping toxic material, and introducing molecules such as pheromones into the immediate environment. Sweat is excreted through sweat glands (apocrine and eccrine glands) strategically located throughout the skin.

Cannabis and Night Sweats

A 2007 study from Fukuoka, Japan, challenges the orthodox hypothesis of body temperature controlled solely by the hypothalamus. Researchers hypothesized that the endocannabinoid system, especially CB1, may regulate body temperature independent of the hypothalamus.[1]

Cannabis, used within the appropriate therapeutic range, is well known for its ability to induce relaxation and, by extension, improve sleep. Now scientists (2008) have tested this age-old knowledge in the context of cancer-induced night sweats. A synthetic orally administered cannabinoid, Nabilone (similar to THC), was effectively used in treating night sweats. Cancer patients who suffered the ill-effects of interrupted sleep experienced an improved quality of life during Nabilone treatment. Further, the cannabinoid positively affected pains, anorexia, and nausea.[2]

Study Summary

Drugs	Type of Study	Published Year, Place, and Key Results	CHI
Nabilone 1 mg 1x daily; and patients with more severe pains 1 mg 2x daily	Case study	2008—University of Toronto, Canada: Significant reduction of night sweats.[2]	3

Total CHI Value 3

Strain-Specific Considerations

CB1 receptors are located primarily in the brain and central nervous system, including the sympathetic nervous system and the hypothalamus, which are both involved in perspiration. The synthetic cannabinoid Nabilone, similar to THC, has been shown to therapeutically influence perspiration patterns in humans. Here, the logic of the available science would suggest a sativa with higher THC:CBD ratios. However, an indica or indica-heavy strain is advised in order to access a balanced and synergistic approach with the body and the mind. Indicas still provide the CB1 activation involved in the mechanism of night sweats, yet also activate CB2 receptors involved in inducing an overall calming and restful state.

Mind-Body Medicine and Night Sweats

Anxiety, intense fears, dread, or guilt are common emotional states that keep the mind running in an endless attempt to control what cannot be controlled. This continuous process can drain every bit of energy and at the same time prevent release, relaxation, and sleep. Even when sleep arrives, these intense emotions may find their expression in the dream world. The body reacts to the dreams with physiological responses. Intense dreams, struggling with uncomfortable topics or nightmares, are commonly associated with night sweats.

Suggested Blessings

May you relax and release all fears.
May you find your antidote to fear.

Suggested Affirmation

There is a place in me where I am completely safe.

Cervical Cancer

Evidence-Based Confidence Level and Therapeutic Potential

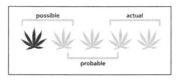

Total Number of Studies Reviewed: 2

CHI Value: 2

Cervix is Latin for "neck." Cancer of the cervix uteri is the development of cancerous cells at the narrow neck of the uterus. The uterus begins at the interior end of the vagina, and together with the fallopian tubes and ovaries comprises the female reproductive system.

Initial symptoms of cervical cancer may include vaginal bleeding, discharge, and painful intercourse. Symptoms of more advanced cancerous development may include lower abdominal pains, pelvic pain, lower back pain, groin pain, and persistent vaginal bleeding. Other general signs often associated with cancer may also be present, such as loss of appetite, weight loss, and low energy.

Orthodox medicine hypothesizes numerous possible causes and co-factors for the development of cervical cancer among higher-risk females. Higher risk is defined by the presence of statistically significant co-factors, such as a family history of cervical cancer, poverty, substance abuse, human papillomavirus (HPV), HIV/AIDS, Herpes simplex, use of pharmaceutical birth control, multiple prior pregnancies, dietary factors, and a high number of sex partners.

Allopathic methods to prevent cervical cancer may include use of the HPV vaccine. Diagnosis involves progressive tests, including pap smears, colposcopies (visual inspection of the cervix using acetic acid), or biopsies. Treatment may include surgery, chemotherapy, or radiation.

Some alternative-leaning physicians may also recommend a diet high in vegetable consumption, especially fruits and vegetables containing lycopene.

Recent studies have shown that lycopene may be protective against HPV persistence.[1] The fruit containing by far the highest amount of lycopene is a Southeast Asian native called *gac* (spiny bitter gourd, *Momordica cochinchinensis*). Other sources of lycopene include tomatoes, watermelon, papaya, pink guava, rosehips, and pink grapefruit.

Cannabis and Cervical Cancer

A Geneva study (2004) demonstrated that anandamide, the body's own cannabinoid, possesses the ability to protect healthy cervical cells from developing cancer via both CB1 and CB2 receptor sites. Beyond protective abilities, anandamide was found to induce apoptosis in cervical cells that had mutated into cancerous forms.[2] By 2008, the Rostock experiment continued to add to our scientific knowledge by confirming anandamide's abilities, as well as that of THC, to significantly decrease cell tumor invasiveness, even at very low dosages.[3]

Study Summary

Drugs	Type of Study	Published Year, Place, and Key Results	CHI
Anandamide analog, methanandamide, and THC	Laboratory test performed on human cervical cancer cells	2008—University of Rostock, Germany: Cannabinoid elicits decrease in tumor cell invasiveness.[3]	1
Anandamide	Laboratory test performed on human cervical cancer cells	2004—University Hospital, Geneva, Switzerland: Anandamide produces apoptosis in cancer cells and exhibits a protective effect via CB1 and CB2.[2]	1

Total CHI Value 2

Strain-Specific Considerations

Pre-clinical experiments suggest a potential mechanism involving both CB1 and CB2 in the destruction of human cervical cancer cells, at least in laboratory tests. Both the body's own anandamide and the plant cannabinoid THC bind with CB1 and CB2. In addition, sativas and indicas contain THC.

Mind-Body Medicine and Cervical Cancer

The uterus is where the fertilized egg nests and develops from an embryo to a fetus. It is a cradle of physical life. The neck of the uterus is narrow but flexible enough to be able to contain and eventually release the fully-grown fetus. The mucosal lining of the uterus sheds monthly in an ancient embodied rhythm of life, death, and rebirth.

See also OBGYN and the introduction to the Cancer section.

Powerful Questions

What are the symptoms keeping you from doing?

How do you feel about that?

Where do these feelings take you?

What scenarios or memories are associated with these feelings?

What is the meaning (messages, unhealthy beliefs/attitudes, etc.) you have given to that scenario?

Suggested Blessing

May you create love and approval for all aspects of yourself.

Suggested Affirmation

I love and appreciate the source of my creativity.

Let Food Be Thy Medicine

Saffron: *Crocus sativus L.* or saffron may possess anticancer activity including activity against ovarian cancer.[4]

Colon Cancer (Colorectal)
Evidence-Based Confidence Level and Therapeutic Potential

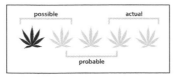

Total Number of Studies Reviewed: 3
CHI Value: 4

The large intestine (colon) absorbs water and salts (electrolytes) from digested matter prior to elimination. In contrast, the small intestine primarily digests and absorbs nutrients. The majority of nutrients have been absorbed by the time the remaining matter reaches the colon. The large intestine consists of the ascending, transverse, and descending colon, followed by the sigmoid colon, closest to the rectum. The colon is lined with a mucous membrane, facilitating the movement of waste and essential gut flora (symbiotic bacteria) involved in the production of vitamins and healthy immune function.

Colon cancer develops in the epithelial cells (lining), which may be found as high up as the junction between the large and small intestine or anywhere following its pathway to the anus. Signs and symptoms depend on location and the spread of the cancer but may include abdominal pain, nausea, vomiting, narrow stools, and unexplained changes in bowel movement, waste color, or texture. However, numerous other bowel diseases exhibit similar symptoms.

Hypothesized causes include cellular mutations by inheritance or dietary exposure to carcinogens. Other known aspects that increase the risk of developing colon cancer are the presence of colon polyps, irritable bowel syndrome, and ulcerative colitis. Additional risk factors include: smoking tobacco, use of alcohol, aged 50 or over, male gender, obesity, a sedentary lifestyle, the presence of other environmental carcinogens, African American heritage, and receiving radiation therapy for cancer.

In 2010, the National Cancer Institute at the National Institutes for Health estimated that the U.S. had over 100,000 new colon cancer patients and more than 50,000 fatalities from rectal and colon cancer combined.[1] Within allopathic medicine, colon cancer is diagnosed by colonoscopies, biopsies, or using imaging technology utilizing ionizing radiation, such as contrast x-rays and CT scans. Treatments include chemotherapy, radiation, or surgery.

Cannabis and Colon Cancer

While other cancer-related studies have shown how cannabinoids can induce cancer cell death through apoptosis, both the Uppsala (2011)[2] and Bristol (2005)[3] experiments indicated another possible mechanism involving the inhibition of the enzyme cyclooxygenase 2 (COX-2). The genetic and pharmacologic studies from Nashville (2008) demonstrated in part that activation of CB1 reduced intestinal tumor growth in mice. It suggests endogenous cannabinoid receptors (CB1) as a possible target of a novel mechanism for prevention and treatment of colon cancer using the body's own anandamide.[4]

Study Summary

Drugs/Study Focus	Type of Study	Published Year, Place, and Key Results	CHI
Tetrahydrocannabinol (Δ^9-THC), tetrahydrocannabinolic acid (Δ^9-THC-A), cannabidiol (CBD), cannabidiolic acid (CBDA), cannabigerol (CBG), and cannabigerolic acid (CBGA)	Laboratory	2011—Uppsala University, Uppsala, Sweden: Cannabinoids inhibited cyclooxygenase enzyme.[2]	1
Endogenous cannabinoid receptor (CB1)	Animal study (mice)	2008—Vanderbilt University Medical Center, Nashville, Tennessee: CB1 expression may reduce intestinal tumor growth.[4]	2
Anandamide	Laboratory	2005—University of Bristol, Bristol, UK: Anandamide-induced colorectal carcinoma cell death produced by neither apoptosis nor necrosis.[3]	1

Total CHI Value 4

Strain- and Form-Specific Considerations

THC, THC-acid, CBD, CBD-acid, CBG, CBG-acid, and endogenous (the body's own) anandamide inhibited colon cancer cell proliferation in the laboratory. CB1 activation has been shown to reduce colon cancer in mice.

Anandamide and THC activate both CB1 and CB2, while CBD has a greater affinity for CB2. Sativa strains with a higher THC:CBD ratio tend to activate CB1 in greater proportions than indica strains with a generally lower THC:CBD ratio.

Juice obtained from fresh leaves of both indica and sativa strains contains non-psychoactive forms of plant cannabinoids, THC-acid, CBD-acid, and CBG-acid. Sativa strains with a higher THC-acid:CBD-acid ratio tend to activate CB1 in greater proportions than indica strains with a generally lower THC-acid:CBD-acid ratio.

Isolated synthetic cannabinoid prescription medications containing THC (such as Sativex, Dronabinol, Marinol, or Nabilone) activate both CB1 and CB2.

Mind-Body Medicine and Colon Cancer

A study conducted by Australian psychiatrists on more than 637 newly confirmed colon cancer patients showed a psychological framework unique to the participants when compared to healthy people of similar age and social situation. The psychological factors included: "... denial and repression of anger, and of other negative emotions, a commitment to prevailing social norms resulting in the external appearance of a 'nice' or 'good' person, and a suppression of reactions which may offend others and the avoidance of conflict."[5]

In summary, aggravating factors may include suppressed emotions, repression of anger, seeking approval from other(s), and suppression of reactions.

Consider appropriate release of emotions, raising self-esteem, and adhering to one's own ideals and standards rather than those of others.

Powerful Questions

What are the beliefs, thoughts, and feelings that I cannot digest, absorb, and eliminate?

Suggested Blessing

May you find a way to replace any beliefs that suppress or inhibit your emotions.

Suggested Affirmation

I can release old feelings and emotions with ease, with fun, and harm to none.

Let Food Be Thy Medicine

Basil ∾ Caraway ∾ Cardamom ∾ Cumin ∾ Nigella Saffron ∾ Turmeric

Basil: Basil thwarted chemical attempts to produce stomach cancer in rodents.[6]

Caraway: Caraway has been used in an experimental model on rats to determine if the spice, commonly used in Ayurvedic medicine for gastrointestinal difficulties, has any impact on the development of chemically induced colon cancer. The researchers determined that dietary caraway (at a dose of 60 mg/kg) indeed has properties that are able to control lipid peroxidation and antioxidant homeostasis, thereby preventing the development of chemically induced colon cancer lesions.[7] Another rodent-based study confirmed these results and further determined that the optimal dose was 60 mg/kg.[8]

Cardamom: Nearby, in the city of Kolkata, researchers at the Chittaranjan National Cancer Institute published results of a cardamom study: "These results suggest that aqueous suspensions of cardamom have protective effects on experimentally induced colon carcinogenesis."[9] These findings echo the time-proven Unani and Ayurvedic application of cardamom as a treatment in certain gastrointestinal diseases.

Cumin: Traditional healers in India have been using cumin for centuries to treat various gastrointestinal complaints. To test the potential therapeutic benefits of cumin, a chemical known to produce colon cancer tumors (called 1,2-dimethylhydrazine, or DMH) was given to rats. For the following 32 weeks, the rats with colon cancer were fed cumin seeds as part of their standard pellet diet.[10] Results showed that dietary cumin significantly suppressed colon carcinogenesis in the test animals.

Another report, this time from New Delhi, suggests similar anti-colon cancer properties of cumin. In a study published in the *Journal of Nutrition and Cancer,* the researchers state: "The results strongly suggest the cancer chemopreventive potentials of cumin seed could be attributed to its ability to modulate carcinogen metabolism."[11]

Nigella: In a University of Mississippi Medical Center study, scientists explored a time-proven technique from the Middle East. They examined the possible therapeutic effects of catechin, found in green tea, and thymoquinone, a major compound from black seed *(Nigella sativa),* on specific colon cancer cells. They compared the effectiveness of both natural substances with that of the current chemotherapeutic drug of choice—5-fluorouracil—against colon cancer cell lines. Scientists determined that both the green tea (catechin) and the thymoquinone from *Nigella sativa* "demonstrated incredible chemotherapeutic responses, thus suggesting that both may have similar chemotherapeutic effects as their pharmacological counterpart 5-fluorouracil, which has known serious side effects, including cardiac toxicity."[12]

Saffron: *Crocus sativus L.* or saffron may possess anticancer activity including against colon adenocarcinoma.[13]

Turmeric: In a meta-analysis, scientists provided an overview of decades of scientific studies on turmeric. They summarized a long list of turmeric's potential therapeutic properties: cancer and diabetic prevention, cancer treatment, promoter of wound-healing, and a therapeutic agent in Alzheimer's, Parkinson's, cardiovascular and pulmonary diseases, arthritis, adenomatous polyposis (multiple polyps in the large intestines—precursor to colon cancer), inflammatory bowel disease, ulcerative colitis (colon inflammation with ulcers), atherosclerosis, pancreatitis, psoriasis, chronic anterior uveitis (inflammation of the middle layer of the eye).[14]

Kaposi's Sarcoma
Evidence-Based Confidence Level and Therapeutic Potential

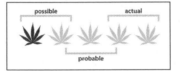

Total Number of Studies Reviewed: 2

Combined CHI Value: 1

Kaposi's sarcoma (KS) is an abnormal connective tissue mass, commonly presenting as multiple lesions on the skin. Moritz Kaposi first described the disease in the late nineteenth century. At that time it was thought to be a cancer, a hereditary condition, or a viral infection. The confusion continued at the beginning of the "AIDS epidemic" in the early 1980s, when doctors considered it the signature disease in people diagnosed with AIDS (especially in the gay community). However, by 1994 it was established that KS is a cancer caused by a virus from the herpes family (the eighth human herpes virus), also called HHV-8 or Kaposi's sarcoma-associated herpes virus (KSHV). The allopathic community no longer considers KS to be an indication of AIDS when combined with a positive HIV test.

Cannabis and Kaposi's Sarcoma

An experiment conducted in Los Angeles (2009) focused on the hypothesis proposed by Peter Duesberg that KS development may be influenced by the use of street drugs, particularly amyl nitrite ("poppers"). The results showed that a potential correlation existed between KS and poppers.[1] An Italian study (2009) discovered that the synthetic cannabinoid WIN55,212-2 was able to inhibit KS growth in the laboratory.[2]

Study Summary

Drugs	Type of Study	Published Year, Place, and Key Results	CHI
Synthetic cannabinoid WIN55,212-2	Laboratory	2009 — University of Catania School of Medicine, Catania, Italy: WIN55,212-2 reduced viability of human Kaposi's sarcoma cells in vitro.[2]	1
Cannabis vs cocaine or amphetamines and poppers	401 HIV- and HHV-8-coinfected homosexual men	2009—Los Angeles, California: Patients with a long-term history of using poppers showed a correlation between poppers (amyl nitrite) and KS. Long-term cannabis use was not correlated with an increased risk of developing KS.[1]	0

Total CHI Value 1

Strain-Specific Considerations

WIN55,212-2 binds with higher affinity to CB2 receptors than CB1 receptors. Indicas and indica-dominant strains tend to present a lower THC:CBD ratio, thus relatively favoring CB2 receptor activation.

Mind-Body Medicine and Kaposi's Sarcoma

The lesions formed by KS often develop around the nose and mouth, neck and chest, and thus are very noticeable. Even though the allopathic community was wrong in painting KS as the signature disease of AIDS, to many it retained the highly charged shame and judgment that was born from it.

KS development suggests that a combination of cancer and viral herpes patterns may be activated.

Powerful Questions

What are the symptoms keeping you from doing?
How do you feel about that?

Where do these feelings take you?

What scenarios or memories are associated with these feelings?

What meaning (messages, unhealthy beliefs/attitudes, etc.) have you given to that scenario?

The answers to these questions can direct your focus to support your capacity for self-healing.

Suggested Blessing

May you realize that you are wholly lovable.

Suggested Affirmation

I allow any shame to be lifted.

Leukemia and Lymphoma (in general)
Evidence-Based Confidence Level and Therapeutic Potential

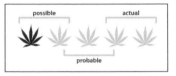

Combined Number of Studies Reviewed: 7

Combined CHI Value: 9

Leukemia is a type of blood cancer that usually begins in the bone marrow. Here, under normal circumstances, production of red and white blood cells and platelets occurs. Cancerous mutations of blood cells at their point of genesis can lead to serious impairment of the functions associated with each type of blood cell.

Lymphomas are cancers that typically form tumors inside lymph nodes. Both white blood cells (natural killer cells, T-cells, B-cells) and lymph nodes (which filter waste and toxins) are important parts of the body's immune system. Therefore, leukemia and lymphoma are closely related and can be considered cancers of the immune system.

A common observation in leukemia is the production of too many poorly functioning white blood cells, which severely reduces natural immunity and increases the risk of infections. Further, this glut of malformed white blood cells can displace red blood cells and platelets, which carry oxygen and are responsible for blood clotting, respectively.

As one would suspect, signs and symptoms of leukemia include a high white blood cell count, anemia, clotting problems leading to opportunistic infections, easy bruising, and spontaneous pinprick bleeds. Depending on severity, anemia symptoms may progress from feelings of weakness to shortness of breath. Other symptoms may mimic the disease, such as malaria or flu, with nausea, vomiting, fever, chills, diaphoresis, bone and joint aches, muscular weakness or pain, and enlarged liver, spleen, and lymph nodes.

Lymphomas are basically classified as Hodgkin's and non-Hodgkin's lymphomas, with dozens of sub-classifications depending on the country or system used. Lymphoma symptoms are similar to those of leukemia, but more commonly include swollen lymph nodes resulting from the backup of unmoved waste materials and tumors inside the nodes.

Depending on the speed of disease development and specific tissues affected, leukemia is generally classified into acute and chronic forms and further broken down as either acute or chronic myeloid or lymphoblastic leukemia. Leukemia can develop in the very young and adults alike. "It is estimated that 43,050 men and women (24,690 men and 18,360 women) will be diagnosed with, and 21,840 men and women will die of, leukemia in 2010."[1] However, of all children suffering from cancers, roughly 1 out of 3 suffers from leukemia.

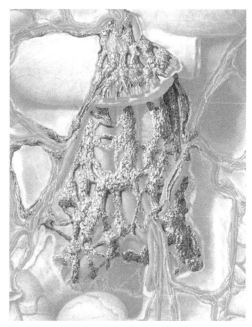

Within the orthodox medical community, the exact causes of the various leukemia types are only partially known, but several risk factors have been identified. Causative relations are found between leukemia and prior chemotherapies for cancer, ionizing radiation, and exposure to benzene, formaldehyde, and other chemical toxins. Risk factors may include genetic predisposition, smoking, viral influences, Down syndrome, and extremely low frequencies (ELF) commonly associated with high-voltage electrical power lines.[2]

Depending on the presence of symptoms, diagnosis occurs by physical examination, lymph node biopsies, or tests of blood and bone marrow. In some cases, doctors perform imaging techniques such as ultrasound, magnetic resonance imaging (MRI), or ionizing radiation via x-rays or CT scan. Allopathic treatments include chemotherapy, bone marrow transplants, and radiation.

Leukemia

Evidence-Based Confidence Level and Therapeutic Potential

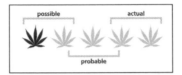

Total Number of Studies Reviewed: 5

CHI Value: 7

The Lymphoma Foundation of America has acknowledged the medical and therapeutic benefits of marijuana and supports its legal use for patients with serious medical conditions.

While a 2005 London study suggested that THC does not work synergistically with chemotherapy agents,[1] a 2008 analysis, also conducted in London, concluded that THC does in fact enhance the effectiveness of anticancer drugs to induce death in leukemia cells.[2]

During this same period (2006), a Columbia, South Carolina, team discovered that CBD, via CB2 pathways, produced apoptosis of leukemia cells, reduced tumor burden, and increased tumor apoptosis, suggesting that CBD may be a novel and highly selective treatment for leukemia.[3]

The London study from 2005[1] and the Virginia experiments (2006)[4] both confirmed THC's ability to induce apoptosis in leukemia cancer cells, and scientists theorized that therapeutic modulation was likely to involve CB1 and CB2 receptors. In addition, Swedish researchers demonstrated the potential of CB1- and CB2-mediated reduction in size and spread of lymphomas.[5]

Study Summary

Drugs/Study Focus	Type of Study	Published Year, Place, and Key Results	CHI
Anandamide analog R(+)-methanandamide (R(+)-MA)	Laboratory and in vivo studies on mice	2008—Karolinska University Hospital, Huddinge, Stockholm, Sweden: Anandamide analog R(+)-methanandamide (R(+)-MA) halts the spread and growth of cancerous tumors in animals with non-Hodgkin's lymphoma.[5]	1+2
THC	Laboratory study on leukemia cell lines	2008—Department of Oncology, St George's University of London, UK: "Clear synergistic interactions between THC and the cytotoxic agents in leukemic cells."[2]	1
CBD	Laboratory and in vivo studies	2006—University of South Carolina School of Medicine, Columbia, SC: CBD, via CB2 pathways, produced apoptosis of leukemia cells, reduced tumor burden, and increased tumor apoptosis.[3]	1
THC	Laboratory	2006—Virginia Commonwealth University, Richmond, VA: Raf-1/MEK/ERK/RSK-mediated translocation played a critical role in THC-induced apoptosis in Jurkat cells (leukemia cells).[4]	1
THC	Laboratory	2005—Multi-institutional, London, UK: THC induces apoptosis in leukemia cancer cells in "test tube."[1]	1

Total CHI Value 7

Suggested Blessing

May your blood bring the joy of life and the balm of forgiveness to every cell of your body.

Suggested Affirmations

I own and express all of my feelings with ease and harm to none.
At the core of my being, I release all fear, replacing it with love.

Let Food Be Thy Medicine

Turmeric ∽ Saffron

Turmeric: The rate for childhood leukemia in Asia is significantly lower than in the West, and researchers increasingly consider environmental factors such as diet to be major contributors. Scientists increasingly focus on turmeric. Over a dozen studies have examined turmeric and leukemia. For instance, studies from Singapore, Chengdu (China), and Bethesda,

Maryland (U.S.), have demonstrated that curcumin, the compound that gives turmeric its bright yellow color, was able to arrest the growth of leukemia in the laboratory.[6] Physicians have treated a total of 50 patients with chronic lymphocytic leukemia and concluded that curcumin may be contributing to a more effective therapy for leukemia patients.[7]

Saffron: *Crocus sativus L.* or saffron may possess anticancer activity including against leukemia.[8]

Lymphoma
Evidence-Based Confidence Level and Therapeutic Potential

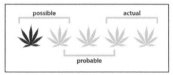

Number of Studies Reviewed: 2

CHI Value: 2

A Swedish study (2009)[1] revealed that the anticancer properties of cannabinoids increased synergistically with the rise of ceramide, a naturally occurring lipid (fat) commonly found in cell membranes. This followed an Italian team's confirmation (2000)[2] that the endocannabinoid anandamide induces apoptosis in lymphoma cancer cells.

Study Summary

Drugs	Type of Study	Published Year, Place, and Key Results	CHI
Endocannabinoid analogue R(+)-methanandamide (R-MA)	Laboratory	2009—Karolinska University Hospital, Huddinge, Stockholm, Sweden: The cannabinoid R-MA produces MCL cell death, and the cytotoxic effect of R-MA is enhanced by modulation of ceramide metabolism.[1]	1
Anandamide	Laboratory	2000—Ministero dell'Università e della Ricerca Scientifica e Tecnologica, Rome, Italy: Anandamide produced apoptosis in human cancer cells (neuroblastoma CHP100 and lymphoma U937 cells).[2]	1

Total CHI Value 2

Strain-Specific Considerations

These pre-clinical laboratory studies and animal experiments highlight the endocannabinoid system in the destruction (apoptosis) of both leukemia and lymphoma cell lines. The body's own anandamide, as well as THC and CBD, have proven to be toxic to these types of cancers, at least in the laboratory. The majority of these studies have been conducted on anandamide and THC, which bind to both CB1 and CB2 receptors. However, one experiment also demonstrated that CBD exhibited the ability to produce apoptosis via CB2 mechanisms.

Sativas or sativa-heavy strains tend to have a higher THC:CBD ratio, binding to both CB1 and CB2, while indicas or indica-heavy strains tend to have a lower THC:CBD ratio, binding to CB1 with a greater affinity.

Mind-Body Medicine and Lymphoma

While no mind-body studies have solely looked at lymphoma, those conducted on leukemia may apply. For instance, consider phrases like *"my flesh and blood," "blood brother,"* and *"blood is thicker than water."* These idioms, similar in many cultures, suggest that health issues with one's blood may be related to family. A study conducted on twenty patients diagnosed with leukemia reported that symptoms occurred while trying to handle multiple stressors from varying sources. Seventeen out of the twenty patients participating in this study claimed significant stress from a common source: the separation of a significant other (father, mother, wife, or other mother-figure) mainly due to death, or separation due to sibling and offspring conflict. Compounding stressors included quick and sudden changes related to work, infection, injury, or surgery.[3]

A study examining potential psychological risk factors for the genesis of acute leukemia discovered that family conflict involving inability to express feelings and emotions (alexithymia) due to guilt, repression, and denial was among the significant risk factors common in those who developed the disease.[4]

See also the passages on "Mind-Body Medicine" in the introductory section for Cancer and under Sickle Cell Disease.

Suggested Blessing

May your blood bring the joy of life and the balm of forgiveness to every
cell of your body.

Suggested Affirmations

I own and express all my feelings with ease and harm to none.
At the core of my being, I release all fear, replacing it with love.

Let Food Be Thy Medicine

Myrrh ∞ Oregano

Myrrh: Based on traditional practice and evidence-based discoveries, one
researcher reported that myrrh's significant antiseptic, anesthetic, and
anti-tumor properties are most likely attributed to a specific alkene called
furanosesquiterpene, present in essential oil of myrrh.[5] University of Texas
scientists discovered that naturally occurring steroids (guggulsterone) from
a closely related species called *Commiphora mukul* could produce apoptosis (destruction of cancer cells), " . . . including leukemia, head and
neck carcinoma, multiple myeloma, lung carcinoma, melanoma, breast
carcinoma, and ovarian carcinoma. Guggulsterone also inhibited the proliferation of drug-resistant cancer cells (e.g., gleevac-resistant leukemia,
dexamethasone-resistant multiple myeloma, and doxorubicin-resistant
breast cancer cells)."[6]

Oregano: Chemists at the University of Central Florida isolated several
compounds from oregano. Studies showed that aristolochic acid I and II
possess cancer-fighting abilities targeted at leukemia.[7]

Liver Cancer

Evidence-Based Confidence Level and Therapeutic Potential

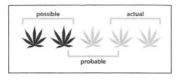

Total Number of Studies Reviewed: 2

CHI Value: 4

Hepatocellular carcinoma (HCC) is the third leading cause of cancer-related death worldwide.[1] While numerous types of liver cancers exist, HCC is by far the most common form. Signs and symptoms may include right upper abdominal distention, tenderness, pain (may be radiating), jaundice (yellow skin, sclera), brown urine, weight loss, nausea, and vomiting.

The allopathic community cannot pinpoint the exact cause of liver cancer. Statistically significant risk factors in the development of liver cancer may include gender (the disease is more common in males), history of chronic hepatitis B or C, cirrhosis, fatty liver, diabetes, toxins, alcoholism, L-carnitine deficiencies, or obesity.

Orthodox diagnosis is conducted via blood tests (examining liver values), imaging tests (x-ray, ultrasound, MRI), or biopsy. Traditional treatment consists of chemotherapy, radiation, surgery (tumor removal or transplant), cold applications (cryoprobe), heat (radiofrequency ablation), and injections of pure alcohol into the tumor sites.

Cannabis and Liver Cancer

In 2009, researchers from Palermo, Italy, wrote: "It has recently been shown that cannabinoids induce growth inhibition and apoptosis in different tumor cell lines." The results confirmed that WIN (a synthetic cannabinoid) produced liver cancer cell death or apoptosis (programmed cell death) in a fashion that was determined to be both dose- and time-dependent. The authors wrote: "... the results seem to indicate a potential therapeutic role of WIN, a synthetic cannabinoid, in hepatic cancer treatment."[2]

Two years later, in another experiment from Madrid, Spain, researchers looking for novel treatment options in cases of liver cancers investigated the effects of the cannabinoids THC and JWH-015 (another synthetic cannabinoid) on various liver cancer cell lines. Results showed that both cannabinoids were able to inhibit liver cancer tumor growth in animal models.[3]

Study Summary

Drugs	Type of Study	Published Year, Place, and Key Results	CHI
THC and JWH-015	Animal and laboratory tests	2011—Alcalá University, Madrid, Spain: Both cannabinoids inhibit liver cancer tumor growth.[3]	1+2
WIN55,212-2 (synthetic cannabinoid receptor agonist)	Laboratory	2009—Università di Palermo, Palermo, Italy: ". . . potential therapeutic role of WIN in hepatic cancer treatment."[2]	1

Total CHI Value 4

Strain-Specific Considerations

The two experiments reviewed here used THC and the synthetic cannabinoids WIN55,212-2 and JWH-015. Each displayed the ability to inhibit liver cancer cell lines or to induce apoptosis (programmed cancer cell death), at least in the laboratory and in animal tests.

THC binds with both CB1 and CB2. WIN55,212-2 binds with higher affinity to CB2 than the CB1 receptor. Similarly, JWH-015 has higher affinity for CB2 than CB1.

Sativa, sativa-heavy strains, indicas, and indica-heavy strains bind to CB1 and CB2, but the latter tend to have a lower THC:CBD ratio, which may favor CB2 activation.

Mind-Body Medicine and Liver Cancer

See the "Mind-Body Medicine" sections under Hepatitis and in the introduction to the Cancer section.[4]

Powerful Questions

What feeling(s) am I unable to let go of?
What feeling(s) am I unable to filter through?

Suggested Blessing

May you release all feelings with ease.

Suggested Affirmations

I release all feelings in fullness.
I release and let go of my anger.

Lung Cancer
Evidence-Based Confidence Level and Therapeutic Potential

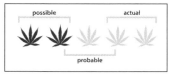

Total Number of Studies Reviewed: 4

CHI Value: 7

Historically, lung cancer was a rare diagnosis until it emerged as a major killer with the advent of the industrial revolution, the introduction of cigarettes (tobacco smoke and second-hand smoke are recognized as the major cause for developing lung cancer), increasing levels of air pollution (e.g., exhaust, asbestos, coal dust, soot), and the cumulative damage of ionizing radiation (x-rays).[1] Lung cancer is now the number-one cancer and leading fatal cancer in the world; some types are highly aggressive and resistant to allopathic treatments. Diagnosis consists of chest x-rays and biopsies, and treatment is limited to chemotherapy, radiation and/or surgery.

Cannabis and Lung Cancer

While inhaling any burned substance is generally bad for the lungs, the cannabinoid THC may prevent lung cancer. As early as 1975, the U.S. government discovered that cannabis plant cannabinoids were able to inhibit lung cancer growth, reduce tumor size, and increase survival rates in animal test subjects.[2] The later studies from Lyon (2006),[3] Rostock (2008),[4] and Harvard (2008)[5] elucidated potential mechanisms: signaling via CB1 and CB2 receptor sites, inducing protection against lung cancer and inducing cancer-infected cells to self-destruct (apoptosis).

Study Summary

Drugs	Type of Study	Published Year, Place, and Key Results	CHI
THC	Animal studies (mice) and laboratory tests	2008—Harvard Medical School, Boston, MA: Tested lung cancer cells contained CB1 and CB2 sites. Significant inhibition of the subcutaneous tumor growth and lung metastasis were found.[5]	1+2
Anandamide analog, methanandamide and delta-9-tetrahydro-cannabinol (THC)	Laboratory test performed on human lung cancer cells	2008—University of Rostock, Germany: Cannabinoid elicits decrease in tumor cell invasiveness.[4]	1
Cannabis	2,252 human subjects	2006—International Agency for Research on Cancer, Lyon, France: Population study found no association between lung cancer and long-term cannabis use.[3]	N/A
Delta-9-tetrahydro-cannabinol, delta-8-tetrahydrocannabinol, cannabinol (CBN), and cannabidiol (CBD)	Animal (mice) and laboratory tests	1975—Virginia Commonwealth University, Richmond, VA: THC and CBN but not CBD retarded lung cancer cell growth, reduced tumor size, and increased survival rates.[2]	1+2

Total CHI Value 7

Strain-Specific Considerations

Lung cancer cells have been shown to contain both CB1 and CB2 receptor sites. The reviewed pre-clinical experiments conducted in the laboratory and on animals revealed that the body's own anandamide and plant cannabinoids THC and CBN produced anti-lung cancer cell activity, ranging from inhibition of growth to initiation of apoptosis (cancer cell self-destruction).

CBN has a higher affinity for CB2, while THC and anandamide bind relatively equally to both CB1 and CB2.

Sativa, sativa-heavy strains, indicas, and indica-heavy strains all bind to CB1 and CB2, but the latter tend to have a lower THC:CBN ratio, which may favor CB2 activation.

Mind-Body Medicine and Lung Cancer

All types of lung cancers affect males significantly more than females. In 1961, scientists explored a hypothesized link between personality constructs and the development of lung cancer. The authors of the study wrote: "The available evidence suggests that lung cancer patients have personality features distinct from the general cigarette-smoking population."[6] By 1984 scientists trying to learn more about the differences between organic and psychological predictors in the development of lung cancer discovered that "Some psycho-social variables, like rationality and anti-emotionality, or long-lasting hope-lessness, were about as relevant as the strongest organic predictors. . . ."[7] In another study, published in 1991, researchers discovered possible predictable psychological conditions in the development of lung cancer that included ". . . low expression of anxiety, and unfulfilled need for closeness. . . ."[8]

Breathing in and breathing out. Taking life in and letting it go again can become a difficult and often painful process, depending on the disease's progression. More often than not, the feelings and emotions we have around the symptoms of lung cancer are a clue to judged emotions and stifled expressions.

Consider learning more about how to value feelings and emotions, express and release emotions, define your feelings and emotions, and feel close with your emotions fostering self-respect.

See also the "Mind-Body Medicine" sections under Cancer (introduction) and Coughing.

Powerful Questions

Do you value feelings or emotions? If not, why not?
What are logic, fact, and reason protecting you from?
What thoughts and feeling(s) are always in the air that must not be allowed in?
What would happen if you were to breathe them in?
What feeling(s) are you hopeless or helpless about?

Suggested Blessings

May your breath and your emotions flow as easy as one, two, three.
May you find the seeds of new vision in the depths of hopelessness.

Suggested Affirmations

I allow all my feelings and emotions to come and go in fullness, and I express them appropriately, with intensity, and with harm to none.
I express and fulfill my need for closeness in healthy ways.

Let Food Be Thy Medicine

Clove ∽ Myrrh

Clove: A study from Kolkata, India, looked at the properties of aqueous solution of clove. It found that the spice could produce apoptosis of lung cancer cells in mice and contains other possible cancer-protective properties.[9]

Myrrh: Based on traditional practice and evidence-based discoveries, one researcher reported that myrrh's significant antiseptic, anesthetic, and anti-tumor properties are most likely attributed to a specific alkene called furanosesquiterpene, present in essential oil of myrrh.[10]

Scientists from the University of Texas discovered that naturally occurring steroids (guggulsterone) from a closely related species called *Commiphora mukul* were able to produce apoptosis. This included: "... leukemia, head and neck carcinoma, multiple myeloma, lung carcinoma, melanoma, breast carcinoma, and ovarian carcinoma. Guggulsterone also inhibited the proliferation of drug-resistant cancer cells (e.g., gleevac-resistant leukemia, dexamethasone-resistant multiple myeloma, and doxorubicin-resistant breast cancer cells)."[11]

Melanoma (Malignant Skin Cancer)

Evidence-Based Confidence Level and Therapeutic Potential

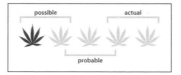

Number of Studies Reviewed: 1

CHI Value: 1

Melanin, produced by specialized skin cells (melanocytes), is the brownish pigment responsible for skin tone variants as well as for the coloring that occurs in tanning, freckles, and moles. Exposure to UV light increases melanin production as a protective mechanism from excessive harmful rays. Melanin converts the majority of UV light to harmless heat, preventing cellular mutation, thus protecting the skin from damage. The darker your skin, the greater your body's protective ability. The majority of melanocytes lie in the base of the epidermis (outer skin layer).

While the majority of skin cancers are non-melanomas, melanomas make up the majority of deaths. Melanoma affects more Caucasians than other ethnicities. While direct sun exposure is healthy, natural and excessive sun exposure can contribute to mutation of DNA in melanocytes. The highest incidence of melanoma occurs in whites living in Australia.

Diagnosis begins with the examination of suspicious tissue, moles, or lesions. Practitioners carefully look at the A, B, C, D, and E's of affected skin. A stands for asymmetry; B for borders (irregularly shaped); C for uneven color(s) presentation (white, pink, red, blue, brown, black); D for diameter (moles larger than 6 mm are more suspicious); and E for evolving or rapid development of shape, color, and size (weeks or months, rather than years). Other signs include pain, itching, scar-like tissue development, a pink growth, a reddish patch, or ulceration with discharge or bleeding.

Allopathic treatment includes surgical removal, chemotherapy and/or radiation.

It's interesting to note that the majority of sunscreens contain ingredients that are considered carcinogenic, or can become carcinogenic in reaction with UV light. Furthermore, using sunblock prevents UVB light-induced vitamin D synthesis, which may protect against certain cancers.[1] This last discovery is especially important to dark-skinned people. Thus, a careful balance between the need for healthy sun exposure and a reduction in excessive sun exposure and associated cancer risk should be maintained.

Ten to fifteen minutes of unclothed exposure to the sun before 10 AM or after 3 PM about three times per week is optimal. This stimulates a gentle and gradual production in melanin for photo protection and supports a healthy immune response mediated in part by the conversion of cholesterol into vitamin D. Dark-skinned people, women who wear veils, and people rarely exposed to the sun may want to consider vitamin D supplementation.

Cannabis and Melanoma

Several studies have confirmed the anti-emetic benefits of cannabinoids on melanoma patients undergoing radiation treatment[2] and chemotherapy.[3]

Indeed, case study reports of successful applications of extracted cannabis oil against melanoma exist, notably from the citizen experiments of Rick Simpson and reports by Cannabis Science, Inc.[4] Still, scientific studies examining the efficacy of cannabis on melanoma are mostly wanting, with the exception of the study conducted by the National Institute of Oncology in Budapest, where researchers proved that CB1 modulation induces apoptosis of human melanoma cells.[5]

Study Summary

Drugs/Study Focus	Type of Study	Published Year, Place, and Key Results	CHI
CB1 receptor agonist, Met-F-AEA, CB1 antagonist, AM251	Laboratory study on human melanoma cell lines	2008—National Inst. of Oncology, Budapest, Hungary: CB1 modulation induces apoptosis of human melanoma cells.[5]	1

Total CHI Value 1

Strain-Specific Considerations

The Hungarian laboratory experiment highlights a potential pathway involving CB1 receptor activation in the destruction of human melanoma cells. The synthetic cannabinoid Met-F-AEA is similar to naturally occurring anandamide, which binds relatively equally to CB1 and CB2.

Sativas and sativa-heavy strains tend to have a higher THC:CBN ratio, which may increase CB1 activation when compared to indicas and indica-heavy strains with lower THC:CBD ratios that may increase CB2 activation.

Mind-Body Medicine and Melanoma

See Skin Cancer (Non-Melanoma) and the introduction to the Cancer section.

Let Food Be Thy Medicine

Bush Tea ∾ Clove ∾ Myrrh

Numerous marijuana patients and advocates alike have reported cases of successful melanoma treatments using highly concentrated solvent extracts of flowers of cannabis.[6]

Bush Tea: Laboratory studies have found that bush tea (rooibos or red tea) contains DNA-protective and antimutagenic properties.[7] South African researchers who discovered that topical bush tea application inhibits skin tumor formation have confirmed the antimutagenic properties of rooibos as well.[8]

Clove: An Indian study determined that aqueous solutions of clove might also have protective properties against skin papillomas (skin tumors).[9]

Myrrh: Based on traditional practice and evidence-based discoveries, one researcher reported that myrrh's significant antiseptic, anesthetic, and anti-tumor properties are most likely attributed to a specific alkene called furano-sesquiterpene, present in essential oil of myrrh.[10] University of Texas scientists discovered that naturally occurring steroids (guggulsterone) from a closely related species called *Commiphora mukul* produced apoptosis (destruction of cancer cells), "... including leukemia, head and neck carcinoma, multiple myeloma, lung carcinoma, melanoma, breast carcinoma, and ovarian carcinoma. Guggulsterone also inhibited the proliferation of drug-resistant cancer cells (e.g., gleevac-resistant leukemia, dexamethasone-resistant multiple myeloma, and doxorubicin-resistant breast cancer cells)."[11]

Pancreatic Cancer

Evidence-Based Confidence Level and Therapeutic Potential

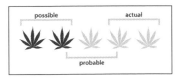

Total Number of Studies Reviewed: 2

CHI Value: 4

One of the most malignant forms of cancer, pancreatic cancer usually has poor outcomes. Onset symptoms may include gastrointestinal difficulties such as abdominal pain (often radiating to the back), lack of appetite, nausea and vomiting, diarrhea, weight loss, jaundice and/or diabetes. Traditional allopathic treatments of surgery and chemotherapy offer meager success rates. "Pancreatic cancer prognosis remains very poor with a five-year survival rate of less than 5% in most reports."[1]

Cannabis and Pancreatic Cancer

The urgency of this particularly aggressive cancer, and the lack of effective treatments, generated a demand for research into new and more successful care. Scientists in Madrid, Spain, took the first steps in 2006 after discovering an increased presence of cannabinoid receptors in pancreatic cancer cells. Experiments in the laboratory and in animals confirmed the potential: cannabinoids effectively induced apoptosis in cancerous cells, leaving normal cells unaffected.[2] That same year, scientists in Pisa, Italy, discovered that a novel endocannabinoid mechanism not regulated via typical CB1 or CB2 receptors was able to destroy pancreatic cancer lines in the laboratory.[3]

Study Summary

Drugs	Type of Study	Published Year, Place, and Key Results	CHI
THC and other cannabinoids	Laboratory and in vivo animal studies	2006—Complutense University, Madrid, Spain: Anti-pancreatic tumor effect via CB2 receptors.[2]	1+2
AM251 (potent CB1 antagonist)	Laboratory	2006—University of Pisa, Italy: Endocannabinoids produce a significant cytotoxic effect via a receptor-independent mechanism.[3]	1

Total CHI Value 4

Strain-Specific Considerations

The results of these pre-clinical trials suggest a CB2-initiated mechanism by which cannabinoids produce toxic effects on pancreatic cancer cell lines.

Indicas and indica-heavy hybrids usually present with a lower THC:CBD/CBN ratio, typically promoting an increased CB2 activation.

Mind-Body Medicine and Pancreatic Cancer

If the heart is metaphorically where we feel our feelings, then the liver is where we process them. The pancreas is where we store these feelings until we put them in proper perspective, "making sense" of them in the larger context of our lives. This metaphor may be echoed in the pancreatic production of insulin where it is needed to utilize sugar. Without it, sugar remains in the blood unused, causing many of the symptoms associated with hyperglycemia (diabetes). Similarly, in emotional terms, feelings flow in the stream of our emotional reality until we transcend them, just like sugar is converted to life-sustaining energy.

See also the sections on Diabetes and Inflammatory Diseases—Pancreatitis, as well as the introduction to the Cancer section.

Powerful Questions

What are the symptoms keeping you from doing?

How do you feel about that?

Where do these feelings take you?

What scenarios or memories are associated with these feelings?

What is the meaning (messages, unhealthy beliefs/attitudes, etc.) you have given to that scenario?

Can the answers to these questions direct your focus to support your capacity for self-healing?

Suggested Blessing

May I learn to provide space for my feelings without letting them control my life.

Suggested Affirmation

I store my feelings only as long as it takes to put them in proper perspective.

Let Food Be Thy Medicine

Turmeric ∾ Nigella

Turmeric: A study from Detroit, Michigan, showed that diflourinated-curcumin, a novel analogue of the turmeric spice component curcumin, was able to inhibit pancreatic cancer tumor growth and aggressiveness in the laboratory.[4]

Nigella: Researchers from Wenzhou, China, report that thymoquinone, a component derived from the medicinal spice *Nigella sativa* (also known as black seed), exhibited inhibitory effects on cell proliferation of pancreatic cell lines in the laboratory and in animal experiments. "Consequently, these results provide important insights into thymoquinone as an antimetastatic agent for the treatment of human pancreatic cancer."[5]

Prostate Cancer
Evidence-Based Confidence Level and Therapeutic Potential

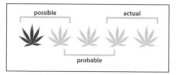

Total Number of Studies Reviewed: 3

CHI Value: 3

The prostate gland is part of the male reproductive system. Located at the outlet of the urinary bladder, the prostate is about the size of a walnut in its healthy state. The urethra, the opening from the bladder, leads through the prostate to the tip of the penis. The gland produces and stores seminal fluids in which sperm originating in the testes move about during ejaculation.

Similarly, females have a glandular tissue called Skene's glands or periurethral glands that produce fluid almost identical to the male version which may be ejaculated during orgasm. However, the "female prostate" is not usually subject to cancerous proliferation.

Prostate cancer is one of the most common cancers in elderly males yet is generally very slow-growing. While many patients never have any particular symptoms, an enlargement of the prostate commonly underlies cancer pathologies. The enlargement exerts pressure on the urethra, making urinating and fully emptying the bladder difficult. Other possible symptoms of prostate cancer include sexual dysfunction, bloody urine, painful urination, or pain in that general region.

In days past, a prostate problem was called "priest's disease," due to the hypothesis that lack of sexual activity may be related to the development of prostate cancer. A significant study conducted over a period of eight years including almost 30,000 males confirmed this association. Results revealed that increased sexual activity (more than 21 ejaculations per month) correlated to a 30% decreased risk of developing prostate cancer over a lifetime when compared to males who ejaculate only four to seven times per month.[1]

More specific causes of prostate cancer remain a mystery to the scientific community. Traditional treatment includes chemotherapy, radiation and/ or surgery.

Cannabis and Prostate Cancer

In 2000, a laboratory experiment conducted in Naples, Italy, demonstrated that the body's own cannabinoid, anandamide, was able to inhibit the growth of both breast cancer and prostate cancer cells.[2] A study from Wisconsin (U.S.) that followed in 2004 found that prostate cancer cells contained significantly higher expressions of both CB1 and CB2 receptors. This in turn led them to suggest a possible novel approach to treating prostate cancer.[3] More insights came in 2009, from Debrecen, Hungary. For the first time, CB1 was identified in epithelial and smooth muscle cells of the healthy human prostate. Researchers confirmed the study results and strongly argued that CB1 possesses a promising future role in the treatment of prostate cancer.[4]

Study Summary

Drugs/Study Focus	Type of Study	Published Year, Place, and Key Results	CHI
Drug receptor CB1	Laboratory study on healthy and cancerous prostate cells	2009—University of Debrecen, Hungary: CB1 found in healthy prostate cells.[4]	1
WIN55,212-2 and SR141716 (CB1) and SR144528 (CB2)	Laboratory study on prostate cancer cells	2004—University of Wisconsin: Prostate cancer cells contained significantly higher expressions of both CB1 and CB2 receptors.[3]	1
Anandamide, HU210, BML-190, SR141716A, SR144528	Laboratory study on prostate and breast cancer cells	2000—Multi-institutional: Anandamide inhibits the growth of breast cancer and prostate cancer cells.[2]	1

Total CHI Value 3

Strain-Specific Considerations

Prostate cancer cells contain significantly higher expressions of both CB1 and CB2 receptors, which has prompted researchers to suggest a possible novel approach in treating prostate cancer. Further, anandamide inhibits the growth of prostate cancer cells in the laboratory. Anandamide and THC bind relatively equally with CB1 and CB2.

While both sativas and indicas as well as hybrids bind with CB1 and CB2, sativas and sativa-dominant strains contain a higher THC:CBD ratio, thus providing an increased similarity to the cannabinoid profile of anandamide.

Mind-Body Medicine and Prostate Cancer

Researchers have discovered a link between psychological stress and healthy prostate function. Results of a study conducted on 83 men diagnosed with benign prostatic hyperplasia (BPH) reveal that stress and hostility influence prostate volume and residual urine volume.[5] Researchers hypothesize that the effect is mediated via the sympathetic nervous system and hypothalamic-pituitary-gonadal axis.

A large-scale and long-term study of 19,730 adults over a period of nine years somewhat confirmed these results. Researchers discovered that anger control and negative affect have a small role in the risk of prostate cancer.[6]

An enlarged male gland applies pressure and strangles the urethra, thus producing the most commonly observed symptom: a struggle to release urine. This pressure can also be metaphorically intuited as psychological pressure on the patient. Derived from the ancient Greek word for "protector" or "guardian," the prostate represents survival, safety, and security. An impaired flow of urine is associated with being "pissed off": "Have I made enough money to live on? Do I have enough for those I love? Am I a good enough provider?"

Other issues include pressure from suppressed anger at old age in connection with male energy, image, or virility: "Am I still hard, strong, tough, or fast enough?" Additionally, pressure from self-judgments about goals never reached or achieved, or pressure from negative self-image or

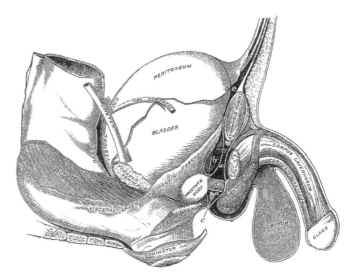

self-talk that says "old is useless, weak, and decrepit" may be present and in need of healing.

Sexual performance pressure is another issue commonly found in patients dealing with prostate enlargement or cancer. Many males address performance pressure by denial, or by looking at outside causes and cures rather than taking an inward look. Blaming a partner or using oral or injectable erectile enhancements does not resolve the underlying psychology. Sexual conflict due to guilt, anxiety, fear, shame, betrayal, or humiliation and past traumatic events all can produce performance pressure, and attention may be required to produce permanent change.

In summary, aggravating factors may include chronic lifelong stress, acute stress, hostility, negative affect, male pressure to be anti-emotional, performance pressure, male guilt, suppressed male anger, and negative older male self-image.

Supporting factors may include stress reduction or management, as well as defining and releasing feelings and emotions around male image, age, and sex and transforming tendencies for negative affect by re-evaluating emotionally limiting beliefs and attitudes.

Powerful Questions

Have I made enough money to live on?
Do I have enough for those I love?
Am I a good enough provider?
Am I still hard, strong, tough, or fast enough?
Where do I feel useless, weak, or decrepit?
What do I think of "the feminine" in me?
What do I think of having feelings?
What feelings or emotions do I hold in?
What else am I holding in?
What blocks a complete release?
Where do I struggle to let go?

Suggested Blessing

May you find a way to forgive and release any pressure(s) surrounding
your masculinity.

I can generate youthful spiritual energy, no matter what age I am.

Let Food Be Thy Medicine

Cayenne ∽ Garlic

Cayenne: After studying cayenne and prostate cancer in the laboratory and in patients, scientists concluded that capsaicin in cayenne "is a promising anti-tumor agent in hormone-refractory prostate cancer, which shows resistance to many chemotherapeutic agents."[7]

Garlic: Applying garlic to rodents, Hong Kong scientists reported significant success in inhibiting primary tumor formation of the prostate, and a reduction of secondary tumor formation. Their study concluded that garlic possesses potent antimetastatic properties (preventing cancer from spreading), which may also apply to other types of cancer.[8]

Rhabdomyosarcoma

Evidence-Based Confidence Level and Therapeutic Potential

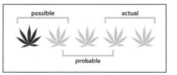

Total Number of Studies Reviewed: 2

CHI Value: 1

This type of cancer is typically a fast-growing and highly malignant tumor found most often in children. It affects the connective tissue and is believed to begin in progenitor cells (similar to stem cells), which later differentiate into muscle cells. The most common location of rhabdomyosarcoma development is the head and neck, followed by the genitourinary tract. Allopaths traditionally suspect hereditary causes, and treatment is limited to chemotherapy, surgery, and radiation. The survival rate in the late 1960s was a mere 10–15%, but by 2000 it had risen to over 70%.[1]

Cannabis and Rhabdomyosarcoma

A 1993 Pittsburgh survey found a possible correlation between a child's development of rhabdomyosarcoma and their birth parent's use of cocaine and marijuana in the year preceding the child's birth. Cannabis use was said to be one potential co-factor, in conjunction with cocaine, in the development of the cancer.[2] To date, no studies have explored whether use of cannabis alone increases the risk of rhabdomyosarcoma.

In fact, sixteen years later, Swiss researchers were able to kill rhabdomyosarcoma cells in a laboratory test using a synthetic cannabinoid. The scientists confirmed the test results in vivo by xenografting rhabdomyosarcoma cancer cells treated with the cannabinoid, which led to a significant suppression of the tumor growth. The Swiss study provides a basis for considering cannabinoids as a new treatment approach for rhabdomyosarcoma.[3]

Study Summary

Drugs	Type of Study	Published Year, Place, and Key Results	CHI
HU210 and THC	Laboratory and animal studies	2009—University Children's Hospital, Zurich, Switzerland: HU210 and THC produced cancer cell death.[3]	1
Cocaine and marijuana	Case-controlled human trial	1993—University of Pittsburgh School of Medicine, Pittsburgh, PA, USA: Survey of parents of 322 patients with rhabdomyosarcoma suggested that parental use of cocaine and marijuana in the year before conception may increase the risk of rhabdomyosarcoma two to fivefold.[2]	0

Total CHI Value 1

Strain-Specific Considerations

To date, two cannabinoids have been tested against rhabdomyosarcoma: HU210, a synthetic cannabinoid with a higher affinity for the CB1 receptors, and THC, which binds relatively equally to CB1 and CB2.

Sativas and sativa-heavy strains tend to present with a higher THC:CBD ratio, thus activating CB1 and CB2 in relatively equal proportions.

Mind-Body Medicine and Rhabdomyosarcoma

Applying the paradigm of co-creation to the dreadful events of often-fatal infant and childhood diseases or accidents remains a very challenging task.

What belief(s) in punishment, what guilt, how much harbored anger, and what responsibility can a baby have?

If we were privy to the intention and choices made beyond the veil of conception or after death's final curtain falls, it would perhaps be easier to understand the elusive why(s). However, discovery may take place in the experiences of present moments, and in the process of finding the most effective road to healing.

Let Food Be Thy Medicine

Saffron: *Crocus sativus L.* or saffron may possess anticancer activity including against rhabdomyosarcoma.[4]

Skin Cancer (Non-Melanoma)
Evidence-Based Confidence Level and Therapeutic Potential

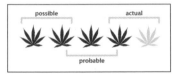

Total Number of Studies Reviewed: 2

CHI Value: 8

The skin is the largest organ of the body. It transmits sensations to the brain, provides temperature regulation, and protects us from environmental toxins and pathogens. Our skin has three basic layers: the outer layer (epidermis), the middle layer (dermis), and lower subcutaneous tissue.

There are two types of non-melanoma skin cancer. Squamous cell carcinoma originates in the outermost layer of the epidermis (which is composed of squamous cells). Basal cell carcinoma originates in the lowest layer (composed of basal cells).

Non-melanoma skin cancers are one of the most common cancers diagnosed to date. With a relatively easy diagnosis and treatment, most non-melanoma skin cancer treatments result in a positive outcome.

During initial stages, a cancerous growth may have a mole-like appearance. To distinguish possible skin cancers from normal moles, practitioners look at the A, B, C, D, and E's of cancerous lesions: A stands for asymmetry; B for borders (irregularly shaped); C for uneven color(s) presentation (white, pink, red, blue, brown, black); D for diameter (melanoma is typically ¼ inch); and E for evolving or rapid development of shape, color, and size (weeks or months rather than years). Other warning signs include pain, itching, scar-like tissue development, a pink growth, a reddish patch, or ulceration with discharge or bleeding.

Allopathic treatment includes forms of surgical removal using type-appropriate tools to shave off the cancerous tissue. The actual slicing may involve using a topical electrical current to stop bleeding and, ideally, to zap the remaining cancer cells. Surgeons may use lasers to vaporize tissue, a wire brush to sand off skin, or freeze the affected tissue (cryosurgery). Depending on the breadth and depth of the cancer, physicians may also use chemotherapies or radiation.

Mohs micrographic surgery is another commonly used method for the removal of non-melanoma skin cancer, especially when found on the nose, ears, or eyelids where it is extremely important to shave off as little tissue as possible. A local anesthetic is injected, and very thin layers of skin are sliced off and immediately examined under a microscope to determine if the last layer removed is free of cancerous cells.

Cannabis and Skin Cancer (Non-Melanoma)

Most Materia Medicas of both the Eastern and the Western healing traditions reference historical applications of whole-plant cannabis topicals for the treatment of skin cancer.

In 2003, a team of researchers from Madrid, Spain, and Clemons, South Carolina, investigated cannabinoids' effectiveness as a non-melanoma skin cancer therapy. The team showed that CB1 and CB2 receptors exist in both healthy and cancerous skin tissue of humans and mice, and that both CB1 and CB2 receptors play a role in the induction of apoptosis of skin tumor cells and the regression of skin carcinomas. Further, they compared the effects of cannabinoids on cell cultures containing normal skin cells and cultures containing cancerous skin cells. Results revealed the destruction of cancerous cells, while normal cells remained unaffected. The authors concluded that: "These results support a new therapeutic approach for the treatment of skin tumors."[1]

Six years later, in 2009, another team of international researchers concluded that the main function of the presence of an endocannabinoid system (ECS) in the skin is to control and balance growth, differentiation, and survival of skin cells, as well as to produce proper immune responses. The team believed that manipulation of the ECS might be beneficial in a multitude of human skin diseases, including acne, dermatitis, dry skin, hair loss (alopecia, effluvium), hirsutism (excessive hair growth), itching, seborrhea, skin tumors, pain, and psoriasis. The authors of the study hypothesized that, in the case of skin cancers, an up-regulation of both ECS receptors CB1 and CB2 would suppress cancerous growths, angiogenesis (blood supply to the tumor), and metastasis (rapid spread of cancer), and even induce apoptosis (cancer cell death).[2]

Study Summary

Drugs/Study Focus	Type of Study	Published Year, Place, and Key Results	CHI
Endocannabinoid system (ECS) and cannabinoids	Meta-analysis	2009—Multi-center international study from Germany, Hungary, United Kingdom, and the United States: "… targeted manipulation of the ECS (…) might be beneficial in a multitude of human skin diseases."[2]	4
JWH-133 (CB2 agonist), WIN55,212-2 (CB1 & CB2 agonist), SR141716 (CB1 antagonist), and SR144528 (CB2 antagonist)	Laboratory cultures, mice and human study	2003—Multi-center international study from Spain and the United States: CB1 and CB2 are present in normal skin and skin tumors of mice and humans. Cannabinoid receptor activation induces skin tumor cell apoptosis.[1]	4

Total CHI Value 8

Strain-Specific Considerations

JWH-133, a CB2 agonist, and WIN55,212-2, a CB1 and CB2 agonist, were tested successfully against non-melanoma skin cancer cells in vitro (cell cultures) and in vivo (animal-tested).

Both sativa and indica strains contain cannabinoids that activate CB1 and CB2 receptors. THC binds with both CB1 and CB2 receptors relatively equally, while CBD has a greater affinity for CB2.

Mind-Body Medicine and Skin Cancer (Non-Melanoma)

The skin is a boundary that lets us know precisely where we end and the outside world begins. It is also the image we present to the world. Since doctors diagnose the majority of skin cancers on the face, neck, back of hands, upper arms, and upper torso, the potential for subjective meaning and understanding varies accordingly. For example, the face communicates emotional states through obvious and subtle micro-expressions. Perhaps more than any other physicality, the face represents the image we present to the world, and the nose leads the way. Scent is processed differently from other senses in that it quickly and directly targets the more ancient part of the brain (limbic system), where emotions such as fear or arousal, rapid hormonal changes, long-term memory, and related behavior are rapidly initiated.

Idioms related to the nose reveal self-controlling judgments and an underlying need for perfection. Brown-nosing. Nose to the grindstone. Cut off your nose to spite your face. Hard-nosed. Don't stick your nose where it does not belong. Nosy. Pay through the nose. Rub his nose in it. Nose up in the air.

The fairytale archetype of the evil witch with the pronounced mole on her nose also springs to mind.

In summary, aggravating factors may include a negative self-image and/or belief in visible punishment, while supporting factors may include the release of any negative self-image, the building of a positive self-image, and a belief in self-forgiveness.

See also Skin Diseases and the introduction to Cancer.

Powerful Questions

Am I comfortable in my own skin?

Do I like my skin?

Which part don't I like?

How do I feel about it, and why?

What part of my skin don't I want anybody to see, and why?

What does that part represent?

What has gotten under my skin that is eating me up?

Suggested Blessing

May you feel safe and secure inside your skin.

Suggested Affirmation

I love and value my boundaries. I love the constant sensual dance between my skin and the world.

Let Food Be Thy Medicine

Bush Tea ～ Clove

Bush Tea: Laboratory studies found that bush tea (rooibos or red tea) contains DNA-protective and antimutagenic properties.[3] South African researchers who learned that topical bush tea application inhibits skin tumor formation have confirmed the antimutagenic properties of rooibos as well.[4]

Clove: One study from Kolkata, India, looked at the properties of aqueous solution of clove and found it to produce apoptosis of lung cancer cells in mice; it also showed other possible cancer-protective properties.[5] Another Indian study determined that aqueous solution of clove might also have protective properties against skin papillomas (skin tumors).[6]

Take Notice: Radiation Protection

See the introduction to Cancer under "Take Notice—Radiation Protection."

Thyroid Cancer
Evidence-Based Confidence Level and Therapeutic Potential

Total Number of Studies Reviewed: 2

CHI Value: 3

Guided by hormones from the pituitary and hypothalamus glands, the thyroid (Greek for "shield") is an integral part of the human endocrine system. Its butterfly-like shape appears to shield or embrace the front of the Adam's apple in males and females alike. It produces thyroid hormones, mainly triiodothyronine (T3) and thyroxine (T4), which are intricately involved in physiological development, growth, and cellular metabolism. In addition, the thyroid enhances and extends the catecholamine effects of adrenalin (increases alertness and "fight or flight" responses).

Minor thyroid diseases fall into two basic categories: hypothyroidism (underproduction of T3 and T4) and hyperthyroidism (overproduction of T3 and T4). The thyroid produces both T3 and T4 by utilizing dietary iodine.

In previous decades, a major cause of thyroid cancer stemmed from orthodox medical procedures involving ionizing radiation. From 1940 to 1960, orthodox medicine used radiation on the necks and heads of many young children to treat relatively mild diseases.[1] Ten to thirty years later, many of those children developed thyroid cancer, which affects women at twice the rate as males. Thyroid's affinity for the element iodine also makes it vulnerable to the ill-effects of numerous iodine isotopes, such as iodine 131, released by nuclear accidents and explosions.

Signs and symptoms may include a feeling of pressure in the throat that will not go away, the physical presence of lumps or nodules, a change in voice, swollen lymph nodes beneath the jaw and neck and/or difficulty swallowing. These symptoms may coexist or be preceded by hyperthyroidism or hypothyroidism, both of which may lead to autoimmune difficulties.

Diagnosis involves a blood test (balance of thyroid hormones), imaging techniques, and a needle biopsy of suspect tissue. Allopathic treatment includes surgery, radiation with iodine 131, and chemotherapy.

Cannabis and Thyroid Cancer

Laboratory tests revealed that thyroid cancer cells are inhibited by cannabinoids. In 2006, Italian scientists from Pozzuoli examined the effects of isolated cannabinoids and cannabis extracts on thyroid cancer cell lines implanted in rodents. Of the five natural compounds tested, scientists discovered cannabidiol and cannabidiol-acid to be the most potent inhibitors of thyroid cancer cells.[2] Test results also revealed that while cannabinoids are toxic to cancer cells, they exert less potent effects on normal cells.

Another laboratory study from Naples, Italy, in 2010 confirmed these initial findings when researchers exposed cancerous thyroid cells to an

Common Signs and Symptoms

Hyperthyroidism	Hypothyroidism
Weight loss with increased appetite	Weight gain with poor appetite
Feeling hot	Feeling cold
Rapid heart beats (tachycardia)	Slow heart beats (bradycardia)
	Dry, coarse hair and/or hair loss, dry skin, brittle fingernails
Toxic goiter (swelling of the lower neck)	Non-toxic goiter (less common)
Protruding eyes	Puffy appearance of face
Diaphoresis (sweating) increased	Diaphoresis (sweating) decreased
Diarrhea	Constipation
Nervousness, anxiety, restlessness	Depression
Tremors (hands and fingers)	Joint and muscle pains/cramps
Feeling weak or easily fatigued	Feeling weak or easily fatigued
Difficulty sleeping	
Mood swings	Slower thinking
Light menses	Heavy menses

analog of anandamide. The exposure inhibited the growth of the cancer cells and led to an increase of apoptosis (death of cancer cells). The scientists also discovered elevated levels of cannabinoid receptor 1 (CB1) expression, thus suggesting that the toxic effect to the mutated cells likely occurred from interaction with the CB1 receptors.[3]

Strain- and Form-Specific Considerations

Scientists tested six cannabinoids against thyroid cancer cells. Significant among them were anandamide, the body's own cannabinoid, which binds relatively equally to CB1 and CB2, and the plant cannabinoids cannabidiol (CBD) and cannabidiol acid (CBD-A). The latter two possess a greater affinity for the CB2 receptor than for the CB1.

Indica or indica-heavy hybrids tend to have a lower THC:CBD ratio, thus increasing the probability of enhanced CB2 activation. Further, CBD-acid is present at higher concentration in fresh, raw leaf. Cannabis-using patients often consume it in juice form.

Mind-Body Medicine and Thyroid Cancer

Hyperthyroidism can cause excess production of thyroid hormones. This excess, also referred to as thyrotoxicosis, can lead to the development of Graves' Disease,[4] an autoimmune disorder due to an overactive thyroid.

Nineteenth- and early twentieth-century observers noticed a correlation between combat stress from the Bohr War and WWI and the development of Graves' Disease. Later, psychosomatic studies described the thyroid as "the gland of the emotions," and thyrotoxicosis as "crystallized fright."[5]

More specifically, early researchers found that thyrotoxicosis was significantly more likely to develop when a patient's emotional stability rested on a particular person in the family. Further, they observed that a threat to or from that person appeared to induce thyrotoxicosis. Participating patients proved to be unduly vulnerable because "... their development had led to overdependence upon parental love and shelter; or fear of repudiation by parents; or excessively high ideals of parenthood, of social and moral duties...."[6]

Another psychiatric study enrolled 200 patients at the Presbyterian Hospital in New York and found that female hyperthyroid patients "... make a desperate and lifelong struggle to win their mother's approval, and to achieve likeness to her, at the same time that they fear her pain.... The men also show fear of deprivation of their mother's comfort, but the fear of loss of approval is less specific, appearing as fear of public disgrace."[7]

The thyroid is centered in the throat, the seat of expression and communication. When individual needs, desires, or feelings are not appropriately expressed and communicated but rather are repressed or harbored,

Study Summary

Drugs	Type of Study	Published Year, Place, and Key Results	CHI
2-methyl-2'-F-anandamide (Met-F-AEA), a metabolically stable analogue of anandamide	Laboratory	2010—University of Naples Federico II, Naples, Italy: Growth inhibition found in cell lines derived from thyroid carcinoma.[3]	1
Cannabidiol (CBD), cannabigerol (CBG), cannabichromene, cannabidiol acid (CBD-A) and THC acid (THC-A)	Laboratory and animal (rat) study	2006—Istituto di Chimica Biomolecolare, Consiglio Nazionale delle Ricerche, Pozzuoli, Italy: Both cannabidiol and the cannabidiol-rich extract inhibited the growth of injected thyroid tumor cells.[2]	2

Total CHI Value 3

throat problems may provide a vehicle to draw attention to these issues of self-expression.

Although lung cancer rates are significantly higher in males, thyroid cancer affects many more women than men. And while researchers point to correlations between lung cancer and rationality and anti-emotionality, a similar case involving thyroid cancer could be made—for instance, women not speaking up for themselves, especially in relation to authority or parental figures.

In summary, aggravating factors may include fear (acute or chronic), fear of loss of parental approval, fear of loss of shelter, overdependence upon parental love and shelter, fear of repudiation by parents, excessively high ideals of parenthood or of social and moral duties.

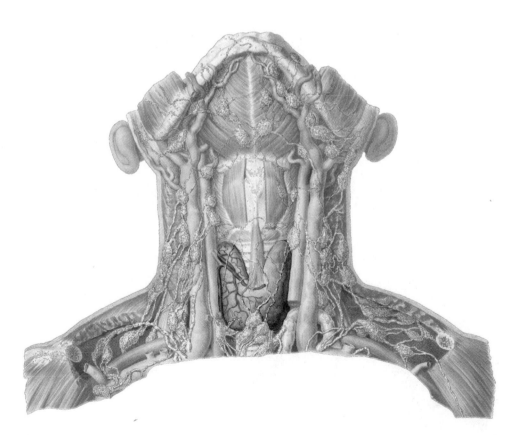

Consider building self-esteem, reducing fear, worry, and stress, releasing the need for perfection, letting mother and father be mere humans with all their quirks and foibles. Know that love is letting go of fear.

See also Colds and Flu, Coughing, and the introduction to the Cancer section.

Powerful Questions

When do I fail to speak up for myself?

How long has this been going on?

When did it start?

How do I feel about it?

What does "not standing up for myself" mean about me?

How important is what my mother/father thinks of me?

How important is what I think of me?

Suggested Blessings

May you realize that it is okay to be who you are right now, no matter what others might think.

May you realize that every feeling retrieved and embraced from the hidden recesses of your mind can serve to reduce the power of cancer.

May you experience the self-respect gained from feeling and releasing all your feelings.

Suggested Affirmations

Right now, I fully accept myself as I am.

No matter what my current limitations are, I love myself as I am and embrace the hope that I can improve in body, mind, and spirit.

I matter.

"No" is an important word for me.

I release all beliefs that keep me from owning and feeling any and all of my human emotions.

I express all my feelings with harm to no one.

Cardiovascular Disease

Heart Disease

Evidence-Based Confidence Level and Therapeutic Potential

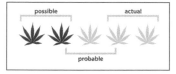

Total Number of Studies Reviewed: 7

CHI Value: 16

The human heart is about the size of a fist. It has four chambers, which it uses in a particular sequence to move blood throughout the entire body. It beats an average of 70 times per minute or more than 100,000 times a day for the duration of a lifetime. It keeps blood flowing constantly, thus taking care of the basic needs of the trillion or so cells that make up each human body.

The heart is a unique muscle that gets its own nourishment from three main vessels called the coronary arteries. In Western medicine's model, when one or more of these coronary arteries is slowly or suddenly blocked (as in the case of a blood clot) or gradually narrows (as in the case of atherosclerosis, a build-up of plaque), the heart muscle begins to ache. If not corrected, this "ache" can progress to tissue death called a myocardial infarction or heart attack. The size of the infarct determines survivability. In 2007, the Centers for Disease Control publicized a report identifying heart disease as the leading cause of death in the U.S., with more than 600,000 victims that year.[1]

Other common causes of damaged hearts or contributing factors include high blood pressure, metabolic syndrome (insulin resistance), excess weight, drug use (especially "uppers" such as cocaine, crack, methamphetamines), stress (especially chronic stress), mineral imbalances, pharmaceutical drugs including those designed to prevent irregular heartbeats, surgical procedures such as bypass or angioplasty, build-up of toxins (such as lead, mercury, etc.), and degeneration from chronic overexposure to free radicals. Whatever the underlying sudden or chronic cause for acute heart pain, in orthodox medicine it boils down to a lack of oxygen. Allopathic treatments include supplemental oxygen, pharmaceuticals, emergency interventions, and surgery.

Cannabis and Heart Disease

In 2004, researchers from Fukuoka City, Japan, reported that the cannabinoids CBN and THC significantly reduced heart attack size in mice. Interpretation of the study data indicated that the neuroprotective effects of THC were mediated via CB1 receptors.[2]

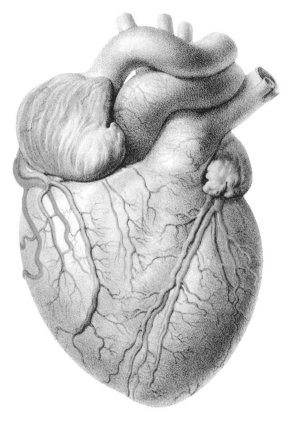

Researchers in Ramat-Gan, Israel (2006), developed a laboratory experiment in part to learn more about THC's mechanism for producing this cardioprotective effect. Results suggested, in a sense, that THC protects heart cells against damage from hypoxia by induction of nitric oxide. THC prepares the heart cells to better withstand hypoxia. The Israeli scientists confirmed that THC has a beneficial effect on the cardio-vascular system during stress conditions.[3]

Discoveries in the same year from Montreal further established the groundwork for a better scientific understanding of the role cannabinoids play in protecting the heart from damage. First, endocannabinoid receptors CB1 and CB2 naturally reside in heart tissue. Second, "This endogenous cardiac canna-binoid system is involved in several phenomena associated with cardio-protective effects." These phenomena include a reduction of infarct (heart attack) size after induced ischemia (restriction of blood flow and oxygen). Third, cannabinoids exert direct cardioprotective effects, which were con-firmed both in vivo and in vitro. The Canadian authors concluded: "Thus, the endogenous cardiac cannabinoid system, through activation of CB2 receptors, appears to be an important mechanism of protection against myocardial (heart muscle) ischemia."[4]

News from Jerusalem (2007) suggested that cannabidiol (CBD) could have significant cardioprotective effects from ischemia and infarct in rats. The authors wrote: "Inasmuch as CBD has previously been administered to humans without causing side effects, it may represent a promising novel treatment for myocardial ischemia."[5]

In 2007 researchers from the island nation of New Zealand conducted a meta-analysis (a review of studies on a topic) of the influence of cannabinoid drugs on the heart. The study revealed that cannabinoids positively influence ". . . vasodilation, cardiac protection, modulation of the baroreceptor reflex in the control of systolic blood pressure, and inhibition of endothelial inflammation and the progress of atherosclerosis. . . ."[6]

A Brazilian research team discovered (2009) that cannabidiol (CBD) calms autonomic responses to stress, such as rapid heart rates, by engaging receptors that select serotonin to achieve such down-regulation (calming effect).[7]

A Geneva study (2009) of trauma or chronic illness in brain and nervous system tissues showed that CB2 activation might also protect ischemic (oxygen-starved) heart cells during angina pectoris or myocardial infarctions (heart attack).[8]

Study Summary

Drugs	Type of Study	Published Year, Place, and Key Results	CHI
Injection of CB2 agonist JWH-133	Animal study (mice)	2009—Geneva, Switzerland: Reduction of infarct size and oxidative stress.[8]	2
Injected cannabidiol (CBD)	Animal study (rats)	2009—São Paulo, Brazil: Cannabidiol (CBD) reduced all stress responses such as anxiety, high blood pressure, and rapid heart rate.[7]	2
Cannabinoid drugs	Meta-analysis	2007—Dunedin, New Zealand: Endocannabinoid receptors are involved in vasodilation, cardiac protection, control of systolic blood pressure, inhibition of endothelial inflammation, and the progress of atherosclerosis.[6]	4
Cannabidiol (CBD)	Animal (rats) and laboratory	2007—Jerusalem, Israel: CBD induces a substantial in vivo cardioprotective effect from ischemia.[5]	2+1
Endocannabinoids and synthetic cannabinoids	Animal study (rats and mice)	2006—Montreal, Canada: Synthetic cannabinoids exert direct cardioprotective effects.[4]	2
THC	Laboratory study	2006—Ramat-Gan, Israel: THC protects cardiac cells against hypoxia.[3]	1
CBD and THC	Animal study (mice)	2004—Fukuoka City, Japan: CBD and THC significantly reduced heart attack size.[2]	2

Total CHI Value 16

Strain- and Form-Specific Considerations

Pre-clinical trials proved that cannabinoids (whether plant, synthetic, or endogenous) have cardioprotective properties. Additionally, research highlighted a yet unknown mechanism for the delivery of CBD's protection.[9]

Sativas and indicas activate CB1 and CB2 receptors; however, indicas or indica-heavy hybrids tend to possess a higher content of the non-psychoactive CBD than do sativas. Raw, fresh leaf or leaf juice contains significantly higher amounts of CBD-acid than heated or processed plant matter does.

Another way to stimulate CB2 receptors, without psychoactive effects, is to ingest plants known to contain significant amounts of the dietary cannabinoid (E)-BCP (See "Let Food Be Thy Medicine," below.)

Mind-Body Medicine and Heart Disease

"From the beginning of our understanding of coronary heart disease, psychological variables have been thought to play an important etiological (causative) role."[10] Researchers who hoped to learn more about this interplay of emotion and heart disease devised a two-fold approach. One involved a meta-analysis of studies correlating emotions with heart disease; the other enrolled 255 medical students, measured their hostility scores, and followed them over a period of 25 years.

Results of the medical student study indicated that those individuals prone to hostility, competitiveness, and impatience were likely to experience "... an attitude which would tend to make one distrustful of and isolated from others."[11] And the higher their hostility scores, the higher their incidence of developing coronary heart disease later in life. The first meta-analysis study also confirmed these conclusions.

Ann Arbor researchers followed 696 men and women between the ages of 30 and 69. During a 17-year period, they examined the relationship between anger-coping responses (suppressive or expressive) and mortality. Results showed that both men and women who suppressed their anger had significantly higher blood pressure, higher rates of cardiovascular disease, and a lower life expectancy.[12]

Two other significant studies examined the effects of suppressed and harbored anger on the development of heart disease. Significant co-factors in coronary mortality included both proneness to anger[13] and suppressed anger.[14]

Besides the tangible connection of unexpressed emotions or propensity to negative affect, researchers discovered one other significant emotional connection. In a 1996 study from Berkeley, California, hopelessness emerged as a predictor in developing ailments such as heart disease and cancer.[15]

A study titled "Is the Glass Half Empty or Half Full?" presented another emotional aspect in the context of developing heart disease. Studying 1,306 males during a 10-year period, researchers discovered that optimism might protect against the risk of coronary heart disease in older men.[16]

While scientifically a heart attack is measured by the size of the infarct, mentally/emotionally it might be measured by a person's reservoir of suppressed emotions and their frequency of responding with negative affect.

In summary, aggravating factors may include negative affect, hostility, competitiveness, impatience, distrust, isolation, suppressed anger, proneness to anger, pessimism, and hopelessness.

Healing may be supported by optimism, tendency for positive affect, emotional release work, feeling all feelings, a sense of humor, love, trusting life, trusting those who are trustworthy, transcending hopelessness, and strong will or determination.

Powerful Questions

What do I think of feelings, period?

What feeling(s) do I tend to avoid?

Which feeling do I have to avoid at all cost?

Where am I afraid to love?

What story or definition of belief is my fear of love connected to?

Where do I believe in punishment?

Where am I hard-hearted with myself?

Where am I hard-hearted with others?

What is unforgivable?

If I cannot forgive the what, can I forgive the why?

How else do I block the flow of my love?

Suggested Blessings

May you learn to love the natural function of your heart: to feel.

May you erase your fear of emotion.

May all hard-heartedness melt away as you feel your feeling.

May you experience the joy of the emotional ebb and flow of life.

Suggested Affirmations

The rhythm of my heart is calm yet strong, bold, and beautiful.

I embrace all my human emotions.

I release all fears.

I feel connected with all humans through the knowledge that we share a capacity for any and all emotions.

Warning: If You Or a Loved One Experiences Any of These Signs and Symptoms, Especially in Combination, Call 911 Right Away.

- Chest pains
- Nausea, sometimes with vomiting
- Weakness
- Sweating
- Pale skin

- Shortness of breath
- Dizziness
- Palpitations (feeling of skipped beats)
- Fainting
- Confusion, altered mental state

Let Food Be Thy Medicine

Acacia ∾ Cacao ∾ Cardamom ∾ Coconut ∾ Garlic
Ginger ∾ Nigella Rosemary ∾ Saffron ∾ Turmeric
(E)-β-Caryophyllene-Containing Spices

Acacia: A study from Riyadh, Saudi Arabia, suggests that gum Arabic/acacia contains cardioprotective properties in the form of superoxide scavengers, which are potent antioxidants.[17]

Cacao: Scientists at the McGill University School of Dietetics and Human Nutrition, Quebec, Canada, cautiously suggest that the consumption of dark chocolate may have a protective impact on heart and vascular illness, and protect against bad cholesterol (LDL).[18]

Cardamom: Scientists from the city of Mysore, India, discovered that cardamom extract protects platelets (blood particles) from aggregation (clotting) and lipid peroxidation (breakdown of fat-like molecules); both may play a part in the development of cardiovascular disease.[19]

Coconut: Researcher Hans Kaunitz correlated data from several laboratory animal studies with findings from the United Nations. He reported that death from ischemic heart disease is lowest where coconut fat intake is highest.[20]

Garlic: Garlic is one of Cuba's most versatile herbs, used for the treatment of peripheral signs and symptoms relevant to heart disease such as water retention, spasms, thrombophlebitis, inflammations, viral infections, and hypertension. Garlic can be used as an overall tonic and to promote healthy veins.[21]

The German Commission E approved garlic as a treatment supportive of dietary measures aimed at reducing elevated levels of lipids in blood and as a preventative measure for age-dependent vascular changes.[22]

For the first time, Japanese researchers have scientifically proven what many traditional practitioners have suspected: garlic, or specifically allicin, contains potent antioxidant properties.[23]

Another Japanese study suggested that odorless garlic powder might play a beneficial role in preventing destructive thrombus (clot) formation such as in heart attacks. Apparently it suppresses the formation of clots by destroying fibrin, a protein involved in the clotting of blood.[24]

A Singapore study determined that S-allylcysteine, an organosulphur-containing compound produced from garlic, offers protection in myocardial infarction (heart attack).[25]

Ginger: Scientists from Jinan, China, reported that components of ginger protect the epithelium (tissue lining inside the arteries) when it is exposed to an environment resulting from a high-fat diet. This rodent-based study confirmed that ginger reduced thickening of the arterial wall as measured by intima-media thickness of the aorta.[26]

Nigella: Two kinds of cardiac hypertrophy exist. One is pathological and produces a variety of heart problems; the other is physiological, usually brought on by regular exercise, and enhances overall heart function. King Faisal University scientists from Dammam, Saudi Arabia, discovered that rats, when fed 800 mg/kg of black seed *(Nigella sativa)* during a two-month period, developed physiological cardiac hypertrophy. This is the first such study to date that examined nigella's potential for overall heart function and health.[27]

Rosemary: In an experiment from Taichung Hsien, Taiwan, scientists concluded that "... rosemary is an excellent multifunctional therapeutic herb; by looking at its potentially potent antiglycative bioactivity, it may become a good adjuvant medicine for the prevention and treatment of diabetic, cardiovascular, and other neurodegenerative diseases."[28]

Saffron: The authors of this study from Tsinghua University, Beijing, China, suggest that *Crocus sativus L.* or saffron can be used to cure coronary heart disease and hepatitis, and to promote immunity.[29]

Turmeric: In a meta-study scientists provide an overview of decade-long scientific studies on turmeric. They summarize a long list of turmeric's potential therapeutic properties: cancer and diabetic preventative, a cancer treatment, promoter of wound-healing, therapeutic agent in Alzheimer's, Parkinson's, cardiovascular and pulmonary diseases, arthritis, adenomatous polyposis (multiple polyps in the large intestines—a precursor to colon cancer), inflammatory bowel disease, ulcerative colitis (colon inflammation with ulcers), atherosclerosis, pancreatitis, psoriasis, and chronic anterior uveitis (inflammation of the middle layer of the eye).[30]

(E)-β-Caryophyllene: Orally administered (E)-β-caryophyllene produced strong anti-inflammatory and analgesic effects in animal studies. (E)-β-caryophyllene or (E)-BCP is a FDA-approved dietary plant-cannabinoid that activates CB2 receptor sites and initiates potent anti-inflammatory actions and protection from oxidative stress, both potential underlying factors in heart disease.

Spice plants known to contain significant amounts of (E)-BCP include (in descending order): Black "Ashanti Pepper" *(Piper guineense)*, White "Ashanti Pepper" *(Piper guineense)*, Indian Bay-Leaf *(Cinnamomum tamala)*, Alligator Pepper *(Aframomum melegueta)*, Basil *(Ocimum micranthum)*, Sri Lanka Cinnamon *(Cinnamomum zeylanicum)*, Rosemary *(Rosmarinus officinalis)*, Black Caraway *(Carum nigrum)*, Black Pepper *(Piper nigrum)*, Basil *(Ocimum gratissimum)*, Mexican Oregano *(Lippia graveolens)*, and Clove *(Syzygium aromaticum)*.

Hypertension
Evidence-Based Confidence Level and Therapeutic Potential

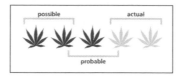

Total Number of Studies Reviewed: 2
CHI Value: 5

Approximately 24% of U.S. adults have high blood pressure or hypertension.[1] Orthodox medicine has no cure for hypertension, nor has it yet to fully understand hypertension's genesis. What we do understand is just how damaging, how dangerous, how deadly it can be, contributing to blindness, kidney failure, heart attacks, strokes, and brain aneurysms. It's as though 24% of Americans keep running red lights at busy intersections and nobody can quite manage to figure out why.

Before we examine high blood pressure let's have a brief look at what blood pressure actually is. Two basic factors determine blood pressure: the amount of blood inside the body and the size of the blood vessels. Smooth muscles, which line the larger blood vessels, regulate blood pressure by expansion or contraction. Blood pressure naturally changes many times during the day in response to different stimuli such as emotions, temperature, or level of physical activity. For instance, when we are getting ready to run a 100-meter race our pressure increases in advance to meet the increased demand for blood, oxygen, and nutrients to the prime muscle groups involved in completing our task. Similarly, when we argue with a spouse and emotions flare up, so does our blood pressure. Conversely, when we sit down to eat a meal, the pressure adjusts downward, as it does when we lie down for a nap. Natural and temporary changes, up or down, are normal and a healthy part of life.

Thus, blood pressure is a necessity of life. However, sustained high blood pressure can be serious in two forms, the chronic and the acute. Both can contribute to all those serious medical conditions, such as heart attacks and strokes we've already mentioned, and many, many others.

While it hasn't really figured out the root causes, modern medicine has identified several observable mental-emotional and physical co-factors.

These include family history, obesity, poor diet, smoking, alcohol abuse, physical inactivity, arteriosclerosis (hardening of the arteries), age, chronic stress, depression, anxiety, insulin resistance, and diabetes.

According to modern medicine, "normal" pressure is 120/80. However, optimal pressure is not clearly defined. Some people are happy and healthy with either lower or slightly higher numbers. However, The Seventh Report of the Joint National Committee on Prevention, Detection, Evaluation, and Treatment of High Blood Pressure suggests that: "The risk of coronary vascular disease, beginning at 115/75 mm Hg, doubles with each increment of 20/10 mm Hg."[2]

The two numbers reflect the pressure that blood exerts against the walls of the arteries as the heart contracts and relaxes, respectively. The more blood the heart moves and the tighter your arteries, the higher your blood pressure rises.

Many patients with chronic but mild or even moderate hypertension demonstrate no signs or symptoms until many years later. When symptoms do appear, they may include dizziness, headaches, blurred vision, nausea, or vomiting.

Orthodox treatment is limited to lifelong pharmaceutical management and intervention during acute phases.

Cannabis and Hypertension

Cannabis has been a folk remedy for hypertension for as long as people and the plant have coexisted. And now, scientific revelations are beginning to provide us with answers to why it works. The presence of endocannabinoid receptors called non-CB1 and non-CB2 in the cells that line arterial blood vessels strongly suggests the system's involvement in balancing and maintaining a healthy blood pressure. And while research into these receptors is in its infancy, other cannabinoid receptors (CB1 and CB2) have been examined and measured in patients with hypertension.

More specifically, researchers from the Glaucoma Clinic at Howard University Hospital in Washington, DC (1976), were the first to look at the relationship between blood pressure and tetrahydrocannabinol (THC), the psychoactive ingredient in cannabis. Results of their study revealed that patients responded to the inhalation of THC with an increase in heart rate (when compared to the control group) followed by a substantial drop in blood pressure (both systolic and diastolic) as well as a drop in intraocular (eye) pressure (relevant to people suffering from glaucoma). Scientists also noted that the increase in heart rate allowed the body to maintain adequate perfusion (cardiac output) while lowering both blood and intraocular pressures in a parallel fashion—potentially good news for patients with hypertension.[3]

An animal trial from the University of Nottingham Medical School, Queen's Medical Centre, Nottingham, UK (2009), conducted on rats, discovered that intravenously administered anandamide (a naturally occurring cannabinoid often referred to as the body's own THC) lowered blood pressure in hypertension but did not affect rats with normal blood pressure. Anandamide achieved the pressure-lowering effects through increased vasodilatation.[4]

Both the Nottingham and the Washington, DC, studies indicated that the plant-based cannabinoid THC and the endocannabinoid anandamide mutually lowered blood pressure without compromising overall perfusion or triggering the commonly associated side effects.

Study Summary

Drugs	Type of Study	Published Year, Place, and Key Results	CHI
Intravenous endocannabinoid anandamide & synthetic cannabinoids WIN55,212-2	Animal study (rats)	2009—University of Nottingham Medical School, Nottingham, UK: Endocannabinoid anandamide and the synthetic cannabinoid WIN55,212-2 lowered high blood pressure through vasodilatation.[4]	2
2.8% THC inhalation	Human clinical trial	1976—Howard University Hospital, Washington, DC: Reduction in blood pressure and intraocular pressure while maintaining adequate perfusion.[3]	3

Total CHI Value 5

Strain- and Form-Specific Considerations

The body's own cannabinoid, anandamide, the synthetic cannabinoid WIN55,212-2, and the plant-based cannabinoid THC have been tested in the context of hypertension. Study results showed that each of these cannabinoids achieved a drop in blood pressure via vasodilation.

Anandamide and THC bind with CB1 and CB2 relatively equally, while synthetic WIN55,212-2 has a higher affinity for CB2 than the CB1 receptors. Cannabinoid research supports the implication of both CB1 and CB2 in activating vasodilation.[5]

Sativas and indicas contain cannabinoids that bind with CB1 and CB2. Indicas and indica-heavy strains present with a lower THC:CBD ratio, thus favoring CB2 expression.

Raw, fresh leaf or juice contains non-psychoactive CBD acid also favoring CB2 activation.

For those wishing to further stimulate non-psychoactive CB2 activation, consider plants known to contain significant amounts of the dietary cannabinoid (E)-BCP (see "Let Food Be Thy Medicine" at the end of this section on hypertension).

Mind-Body Medicine and Hypertension

The physicians Grace and Graham at the New York Hospital–Cornell Medical Center (1952) were the first to study a link between attitude and hypertension. In their publication the scientists wrote: "Arterial hypertension occurred when an individual felt that he must constantly be prepared to meet all possible threats." Typical statements were: "I had to ready for anything. . . . Nobody is ever going to beat me; I'm ready for everything. . . . It was up to me to take care of all the worries."[6]

Scientists from the U.S. Centers for Disease Control and Prevention, Atlanta, GA (2000), conducted a long-term experiment on 3,310 initially normotensive and chronic disease-free persons. During a period of 22 years, doctors measured and recorded participants' blood pressure. Each participant cooperated in evaluations using two basic emotional scales— the "Relaxed vs. Anxious" scale (GWB-A), which assesses nervousness, stress, strain, pressure, anxiety, worry, and tension, and the "Cheerful vs. Depressed" scale (GWB-D),[7] which assesses unhappiness, sadness, discouragement, hopelessness, and lack of cheerfulness. After adjusting for co-factors, the analysis revealed that those participants rating high on depression and anxiety developed hypertension at a rate greater than those who rated high on the relaxed and cheerfulness ends of the scales.[8] These results confirmed anxiety and depression as predictive signs for the future development of hypertension.[9]

Another large population study conducted by a team from numerous U.S. universities (published in the *Journal of the American Medical Association,* 2003) on 3,308 adults between the ages of 18 and 30 shared similar findings at 15-year follow-ups. These researchers concluded that tendencies for impatience and hostility suggested a future risk for developing hypertension.[10]

Another study from the University of Texas (2006) enrolled 2,564 Mexican Americans aged 65 and older and evaluated possible correlations between primary measures of blood pressure values and a positive emotion score. Results suggested that subjects were less likely to be hypertensive if they identified with the feeling that "I am just as good as other people," felt happy, felt hopeful about the future, and enjoyed life.[11] Echoing these results, a Harvard study entitled "Positive Emotion and Health: Going Beyond the Negative" discovered an association between higher levels of curiosity and hope with the decreased likelihood of hypertension.[12]

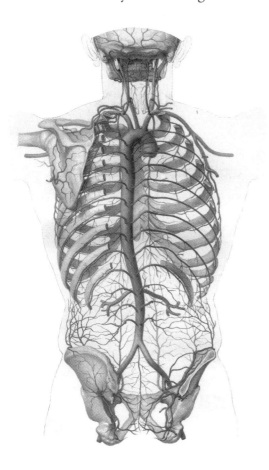

The orthodox medical tradition acknowledges effects of certain emotional stressors such as fear, anxiety, and depression. These emotions trigger the release of adrenalin, which in turn speeds up the heart and signals the smooth muscles in the arteries to constrict, thus increasing blood pressure.

Furthermore, in the chronically stressed state, the same adrenal glands that discharge adrenalin also release corticosteroids. Unchecked release of corticosteroids weakens the immune system, making the patient more vulnerable to other diseases. The increased hormonal (adrenalin) and steroidal impact on the body can lead to a host of problems including sexual dysfunction, muscle spasms and/or hair loss. Each of these consequences can develop into reasons for more stress, fueling the vicious cycle.

Preventive measures such as dietary changes, stress reduction (meditation, noise reduction, dimming of lights, breathing techniques, watching an aquarium), appropriate exercise, quitting smoking, and reducing heavy alcohol use have all proven to significantly assist in reducing hypertension.

However, release from chronically constricting emotions such as fears, anxieties, worries, stress, strain, impatience, hostility, and harbored or suppressed anger may be a more lasting solution to hypertension as root causes are identified and transcended.

In summary, aggravating factors may include anxiety, nervousness, stress, strain, pressure, anxiety, worry, unhappiness, sadness, discouragement, hopelessness, lack of cheerfulness, impatience, hostility, and constant threat perceptions.

Conversely, consider working on feeling okay about oneself, feeling happy, feeling joyful, feeling hopeful about the future, and stimulating hope and curiosity.

Powerful Questions

What family-related pressure am I aware of?
Which fears are my constant companions?
How long have I had them?
Where did they come from?
Why am I maintaining them?
What definitions or beliefs are they rooted to?
Why won't I release these roots?
What positive effects do I derive from these roots?
Can I replace these effects with something else so I can let go of the root?
What am I going to plant instead?

Suggested Blessings

May our flowers assist you in rooting out your fears, anxieties, and the stressors of the unresolved and unforgiven.
May an inner ease reign supreme.

Suggested Affirmation

I can replace all definitions and beliefs that cause me fear. Only I can replace them.

A CASE STUDY ON REPRESSED EMOTIONS AND HYPERTENSION
(FROM CORNELL MEDICAL CENTER)

Not every case of hypertension can be connected to measurable propensity for negative affect. An additional perspective is demonstrated by the case of a 43-year-old African American woman who suffered from chronic and severe hypertension with complications that could not be controlled, even with aggressive pharmaceutical interventions.[13] There was no reported stress or distress other than that associated with her blood pressure. Despite employing multiple blood pressure medications for about a decade, her hypertension remained dangerously uncontrollable.

Then, after an apparently normal conversation with her nephew, she began experiencing recurring nightmares. She dreamed that a man was approaching her from behind and grabbing her, which caused her to wake up screaming. She was terrified to go to bed. Her physician asked if she had ever been attacked. Hesitantly, the patient reported that since the nightmares' onset, she had started to recall fragmented memories of rape by her uncle. She remembered telling only her father, who promised, "I'll take care of it, baby." He never did. The rapist had long since left the family. She had suppressed the episode for 30 years until her now-grown nephew, who resembled her uncle, triggered the emergence of the event.

In the past she had remembered bits and pieces of the rape but felt only numb and detached. Now, however, she was very agitated recalling the event and kept repeating: "He hurt me, he hurt me." She agreed to counseling and after several sessions also revealed that her abusive ex-husband attempted to strangle her while her father, whom she adored, was present but did nothing to protect her. In subsequent sessions, the emotional intensity of her memories strengthened. For the first time, the patient reported feeling powerlessness, betrayal, and rage at her uncle and her father. By processing her emotions, she started to identify first as a victim, and then as a survivor. By ending her own silence about the abuse she had suffered, she took back some of her own power. With new energy and insight, she was then able to explore how best to protect herself as a self-aware adult.

These changes were followed by a dramatic and sustained improvement in her blood pressure. Over a period of 18 months, her blood pressure returned to normal, and there was no recurrence of nightmares despite a gradual reduction of pharmaceuticals.

Let Food Be Thy Medicine

Bush Tea ∾ Cacao ∾ Caraway ∾ Garlic
(E)-β-Caryophyllene-Containing Spices

Bush Tea: A study from Karachi, Pakistan (2006), determined why bush tea (rooibos or red tea) is effective in treating hyperactive gastrointestinal problems, respiratory difficulty, and high blood pressure. Bush tea is a bronchodilator and antispasmodic with blood pressure-lowering properties. It apparently achieves this by potassium (ATP) channel activation with a selective bronchodilatory effect.[14]

Cacao: Scientists at the McGill University School of Dietetics and Human Nutrition in Quebec, Canada (2007), cautiously suggest that the consumption of dark chocolate may have a protective impact on heart and vascular illnesses and their connections to oxidized bad cholesterol (LDL).[15]

A meta-analysis of similar studies from Köln, Germany (2007), looking at dietary intake of cacao and the reduction in blood pressure, suggests that food rich in cacao may contribute to a reduction of high blood pressure.[16]

Caraway: North African traditional healers from Fez, Morocco, use caraway as a diuretic for patients experiencing water retention, difficulty passing urine, and in some cases high blood pressure. Through an animal study (2007), Moroccan scientists determined that caraway does possess strong diuretic properties,[17] which apparently work similarly to the commonly used anti-hypertensive pharmacological drugs Lasix and Hydrochlorothiazide.

Garlic: Garlic is one of Cuba's most versatile herbs, used for the treatment of peripheral signs and symptoms relevant to heart disease, such as decreased water retention, spasms, thrombophlebitis, inflammations, viral infections, and hypertension. It is used as an overall tonic and promoter of healthy veins.[18]

In 1994 the German Commission E approved garlic as being "supportive to dietary measures at elevated levels of lipids in blood. Preventative measures for age-dependent vascular changes."[19]

For the first time, Japanese scientists from Kyorin University (2006) were able to scientifically prove what many traditional practitioners have suspected—garlic, or specifically allicin, contains potent antioxidant properties.[20] Another study from Kurashiki Sakuyo University, Japan (2007), suggests that odorless garlic powder can play a beneficial role in preventing destructive thrombus (clot) formation, such as in heart attacks. Apparently it suppresses the formation of clots by destroying fibrin, a protein involved in blood clotting.[21]

(E)-β-Caryophyllene: (E)-β-Caryophyllene or (E)-BCP is a FDA-approved dietary plant-cannabinoid that activates CB2 receptor sites, which have been shown to be involved in the modulation of blood pressure, inflammation, and oxidative stress common in patients with hypertension. Spice plants known to contain significant amounts of (E)-BCP include (in descending order): Black "Ashanti Pepper" *(Piper guineense),* White "Ashanti Pepper" *(Piper guineense),* Indian Bay-Leaf *(Cinnamomum tamala),* Alligator Pepper *(Aframomum melegueta),* Basil *(Ocimum micranthum),* Sri Lanka Cinnamon *(Cinnamomum zeylanicum),* Rosemary *(Rosmarinus officinalis),* Black Caraway *(Carum nigrum),* Black Pepper *(Piper nigrum),* Basil *(Ocimum gratissimum),* Mexican Oregano *(Lippia graveolens),* and Clove *(Syzygium aromaticum).*

Stroke (Cerebrovascular Accident or CVA)
Evidence-Based Confidence Level and Therapeutic Potential

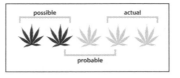

Total Number of Studies Reviewed: 3

CHI Value: 8

A stroke (cerebrovascular accident or CVA) is a loss of brain function. There are two types of strokes: ischemic and hemorrhagic. In an ischemic stroke, an obstruction (thrombosis, embolism) prevents blood from reaching the brain cells on the other side of the obstruction; thus, it blocks oxygen and may cause tissue damage or death. A hemorrhagic stroke, which results from a ruptured blood vessel causing blood leakage, produces the same consequences.

Epidemiological and clinical studies have identified common modifiable and non-modifiable predictors or co-factors in the development of stroke.

Modifiable co-factors include alcohol abuse, smoking, inactivity, diabetes, obesity, and hypertension, while non-modifiable co-factors include age, race, and hereditary factors.

Depending on the size of the stroke and where it occurs, the loss of certain brain function may be limited and self-correcting, as in transient ischemic attacks (TIA), or it can be massive (CVA), involving loss of major motor function. A massive stroke may cause complete flaccidity in one half of the body. High blood pressure is considered the main contributing factor in stroke. A stroke in the lower parts of the brain, which regulate heartbeat and breathing, can rapidly lead to death. Therefore, time is of great importance. The sooner an effective treatment begins, the fewer brain cells will die.

Allopathic treatment of an ischemic stroke includes either thrombolysis, where doctors use pharmaceuticals (anticoagulants and thrombolytics) to break the clot apart, or a thrombectomy, a mechanical means to remove the clot. Hemorrhagic stroke cannot be treated by anticoagulants and thrombolytics as they might exacerbate the bleed. Instead, doctors may opt for surgery to relieve pressure caused by the leaking blood. The majority of fatal strokes are hemorrhagic strokes, and presently there is no way to fix a leaking blood vessel in the brain. However, since the symptoms of both types of strokes are basically the same, perhaps the biggest challenge for the treating physician is determining which type of stroke occurred.

Signs and symptoms may come and go, especially in TIAs. However, in a massive stroke, they are usually sudden and noticeable. Symptoms in massive strokes include headache, nausea, vomiting, slurred speech, expressive aphasia (not finding proper words), dizziness, blurred vision, unequal grips or facial expressions, weakness on one side of the body, numbness, ataxia (inability to walk), high blood pressure (or history of hypertension) altered mental status (confusion, irritability, aggression), loss of consciousness, incontinence and/or drooling.

If you notice symptoms of stroke, call 911 or visit the nearest emergency room. Clearly, the first hour following the onset of symptoms is crucial. To get the most out of the limited allopathic treatment options currently available, it helps to immediately start the process of differentiating the underlying type of stroke, followed by the appropriate treatment.

Cannabis and Stroke

In 2003, the U.S. federal government issued itself a patent on a newly found property of cannabis making it "...useful in the treatment and prophylaxis of a wide variety of oxidation-associated diseases, such as ischemic,

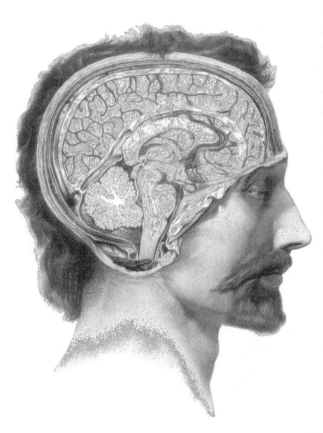

age-related, inflammatory, and auto-immune diseases. Cannabinoids have particular application as neuroprotectants, for example in limiting neurological damage following ischemic insults, such as stroke and trauma, or in the treatment of neurodegenerative diseases, such as Alzheimer's disease, Parkinson's disease, and HIV dementia."[1]

Researchers from Fukuoka, Japan, further elucidated the U.S. government's patented findings on the plant's neuroprotective properties. Examining strokes in animals, scientists compared the effects of two cannabinoids (THC and CBD). The discoveries offered promise. THC treatment administered prior to a stroke in mice reduced the resulting infarction, which was measured at intervals up to 3 days. Even more promising, cannabidiol treatment offered before and after resulted in potent and long-lasting neuroprotection. Scientists concluded: "Cannabidiol provides potent and long-lasting neuroprotection through an anti-inflammatory CB(1) receptor-independent mechanism, suggesting that cannabidiol will have a palliative action and open new therapeutic possibilities for treating cerebrovascular disorders."[2]

The same team of scientists from Fukuoka also concluded that 24 hours after the induced stroke in mice, THC significantly increased the expression of CB1 receptors in both the striatum and cortex but not in the hypothalamus (responsible for body temperature regulation). These and other observations led the team to conclude that THC prevents stroke by producing a lower body temperature independent of the hypothalamus.[3] These findings describe a new mechanism of body temperature control.

The U.S. government's patent on the neuroprotective properties of cannabinoids presents a scientific foundation for the use of cannabinoids in patients with stroke. If the Japanese results can be confirmed in humans, cannabinoids, especially cannabidiol, may one day be used as neuroprotective agents in patients prone to stroke as well as a first-line drug treatment in patients with an acute stroke.

Study Summary

Drugs	Type of Study	Published Year, Place, and Key Results	CHI
THC and CBD	Animal study (mice)	2007—Fukuoka, Japan: Increased CB1 receptors in striatum and cortex, but not in hypothalamus. THC is neuroprotective when given before CVA. Cannabidiol is neuroprotective when given before and after CVA.[2]	2
THC and CBD	Animal study (mice)	2007—Fukuoka, Japan: THC prevents stroke by reducing body temperature not mediated via the hypothalamus; cannabidiol provides potent and long-lasting neuroprotection through an anti-inflammatory CB(1) receptor-independent mechanism.[3]	2
Cannabinoids	Meta-analysis	2003—United States government: Cannabinoids neuroprotective in stroke.[1]	4

Total CHI Value 8

Strain- and Form-Specific Considerations

The results of these pre-clinical studies suggest the possibility that THC is neuroprotective before a stroke; that CBD is neuroprotective when used before and after a stroke; and that CBD may provide neuroprotection independently of the currently known cannabinoid receptor system. CBD has a higher affinity for CB2, while THC binds relatively equally to CB1 and CB2. Clinical trials conducted on humans will ultimately prove whether or not the pre-clinical results translate directly to the human condition.

Both basic strains provide biologically active full-spectrum cannabinoid and non-cannabinoid plant materials. Indicas and indica-heavy hybrids contain a lower THC:CBD ratio favoring CB2 expression when compared to sativas or sativa-heavy strains.

Raw, fresh leaf or juice contains non-psychoactive CBD-acid at higher concentrations, thereby increasing CB2 activation.

Mind-Body Medicine and Stroke

A multi-institutional study from Texas involving 2,478 elderly people studied participants during a period of six years. They were asked to fill out questionnaires (see the following CES-D scale questions[4]) prompting yes or no answers leading to indicative feelings or symptoms during each preceding week.

Those who scored higher on reporting "negative feelings" were significantly associated with an increase in stroke, while those who scored higher on "positive feeling" seemed to be protected against stroke.[5] (See also the story of Jill Bolte Taylor on page 498.)

"I felt that I could not shake off the blues even with help from my family and friends."

"I felt depressed."

"I thought my life had been a failure."

"I felt fearful."

"I felt lonely."

"I had crying spells."

"I felt sad."

"I was bothered by things that usually don't bother me."

"I did not feel like eating; my appetite was poor."

"I had trouble keeping my mind on what I was doing."

"I felt everything I did was an effort."

"My sleep was restless."

"It seemed that I talked less than usual."

"People were unfriendly."

"I felt that people disliked me."

"I could not get going."

The remaining items made up the positive-affect measure. A high score on this scale indicated positive affect. Researchers concluded that positive affect seems to play a role in protecting against stroke in older adults.[6]

"I felt that I was just as good as other people."

"I felt hopeful about the future."

"I was happy."

"I enjoyed life."

Powerful Questions

What is my blood pressure trying to tell me?

Where am I hard and inflexible?

Where do I resist change?

Where am I consistently or deadly stubborn?

What belief or definition fuels my stress?

The brain is divided into two hemispheres (halves). While both halves can generally complete all tasks, each side varies in its strengths. The right half of the brain governs the left side of the body associated with intuition, art, focus on the big picture, creativity, and emotion (considered female characteristics). The left half of the brain governs the right side of the body associated with logic, language, reason, focus on detail, and analytical thinking (considered male characteristics). In cases of one-sided loss of function, patients are helpless. Patients are confined to bed because their other half is gone. The affected half is lifeless, simply being lugged along by the healthy side. In such instances, it appears that the body is a mirror for the mind's routine of numbing or ignoring the male or female side.

Which side was taken from me?

What is my relationship to my male/female characteristics?

Did I judge, hate, or ignore those characteristics?

Where am I a one-sided person?

Can I make peace with my lost side and breathe new life into it?

What am I going to use to build my new other half?

Stroke survivors face many developmental tasks. They must re-learn how to speak, do, and think. They will be different than their former selves.

Suggested Blessings

May you ease the pressure in your body and your mind.

May you relax and release all that is stubborn and inflexible.

May you protect both halves of your brain.

May you integrate your previously hidden or oppressed half and emerge
more balanced and anew.

Suggested Affirmations

Life is change, and I can relax by choosing to believe that I can handle whatever comes my way. I trust life.

I am part of life and I trust myself.

Let Food Be Thy Medicine

Bush Tea ∾ Cacao ∾ Garlic ∾ Ginger
(E)-β-Caryophyllene-Containing Spices

Bush Tea: A study from Karachi, Pakistan, determined why bush tea (rooibos or red tea) is effective in treating hyperactive gastrointestinal problems, respiratory difficulty, and high blood pressure. Bush tea is a bronchodilator and antispasmodic, with blood pressure-lowering properties. It operates by potassium (ATP) channel activation with a selective bronchodilatory effect.[7]

Cacao: Scientists at the McGill University School of Dietetics and Human Nutrition, Quebec, Canada, cautiously suggest that the consumption of dark chocolate may have a protective impact on heart and vascular illness and their connection to oxidized bad cholesterol (LDL).[8]

Garlic: Garlic is one of Cuba's most versatile herbs, used for the treatment of peripheral signs and symptoms relevant to heart disease such as water retention, spasms, thrombophlebitis, inflammations, viral infections, and hypertension. It is also considered an overall tonic and promoter of healthy veins.[9]

The German Commission E approved garlic as being "supportive to dietary measures at elevated levels of lipids in blood. Preventative measures for age-dependent vascular changes."[10]

For the first time, Japanese scientists were able to scientifically prove what many traditional practitioners have suspected—that garlic, or specifically allicin, has potent antioxidant properties.[11]

Another study from Japan suggests that odorless garlic powder can play a beneficial role in preventing destructive thrombus (clot) formation such as in heart attacks. Apparently it suppresses the formation of clots and destroys fibrin, a protein involved in the clotting of blood.[12]

Ginger: Scientists from Jinan, China, have shown that components of ginger protect the epithelium (tissue lining inside the arteries) when it is exposed to an environment resulting from a high-fat diet. This rodent-based study confirmed that ginger reduced the thickening of the artery wall as measured by intima-media thickness of the aorta.[13]

(E)-β-Caryophyllene: (E)-β-Caryophyllene or (E)-BCP is a FDA-approved dietary plant-cannabinoid that activates CB2 receptor sites, which have been shown to be involved in the modulation of blood pressure, inflammation, and oxidative stress common in patients with hypertension. Spice plants known to contain significant amounts of (E)-BCP include (in descending order): Black "Ashanti Pepper" *(Piper guineense),* White "Ashanti Pepper" *(Piper guineense),* Indian Bay-Leaf *(Cinnamomum tamala),* Alligator Pepper *(Aframomum melegueta),* Basil *(Ocimum micranthum),* Sri Lanka Cinnamon *(Cinnamomum zeylanicum),* Rosemary *(Rosmarinus officinalis),* Black Caraway *(Carum nigrum),* Black Pepper *(Piper nigrum),* Basil *(Ocimum gratissimum),* Mexican Oregano *(Lippia graveolens),* and Clove *(Syzygium aromaticum).*

See also Heart Disease, Hypertension, and Inflammatory Diseases.

Diabetes Mellitus
Evidence-Based Confidence Level and Therapeutic Potential

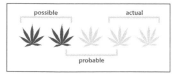

Total Number of Studies Reviewed: 6

CHI Value: 11

Ancient physicians used the Greek word *diabetes,* which translates as "fountain," due to their observation of frequent urination in diabetic patients (the body's natural means to rid itself of excess sugar). They also noticed that their urine tasted quite sweet, as evidenced by the many ants collecting about it. *Mellitus* derives from the Greek word for "honey"; thus, *diabetes mellitus.*

Diabetes is a disease related to the pancreas, a relatively small gland located behind the stomach and in front of the spine that opens into the duodenum (neck of the small intestine). Of all the glands in the endocrine system, the pancreas, along with the adrenals, sits directly in the body's center. The pancreas produces hormones such as insulin and glucagon as well as digestive enzymes that break down food into basic sugar molecules usable as food/energy by each cell of the human body.

Between the years 1958 and 1993, the number of diabetic patients in the U.S. increased five-fold.[1] Therefore, diabetes emerged as a major public-health concern of the twenty-first century. Still, the number of insulin-controlled diabetic patients varies greatly among different countries. "On average, less than one per 100,000 people in Shanghai, China, has diabetes; while, for example, whites in Allegheny County, Pennsylvania, have been diagnosed with diabetes at a rate 26 times higher. Populations in Finland fare even worse with a more than 50 times greater incidence of the disease."[2]

Orthodox medicine lacks a cure and has not yet located the exact origins of the illness. However, mainstream science considers a likely cause to be genetic predisposition in conjunction with some form of environmental trigger(s) or life stressor(s). One primary environmental cause is likely the emergence of industrial food production with its decline in nutrient densities and the widespread use of pesticides and hormones and/or modern food processing and storage methods that contain endocrine disruptors. Other potential causes include certain pharmaceutical drugs, infectious pathogens, lifestyle factors (poor diet, lack of exercise, chronic stress), or an overzealous immune system that turns on itself. Higher maternal age at birth or the lack or duration of breastfeeding are also cited as possible causes, particularly in cases of pediatric diabetes.

Alternatively, some researchers consider diabetes a metabolic disease involving cellular resistance to two specific hormones: insulin, which is produced by the pancreas, and leptin, which is made by adipose tissue (fat cells). Leptin signals the brain to reduce hunger. Leptin-sensitive people will feel satiated sooner and convert fat faster, while leptin-resistant individuals will eat longer and keep energy stored in fat.

Insulin tells individual cells when to turn fat or sugar into energy. Insulin-sensitive people easily convert fat and sugar into energy. In insulin-resistant people, cells do not get the message and the sugar remains poorly used, thus fat accumulates.

Other recent scientific discoveries suggest still another cause for the early genesis of diabetes—fatty livers. Some scientists propose that eating excessive or unhealthy sugar induces the liver to convert sugar into unhealthy types of fats, which are deposited in the liver, among other places. Fatty livers produce insulin resistance (metabolic syndrome) in both obese and healthy people alike, increasing the risk of cancer and heart disease. Evidence suggests that avoiding sugar and eating low-glycemic foods quickly rids the body of liver/abdominal fat, and insulin resistance disappears.

Traditionally, orthodox medicine categorizes diabetes into three kinds: Type I, Type II, and gestational diabetes. Type I diabetes was once called juvenile diabetes because it occurred mostly in children or adolescents. In Type I, the pancreas stops producing the hormone insulin. Without insulin the body cannot use the food life depends on, cellular sugar. Treatment in the orthodox paradigm consists of daily insulin injections, normally administered by the patients themselves.

Type II diabetes, or adult-onset diabetes, is the most common form of the disease. In Type II the pancreas does not produce enough insulin, or the body's cells are insensitive to the presence of insulin and ignore it. This prevents the body from converting sugar into energy. Early Type II usually does not require the use of insulin; modern medical practitioners generally prescribe oral pharmaceuticals instead.

Diabetes, especially Type I or advanced Type II, is potentially life-threatening. Complications diminish one's life expectancy and quality of life.

Gestational diabetes (diabetes that occurs during some pregnancies) most often self-corrects after delivery. While not very well understood, it is hypothesized that hormonal changes during pregnancy may produce a temporary resistance to insulin, thereby producing higher than normal blood sugar levels.

Early signs and symptoms of diabetes include frequent urination, sweet-smelling urine, and increased thirst and hunger. Over long periods of time, symptoms may progress to cold, pale, and clammy skin, altered levels of consciousness, unconsciousness, neuropathies, skin ulcers, peripheral vascular diseases, kidney problems, acute metabolic problems (diabetic ketoacidosis, hypoglycemia, diabetic coma, lactic acidosis), loss of vision, heart disease, stroke, infections, sepsis, and periodontal disease.

Diagnostic tools include a simple blood test used to measure sugar content. Measurements between 80 and 120 are considered normal. Orthodox disease management is limited to pharmaceutical treatments (oral or injections), nutritional and dietary recommendations, and lifestyle changes.

Cannabis and Diabetes

While cannabis oil has been used historically in the treatment of diabetes, and while many diabetic patients claim that cannabis lowers high blood sugar levels and stabilizes mood changes and mental irritability, to date no human studies have been conducted to examine the general effects of cannabinoids on diabetic patients. However, the known anti-inflammatory and immunomodulating properties of the plant have prompted the following experiments relevant in the context of diabetes.

Israeli scientists demonstrated a potential link between endocannabinoid receptor sites and diabetes. The Jerusalem studies (2006 and 2008) suggest that the cannabinoid cannabidiol (CBD) might possibly be a novel therapeutic agent for treatment of Type I diabetes.[3] An Edinburgh laboratory study (2009) discovered a synthetic cannabinoid's ability to grow nerve extensions in a glucose-rich environment, thus providing a basis for potentially novel neuroprotective drugs for diabetic patients.[4] Two U.S. studies from Augusta, Georgia (2006),[5] and East Lansing, Michigan (2001),[6] conducted on rodents demonstrated that the cannabinoids THC and CBD could reduce diabetic neuropathies. Scientists carrying out the Augusta study observed a reduction in retinal oxidative stress with an additional attenuation of autoimmune diabetes in the mice. A Polish research team (2008) learned more about the mechanism by which cannabinoids ease diabetic neuropathies (nerve pain), discovering that certain pharmaceutical medications (COX-1 inhibitors such as indomethacin) work synergistically to further ease such pains.[7]

Strain-Specific Considerations

In these studies, the synthetic cannabinoids WIN55,212-2, AM1241, and HU210 and the plant cannabinoids THC but especially CBD underwent testing relevant to diabetes.

WIN55,212-2 and AM1241 bind with higher affinity to CB2, while HU210 has a higher affinity for the CB1 receptors. THC binds relatively equally to CB1 and CB2, while CBD has a greater affinity for CB2.

Study Summary

Drugs	Type of Study	Published Year, Place, and Key Results	CHI
Synthetic cannabinoid HU210	Laboratory	2009—School of Life Sciences, Edinburgh Napier University, Scotland, UK: Neurite growth may play a therapeutic role in reversing neuropathies.[4]	1
CB-1 and CB-2 receptor agonists WIN55,212-2; Met-F-AEA; and AM1241	Animal study (mice)	2008—Department of Pharmacodynamics, Medical University of Warsaw, Poland: CB1 & CB2 agonists reduce sensitivity to pain in a dose-dependent fashion, and COX-1 inhibitors (e.g., indomethacin) may increase these cannabinoid properties at low dosages.[7]	2
Cannabidiol (CBD)	Animal study (mice)	2008—Department of Bone Marrow Transplantation and Cancer Immunotherapy, Hadassah Hebrew University Hospital, Jerusalem, Israel: CBD reduced the manifestations of diabetes and exhibited more intact islets of Langerhans than a control group.[3]	2
Cannabidiol (CBD)	Animal study (mice)	2006—Department of Bone Marrow Transplantation and Cancer Immunotherapy, Hadassah Hebrew University Hospital, Jerusalem, Israel: CBD treatment significantly reduced the incidence of diabetes in non-obese diabetic mice.[3]	2
Cannabidiol (CBD)	Animal study (rats)	2006—Multi-institutional Research Team, Augusta, Georgia: Rats treated with cannabidiol (CBD) experienced significant protection from developing diabetic retinopathy.[5]	2
Delta-9-THC administered orally in corn oil at 150 mg/kg for 11 days	Animal study (mice)	2001—Michigan State University, East Lansing: Delta-9-THC is capable of attenuating the severity of autoimmune diabetes in mice with the induced disease.[6]	2

Total CHI Value 11

Indicas and indica-heavy strains contain lower THC:CBD ratios, which tends to result in activation of both CB1 and CB2; but it initiates more CB2 than sativa strains do.

Mind-Body Medicine and Diabetes

Results from a Harvard study entitled "Positive Emotion and Health: Going Beyond the Negative" alluded to the role that emotions play in the genesis of diabetes. Scientists discovered an association of higher levels of curiosity and hope with a lower incidence of diabetes.[8]

Becoming an insulin-dependent diabetic poses a serious demand for change and forces a significant shift in lifestyle, with a focus on attention to details. The individual must now seriously monitor sugar levels, carefully determine when and how to nurture the body, and understand when and how to exercise. Depending on the progression of the disease, the patient must become sensitive to the early signals, subtle sensations, and internal experiences that indicate hypoglycemia if s/he wants to avert an acute event. The body plays out the core issues of diabetes. The patient appears locked in a constant struggle to gain access to the energy that fuels and sustains physical life.

In the diabetic patient, sugar is not converted into cellular energy, thus keeping individual cells from operating efficiently. As a result, a wide variety of diabetic symptoms ensue. In hyperglycemia, sugar remains suspended in blood, available but not utilized. In other words, there is plenty of food in the pantry but the key to the locked door—insulin—is missing. In severe cases of hyperglycemia, the patient initially presents with thirst and frequent urination, which when left untreated can progress to lethargy and confusion until s/he slips into a silent diabetic coma.

In the self-treating insulin-dependent diabetic patient, a delicate daily balance between insulin dose and measured blood sugar levels is essential to maintain healthy bodily functions. A simple error can quickly lead to too much insulin in the bloodstream, causing hypoglycemia, where sugar absorbs at such a rapid pace that too little remains for sustained cellular function. The hypoglycemic symptoms, including expressions of irritability, anger, confusion, and pale and very moist skin, often lead to a variety of expressions. These range from a quiet fury or rage to physical combativeness when approached by caregivers such as paramedics.

Thus, paradoxically, a diabetic person may be physically either too sweet or not sweet enough but at its cellular core in both cases exists a struggle to convert sugar or fat into life-sustaining energy or power. The central emotion observed in both hypoglycemia and hyperglycemia appears as a rage turned inward. This rage, focused on the center organ of the body, the pancreas, effectively renders the whole body useless in activating available power.

In the context of diabetes, rage is not simply louder anger. Rage is a complex and paradoxical emotion that can be empowering or disempowering; it can be destructive or instructive; it can be imprisoning or liberating. Rage can be a vicious enemy or a protective ally, and in the context of diabetes, it finds association with the inappropriate use of powers or unwillingness to be truly powerful.

In juvenile diabetes, the source of disempowering rage can often be traced to family power dynamics; in adult-onset diabetes, this disempowering rage is often connected to societal issues.

"Many patients believe that their diabetes has been caused by stress or an adverse life event."[9] When thinking back to the first appearance of diabetes, patients might recall experiencing "trigger events" such as the violation of deeply valued ideals, a defiling of one's sense of worth, the removal of power, or the crushing of one's spirit. There may have been a single event of great intensity or an onslaught of repeated events that caused damage over time.

In addition to the notion of trigger events, researchers have noted that interventions aimed at reducing family conflict and improving caregiver involvement garnered positive results in improving diabetes' outcome.[10]

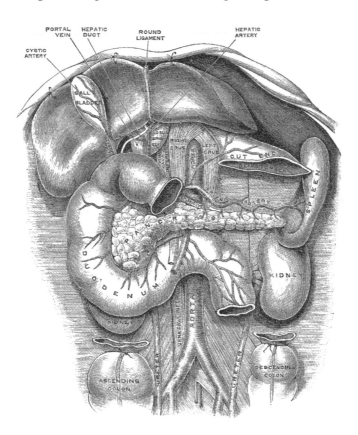

These beliefs and findings indicate that psychosomatic origins of diabetes likely occur in power dynamics involving conflict, anger, fury, resentment, and rage where the person feels hopeless and resigned or unable to change anything.

Power-Rage Dynamics: Lacking the will to be powerful or perceiving oneself as powerless may be a psychosomatic link to diabetes.

When a child must assume responsibilities that require adult powers, childhood ends prematurely. Intense longing for this stolen childhood and rage about having to be the grown-up in the family may result for the child or juvenile. Diabetes may emerge as an unconscious strategy to reclaim childhood. While it may work to shift the power-responsibility dynamic of the family, such a well-intentioned and initially helpful strategy, left unhealed, can ultimately evolve into a serious liability.

Alternatively, a caregiver may be over-reaching or actively suppressing growth, age-appropriate responsibility, and emerging power of the developing child/person in an attempt to retain control, driven by fear of losing them. Sick and unable to attend school or having diabetes may be a child's attempt to provide a troubled parent with the control they seek.

Nature automatically takes the body from infancy through adolescence and into adulthood. However, the maturing of the mind is a process involving conscious growth, engagement, and work. Rage at having to do this work is a rage directed at the source of life itself. The refusal to be responsible and the implicit entitlement in "I should not have to do this work" emerge in the diabetic expression of not wanting to utilize the energy or power to be responsible for one's own growth and well-being.

When a person in a position of power demands blind loyalty from others, or when a subordinate provides blind loyalty to an unprincipled or unscrupulous leader, a fertile and vast breeding ground unfolds for abusive behavior or the condoning of abuse. While both will have a reason or justification for such a misuse of power, neither will truly be able to utilize the available powers, strengths, or talents inherent in every human, including their own.

Somewhere hidden in this depth of rage, patients can discover root beliefs from which such rage was born. Examples may include: power cannot be trusted; power corrupts; I am safe when I am powerless; I cannot be trusted with power; I am resigned to letting others have power; others cannot be trusted with power.

In summary: Hypoglycemia—not sweet enough (being hard on self, believing that one is undeserving). Hyperglycemia—being too sweet (over-caring, helping others but suffering to do so).

Consider developing a caring that does not involve personal suffering. For example, gratitude makes it difficult to be hard on oneself, feel undeserving, to over-care, or to help others while suffering. Embrace hope and curiosity.

See also Pain/Neuropathies.

Powerful Questions

Think back: what was going on when you first started to have symptoms?

Was there a feeling of loss for a private treasure (self, power, value, self-worth)?

Which treasures does my rage hold for me?

What have I given to my rage?

Where am I too sweet with an abusive person?

Where can I not speak truth to power?

In what situation am I a "yes" wo/man?

How can I respond consciously and constructively to the power in my family?

How can I express my rage (fury, resentment, anger) constructively but without hurting anyone?

What are my feelings about receiving nourishment from others?

How do I feel about nourishing myself?

Do I want to nurture myself?

Does this power/rage apply to me?

If so, how can I answer the power/rage dynamic?

How do I feel about nurturing myself with constant attention to details?

Suggested Blessing

May you find your answer to the paradox of rage.

Suggested Affirmations

I am worth every loving attention to detail.

I am able to heal.

I am willing to heal.

I deserve to heal.

I can take responsibility for my health and well-being.

I love myself in every single cell of being and as a whole organism just as I am right now.

Power is a force for good when informed by ideals and guided by the constant application of principles.

Let Food Be Thy Medicine

Cacao ∾ Caraway ∾ Cayenne ∾ Cinnamon ∾ Clove ∾ Cumin
Garlic ∾ Ginger ∾ Nutmeg ∾ Oregano ∾ Rosemary ∾ Turmeric
(E)-β-Caryophyllene-Containing Spices

Cacao: Although traditional practitioners use cacao in their work with diabetic patients, cacao's exact working mechanism remains a mystery. However, University of Putra scientists in Selangor, Malaysia, have confirmed that cacao extract may indeed possess dose-dependent hypoglycemic and hypocholestrolemic properties.[11]

Caraway: Moroccan scientists from the city of Errachidia determined in animal-based studies that caraway could lower blood sugar levels without increasing the body's production of insulin.[12]

Cayenne: Fat- and sugar-balancing effects of cayenne (among other herbs) have been documented at the Johann Wolfgang Goethe University in Frankfurt, Germany. Results of this study suggest a rationale for the use of cayenne in diabetic treatment.[13]

Doctors from Bangkok, Thailand, noted an increase in metabolic rates and a slowing of sugar (glucose) uptake after giving 5 gm each of fresh cayenne to a group of women. This, in turn, may provide scientists with an appreciation for traditional healers worldwide who use cayenne as a means to treat certain forms of diabetes.[14]

Cinnamon: Canadian researchers have determined that cinnamon may be a valuable candidate for new antidiabetic medications.[15] The spice is widely used in Ayurvedic medicine in the treatment of diabetes. Studies from Tamil Nadu indicate that cinnamon contains hypoglycemic and hypolipidemic properties[16] and improves glucose metabolism.[17]

Clove: Scientists at Vanderbilt University School of Medicine in Nashville, Tennessee, explored clove because it has insulin-like effects, which may prove beneficial in the treatment of diabetes.[18] The data revealed that clove, much like insulin, stimulates a certain gene sequence expression and thereby sets in motion chemical reactions important in effective sugar metabolism.

Cumin: A meta-analysis from Mysore, India, conducted animal and clinical trials to determine that cumin, among other select spices, contains beneficial antidiabetic food adjuncts.[19]

Garlic: Scientists at the Russian Academy of Medical Sciences conducted a live double-blind, placebo-controlled study on 60 Type II diabetic patients.[20] Using time-controlled garlic powder tablets, they found that garlic produced improved metabolic control in patients due to lowered blood glucose and triglyceride levels. These scientists now recommend garlic in conjunction with dietary control and other measures in the treatment of adult-onset diabetes. Scientists believe that garlic helps make glucose and fat metabolism more efficient, thereby contributing to the prevention of long-term complications such as heart attacks.

Ginger: Scientists in Safat, Kuwait, examined the effectiveness of ginger to alleviate diabetic rats' inability to break down sugar and convert it to usable energy. They discovered that ginger dosed at 500 mg/kg could lower blood glucose, cholesterol, and triacylglycerol levels when compared to the control group of rats not receiving the treatment.[21]

Research from Durban, South Africa, supports the time-proven use of ginger by traditional African healers as an effective means to treat painful and chronic arthritic inflammatory conditions and to achieve better metabolic control in patients with Type II adult-onset diabetes.[22]

Nutmeg: Korean scientists from Yusong-gu explored the use of an isolated nutmeg extract in the treatment of Type II diabetes and obesity. They discovered that the extract inhibited a certain protein expression, thereby enhancing insulin signals inside the cells.[23]

Oregano: Endocrinologists in Errachidia, Morocco, examined the potential of a water-based extract of oregano as a therapeutic agent in treating hyperglycemia. They found, in an animal model, that the extract could reduce sugar levels without increasing blood insulin concentrations.[24]

Rosemary: University scientists from Taichung Hsien, Taiwan, concluded that "... rosemary is an excellent multifunctional therapeutic herb; by looking at its potentially potent antiglycative bioactivity, it may become a good adjuvant medicine for the prevention and treatment of diabetic, cardiovascular, and other neurodegenerative diseases."[25]

Turmeric: In this meta-study, scientists from Dallas, Texas, provided an overview of decades of scientific studies on turmeric. Researchers summarized a long list of turmeric's potential therapeutic properties, including as a diabetic and pancreatitis preventative.[26]

(E)-β-Caryophyllene-containing spices: Researchers suggest that activation of CB2 receptors via (E)-β-caryophyllene-containing spices may present a new and additional therapeutic strategy in the treatment of a multitude of diseases associated with inflammation and oxidative stress; both are underlying factors in diabetes.[27] This dietary cannabinoid is approved by the U.S. government (FDA). Key (E)-β-caryophyllene-containing organic spices are relatively easy to obtain. Spices that contain β-caryophyllene include (in descending order): West African Black "Ashanti Pepper" *(Piper guineense),* White "Ashanti Pepper" *(Piper guineense),* Indian Bay-Leaf *(Cinnamomum tamala),* Alligator Pepper *(Aframomum melegueta),* Basil *(Ocimum micranthum),* Sri Lanka Cinnamon *(Cinnamomum zeylanicum),* Rosemary *(Rosmarinus officinalis),* Black Caraway *(Carum nigrum),* Black Pepper *(Piper nigrum),* Basil *(Ocimum gratissimum),* Mexican Oregano *(Lippia graveolens),* and Clove *(Syzygium aromaticum).*

Improve Cellular Fat and Sugar Metabolism Naturally

- Eat foods with a low glycemic index.
- Avoid toxic sugars: aspartame (NutraSweet®), sucralose (Splenda® and Splenda® Essentials, a newer form of Splenda® dressed up as a health food with added vitamins, fiber, minerals), saccharin (Sweet'n Low®), and high-fructose corn syrup. Agave nectar is *not* a traditional, natural, low-glycemic sugar, despite being marketed as such. It is a highly processed chemical product to be avoided.
- Use healthy sugars such as fructoligosaccharides (FOS) or stevia.
- Organic honey and maple syrup can be used in very small dosages. While they are natural sweeteners, both have a high glycemic index and as such require a significant amount of insulin to digest.

Eye Disease and Eye Function
Age-Related Macular Degeneration
Evidence-Based Confidence Level and Therapeutic Potential

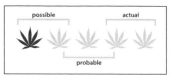

Number of Studies Reviewed: 1

CHI Value: 1

This painless eye disease is characterized by loss of accurate sight in the center of the field of vision. Most common in seniors, age-related macular degeneration is due to damage of the retina (the tissue lining the inner surface of the eye). It exists in wet or dry forms. Orthodox medicine has no cure and does not know the exact mechanism causing the disease's development. Possible causes include aging, family history, plaque build-up, high glycemic index food consumption, high blood pressure, smoking, and damage from oxidative stress.

Signs and symptoms may include but are not limited to drusen (tissue build-up on the eye), sudden loss of visual accuracy, blurred vision, and loss of central vision. The disease will not cause blindness, and many people learn to function with peripheral vision alone. However, patients might lose the ability to drive or see faces. Various treatments exist. The more orthodox of these involves injections of pharmaceutical agents directly into the eye. Presently scientists are testing experimental treatments using stem cells. In addition, natural treatments currently practiced include dietary changes and nutritional supplements such as lutein, carotenoids, and omega-3 fatty acids.

Cannabis and Age-Related Macular Degeneration

Researchers widely agree that cannabinoid receptors are present in nerve cells. The endocannabinoid system plays an important role as a potential therapeutic agent in neurodegenerative diseases. However, until 2009, it remained uncertain whether receptors existed in human retinal pigment epithelial cells and, more importantly, what role they might play in age-related macular degeneration.

Results from a study in Shanghai, China (2009), showed that retinal pigment epithelial cells indeed contain cannabinoid receptors CB1 and CB2. In fact, these researchers note that the presence of cannabinoids triggers a cellular response in retinal pigment epithelial cells in such a way as to significantly protect them from oxidative damage, considered one of the possible causes of age-related macular degeneration.[1]

Study Summary

Drugs	Type of Study	Published Year, Place, and Key Results	CHI
Cannabinoid receptors and one enzyme responsible for endocannabinoid hydrolysis, fatty acid amide hydrolase (FAAH)	Laboratory test	2009—Department of Ophthalmology, Ruijin Hospital, Shanghai Jiaotong University School of Medicine, Shanghai, People's Republic of China: Retinal pigment epithelial cells contain CB1 & CB2. Cannabinoids may protect the retina from oxidative stress—one of the causes of age-related macular degeneration.[1]	1

Total CHI Value 1

Strain-Specific Considerations

Retinal pigment epithelial cells contain CB1 and CB2 receptors. Sativas and indicas, as well as their varied hybrids, contain cannabinoids that will activate CB1 and CB2.

Powerful Questions

What is at the center of my life that I do not want to see?
Why do I want to focus only on the periphery of my world?
Why do I not want to see your face?
What is going to happen if I see clearly?
What don't I want to see?
Might I have difficulty facing you on an emotional level?

Suggested Blessing

May a pristine focus and crisp clarity inform everything you see.

Suggested Affirmation

I can create a life that is wondrous to see no matter what perspective I choose.

Let Food Be Thy Medicine

Oxidative Stress Reduction: Acacia ∾ Cacao ∾ Cinnamon ∾ Clove Cumin ∾ Fennel ∾ Ginger ∾ Oregano ∾ Turmeric

Acacia: Gum Arabic/acacia protects from oxidative stress by means of superoxide scavengers (potent antioxidants).[2]

Cacao: University Hospital doctors from Zürich highlight the antioxidant properties of cacao, among other therapeutic effects.[3]

Cinnamon: An Indian study from Mysore revealed that a cinnamon fruit powder water extract contains potent antioxidant properties.[4]

Clove: Scientists from Vienna discovered more about the mechanism by which the essential oil of clove's potent antioxidant properties work.[5]

Cumin: A study from Andhra Pradesh, India, compared the antioxidant activity of aqueous extract of cumin with that of ascorbic acid (vitamin C). Researchers determined that cumin scavenges superoxide radicals while inhibiting lipid peroxide and hydroxyl radicals to perform the same tasks.[6]

Fennel: Researchers examined the antioxidant properties of fennel in an animal experiment from Afyon, Turkey.[7]

Ginger: Indian scientists from Mysore determined that ginger protects the body by multiple means, including scavenging of free radicals (i.e., ginger contains strong antioxidants).[8]

Oregano: Scientists from the Department of Pharmacology and Biochemistry at the University of Medicine, Varna, Bulgaria, conducted studies following the model of traditional Bulgarian herbalists. Using a tea preparation of oregano, they discovered that it has a high phenolic content as well as significant antioxidant properties.[9]

Turmeric: Based on the evidence of numerous laboratory and animal trials, scientists from Vandoeuvre-Lès-Nancy, France, contend "... that curcumin plays a protective role in numerous diseases; its therapeutic action being on the prevention or modulation of inflammation and oxidative stress."[10]

In a meta-study from Dallas, Texas, scientists gave an overview of decades of scientific studies on turmeric. They summarize a long list of turmeric's potential therapeutic properties, including protection from chronic anterior uveitis (inflammation of the middle layer of the eye).[11]

Glaucoma
Evidence-Based Confidence Level and Therapeutic Potential

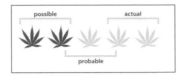

Total Number of Studies Reviewed: 9

CHI Value: 19

Glaucoma can be classified as a group of eye diseases in which vision can be partially or completely lost, sometimes without warning. Early glaucoma patients may not even be aware of the disease's progress. Ultimately, glaucoma damages the optic nerve leading from the eye to the brain, resulting in partial or complete blindness. While other factors may play a role in the disease's development, chronic or acute increased intraocular pressure is commonly present, although some glaucoma patients maintain normal intraocular pressure. Normally aqueous humor (fluid inside the eye) flows through channels to maintain eye health and function. In glaucoma patients this fluid becomes blocked.

Allopathic medicine has neither a cure for glaucoma nor the ability to restore lost vision due to glaucoma. Instead, doctors focus on surgery and prescription medications to slow the disease's progression. While glaucoma is commonly observed in the senior population, it may develop at any age.

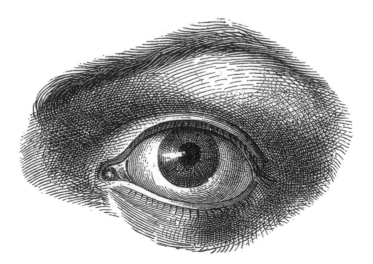

Statistically, people over 40, those with a family history of glaucoma or vision problems, diabetic patients, and people taking corticosteroid prescription medications are at increased risk for glaucoma. In addition, the following ethnic groups are at increased risk: African American, Hispanic, Inuit, Irish, Japanese, Russian, and people of Scandinavian descent.

Symptoms may include loss of peripheral vision, red sclera (white of eye), loss of visual acuity, eye aches, tunnel vision, or (in some cases) nausea and vomiting.

To diagnose glaucoma, an ophthalmologist (eye doctor) will test vision and then examine the eyes after administering a medicated eye drop that dilates the pupil.

Cannabis and Glaucoma

Cannabis has been part of traditional medicine's treatment of eye disease for millennia. Most historical Materia Medicas include cannabis prescriptions for the treatment of eye problems. Of late, the discovery of ocular cannabinoid receptors has stimulated a new round of ophthalmic cannabinoid research. Potential areas of investigation include the neuroprotective properties of cannabinoids, the stimulation of neural microcirculation, and the suppression of both apoptosis (cell death) and damaging free-radical reactions.

Modern scientists showed interest in cannabis in 1971 when it was first noted in scientific literature that smoking marijuana lowered intraocular pressure. In this first study, modern researchers enlisted 11 healthy youths to smoke 2 gm of cannabis with a 0.9% THC content provided by the National Institute for Mental Health. Prior to and one hour following smoking cannabis, complete ocular examinations were performed, and a substantial decrease in intraocular pressure was observed in 9 of 11 subjects.[1]

A 1976 Washington, DC, study further examined the impact of THC. It revealed that patients responded to the inhalation of 2.8% THC with an increase in heart rate (when compared to a control group), followed by a substantial drop in blood pressure (both systolic and diastolic), and a drop in intraocular pressure. Scientists also noted that increased heart rate allowed the body to maintain adequate perfusion (cardiac output) while lowering both blood and intraocular pressures in parallel fashion.[2] Risk versus benefit analyses were conducted between 1977 and 1998. These studies concluded that intraocular pressure (IOP) follows a parallel course to that of arterial blood pressure. While some scientists considered an increased heart rate an adverse effect, other researchers considered it a balancing mechanism protecting the patient from the effects of hypotension (low blood pressure).

New insights emerged from an animal study in Louisville, Kentucky (2000). Results indicated that the reduction of IOP is mediated by CB1 cannabinoid receptors in the eye itself, and that the synthetic cannabinoid WIN55,212-2 (like natural cannabinoids) can also reduce IOP.[3] Scientists at Oxford followed this work in 2006 with a randomized, double-blind, placebo-controlled, four-way crossover human study on patients with increased intraocular pressure (ocular hypertension). Subjects received a single dose of 5 mg Delta-9-THC, or 20 mg CBD, or 40 mg CBD, or a placebo. The authors wrote: "A single 5-mg sublingual dose of Delta-9-THC reduced the IOP temporarily and was well tolerated by most patients. Sublingual administration of 20 mg CBD did not reduce IOP, whereas 40 mg CBD produced a transient increase IOP rise."[4] The apparent differing effects of isolated cannabinoids may point to the complex yet synergistic mechanisms by which these cannabinoids naturally combine to achieve therapeutic effects.

In Aachen, Germany (2007), scientists gave THC in the form of Marinol to healthy physicians to test its impact on blood circulation of the eye, as well as its effect on intraocular pressure (IOP). Two hours after ingestion, the drug reduced IOP and retinal arteriovenous passage time. The authors concluded that this effect may be beneficial in ocular circulatory disorders, including glaucoma.[5]

Strain-Specific Considerations

The majority of clinical studies have examined the impact on glaucoma of cannabinoids primarily in the form of THC. THC binds relatively equally with both CB1 and CB2. Both sativas and indicas contain CB1- and CB2-binding cannabinoids.

Mind-Body Medicine and Glaucoma

A Yale University School of Medicine study conducted on seven glaucoma patients and a healthy control group concluded that hypnosis could be an important tool in reducing objective and subjective symptoms of glaucoma. All patients showed a significant reduction in intraocular pressure. Subjective

Study Summary

Drugs	Study Subjects	Published Year, Place, and Key Results	CHI
THC as Marinol (7.5 mg)	8 healthy physicians	2007—RWTH Aachen University, Department of Ophthalmology, Aachen, Germany: THC reduced intraocular pressure and improved blood circulation of the eye.[5]	4
Single daily dose of one of the following: 5 mg Delta-9-THC, 20 mg CBD, 40 mg CBD, or placebo	6 patients with increased intra-ocular pressure	2006—Department of Ophthalmology, Aberdeen Royal Infirmary, School of Medical Sciences, Institute of Medical Sciences, University of Aberdeen, UK: Dose-specific therapeutic effect (5 mg THC by mouth).[4]	5
Synthetic cannabinoid 1WIN55,212-2	Animal study (rabbits)	2000—Department of Pharmacology and Toxicology, University of Louisville School of Medicine, Louisville, Kentucky, U.S.: WIN55,212-2 also reduces intraocular pressure, and IOP reduction is mediated by CB1 cannabinoid receptors in the eye.[3]	
Smoked cannabis v. cannabinoids	Discussion/analysis	1998—Department of Ophthalmology, Medical College of Georgia, Augusta, U.S.: Benefits do not outweigh adverse effects.[6]	0
Topical solution of 0.05% and 0.1% THC in light mineral oil	6 glaucoma patients	1981—Smoked THC lowers occular and systolic pressure. Topical treatment ineffective.[7]	3
Smoked cannabis	18 glaucoma patients	1980—Increased heart rate, decreased blood pressure, and IOP with side effects.[8]	0
2.8% THC inhalation	Human clinical trial	1979—Glaucoma Clinic at Howard University Hospital, Washington, DC: Reduction in blood pressure and intra-ocular pressure while maintaining adequate perfusion.[2]	3
THC intravenously. Two strengths were used—0.022 mg/kg of body weight and 0.044 mg/kg of body weight	10 people with normal IOP	1977—Increased heart rate (22% to 65%), decreased IOP (average 37%).[9]	0
2 gm inhaled cannabis (THC 0.9%)	A group of 11 healthy youthful subjects	1971—Substantial decrease in intraocular pressure observed in a large percentage of subjects.[1]	3

Total CHI Value 19

improvements were reported as follows: fewer headaches, less tearing, feeling generally more relaxed, and sleeping better. The authors suggested that "these findings serve to emphasize the significant role of the emotions in glaucoma, although the mechanisms involved remain obscure."[10]

In glaucoma, the fluid of the eye is under too much pressure with no release in sight.

In summary, consider emotional pressure building up over long periods of time.

Healing factors may include forgiving oneself for the iron-willed determination to hold on to emotional baggage.

Powerful Questions

What tears have I refused to shed?
What past hurt is still in need of healing?
What am I refusing to release?
Where can I apply forgiveness to bring about release?

Suggested Blessings

May you find a way to ease all that is hard and stubborn in you.
May old hurts be released and be replaced by a present love.

Suggested Affirmation

May the salt and substance of my tears bring gentle relief, tenderness, and freedom from the hurts of the past.

Let Food Be Thy Medicine

See "Let Food Be Thy Medicine" in the sections on Hypertension (under Cardiovascular Disease) and Age-Related Macular Degeneration (under Eye Disease and Eye Function).

Improved Night Vision
Evidence-Based Confidence Level and Therapeutic Potential

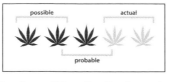

Number of Studies Reviewed: 1

CHI Value: 3

A team of international researchers from the United States, Spain, and Morocco "... have documented (2004) an improvement in night vision among Jamaican fishermen after ingestion of a crude tincture of herbal cannabis, while two members of this group noted that Moroccan fishermen and mountain dwellers observe an analogous improvement after smoking kif, sifted *Cannabis sativa* mixed with tobacco *(Nicotiana rustica)*." To field-test these anecdotal reports, researchers devised a placebo-controlled double-blind trial using volunteers. Volunteers were given either placebo or oral THC in the form of Marinol or smoking kif. Improvements in night vision were noted after the ingestion of THC and after the smoking of kif. The authors write: "It is believed that this effect is dose-dependent and cannabinoid-mediated at the retinal level. Further testing may assess possible clinical application of these results in retinitis pigmentosa or other conditions."[1]

Study Summary

Drugs	Study Subjects	Published Year, Place, and Key Results	CHI
Marinol (THC) 20 mg and smoked kif	4 healthy subjects	2004—International research team: Improved night vision.[1]	3

Total CHI Value 3

Mind-Body Medicine and Improved Night Vision

Deep relaxation increases parasympathetic tone and with it the dilation of the pupils, allowing more light to enter.

Uveitis
Evidence-Based Confidence Level and Therapeutic Potential

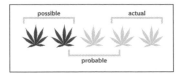

Total Number of Studies Reviewed: 3

Total CHI Value: 6

This disease is an inflammation of the uvea (the middle layer of the eye). Uveitis is primarily defined by which side of the uvea is affected. Anterior uveitis (aka iritis) refers to the inflammation being on the outermost side, while posterior uveitis (aka choroiditis) describes the affected inside layer. When both sides of the uvea are inflamed it is called pan-uveitis. No matter which form the illness takes, inflammatory cells can enter the gelatinous-like center of the eye and spread. In most case scenarios the infection occurs suddenly and spreads quickly. Uveitis can affect one or both eyes and depending on cause can be infectious or non-infectious.

Symptoms may include pain, redness, blurriness of the eye, photophobia (light is unpleasant), the presence of floaters (dark spots seem to float in your field of vision), and headaches.

The illness is poorly understood and can have serious consequences such as blindness. Orthodox medicine suggests that the disease is a secondary development due to certain underlying conditions including microbial infections (syphilis, herpes, TB), injuries to the eye, autoimmune diseases (e.g., sarcoidosis—a concentration or nodule of inflammatory cells), chronic inflammatory illnesses (e.g., Crohn's disease, IBS), pharmaceutical drugs (e.g., Rifabutin), or the presence of certain cancers (e.g., leukemia, lymphoma).

Diagnosis primarily includes a complete eye examination and laboratory test looking at possible underlying illness. Treatment, depending on underlying findings, often includes anti-inflammatory medication (e.g., cortisol), antibiotic or antiviral medication and/or surgery.

Cannabis and Uveitis

An animal experiment conducted at Dalhousie University in Halifax, Canada (2014), used a synthetic CB2 agonist to explore its influence on rats with toxin-induced uveitis. Results showed that CB2 receptors mediated therapeutic immune responses by reducing transcription factors (e.g., AP-1) and inflammatory mediators (e.g., cytokines). The study's authors suggest that "CB2 receptors may be promising drug targets for the development of novel ocular anti-inflammatory agents."[1]

An additional study from the Medical College of Georgia, Augusta, Georgia (2008), focusing on the deterioration of uveitis by oxidative stress, discovered that CBD exerts an anti-inflammatory and neuroprotective effect.[2] And, another experiment conducted on mice by the University of Aberdeen, UK, similarly confirmed a potent ability of CB2 activation on inflammation, but this time related to autoimmune uveoretinitis, suggesting broad therapeutic application potential in cases of uveitis.[3]

Study Summary

Drugs	Type of Study	Published Year, Place, and Key Results	CHI
Synthetic CB2 receptor agonist, HU308 (1.5% topical)	Animal study (rats)	2014—Department of Pharmacology, Dalhousie University, Halifax, NS, Canada: Activation of CB2 receptors was anti-inflammatory in a model of acute EIU and involved a reduction in NF-κB, AP-1 and inflammatory mediators.[1]	2
CBD	Animal study (rats)	2008—Department of Ophthalmology, Medical College of Georgia, Augusta, GA: CBD exerts anti-inflammatory and neuroprotective effects by a mechanism that involves blocking oxidative stress and activating p38 MAPK and microglia.[2]	2
CB2 agonist JWH-133	Animal study (mice)	2007—Department of Ophthalmology, School of Medicine, Institute of Medical Sciences, University of Aberdeen, Foresterhill, Aberdeen, UK: The cannabinoid agonist JWH-133 has a high in vivo, anti-inflammatory property and may exert its effect via inhibiting the activation and function of autoreactive T cells and preventing leukocyte trafficking into the inflamed tissue.[3]	2

Total CHI Value 6

Strain-Specific Recommendations

Combined these three studies suggest a broad therapeutic potential for CB2 rich strains.

Mind-Body Medicine and Uveitis

Depending on underlying cause, you may want to consult the sections in this book on inflammation, certain cancers (leukemia, lymphoma), or microbial infections (e.g., herpes).

Powerful Questions

What is irritating to see?

How do you feel about that irritation?

What hurts to see?

What is frustrating to see?

Where do these feelings take you?

What scenarios or memories are associated with these feelings?

What is the meaning (messages, unhealthy beliefs/attitudes, etc.) that you have given to that scenario?

Suggested Blessings

May you look upon the world anew with ease.

May you infuse your sight with gentleness, empathy, and compassion.

Suggested Affirmations

I can see clearly now.

I allow all irritation to be lifted so I can see clearly now.

I can look upon anything in balance and in harmony.

Fever/Temperature Regulation

Fever

Evidence-Based Confidence Level and Therapeutic Potential

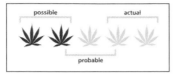

Number of Studies Reviewed: 2

CHI Value: 4

The body's temperature changes all the time. Things like clothing, exertion and exercise, environmental conditions, and hormonal changes (for example, during female menopause) can all affect the body's temperature.

A normal body temperature is generally considered to be about 37°C or 98.5°F; a mild fever between 99°F and 101°F; and a high fever above 103°F. Body temperatures above 42°C/108°F are potentially fatal.

The body's immune system induces fever in an attempt to rid itself of an invader. This invader could be as simple as a cold virus or as exotic as a malarial parasite. The body's rise in temperature is designed to destroy these invading armies of microbes while simultaneously recruiting production of the body's police force, the white blood cells. Therefore, fever is actually a good thing when it remains low and lasts only for a short time.

Most fevers tend to lessen in a day or two. If you have a fever for more than two days or higher than 101 degrees, consult a physician to find the underlying causes and to discuss an appropriate treatment plan. Remember, mild short fever can help in healing the body, but high fevers, especially long-term high fevers, can kill.

Warning

Aspirin is a common medication that people use quite effectively to treat minor pains and fevers. Salicin, the active ingredient in aspirin, was originally isolated from willow bark but is now produced synthetically. Long ago, willow bark was used as effectively and in the same way that we use aspirin today.

However, use caution when considering aspirin for young children and young adults (younger than 19 years). It is recommended to never give a child or adolescent aspirin or other medication containing salicin if they may have a viral infection such as a cold, flu, or other common childhood disease like chickenpox together with a fever. Why? Under those conditions salicin can be fatal to a child/young adult. It is called Reye's syndrome.

Reye's Syndrome

While the exact cause of Reye's syndrome remains unknown, it has been noted that a very high percentage of youngsters who develop the condition previously had taken aspirin (or other medications containing salicin) during a viral infection. Reye's syndrome is a potentially deadly condition that affects the liver and brain. Those who survive Reye's syndrome are often left physically and mentally handicapped.

Signs and symptoms of Reye's syndrome include nausea and vomiting, increased generalized weakness, bizarre behavior, altered mental status, acting as if drunk, loss of consciousness, and seizures.

Western medicine has no cure. Treatment is usually performed in intensive care units and is focused primarily on reducing swelling of the brain or preventing liver damage or a score of other potentially severe complications.

Febrile Seizures

A seizure may occur while a child of three months to four years has a fever.

The precise reasons for febrile seizures are not known. One hypothesis: When a child is born, the brain is not finished growing. During the subsequent months and even years, the brain and nervous system continue to expand and develop. However, the part of the brain responsible for temperature regulation in the body sometimes develops at a slower pace. Therefore, it is argued that during times of fever, an "overload" to the neurological system occurs, producing a seizure. Once the temperature-regulating part of the brain is fully developed, seizures during fevers cease.

What should you do when you have a child between three months and four years who suddenly has a seizure? Put the child on a bed or clean flat surface. Roll the child onto his side so as to avoid any mucus (spit) or vomit entering the lungs. Protect the child from hitting his head against the floor or other standing objects. Have someone call 911 immediately. In most places in the U.S., a paramedic should arrive within a few minutes. Most febrile seizures will stop by themselves in a few seconds or a few minutes.

An emergency-room definition for status epilepticus is continuous seizure activity lasting longer than five minutes, or multiple seizures without regaining consciousness between seizures. This is considered a true emergency. Status epilepticus is a potentially life-threatening condition in which the brain and by extension the entire nervous system enter into excessive nerve cell activity.

Cannabis and Seizures

To date, two studies exist examining the potential properties of cannabinoids relevant to fever genesis and pediatric fever-induced seizures. In 2006, Philadelphia scientists attempted to induce fevers by injecting rats with lipopolysaccharide, a component of the outer membrane of Gram-negative bacteria. Results showed that "... cannabinoids interact with systemic bacterial lipopolysaccharide injections and indicate a role of the CB1 receptor subtype in the pathogenesis of lipopolysaccharide fever."[1]

A 2007 study in Fukuoka, Japan, concluded that the endocannabinoid system, especially CB1, may regulate body temperature independently of the hypothalamus, which was previously assumed to be solely responsible for body temperature regulation.[2]

See also Neurological Diseases/Epileptic Seizures.

Study Summary

Drugs	Study Subjects	Published Year, Place, and Key Results	CHI
THC and cannabidiol	Animal study (mice)	2007—Department of Neuropharmacology, Faculty of Pharmaceutical Sciences, Fukuoka University, Fukuoka, Japan: Increased CB1 receptors in striatum and cortex, but not in hypothalamus. Indications that CB1 may play a role in fever.[2]	2
WIN55,212-2	Animal study (rats)	2006—Multi-institutional research team: CB1 may play a role in fever.[1]	2

Total CHI Value 4

Strain-Specific Considerations

THC binds with CB1 and CB2 relatively equally. CBD and WIN55,212-2 have a higher affinity for CB2.

Sativas or sativa-dominant strains tend to present with a higher THC: CBD ratio.

Mind-Body Medicine and Fever

The body commonly responds to an invasion of pathogens with a fever to "boil off" the pathogens. In cases of a mild invasion, a low-grade fever will suffice to regain health and well-being. If the threat is more serious, the body will try to meet the challenge by raising the temperature and extending the length of the fever.

However, in some cases a high fever may begin to depress the level of consciousness of the patient, produce hallucinations, seizures, loss of consciousness, and sometimes results in death.

It is as if a door to the unconscious has opened and unleashed a series of uncontrollable experiences similar to the physical response to microbial invaders. For instance, conflicting or opposing beliefs may generate invasive, intense, and paradoxical thoughts and emotions, thus creating overwhelming friction to a mind unprepared and without the skill set to release and transcend the tension constructively.

For more information, go to the section on Neurological Diseases—Epileptic Seizure and/or the introduction to the Cancer section, as well as "Cancer-Induced Night Sweats."

Fibromyalgia

Evidence-Based Confidence Level and Therapeutic Potential

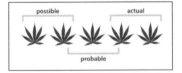

Total Number of Studies Reviewed: 3

CHI Value: 14

Fibromyalgia, an illness characterized by chronic pain combined with some form of psychiatric diagnosis, still lacks an observable underlying pathology. The disease picture of fibromyalgia usually includes widespread chronic pains in muscles and connective tissue, joint stiffness, general weakness, exhaustion, depression, anxiety, and insomnia. "Nearly 2 percent of the general population in the United States suffers from fibromyalgia, the majority of them being middle-aged females."[1]

No specific test exists to determine an exact diagnosis. Symptoms are often similar to those of rheumatism, osteoporosis, or arthritis. Physicians try to diagnose by process of elimination. Diagnostic criteria established by the American College of Rheumatology include the following: a history of diffused and chronic pains for more than three months and present in all four quadrants of the body, and the presence of pain in at least 11 of 18 specific trigger points.

Orthodox pharmaceutical treatment includes muscle relaxants, pain medication (opioids), antidepressants, anti-seizure medication, dopamine agonists, and cannabinoids.

Cannabis and Fibromyalgia

In 2007, researchers in Winnipeg, Canada, enrolled 40 fibromyalgia patients to measure the effects of Nabilone, a synthetic cannabinoid, on pain and quality of life. The results of this randomized, double-blind, placebo-controlled trial showed that "Nabilone appears to be a beneficial, well-tolerated treatment option for fibromyalgia patients, with significant benefits in pain relief and functional improvement."[2]

While most studies have focused on using cannabis for the treatment of fibromyalgia pains, another randomized, double-blind, placebo-controlled, crossover clinical trial from Montreal, Canada (2008), examined the effects of this synthetic cannabinoid on insomnia. Twenty-nine patients with the disease completed a course in which they received either Nabilone (0.5–1.0 mg before bedtime) or the tricyclic antidepressant amitriptyline (10–20 mg before bedtime), the latter commonly prescribed for insomnia with fibromyalgia. Each patient took the medicine for a period of two weeks with a two-week period of no medication in between. The results showed that while both medications significantly improved people's sleep, Nabilone was superior.[3]

In 2009, scientists from Worcester, Massachusetts, conducted a meta-analysis of recent and relevant studies and found that ". . . all classes of cannabinoids, including the endogenous cannabinoids such as anandamide, related compounds such as the elmiric acids (EMAs), and non-cannabinoid components (200–250 constituents) of cannabis, show anti-inflammatory action."[4] The analysis demonstrated that all types of cannabinoids as well as non-cannabinoid parts of the plant are effective in reducing pain from inflammation, as in post-surgery conditions and cases of rheumatism, rheumatoid arthritis, chronic neuropathic pain, and fibromyalgia.

Study Summary

Drugs	Type of Study	Published Year, Place, and Key Results	CHI
All types of cannabinoids (endogenous, plant-based, and synthetic)	Meta-analysis (2004–2009)	2009—University of Massachusetts Medical School, Worcester: Cannabinoids effective in pain from post-surgery, rheumatism, rheumatoid arthritis, chronic neuropathic pain, and fibromyalgia.[4]	4
Synthetic cannabinoid Nabilone, 0.5–1.0 mg at night	29 patients with fibromyalgia	2008—Pain Clinic, McGill University Health Centre, Montreal, Quebec, Canada: Improved sleep.[3]	5
Synthetic cannabinoid Nabilone, 2 mg orally	40 patients with fibromyalgia	2007—Section of Physical Medicine and Rehabilitation, University of Manitoba, Rehabilitation Hospital, Health Sciences Centre, Winnipeg, Manitoba, Canada: Significant reduction of pain and improvement of quality of life.[2]	5

Total CHI Value 14

Strain-Specific Considerations

Two of the studies reviewed used primarily the synthetic cannabinoid Nabilone (similar to THC), which binds relatively equally to CB1 and CB2.

Both sativa and indica strains contain cannabinoids that activate CB1 and CB2. However, sativas or sativa-heavy strains tend to produce higher THC:CBD ratios than indica strains.

Mind-Body Medicine and Fibromyalgia

While examining the differences between fibromyalgia patients and healthy people using functional brain-imaging studies, neurotransmitter studies, and brain anatomy studies, researchers discovered "... that fibromyalgia patients have alterations in central nervous system (CNS) anatomy, physiology, and chemistry that potentially contribute to the symptoms experienced by these patients." The report's authors go on to say: "The frequent comorbidity of fibromyalgia with stress-related disorders, such as chronic fatigue, post-traumatic stress disorder, irritable bowel syndrome, and depression, as well as the similarity of many CNS abnormalities, suggests at least a partial common substrate for these disorders." The authors further conclude: "Despite the numerous cerebral alterations, fibromyalgia might not be a primary disorder of the brain but may be a consequence of early life stress or prolonged or severe stress, affecting brain modulatory circuitry of pain and emotions in genetically susceptible individuals."[5]

Arizona researchers studying fibromyalgia patients discovered that low positive affect, especially during stressful weeks, was a key component in the syndrome. This insight provided a new direction away from the commonly held notion that negative affect was a significant factor. Interventions that focus on improving positive affective resources, especially during times of stress, could thus provide a more positive therapeutic experience.[6]

Research also revealed that fibromyalgia patients experienced improved psychological well-being and a reduction in pain and fatigue through emotional expression of personal traumatic experiences simply by writing about them for 20 minutes, three times a week.[7]

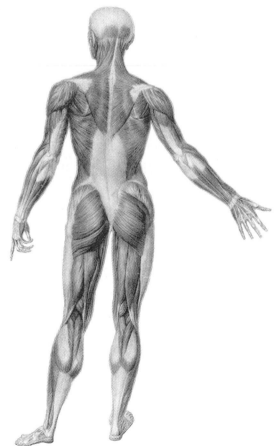

Another study conducted by researchers from the University of Washington concluded: "Fibromyalgia seems to be associated with increased risk of victimization, particularly adult physical abuse. Sexual, physical, and emotional trauma may be important factors in the development and maintenance of this disorder and its associated disability in many patients."[8]

In summary, contributing factors may include early life stress, prolonged severe stress, low levels of positive emotions (affect) especially during times of stress, increased risk of victimization particularly adult physical abuse, and sexual, physical, and emotional trauma.

Consider that by expressing and releasing personal traumatic experiences, we increase positive affect during times of stress.

Powerful Questions

Why does it hurt to move in life?

What age-old pains are still stressing me?

What does the pain remind me of?

What purposes do my aches and pains serve?

How do I release pain?

Are there other ways to release pain?

What is keeping me from reaching my potential?

Can I employ forgiveness?

Suggested Blessings

May our flowers bring ease and healing into your nights.

May our flowers assist you in moving, reaching, and more fully participating in all the beauty that life has to offer.

Suggested Affirmation

The past is gone and I am free to be me.

Take Notice: Tai Chi

Researchers conducted a single-blind, randomized trial of classic Yang-style tai chi, comparing stretching exercises to wellness education as put forth by the American College of Rheumatology 1990 criteria. Results showed that of the 66 enrolled patients with fibromyalgia, those 33 who were included in the tai chi group showed measurable clinical improvement and a general increase in quality of life. The investigators of the study noticed that the benefits of tai chi were still present after six months, and no adverse effects were observed.[9] So it would appear with a little effort and gentle daily practice, symptoms will diminish and life will improve, with no worries about side effects.

Hemorrhoids

No modern cannabis studies available

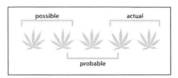

The structures of the anus contain channels or hemorrhoids, which are composed of connective tissues filled with small arterial and venous blood vessels that function to make the passing of stool easier. Only when they become inflamed, swollen, or begin to bleed are they cause for concern. In the Western world, about half of the population has had some form of symptomatic hemorrhoidal issue. Symptoms include itching, pain, bleeding, external and internal protrusion of hemorrhoids, minor anal leakage, and painful bowel movements.

Hemorrhoidal swelling and inflammation occurs due to pressure in the anal region via pregnancy, chronic constipation or diarrhea, long periods of sitting in the same position, or severe straining during bowel movements.

Allopathic medicine uses pharmaceutical and surgical procedures in the treatment of hemorrhoids. Medicated creams, oils, ointments, and suppositories aim to relieve pain, inflammation, or itching and to produce easier elimination. Minor procedures include rubber band ligation, injections, or coagulation using a laser. Surgical procedures include stapling and hemorrhoidectomies.

Cannabis and Hemorrhoids

In 1845, European medical literature described hemp leaf oil as being effective at reducing inflammation and managing neuralgic pains in cases of hemorrhoids.[1] A paste of cannabis leaves was reportedly used for treatment in India.[2] No modern studies exist to verify efficacy.

However, case reports from patients suffering from hemorrhoids suggest potential benefits of cannabis-infused oils such as hemp or almond oil in the care of inflamed hemorrhoidal tissues. Basic food-grade hemp oil (with its lubricating and tissue-soothing properties) infused with cannabis flowers potentially combines anti-inflammatory, antiseptic, and analgesic properties.

Mind-Body Medicine and Hemorrhoids

Grace and Graham write: "Constipation occurs when an individual was grimly determined to carry on even though faced with a problem he could not solve." Typical statements were (17 patients with constipation): "I have to keep on with this, but I know I'm not going to like it." "It's a lousy job but it's the best I can do." "This marriage is never going to get any better but I won't quit." "I'll have to keep on with this but I'm not going to like it." "I'll stick with it even though nothing good will come of it." The authors concluded: "Constipation is a phenomenon of holding on without change."[3] This corresponds to the patients' attitude of trying to continue with circumstances as they are, without hope of immediate improvement despite definite desire to do something different.

One of the main functions of the colon is to retrieve water from chyme (waste). The element water is commonly associated with feelings and emotions. The dryer the stool, the harder it is to release. Chronic or acute constipation often results in inflamed and protruding hemorrhoids. Dry paper worsens inflammation, and moist towelettes ease the pain. While holding on to every bit of water may be the body's signal of dehydration, for some it may also mirror a psychological structure indicative of a lack of emotional ownership. Some describe it as being stingy with one's feelings or emotional release. Hemorrhoids may also represent fear of letting go or the fear of getting hurt when letting go.

Emotionally speaking, constant irritation, inflammation, and associated pains may be messages to pay attention throughout the day and relax rectal sphincter muscles. Until the pain sets in, many hemorrhoid sufferers are simply unaware that they carry a lot of tension in the form of anxiety (often undefined fears or aggression) in the rectal region, thus contributing to constant strain of the tissue affected. Becoming more conscious of the tension and choosing instead to gently relax the region can bring relief.

In summary, aggravation factors may include holding on to something we don't like, while lacking desire or ability to change it; fear of letting go, or the fear of getting hurt when letting go; and chronic irritation or inflamed thinking around the topics of safety and security.

Consider emotional release work that gently addresses issues around safety and security; and think of "Impossible" as "I am possible."

Powerful Questions

Do I hold tension in my buttocks or rectum?

What is the feeling or emotion associated with the tension?

Can I gently release these feelings?

Can I choose to relax the region whenever I become aware of tension?

Where do I believe I have to hold back on feeling?

Do I have to ration my emotions?

Why does it hurt to let go?

Why is it a struggle to let go?

Do I believe that it hurts to let go?

Suggested Blessing

May you release with ease all that is not serving your health and your healing.

Suggested Affirmation

I easily release all that is burdensome and stagnant.

Anecdote

Johnny used to have hemorrhoid flare-ups with different intensities. Sometimes it was just a painless bleed after a bowel movement. Other times his hemorrhoids were excruciatingly painful while bearing down. In such cases the pain would last for hours. He tried the usual herbal and pharmaceuticals to ease his pain and discomfort without much success. After a bit of research on the adverse effects of a surgical procedure, Johnny opted against it.

He tried cannabis oil topically before and after a bowel movement. This provided significant relief by reducing the inflammation and the time it took to feel better after strain-induced flare-ups. However, while the oil reduced symptoms, his hemorrhoidal condition remained a chronic issue until he began noticing the same emotional state every time he decided to go to the bathroom.

Johnny used some of the oil internally and allowed his emotions to come to the forefront of his awareness. He felt anxious, dreading a bowel movement, anticipating the struggle and the burning pains. He allowed the feeling to take him deeper and noticed that he was feeling the same way about his financial situation.

Johnny bought whatever he wanted in the moment, even if it meant falling deeper into credit card debt. For years he spent today, not thinking about tomorrow. Soon he was in over his head, using one credit card to pay the monthly debt on another. He was late more and more often. He dreaded the debt collector's calls, feeling anxious with each ring of the telephone. He realized that his poor financial choices and poor dietary choices led to the same emotional states.

Johnny started to make better food choices, taking into account the delayed effect of his food choices. However, while drinking more water and eating more fiber helped to ease his symptoms, his hemorrhoids did not cease to be an issue until he began making serious changes in his financial life as well.

He designed a budget and stuck to it. He stopped using his cards and began the process of digging himself out of debt. He made purchasing choices with tomorrow in mind. And it was here that Johnny noticed his anxieties had lifted and his hemorrhoids stopped being an issue for him.

For Johnny, the message of the hemorrhoids was to start caring more for himself by considering the long-term emotional impact of his financial and dietary choices. Once he understood the message the disease had for him and answered it, his hemorrhoids ceased to be an issue at all.

Let Food Be Thy Medicine

Acacia ∽ Clove ∽ Garlic

Acacia: Acacia improves stool consistency and reduces the occurrence of fecal incontinence in adults.[4] Some alternative practitioners in the U.S. have begun to use this highly soluble fiber to ease symptoms of irritable bowel syndrome (IBS). Further studies are under way to determine the mechanism whereby acacia appears to reduce sugar-induced weight gain.

Clove: Patients suffering from chronic anal fissures were given a clove oil 1% cream preparation. Healing occurred in five times as many patients as in the control group. The 1% clove cream patients also had a greater reduction in resting anal pressure than those in the control group.[5]

Garlic: One of Cuba's most versatile herbs, garlic is used in the treatment of asthma to bring up phlegm, to prevent and treat infections caused by bacteria, and to decrease water retention, spasms, and thrombophlebitis. Used to treat fungal infections, garlic also works as a tonic, promotes healthy veins, and prevents parasites, inflammation, hemorrhoids, bacterial infections, viral infections, hypertension, muscular pains, back pains, synovitis (inflammation of a membrane in the knee joint), and varicose veins.[6]

Hemorrhoids May Demand New Eating Habits

Animal products contain no fiber, while all vegetable matter is essentially fiber, soluble or non-soluble. Consider leaning more and more toward a vegan diet.

Increase water intake. If the body does not receive enough water it will take its needed portions from chyme, causing harder stool, forcing us to struggle with elimination.

Stop using dry tissue paper. Instead, use moist towelettes without any irritating additives, or simply use water to clean the rectum (bidet or shower). Use cold water to ease the inflammation and burning sensation. Use a topical astringent (which contracts swollen tissue) such as witch hazel. Use continuous proper hygiene.

After each cleansing, use a couple of drops of cannabis-infused hemp or coconut oil to keep the area slightly lubricated.

In cases of constipation, use a bulb syringe filled with warm organic coconut oil to lubricate the anal passage. This allows for easy stool passage and reduces strain.

Avoid long periods of sitting. Get the body moving frequently.

Rapid eating and poor food choices ought to be replaced by relaxed eating and a healthy diet with plenty of fiber. Relax your bottom when eating. Try to check for aggression and anxieties before eating. If they are present, try to let it be okay that they are there, or relax in spite of them.

Inflammatory Diseases (in general)

Combined Evidence-Based Confidence Level and Therapeutic Potential

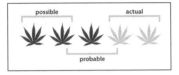

Total Number of Studies Reviewed: 28

Combined CHI Value: 79

Inflamed tissue is a natural and necessary response of the healing process. Without inflammation, injuries would not heal. Inflammation occurs in response to the invasion of an organism, exposure to a toxin, or the presence of impaired or injured cells. The inflammatory response is a general intervention and not as specific as, for example, the production of antibodies aimed to destroy a specific invader or threat. This general response involves swelling (accumulation of fluids), heat, redness (increased micro-blood supply), and the impairment of function and pain at the affected site, which serves as a constant reminder to guard the site until the healing process is complete.

Inflammation is classified as either acute or chronic. An acute inflammation is a temporary reaction to an organism's injury and ends when the affected tissue is healed. Chronic inflammation varies. It can result from the existence of a maintaining cause, such as the presence of a foreign object; when an invading organism or toxin cannot be expelled or continuously reappears; when an injury is not allowed to heal and instead is constantly agitated; or, lastly, from an over-reactive immune system that attacks itself, such as in Crohn's Disease.

Let Food Be Thy Medicine

Caryophyllene: (E)-β-Caryophyllene or (E)-BCP is a FDA-approved dietary plant-cannabinoid that activates CB2 receptor sites and initiates potent anti-inflammatory actions.[1] For more information on these specific spices see Chapter I, "Four Prime Cannabinoids/(E)-BCP."

OTHER SPICES THAT MAY AID THE INFLAMMATORY CONDITION
Cayenne ∾ Garlic ∾ Myrrh ∾ Nigella ∾ Turmeric

Cayenne: Cayenne stimulates peripheral circulation. In Cuba, a topical tincture and cream are used to treat chronic aches and pains of lumbago, arthritis, and rheumatism.[2]

Garlic: The bulb is used in Cuba for the treatment of thrombophlebitis and other inflammations.[3]

Myrrh: A study from the University of Cincinnati, Ohio, confirmed the physiological benefits of myrrh, used for thousands of years in the treatment of arthritis. Myrrh modulates inflammatory responses.[4]

Nigella: An experiment from Yüzüncü Yil University, Turkey, demonstrated that the volatile oil of nigella can suppress artificially induced arthritis in rats. Nigella has historically been used in the treatment of arthritis and other chronic inflammatory conditions.[5]

Turmeric: In a meta-study, scientists gave an overview of decades of scientific studies on turmeric. They found that turmeric's anti-inflammatory properties effectively supported the healing of wounds, arthritis, inflammatory bowel disease, ulcerative colitis (colon inflammation with ulcers), atherosclerosis, pancreatitis, psoriasis, chronic anterior uveitis (inflammation of the middle layer of the eye).[6]

Arthritis
Evidence-Based Confidence Level and Therapeutic Potential

Total Number of Studies Reviewed: 3
CHI Value: 6

Arthritis is inflammation of a joint connecting two bones such as the fingers, wrists, hips, back, and knee joints. People suffering from arthritis often complain of pain in the affected joint, which is commonly accompanied by redness, a sensation of heat, and minor swelling. Arthritis typically develops gradually over many years. Initially, it presents as an occasional mild ache in the joints which progresses into chronic pains, stiffness, and swelling. The arthritis sufferer begins to avoid certain painful movements so as to guard against the pain, resulting in further stiffness, limited range of motion, and decreased mobility. Arthritis has become the leading cause of disability in the U.S., with more than 46 million people suffering various forms of physical difficulties.[1]

Western medicine claims little specific knowledge of the causes or cures of this ailment. However, more than one hundred different causes for arthritis are considered, including gout and scleroderma, and viral, bacterial, or fungal infections. Limited treatments focus on suppressing pain and/or diminishing inflammation flare-ups.

One of the major classes of pharmaceutical drugs for arthritis, nonsteroidal anti-inflammatory drugs (NSAIDs), can result in serious consequences and should be taken with caution. "Each year 41,000 older adults are hospitalized [from], and 3,300 of them die from ulcers caused by NSAIDs. Thousands of younger adults are hospitalized."[2]

Cannabis and Arthritis

In one animal study, researchers from the UK, U.S., and Israel (2000) discovered that cannabidiol (CBD) treatment in rats effectively blocked progression of both acute and chronic arthritis.[3]

In a variety of animal assays (a procedure for testing effectiveness of a drug), cannabinoid-derived ajulemic acid showed efficacy in models for pain and inflammation. In a Worcester, Massachusetts, study (2004) on rat adjuvant arthritis, ajulemic acid displayed a remarkable action in preventing destruction of inflamed joints.[4]

Researchers from Calgary, Canada (2011), injected the synthetic cannabinoid URB597 into the osteoarthritic knees of rodents and discovered that it significantly reduced pain. This mechanism was mediated via CB1 receptors. Scientists consider cannabinoids a possible novel approach to treating osteoarthritis pain.[5]

Strain-Specific Considerations

Pre-clinical trials have explored URB597, cannabinoid-derived ajulemic acid (HU239), and the plant cannabinoid CBD to reduce arthritis in rodents.

Study Summary

Drugs	Type of Study	Published Year, Place, and Key Results	CHI
URB597	Animal study (rodents)	2011—University of Calgary, Canada: Injecting URB597 into the osteoarthritic knees of rodents significantly reduced pain.[5]	2
Cannabinoid-derived ajulemic acid	Animal study (rats)	2005—Worcester, University of Massachusetts Medical School: Cannabinoid-derived ajulemic acid reduced pain and inflammation and protected joints from damage in arthritis.[4]	2
Cannabidiol (CBD)	Animal study (rats)	2000—International scientific institutions: Protection of joints from damage. Cannabidiol (CBD) at 25 mg/kg per day orally was optimal in blocking progression of disease.[3]	2

Total CHI Value 6

URB597 is an inhibitor of an enzyme (fatty acid amide hydrolase or FAAH) that breaks down anandamide, thereby increasing anandamide presence and activity in the body. The endocannabinoid anandamide binds relatively equally to CB1 and CB2. Ajulemic acid (HU239) is a synthetic cannabinoid hypothesized to be a CB1 agonist, while CBD has a greater affinity for CB2 than CB1.

The sativa and indica strains all contain CB1- and CB2-activating cannabinoids. Indicas and indica-heavy strains usually contain lower THC:CBD ratios, thereby favoring CB2 activation.

Mind-Body Medicine and Arthritis

For many years, psychosomatic theories have emerged to suggest the mind's impact on the genesis, progression, and management of arthritis. One study considered psychological stress factors as a causative influence in the development of rheumatoid arthritis. In this model researchers attribute the loss of muscle tone to increased muscle tension associated with psychosomatic stress. Stress reportedly interferes with signals from a central nervous system-based (CNS) neurological feedback loop (fusimotor frequency) necessary in maintaining muscle tone.[6]

In another experiment, researchers examined 266 osteoarthritis (OA) patients for possible correlations between their mental health and OA affecting the knees and/or the hips. Researchers discovered that the intensity and type of pain experienced by patients related directly to the quality of their mental health. The authors of the study suggested that mental health measures could be employed to manage chronic and flare-up pain associated with the disease.[7]

In summary, consider psychological stressors, repressed emotions, suppressed emotions, hurt, and anger in combination.

Support may come from discovering and releasing repressed or suppressed feelings and emotions, along with developing an appreciation of our emotional nature and the entire emotional spectrum of which humans are capable.

Powerful Questions

What is tucked away inside the affected joint?

Why does it hurt to reach and stretch to become taller than I really am?

What limiting belief(s) is keeping me contracted?

What belief says it hurts to reach and stretch?

Where am I emotionally inflexible?

What feeling is keeping me from reaching for the stars?

Where am I inflexible in my thinking?

What thoughts are limiting my reach?

Suggested Blessing

May the spirit of reconciliation and forgiveness grease your joints so you can reach and stretch for your dreams and for the stars.

Suggested Affirmation

I can feel and release all my feelings with ease, have fun, and harm no one.

Anecdote

Karl was diagnosed with arthritis by age 53. It started with an occasional stiffness in his left knee but over time graduated into a pain he felt deep inside his joint. He would have occasional flare-ups and swelling, especially after sitting for a longer period or when the temperature dropped. He had been given numerous pharmaceutical medications over the years, including steroid injections into the joint, but no intervention really touched the pain. On top of that he began feeling depressed.

One winter night the pain escalated, and a friend suggested he try some cannabis. At this point, willing to try anything, he did something he had never thought he would do. He inhaled. After a few minutes, Karl felt relaxed and, to his surprise, the pain diminished. He noticed more flexibility in his joint and was able to enjoy a deep and restful night's sleep. An experience with cannabis a few months later helped move him beyond mere pain management toward deeper healing.

This time, when Karl treated himself for the pain as usual, he felt his visual attention drawn into his left knee. He saw the lining of the joint covered in a sand-like dirty dust. He was curious and his imagination drew ever closer to the dusty residue. He felt himself entering a single grain of dust and instantly felt tense. Somehow, his sense of wonder kept him exploring rather than retreating from the unpleasant sensation. He felt hurt. But it was a hurt from long ago, a vivid memory of a friend telling his secret to another. He remembered it like it was yesterday. Karl felt that it was right to stay with the hurt for what must have been perhaps 10 or 20 minutes. Suddenly, the hurt released. He was left feeling lighter and with what he considered his "real hurt."

He subsequently turned this experience into a healing meditation where he would imagine himself (without the help of cannabis) enter his left knee, visualize the dirty dust, select an individual grain and enter it. Each time he would find another scene, another hurt, or sometimes a sensation of anger. Each time he would let himself feel it until it was no more. Little by little, Karl noticed a significant and sustained improvement, not just with the arthritic knee but also in how he felt about himself. His depression

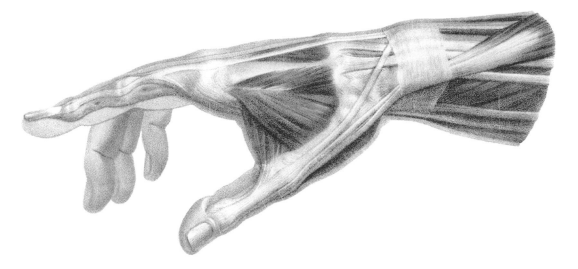

began to lighten, and he described himself as happier and more confident in dealing with whatever feeling or emotion came his way.

Let Food Be Thy Medicine

Cayenne ∾ Myrrh ∾ Nigella ∾ (E)-β-Caryophyllene

Cayenne: The plant stimulates peripheral circulation. In Cuba, a topical tincture and cream are used to treat chronic aches and pains of lumbago, arthritis, and rheumatism.[8]

Myrrh: A study from the University of Cincinnati, Ohio, discovered physiological benefits of myrrh, used for thousands of years in the treatment of arthritis. Myrrh modulates inflammatory responses.[9] Scientists from the King Saud University, Kharj, Saudi Arabia, confirmed that myrrh treatment via drinking infused water increased white blood cell count.[10] These results may serve as an explanation for the time-proven efficacy of myrrh in the treatment of wounds and inflammation.

Nigella: An experiment from Yüzüncü Yil University, Turkey, demonstrated that the volatile oil of nigella can suppress artificially induced arthritis in rats. Nigella has historically been used in the treatment of arthritis and other chronic inflammatory conditions.[11]

(E)-β-Caryophyllene or (E)-BCP: This FDA-approved dietary plant-cannabinoid activates CB2 receptor sites and initiates potent anti-inflammatory actions. Spice plants known to contain significant amounts of (E)-BCP include Black "Ashanti Pepper," White "Ashanti Pepper," Indian Bay-Leaf, Alligator Pepper, Basil, Cinnamon, Rosemary, Black Caraway, Black Pepper, Mexican Oregano, and Clove. For more information on these specific spices see Chapter I, "Four Prime Cannabinoids/ (E)-BCP."

Atherosclerosis

Evidence-Based Confidence Level and Therapeutic Potential

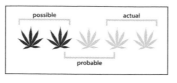

Total Number of Studies Reviewed: 3

CHI Value: 6

In the past, atherosclerosis was largely defined in terms of the accumulation of plaque or bad cholesterol (LDL) within the arterial walls, leading to obstructions. However, it is now understood to be more than a simple build-up of plaque. This obstruction is actually a physical response to injuries in the walls' lining. Causes of arterial wall injuries include high blood pressure, infectious microbes, or excessive presence of a certain amino acid called homocysteine. Studies have demonstrated that inflammatory molecules stimulate events leading to the development of atherosclerotic lesions. Some researchers consider atherosclerosis a natural type of band-aid approach to cover an injury or inflammation. When the band-aid becomes too thick or breaks loose, symptoms of a chronic or acute nature occur. In mild cases, this can lead to diminished oxygen supply to the tissue on the other side of the occlusion; in acute cases, it can cause severe strokes or heart attacks.

Atherosclerosis develops slowly over many years. If present in the limbs (called peripheral artery disease), it may present as a pain in the legs or arms, especially when exercising. Atherosclerosis in arteries in the torso may produce signs and symptoms similar to heart disease or strokes: primarily chest pain, shortness of breath, or loss of sensation and function (speech and movement of limbs).

In addition to a careful examination and patient history, physicians may request several tests to determine the risk of atherosclerosis. Doctors may scan blood samples for levels of cholesterol(s), the concentration of fibrinogen (a blood protein involved in clotting—too much fibrinogen may mean atherosclerosis), homocysteine (too much may contribute to atherosclerosis), and C-reactive protein produced by the liver. These factors could indicate the presence of inflammation and might be associated with atherosclerosis. Other diagnostic examinations range from such safe tests as stress tests, ultrasound, the ankle-brachial index (a test that helps to determine if atherosclerosis is present in the legs), or electrocardiogram (EKG) to those tests with the potential for severe side effects such as CT-scans, cardiac catheterization and angiograms involving arterial invasion, injection of dye, and the use of x-rays (ionizing radiation).

Orthodox treatment includes surgery and numerous pharmacological interventions. Lifestyle recommendations may include stress reduction, appropriate exercise, and the control of contributing factors such as weight, food choices, and smoking.

Cannabis and Atherosclerosis

In 2006 researchers acknowledged some important benefits of cannabis use. "Habitual cannabis use has been shown to positively affect the human immune system, and recent advances in endocannabinoid research provide a basis for understanding these immunomodulatory effects. Cell-based experiments or in vivo animal testing suggest that regulation of the endocannabinoid circuitry can impact almost every major function associated with the immune system." The scientists tested numerous novel molecules that exert their biological effects through the endocannabinoid system. The result of this exploration suggested the therapeutic potential of cannabinoids on inflammatory diseases such as atherosclerosis.[1]

Researchers observed that the enzyme 15-LOX could oxygenate low-density lipoprotein (LDL), which leads to the production of oxidized LDL. They understood that this in turn might play a factor in developing atherosclerosis. So in 2009, researchers from Kanazawa, Japan, conducted an experiment examining the impact of cannabinoids on 15-LOX. Results indicated that the cannabinoids cannabidiol (CBD) and its derivatives CBD-2'-monomethyl ether and CBD-2',6'-dimethyl ether (CBDD) inhibit 15-LOX enzyme activity to varying degrees. Researchers thus suggested that CBDD, which had the strongest enzyme inhibitory effects, could be a useful prototype for producing medicines for atherosclerosis.[2]

A group of scientists from Shaanxi, China (2010), examined the impact of a synthetic cannabinoid (WIN55,212-2) on the development of atherosclerosis in an animal study using mice. Results revealed a significant and direct reduction in the size of aortic atherosclerotic lesions.[3]

Study Summary

Drugs	Type of Study	Published Year, Place, and Key Results	CHI
Synthetic cannabinoid (WIN55,212-2)	Animal study	2010—Department of Cardiovascular Medicine, First Affiliated Hospital of Medical School, Xi'an Jiaotong University, Shaanxi, China: Significant and direct reduction in the size of aortic atherosclerotic lesions.[3]	2
The cannabinoids cannabidiol (CBD) and its derivatives CBD-2'-monomethyl ether and CBD-2',6'-dimethyl ether (CBDD)	Laboratory	2009—Department of Hygienic Chemistry, Faculty of Pharmaceutical Sciences, Hokuriku University, Kanazawa, Japan: CBDD may be a useful prototype for producing medicines for atherosclerosis.[2]	1
Cannabinoids	Laboratory and animal	2006—Center for Drug Discovery, Northeastern University, Boston, MA: Potential reduction of inflammation.[1]	1+2

Total CHI Value 6

Strain- and Form-Specific Considerations

In two pre-clinical studies, researchers examined the synthetic cannabinoid WIN55,212-2, the plant cannabinoid cannabidiol (CBD), and its derivatives CBD-2'-monomethyl ether and CBD-2',6'-dimethyl ether (CBDD) in the context of atherosclerosis.

WIN55,212-2 binds to both receptors but with higher affinity to CB2 than CB1. The same is true for CBD. Indica and indica-heavy strains tend to possess a lower THC:CBD ratio, thus favoring CB2 expression. Raw cannabis, fresh leaf, and leaf juice contain CBD-acid and thus favor CB2 activation.

Mind-Body Medicine and Atherosclerosis

While the connection between psychological factors and cardiovascular disease has been well demonstrated in numerous meta-analyses,[4] fewer experiments exist to date to elucidate this connection in the context of atherosclerosis. In fact, those available show different results. One such study conducted on 1,592 men and women during a period of five years determined that social deprivation and hostility were significantly associated with the progression of atherosclerosis.[5] Data used from the Multi-Ethnic Study of Atherosclerosis, a study of 6,814 persons aged 45 to 84 years with no history of clinical cardiovascular disease, revealed that pessimism relates to higher levels of inflammation.[6] Opposing study results failed to find connections between psychological factors and the disease's development.[7]

One theory holds that if plaque build-up is a response to an inflammation of the artery lining that caused the body to respond with deposits in a "band-aid" attempt to contain the damage, the original inflammation likely still lingers beneath it. Thus, an underlying emotional architecture of social deprivation/isolation or loneliness could be a wall we build around ourselves to keep away emotions such as pain and shame that seem too difficult to confront. While initially the wall of isolation may be effective as a protective barrier, over time it can become a problem larger than the one it was built to contain.

Alternatively, it can be argued that blood has to do with family, and since veins and arteries serve to carry blood, it may be helpful to look for intolerable emotions and experiences related to family.

In summary, aggravation factors may include social deprivation and hostility, loneliness, isolation, and pessimism.

Consider undoing the internal architecture of loneliness, social isolation, and deprivation, and seek the following: optimism, safe and meaningful social interaction, social contact and mutual support in problem solving, releasing suppressed and repressed emotions, and developing tendencies for positive affect.

Powerful Questions

How does your family respond to the presence of something intolerable?
How do I respond to the presence of something intolerable?
Does your family brush intolerable experiences under the carpet?
Do I use the barrier of loneliness to shelter myself from pain?
Where is belonging associated with pain or shame?
What resource do I have today that allows me to deal with what before was intolerable?

Suggested Blessing

May your need to cover up or hide perceived past transgressions or mistakes transcend into the experience of complete safety and trust.

Suggested Affirmations

I now choose to heal instead of judging.

I now choose to flush all hurt, pain, and shame from the core of my being.

Let Food Be Thy Medicine

Cacao ∾ Cardamom ∾ Coconut ∾ Garlic ∾ Rosemary ∾ Turmeric (E)-β-Caryophyllene

Cacao: Scientists at the McGill University School of Dietetics and Human Nutrition in Quebec, Canada, cautiously suggest that the consumption of dark chocolate may have a protective impact on heart and vascular illness and their connection to oxidized bad cholesterol (LDL).[8]

Cardamom: Scientists from the city of Mysore, India, discovered that cardamom extract protects platelets (blood particles involved in clotting) from aggregation and lipid peroxidation associated cardiovascular disease.[9]

Coconut: Researcher Hans Kaunitz correlated data from several laboratory animal studies with findings from the United Nations. He reported that death from ischemic heart disease is lowest where coconut fat intake is highest.[10]

Garlic: The plant may be helpful when peripheral signs and symptoms of heart disease are present. These include water retention, spasms, thrombophlebitis, inflammations, viral infections, and hypertension.[11]

The German Commission E approved garlic as a treatment for vascular concerns: "Supportive to dietary measures at elevated levels of lipids in blood. Preventative measures for age-dependent vascular changes."[12]

Japanese scientists were the first to scientifically prove what many traditional practitioners have suspected, namely that garlic, or specifically allicin, has potent antioxidant properties.[13]

Another study from Japan suggests that odorless garlic powder can play a beneficial role in preventing destructive thrombus (clot) formation such as in heart attacks. It apparently does so, according to the researchers, by suppressing the formation of clots and by destroying fibrin, a protein involved in the clotting of blood.[14]

Rosemary: In an experiment from Taichung Hsien, Taiwan, scientists concluded that ". . . rosemary is an excellent multifunctional therapeutic herb;

by looking at its potentially potent antiglycative bioactivity, it may become a good adjuvant medicine for the prevention and treatment of diabetic, cardiovascular, and other neurodegenerative diseases."[15]

Turmeric: In this meta-study, scientists presented an overview of decades of scientific studies on turmeric. A long list of turmeric's potential therapeutic properties included beneficial effects in cardiovascular disease.[16]

(E)-β-Caryophyllene or (E)-BCP: This is a FDA-approved dietary plant-cannabinoid that activates CB2 receptor sites and initiates potent anti-inflammatory actions. Spice plants known to contain significant amounts of (E)-BCP include: Black "Ashanti Pepper," White "Ashanti Pepper," Indian Bay-Leaf, Alligator Pepper, Basil, Cinnamon, Rosemary, Black Caraway, Black Pepper, Mexican Oregano, Clove. For more information on these specific spices see Chapter I, "Four Prime Cannabinoids/(E)-BCP."

(Interstitial) Cystitis
Evidence-Based Confidence Level and Therapeutic Potential

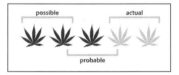

Total Number of Studies Reviewed: 1

CHI Value: 3

Interstitial cystitis (IC; painful bladder syndrome) predominantly affects women. The disease presents with chronic burning bladder pains due to inflammation and thinning of the urinary bladder lining. Other common symptoms include pain in the pelvic region (vagina, perineum), the chronic sensation of having to urinate or having voided incompletely, painful burning upon urination, and polyuria (high frequency of urination). The chronic pain may also present as acute flare-ups, which are often triggered by stress, menses, bacteria, or sex. Cystitis can be a debilitating condition that may severely reduce the quality of life in patients who are often depressed, have relationship and emotional difficulties, or are unable to sleep or work but otherwise function normally.

Bacteria do not typically cause IC. Within orthodox medicine, the cause of the infection remains unknown; but it is hypothesized that IC is an autoimmune disease where the body's own defenses attack the lining of the bladder. Diagnostic tests may include a physical examination, a careful patient history, urine testing, cytoscope (a camera tube inserted into the urethra and extended into the bladder), and bladder tissue biopsies.

IC has no known cure within orthodox medicine. Management techniques include pharmaceuticals, external nerve stimulation (TENS units), physical bladder stretching (using water or a gas), and surgery. Urologists may also use a wood pulp by-product, dimethylsulfoxide (DMSO), injected into the bladder to alleviate symptoms.

Cannabis and Cystitis

Researchers (2003) reported on the case of a 31-year-old female patient suffering for 20 years from chronic cystitis.[1] Her persistent burning sensation grew so great that it interfered with sleeping. She tried pharmaceutical pain control (opioids and others) and a variety of alternative treatments, all without success. She was given Nabilone (1 mg by mouth), which significantly reduced her burning pain by about a third but also caused confusion, psychotic sensations, and bad dreams. Dose reduction did not resolve the adverse effects. Doctors switched to Dronabinol (2.5 mg by mouth), which further reduced her pain by another third without adverse effects, with the exception of "feeling strange." She was able to sleep and function without impediment. The dose, reduced to 2.5 mg by mouth every other day, continued to manage her pain without any side effects. After a period of six months, the therapeutic progress appeared well maintained.

Study Summary

Drugs	Type of Study	Published Year, Place, and Key Results	CHI
Nabilone and Dronabinol	One female patient with chronic cystitis	2003—Nabilone reduced pain but caused adverse effects. Dronabinol reduced pain further without adverse effects.	3

Total CHI Value 3

Strain-Specific Considerations

Dronabinol is a synthetic cannabinoid very similar to THC (isomer), while Nabilone is a synthetic cannabinoid with some of the same properties as THC.

Mind-Body Medicine and Interstitial Cystitis

One experiment conducted on patients with interstitial cystitis showed significantly greater startle responses during non-imminent threat conditions when compared to healthy human subjects.[2] The enhanced responsiveness in IC patients was associated with affective (feeling/emotion) circuits that included the amygdala, the portion of the limbic brain that is responsible for intense emotions and emotional memory. It is this discovery that suggests a possible psychosomatic connection related to an intense and likely early traumatic memory or experience.

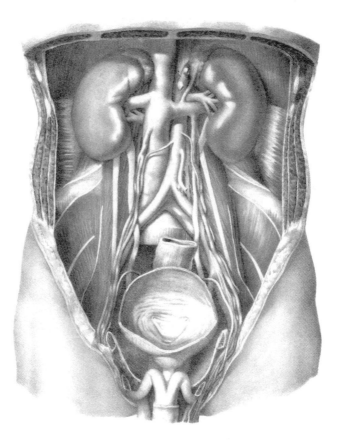

Researchers at Tufts University School of Medicine conducted a meta-analysis of 713 mostly original papers published between 1990 and August 2008. One of the resulting discoveries suggested that stress played a significant role in IC and should be targeted to better understand and manage the disease.[3]

The location of the primary symptoms of IC (the bladder), and its function of storing and voiding urine, as well as chronic burning and ineffective void, all lend themselves to possible interpretations from a psychosomatic perspective.

In summary, aggravating factors may include stress and suppressed or repressed emotions.

Consider working with stress prevention, stress management, learning positive coping skills, and emotional release work.

Powerful Questions

How do I feel when I cannot completely void my urine?

What am I holding on to that hurts or burns?

What burning anger will not end?

Is there an emotion or memory that is constantly irritating me?

Which anger is causing me so much pain not to feel?

What feeling is starting to dribble out of me? Can I let it flow?

Suggested Blessing

May you relax enough to realize that anger, hurt, rage, or shame only cause lasting damage when you pretend they do not exist.

Suggested Affirmation

It is okay to be pissed off.

I can release my anger with ease and harm to none. I can change any belief that says, "It's not okay to be angry."

I can change any belief that says, "It hurts to be angry."

Take Notice

For more information on alternative medical perspectives and natural treatment possibilities, consider looking at a book written by Amrit Willis, RN, entitled *Solving the Interstitial Cystitis Puzzle: A Guide to Natural Healing.* Published by Holistic Life Enterprises, Beverly Hills, California, 2001 & 2003.

Rheumatoid Arthritis
Evidence-Based Confidence Level and Therapeutic Potential

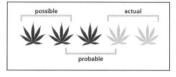

Total Number of Studies Reviewed: 3

CHI Value: 10

Rheumatoid arthritis is the most crippling form of arthritis, deforming joints and bending bodies. It is considered an autoimmune disorder, which apparently occurs when something goes wrong with the body's immune system and it attacks healthy parts of the body such as joints. One can tell long-time rheumatoid arthritis sufferers from a distance—their joints take on a gnarly appearance.

Cannabis and Rheumatoid Arthritis

In 2006, researchers from the UK enrolled 58 patients with rheumatoid arthritis in a double-blind, placebo-controlled study to determine the effect of cannabinoids on pain and other symptoms. The results indicated that patients who received the cannabinoids slept better and experienced a reduction in pain when compared to the placebo group. Researchers wrote: "In the first ever controlled trial of a CBM in RA [rheumatoid arthritis], a significant analgesic effect was observed and disease activity was significantly suppressed following Sativex treatment."[1]

Boston scientists (2006) acknowledged that "Habitual cannabis use has been shown to [positively] affect the human immune system, and recent advances in endocannabinoid research provide a basis for understanding these immunomodulatory effects. Cell-based experiments, or in vivo animal testing, suggest that regulation of the endocannabinoid circuitry can impact almost every major function associated with the immune system." After testing numerous novel molecules that exert their biological effects through the endocannabinoid system, the researchers suggested the therapeutic potential of cannabinoids on inflammatory diseases such as rheumatoid arthritis.[2]

A 2009 Worcester, Massachusetts, meta-analysis of studies on cannabinoids in the context of pain is instructive.[3] Results showed that all types of cannabinoids as well as non-cannabinoid parts of the plant effectively reduce pain from inflammation found in post-surgery patients, rheumatism, rheumatoid arthritis, chronic neuropathic pain, and fibromyalgia.

Study Summary

Drugs	Type of Study	Published Year, Place, and Key Results	CHI
All types of cannabinoids (endogenous, plant-based, and synthetic)	Meta-analysis (2004–2009)	2009—University of Massachusetts Medical School: Cannabinoids effective in reducing pain from rheumatoid arthritis.[3]	4
Cannabinoids	Laboratory	2006—Center for Drug Discovery, Northeastern University, Boston, MA: Potentially useful in reduction of inflammation.[2]	1
Sativex (sublingual spray) daily in the evening		2006—Multi-institutional study: Randomized, double-blind, parallel group study on patients with RA. Improvement in sleep and reduction in pain.[1]	5

Total CHI Value 10

Strain-Specific Considerations

Sativex, produced by a large pharmaceutical corporation, is an oromucosal mouth spray consisting of roughly equal parts of THC (2.7 mg) and CBD (2.5 mg). Sativex is not synthetic, but rather made from cannabis. However, the formulation ratios are very similar when compared to actual *Cannabis sativa* ratios.

Sativa and sativa-prominent hybrids contain relatively higher THC:CBD ratios and thus activate CB1 and CB2.

Mind-Body Medicine and Rheumatoid Arthritis

Researchers from Ann Arbor looking at psychological factors in the development of rheumatoid arthritis "... suggested that the rheumatoids communicate poorly with their relatives about their hurt feelings."[4]

Autoimmune diseases may mirror an intense and likely longstanding conflict of belief and the dueling emotions this elicits. H. Levitan, MD, studied onset situations in rheumatoid arthritis.[5] A case study of three female patients with the disease revealed that two shared mental/emotional denominators. First, upon onset of the disease, each woman was in a relationship that produced at once intense rage and love for her partner. These patients hated their relationships but were too dependent to leave them behind. Second, neither woman acted out her anger but had to endure the abuse that elicited the rage and also the impact of her own unexpressed feelings. Thus, the unexpressed intense emotions produced by conflicting beliefs such as 'without my husband I am on the street' or 'it is not okay to feel angry' might have contributed to an internal experience of dependency misinterpreted as love and silent rage, respectively.

In another study of 33 patients (4 male, 29 female) with rheumatoid arthritis, researchers concluded, "In these cases the general psychodynamic background is a chronic inhibited hostile aggressive state as a reaction to the earliest masochistic dependence on the mother that is carried over to the father and all human relationships, including the sexual. The majority of these personalities learn to discharge hostility through masculine competition, physical activity, and serving, and also through domination of the family."[6]

In summary, aggravating factors may include having to endure abuse perpetrated by a perceived authority (God, priest, leader, husband), leading to suppressed hurt and unexpressed rage with both, combining to form hostility; unexpressed feelings; conflicting beliefs; and hostility composed of anger and hurt directed at oneself.

Consider working to discover and release repressed and/or suppressed feelings and emotions; develop an appreciation of our emotional nature and the entire emotional spectrum of which humans are capable; replace conflicting and unhealthy belief(s) with those that will engender love, caring, and compassion; and find, embrace, feel, release, and forgive all lingering hurt and angers.

Also see Arthritis, above.

Powerful Questions

What is eating away at me (in my affected joints)?

Suggested Blessing

May the spirit of reconciliation and forgiveness grease your joints so that you can reach and stretch for your dreams and for the stars.

Suggested Affirmations

I can feel and release all my feelings with ease and fun and harm to none. I can forgive myself for anything.

Let Food Be Thy Medicine

Cayenne ∾ Myrrh ∾ Nigella ∾ Rosemary ∾ Turmeric (E)-β-Caryophyllene-Containing Spices

Cayenne: Cayenne stimulates peripheral circulation. In Cuba, a topical tincture and cream are used to treat chronic aches and pains of lumbago, arthritis, and rheumatism.[7]

Myrrh: This study conducted by the University of Cincinnati, Ohio, confirmed physiological benefits of myrrh, used for thousands of years in the treatment of arthritis. Myrrh modulates inflammatory responses.[8]

Nigella: A study conducted at the Yüzüncü Yil University, Turkey, demonstrated that the volatile oil of nigella can suppress artificially induced arthritis in rats. Nigella has historically been used in the treatment of arthritis and other chronic inflammatory conditions.[9]

Rosemary: The German Commission E has approved rosemary for "External: Supportive therapy for rheumatic diseases, circulatory problems."

Turmeric: The World Health Organization Monographs on selected Medicinal Plants describe the uses of turmeric in pharmacopoeias and traditional systems of medicine: "Treatment of . . . pain and inflammation due to rheumatoid arthritis. . . ."

(E)-β-Caryophyllene: This FDA-approved food-based plant-cannabinoid activates CB2 receptor sites and initiates potent anti-inflammatory actions. Spice plants known to contain significant amounts of (E)-BCP include

Black "Ashanti Pepper," White "Ashanti Pepper," Indian Bay-Leaf, Alligator Pepper, Basil, Cinnamon, Rosemary, Black Caraway, Black Pepper, Mexican Oregano, and Clove. For more information on these specific spices, see Chapter I, "Four Prime Cannabinoids/(E)-BCP."

Gastrointestinal Inflammatory Diseases

Gastro-Esophageal Reflux Disease (GERD)

Evidence-Based Confidence Level and Therapeutic Potential

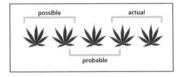

Total Number of Studies Reviewed: 1

CHI Value: 5

Commonly known as heartburn and acid reflux disease, this illness is due to damage of the esophageal mucous membrane and the esophageal sphincter. Damage occurs when stomach acid reaches the lower part of the esophagus. Under normal conditions, the esophageal sphincter opens to allow food and drink to enter the stomach but closes right after to prevent stomach acid from affecting the tissue above. In GERD, however, the closing action is temporarily incomplete, allowing acid to reach unprotected tissue and cause damage. This mechanism is also referred to as transient lower esophageal sphincter relaxations. Symptoms include heartburn, regurgitation (tasting one's stomach contents), pain when swallowing, nausea, vomiting (especially in children), and chest pains (often with burning sensation).

GERD-produced damage can lead to long-term problems and acute episodes. Allopathic treatments include pharmaceuticals and surgery, each with their own risks and side effects.

Effective management may include lifestyle changes such as not eating for two hours before lying down, sleeping slightly elevated, and a more alkaline diet.

Cannabis and GERD

The effects of cannabinoids appear to have a dose-specific therapeutic window warranting a cautious and gradual approach to their use for treatment of GERD. Dutch researchers (2009) noted that 10-mg doses of THC given to the study subjects (dogs and humans) significantly reduced symptoms of GERD such as meal-induced transient lower esophageal sphincter relaxations and spontaneous swallowing, while dosage levels of 20 mg caused some volunteers to experience nausea, vomiting, hypotension, rapid heart rates, and other central effects. To protect the participants from the dose-dependent side effects, scientists discontinued dosage tests at 20 mg before the study design reached its parameters.[1]

Study Summary

Drugs	Type of Study	Published Year, Place, and Key Results	CHI
THC (dogs), THC (humans); 10 mg and 20 mg	Trial on healthy human (placebo-controlled) volunteers and dogs	2009—Academic Medical Centre, Department of Gastroenterology and Hepatology, Amsterdam, The Netherlands: THC significantly inhibited the increase in meal-induced transient lower esophageal sphincter relaxations and reduced spontaneous swallowing in both dogs and humans. High doses produced side effects.[1]	5

Total CHI Value 5

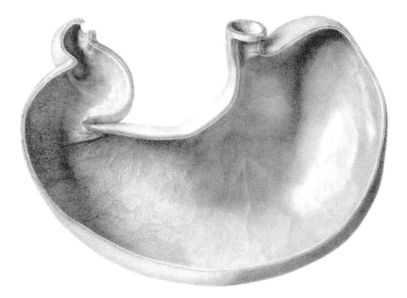

Strain-Specific Considerations

Both CB1 and CB2 may be involved in triggering transient lower esophageal sphincter relaxations in humans. THC binds with both CB1 and CB2 relatively equally. Both sativas and indicas contain cannabinoids that activate CB1 and CB2.

Mind-Body Medicine and Gastro-Esophageal Reflux Disease (GERD)

One study conducted on 60 patients diagnosed with heartburn concluded that, "As with other chronic conditions such as irritable bowel syndrome (IBS), heartburn severity appears to be most responsive to major life events and not an accumulation of more minor stressors or fluctuations in mood. In addition, vital exhaustion, which may in part result from sustained stress, may represent the psychophysiological symptom complex most closely associated with heartburn exacerbation."[2]

Another experiment using 19 healthy volunteers demonstrated that the introduction of anxiety increases acid-induced esophageal hyperalgesia (increased sensitivity to pain).[3]

Aggravating factors may include major life events and vital exhaustion due to sustained stress or anxiety.

Consider working with healing the damage done by major life events, getting rest, trying anxiety intervention, and reducing fear, worry, and stress.

Powerful Questions

What hurts to swallow?
What burns to break down?
What about nurturing is difficult?
Is there anything about nurturing that is unsafe?

Suggested Blessing

May I release all that is fear.
May you replace all that is fear with a deep and nurturing love.

Suggested Affirmation

I trust appropriately.

Inflammatory Bowel Disease (IBS)

Evidence-Based Confidence Level and Therapeutic Potential

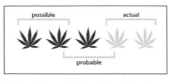

Total Number of Studies Reviewed: 3

CHI Value: 8

Like the name suggests, this disease primarily affects the gastrointestinal tract but is also associated with inflammation. Orthodox medicine struggles to understand the causes for IBS and, to date, offers no cure. Possible reasons for developing IBS may include stressful life events (mind-bowel axis), infections by yet-to-be-identified pathogens or toxins, immune dysfunction, or unhealthy gut environment.

IBS is classified according to the primary symptoms displayed by each patient. Thus diarrhea, constipation, and alternating diarrhea with constipation and infection become the basis for diagnosing the disease as IBS-D, IBS-C, IBS-A, or post-infectious IBS-PI, respectively. Ulcerative colitis is a form of IBD that can affect other body parts as well. Crohn's disease, another form of IBD, is an autoimmune disorder affecting the gastrointestinal tract.

Other frequently observed symptoms may include abdominal discomfort (gas, bloating, cramps), the sensation of incomplete void of stool, gastroesophageal reflux disease (GERD), anxiety, depression, pain (abdominal, back, head, muscle), increased generalized weakness, and lack of energy.

Orthodox diagnoses are performed by elimination. Doctors run a variety of tests to rule out diseases with similar symptoms. These may include colonoscopies, screening for parasites (blood or stool tests), testing for lactose intolerance (hydrogen breath test) or the presence of infections (stool examinations), as well as tests for celiac disease (blood test screening for antibodies). If none of these diseases are responsible for the patient's symptoms, practitioners may follow one of several possible established diagnostic algorithms (a list of questions related to the patient's symptoms).

Physicians manage the disease with dietary modifications, pharmaceutical medications, and referrals to psychotherapy. Canadian researchers conducted a meta-analysis of all randomized controlled trials published on Medline, Embase, and the Cochrane register up through April 2008. They reported that fiber, antispasmodics, and peppermint oil exhibited greater effectiveness than a placebo in the treatment of irritable bowel syndrome.[1]

Cannabis and Inflammatory Bowel Disease (IBD) or Syndrome (IBS)

Case reports from cannabis-using IBS patients suggest that cannabis may be effective in managing some symptoms, especially nausea, diarrhea, stress, cramps, and lack of appetite. Human studies remain underway to determine a scientific basis for the use of marijuana in the treatment of IBS.

However, Italian researchers (2010) conducted a meta-analysis/review of the available pre-clinical studies related to cannabinoids and the gut. The authors wrote: "Anatomical, physiological, and pharmacological studies have shown that the endocannabinoid system is widely distributed throughout the gut, with regional variation and organ-specific actions.

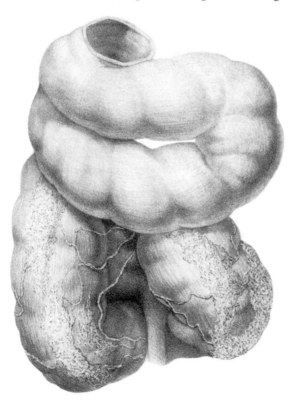

It is involved in the regulation of food intake, nausea and emesis, gastric secretion and gastroprotection, GI motility, ion transport, visceral sensation, intestinal inflammation and cell proliferation in the gut."[2] Three pre-clinical studies give us more insights.

In 2006 Boston researchers tested numerous novel molecules that exert their biological effects through the endocannabinoid system. The results suggested a therapeutic potential of cannabinoids on inflammatory diseases such as IBD.[3]

Two years later, researchers from Alberta, Canada, similarly showed that cannabinoids reduced colitis in test animals. The scientists concluded that ". . . drugs targeting EC degradation offer therapeutic potential in the treatment of inflammatory bowel diseases."[4]

Another experiment conducted in 2008 in Naples, Italy, indicated that CBD could reduce hypermotility in mice. Based on these observations, scientists hypothesized that CBD normalizes motility in cases of inflammatory bowel disease.[5]

Study Summary

Drugs	Type of Study	Published Year, Place, and Key Results	CHI
CBD	Animal study (mice)	2008—University of Naples, Italy: CBD could reduce hypermotility in mice.[5]	2
Fatty acid amide hydrolase (FAAH) blocker URB597	Animal and laboratory (mice and human DNA)	2008—Division of Gastroenterology, Department of Medicine, University of Calgary, Alberta, Canada: EC membrane transport inhibitor VDM11 enhances the action of the ECS. Cannabinoids reduce colitis.[4]	1+2
Cannabinoids	Laboratory and animal	2006—Center for Drug Discovery, Northeastern University, Boston, MA: Potential reduction of inflammation.[3]	2+1

Total CHI Value 8

Strain-Specific Considerations

While research has discovered both CB1 and CB2 in parts of the gastrointestinal tract, patients with Crohn's disease reported that indica strains worked especially well for them in reducing pain, nausea, vomiting, depression, low energy, and lack of sleep. This observation may be supported, in part, by the aforementioned pre-clinical trial from Naples, which showed that CBD could reduce hypermotility (abnormally high activity) in the guts of mice.

Indicas or indica-heavy strains tend to have a lower THC:CBD ratio when compared to sativas, resulting in a relative increase in CB2 activation.

Mind-Body Medicine and Inflammatory Bowel Disease (IBD) or Syndrome (IBS)

Two studies conducted by international teams of scientists using placebos demonstrated the significant therapeutic potential of belief in relieving IBS symptoms.[6] Similarly, a meta-analysis of studies on IBS revealed that "Psychiatric disorders, especially major depression, anxiety, and somatoform disorders, occur in up to 94% of patients with IBS."[7]

In cases of IBS-C, consider the following observations: "Constipation occurs when an individual was grimly determined to carry on even though faced with a problem he could not solve." Typical statements were (17 patients with constipation): "I have to keep on with this, but I know I'm not going to like it. . . . It's a lousy job but it's the best I can do. . . . This marriage is never going to get any better but I won't quit . . . I'll stick with it even though nothing good will come of it."[8] The authors concluded: "Constipation is a phenomenon of holding on without change." This corresponds to the patients' attitude of trying to continue with things as they are, without hope of immediate improvement or definite desire to do something different.

In cases of IBS-D, consider the following observations: "Diarrhea occurred when an individual wanted to be done with a situation or to have it over with, or to get rid of something or somebody." One man who developed severe diarrhea after he had purchased a defective automobile said: "If I could only get rid of it. . . . I want to dispose of it." Typical statements of others were: "If the war was only over with. . . . I wanted to get done with it. . . . I wanted to get finished with it."[9]

If nausea or vomiting is a persistent problem, consider the following observations: "Nausea and vomiting occurred when an individual was thinking of something which he wished had never happened. He was preoccupied with the mistake he had made, rather than with what he should have done instead. Usually he felt responsible for what happened." Typical statements: "I wish it hadn't happened. . . . I was sorry I did it. . . . I wish things were the way they were before. . . . I made a mistake. . . . I shouldn't have listened to him."[10] The authors concluded that "Vomiting is a way of undoing something which has been done. It thus corresponds with the patients' wishes to restore things to their original situation, it is as if nothing ever happened."

In summary, aggravating factors may include major depression, anxiety, somatoform disorders, tendency for negative affect. IBS-C: holding on without change. IBS-D: wanting to get rid of something or somebody, hyper-focus on regret or remorse.

Consider engaging antidepressive measures, anti-anxiety measures; working to decipher any message(s) of the physical symptoms; improving tendency for positive affect. IBS-C: work on releasing with ease. IBS-D: work on reducing fear, worry, and stress; focus instead on forgiveness, learning from the situation, and initiating positive action.

Suggested Blessing

May you discover your internal point of peace. May you feel the safety and security that you desire.

Suggested Affirmations

I compost all that is fear, worry, and stress.

I now believe—the source and genesis for feeling safe and secure lie within me.

Let Food Be Thy Medicine

Acacia ∾ Turmeric ∾ (E)-β-Caryophyllene

Acacia: Research from Minneapolis, Minnesota, suggests that acacia improves stool consistency and reduces the occurrence of fecal incontinence in adults.[11] Alternative practitioners in the U.S. have begun to use the highly soluble fiber to ease symptoms of irritable bowel syndrome. Further studies are underway to determine the mechanism whereby acacia appears to reduce sugar-induced weight gain.

Turmeric: In this meta-study, scientists gave an overview of decades of scientific studies on turmeric. Turmeric showed promise as a treatment for adenomatous polyposis (multiple polyps in the large intestine—precursor to colon cancer), inflammatory bowel disease, and ulcerative colitis (colon inflammation with ulcers).[12]

In a double-blind randomized placebo-controlled human study from Hamamatsu, Japan, scientists examined turmeric's ability to prevent relapse in patients with a history of dormant ulcerative colitis. They concluded that curcumin, an active ingredient in turmeric, seemed to be a safe medication for maintaining remission from ulcerative colitis.[13]

(E)-β-Caryophyllene: This FDA-approved dietary plant-cannabinoid activates CB2 receptor sites and initiates potent anti-inflammatory actions. Spice plants known to contain significant amounts of (E)-BCP include: Black "Ashanti Pepper," White "Ashanti Pepper," Indian Bay-Leaf, Alligator Pepper, Basil, Cinnamon, Rosemary, Black Caraway, Black Pepper, Mexican Oregano, and Clove. For more information on these specific spices, see Chapter I, "Four Prime Cannabinoids/(E)-BCP."

Pancreatitis
Evidence-Based Confidence Level and Therapeutic Potential

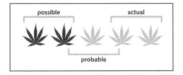

Total Number of Studies Reviewed: 2

CHI Value: 3

The pancreas is both an endocrine gland secreting hormones such as insulin, glucagons, and somatostatin, and a digestive organ producing digestive juices containing enzymes vital to the breakdown of food particles and their molecular absorption in the small intestine. Pancreatitis, an inflammation of the pancreas, occurs when the digestive enzymes are activated while still in the pancreas, causing the breakdown of cells while still inside the organ. The resulting irritation and inflammation cause the symptoms associated with the disease.

The pancreas is a vital organ and the human body cannot exist without it. A damaged or impaired pancreas can lead to digestive difficulties and the development of diabetes. Orthodox medicine identifies numerous reasons for pancreatitis. The chief culprits leading the way are alcoholism and gallbladder stones. Other causes include toxic pharmaceutical medication such as those used to treat AIDS, abdominal surgeries or injuries, and high concentrations of minerals, fats, or parathyroid hormones.

Symptoms may vary between acute and chronic versions of the disease but usually include upper abdominal pains. Diagnostic tools may include physical examinations, blood tests screening for concentrations of pancreatic enzymes, stool samples determining the presence of undigested fat, the use of imaging devices such as magnetic resonance imaging (MRI), CT scans utilizing ionizing radiation (x-rays), ultrasound, and endoscopic ultrasound. Treatment plans unfold depending on the underlying cause and may include intravenous fluids, pharmaceutical medications, surgeries and/or dietary restrictions (no alcohol, smoking, or fat).

Cannabis and Pancreatitis

While cannabinoids have been shown to ameliorate liver fibrosis, their effects in chronic pancreatitis and on pancreatic stellate cells mostly remain unknown. However, during recent investigations, an international group of scientists discovered that CB1 and CB2 receptors are found in the human pancreas and that the administration of synthetic cannabinoids constituted a novel option in treatment of inflammation and fibrosis in chronic pancreatitis.[1]

Study results are inconsistent: it would appear that in some cases, cannabinoids such as anandamide have a therapeutic effect on acute pancreatitis; at other times, their treatment produced an aggravation of the acute inflammation. This international team of researchers (2008) explained the apparently paradoxical nature of earlier study results. They wrote: "... the effect of anandamide on the severity of acute pancreatitis depends on the phase of this disease. Administration of anandamide, before induction of pancreatitis, aggravates pancreatic damage; whereas anandamide administered after induction of pancreatitis reduces the severity of acute pancreatitis."[2]

Study Summary

Drugs	Type of Study	Published Year, Place, and Key Results	CHI
Synthetic cannabinoid	Laboratory	2008—Various international scientific institutions: Positive treatment option for inflammation and fibrosis in chronic pancreatitis.[1]	1
Anandamide	Animal study (rats)	2008—Department of Physiology, Jagiellonian University Medical College, Krakow, Poland: Effect of anandamide on the severity of acute pancreatitis depends on the phase of this disease.[2]	2

Total CHI Value 3

Strain-Specific Considerations

CB1 and CB2 receptors are present in the human pancreas. Research has shown that CB1 and CB2 activation may positively affect pancreatitis—at least in pre-clinical animal trials. Anandamide binds relatively equally to both CB1 and CB2, as does THC.

Sativa and sativa-dominant strains contain higher THC:CBD ratios when compared to indicas or indica-heavy hybrids.

Mind-Body Medicine and Pancreatitis

In a Japanese study conducted on 69 patients with chronic pancreatitis, researchers used a comparative analysis to examine potential psychosomatic influences.[3]

Suspicious type	Definite type
Suspicious type (actual psychosomatic disease)—primarily related to psycho-somatic factors.	Definite type (character psychosomatic disease)—primarily manifested as chronic alcohol-drinking habits.
Significantly more psychological complaints, including neurotic reactions.	Significantly more compulsive tendencies and incidences of stern discipline, compulsive parents, dominant fathers, and separation experiences.

If the heart is where we feel our emotions and the liver where we process them, then the pancreas represents the space where we gather, collect, and store them. Difficulty with this organ may arise when we refuse to put our emotional life into perspective. Refusing to integrate our emotional experiences or being irritated/inflamed by the idea of having to give dimensions to our emotional reality may warrant a message. Emotions are central to the human experience. Emotions are normal and natural, and the degree to which we diminish their importance in life is the degree to which we diminish self-respect.

In summary, aggravating factors may include devaluing emotions and ignoring the importance of our emotional experience.

Consider learning to feel and express all emotions appropriately, without hurting anyone.

Powerful Questions

Do I feel like a victim of my feelings and emotions?
Do I place any value on feelings and emotions?
Do I want to numb myself to my emotions?

Suggested Blessing

May I discover a new depth of self-respect.

Suggested Affirmation

I honor all my emotions safely and appropriately.

Let Food Be Thy Medicine

Turmeric: In a large meta-study, scientists provided an overview of decades of scientific analysis on turmeric. Turmeric's potential therapeutic value in the treatment of pancreatitis was noted.[4]

Periodontitis

Evidence-Based Confidence Level and Therapeutic Potential

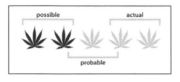

Number of Studies Reviewed: 1

CHI Value: 2

Periodontitis is an inflammation of the tissues that support the teeth. Thought to be caused by oral microbes and an overzealous immune response, it leads to the reduction of tissue support and alveolar bone loss. The process of resorption initiates this deficiency where bone cells leak substances and become weak.

Symptoms may include painful swelling of the gums and tissue surrounding the teeth, tissue reduction, deep pockets around the teeth, bad breath (halitosis), and loose teeth. Periodontitis may also be implicated in the development of heart attacks, strokes, and atherosclerosis.

Orthodox medical treatments include deep cleaning, surgical cleaning, and interventions. Alternative treatments may involve solutions of hydrogen peroxide or other oral oxidants.

Cannabis and Periodontitis

The first known study to examine the therapeutic effects of cannabidiol on resorption-produced periodontitis took place in Brazil in 2009. The analysis demonstrated that CBD-treated rats presented a reduction of alveolar bone loss. The authors wrote: "These results indicate that CBD may be useful to control bone resorption during progression of experimental periodontitis in rats."[1]

Study Summary

Drugs	Type of Study	Published Year, Place, and Key Results	CHI
Cannabidiol (CBD)	Animal study (rats)	2009—Laboratory of Molecular Biology, University of Uberaba, Brazil: CBD may be useful to control bone resorption.[1]	2

Total CHI Value 2

Strain-Specific Considerations

CB1 and CB2 receptors are found in bone tissue. Anandamide is produced in bone and synovial tissue. A pre-clinical trial conducted on animals discovered that CBD aided in mitigating periodontitis, at least in animals. CBD has a greater affinity for CB2.

Indica and indica-dominant stains tend to contain a lower THC:CBD ratio, resulting in a relatively higher activation of CB2.

Mind-Body Medicine and Periodontitis

Studies have identified possible psychological, behavioral, physiological, and demographic risk factors implicated in the progression of simple gingivitis to the development of periodontitis. Relationships have been

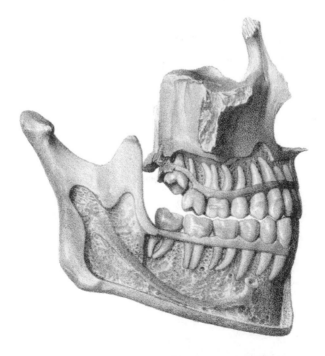

observed between ongoing stressors such as financial difficulties, grief, caring for a spouse with Alzheimer's disease (or other dementias), depressed mood, and general perceived and ongoing stress or hassles. Physiological responses included elevation in pro-inflammatory cytokines and a reduction of salivary flow. Both contributed to reducing the body's ability to properly respond to bacterial infection, which increases the risk for periodontitis.[2]

Taking a bite out of the apple of life has become an impossible or painful experience. Similarly, being able to chew and enjoy solid foods has become an irritation or a thing of the past. Chronic stressors are eroding the substance of once-solid bone tissue. Bones are a physiological foundation on which the layers of the body build and rely. When this foundation erodes, it may help to examine foundational issues related to family.

It is easy to imagine the chronic stress that comes with seeing your spouse slip away into the void. Scientists have determined that caregivers of spouses who suffer from dementia are more than twice as likely to develop oral bone loss as non-caregivers.[3] Studies of this nature may speak to the emotional impact of an eroding foundation of a family union.

In summary, aggravating factors may include chronic mental and emotional stressors, particularly stress to family foundations (past or current).

Consider working with reducing fear, worry, and stress. Apply positive affect-producing qualities such as forgiveness, acceptance, gratitude, etc., to the process involving significant life changes.

Powerful Questions

Can I identify any ongoing stressors eroding my sense of foundation/family?

Are the stressors man-made or unavoidable?

If they are unavoidable, where can I ask for help through these trying times?

Could I infuse acceptance, forgiveness, or gratitude into my process?

What new choice(s) may provide a safe and new direction?

Suggested Blessing

May you reach for new depth, new horizons, and an expanded sense of belonging.

Suggested Affirmation

I release all that is not love from the core of my life.

Take Notice

Floss your teeth regularly and consider the following homemade, anti-inflammatory, antibacterial tooth powder for brushing your teeth after each meal:

Mix equal parts of the following: xylitol, a "tooth friendly" sugar, ideally made from birch bark, included for caries prevention and its antibacterial properties, and sodium bicarbonate ($NaHCO_3$/baking soda), used to increase oral pH, which acts as an antiseptic and neutralizes the acidic environment of the mouth. Add cinnamon, cardamom, nutmeg, or ginger for taste and for their combined antibacterial, anti-caries,[4] and anti-inflammatory properties. Moisten your toothbrush, dip it into the mixed powder, and brush your teeth.

Insomnia

Evidence-Based Confidence Level and Therapeutic Potential

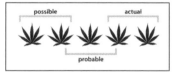

Total Number of Studies Reviewed: 1

CHI Value: 5

Insomnia is difficulty or inability to fall or stay asleep. While many possible causes exist for insomnia, it is interesting to note that its preceding symptoms mirror the condition's effects. Depending on the severity, insomnia affects mental and physical performance as well as emotional expressions (sufferers become moody or irritable). Insomnia may produce symptoms of anxiety, depression, low energy and affect, fatigue, hallucinations, lowered immunity, and hormone disruption—each with its own set of possible complications (i.e., hypertension or heart disease).

If insomnia follows acute pain, jet leg, or a new work schedule, it is usually self-correcting with time. Insomnia due to other causes is more complex.

Insomnia caused by anxiety or use of addictive substances (such as methamphetamines) requires more time and active intervention to resolve.

Orthodox medicine's approach to insomnia includes diagnostics to determine underlying causes. Common pharmacological treatments for insomnia include psychoactive benzodiazepines such as Valium (can be addictive), sedative-hypnotic drugs like Ambien (can be addictive), opiates for the co-treatment of pain (can be addictive), and antidepressants (possible serious side effects). While these agents help manage the symptoms, none of these medications cure chronic insomnia, which usually returns once the medication is stopped.

Cannabis and Insomnia

Like cannabis, the majority of common pharmacological treatments for insomnia affect both body and mind. Most studies on the effects of cannabis and sleep took place in the 1970s and 1980s.[1] These early studies revealed that cannabis had a varied impact on sleep. The plant seemed to act like a sedative in some ways but also reduced deep sleep. None of the early studies explained this paradoxical influence. However, the Farnborough study[2] revealed an apparent self-balancing mechanism between CBD and THC. Dose-dependent THC appears to have sedative effects, while dose-dependent CBD appears to have some alerting properties.

Study Summary

Drugs	Type of Study	Published Year, Place, and Key Results	CHI
4 treatments were an oromucosal spray of either placebo or 15 mg THC or 5 mg THC with 5 mg CBD or 15 mg THC with 15 mg CBD	8 healthy human volunteers (4 males, 4 females; 21 to 34 years old)	2004—QinetiQ Ltd, Centre for Human Sciences, Farnborough, Hampshire, UK: THC appears to have some sedative effects. CBD appears to have some alerting properties.	5

Total CHI Value 5

Strain-Specific Considerations

Practical reports from patients using cannabis to improve their sleep have shown that the use of indica and indica-dominant strains with their particular mix of cannabinoid ratios, namely a relatively lower THC:CBD combination, encourages sedation, relaxation, and grounding effects.

Mind-Body Medicine and Insomnia

Researchers discovered that insomniac patient populations appear to have two characteristic traits that may make them vulnerable to developing the disorder but also provide a potential basis for therapeutic interventions. Commonly noted traits of insomniacs include a poor mechanism for managing stress, and states of cognitive-emotional hyperarousal (exaggerated mental-emotional responses and/or tensions).[3] Since both insomnia and hyperarousal are frequently present in post-traumatic stress disorders, some clinicians suggest a potential similar connection with past traumatic events in cases of insomniacs.

Whatever the physical reasons for insomnia may be, a commonly observed thread is the inability to let go and relax. The mind is constantly engaged in thinking to a point where it could be considered excessive, suggesting a belief(s) that forces the mind to control and dominate the thinking process itself. Relaxation and surrender to sleep can happen only when everything is worked out perfectly, which of course will never happen. The mind can always come up with another thing that could go wrong. Within the insomniac's mind, undefined feelings produce ongoing anxieties; omnipresent fears create the constant need for control; guilt induces the constant threat of imagined punishment and the need to protect oneself; and deprecating self-talk runs in endless loops.

Regular, deep, and restful sleep usually returns once the person learns to trust the process of life.

Aggravating factors may include chronic stress, poor mechanisms for managing stress, unresolved past traumatic events (consider insomnia in the context of PTSD), fear-based belief(s), or inappropriate trust.

Consider reducing fear, worry, and stress; developing appropriate stress-management skills; changing fear-based beliefs; and developing appropriate trust with self and people who are trustworthy.

Powerful Questions

What is going to happen if I let go and fall asleep?

I cannot trust myself because . . . ?

I cannot trust life because . . . ?

Can I let go of these definitions or beliefs?

What must I believe to have a peaceful slumber and restful sleep?

Suggested Blessings

May our flowers help you to retrieve your imagination from the cesspool of fear.

May you remember that you are the director of your internal experiences.

Consider taking your imagination and boldly going where fear does not dare to tread.

Suggested Affirmations

The day is over, this day is gone. I release the day and all the good and bad that may have come with it.

Libido

Evidence-Based Confidence Level and Therapeutic Potential

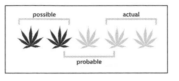

Number of Studies Reviewed: 1

CHI Value: 2

Sigmund Freud and Carl Jung introduced the term "libido" into common usage via psychological theory. Today it is used to describe sexual virility and desire, biological drive, or psychic-emotional force.

While some people with low libido may simply be asexual (not really interested in sex at all), others describe it as reduced frequency or complete absence of "normal" desire. It's no wonder researchers spend so much time and energy seeking to discover the potential underpinnings of people complaining of low libido. Psychiatry even has a name for it: low libido hypoactive sexual desire disorders. Non-physical or psychosomatic causes of the pathological type of low libido may include subjective emotional reasons, anxieties, guilt, shame, stress, worry, chronic fears, sexual abuse, and post-traumatic stress syndrome.

Orthodox medicine suggests the following as underlying physical reasons for a low libido: pathological sexual desire disorders, erectile dysfunction, impotence (in males), frigidity (in women), female sexual arousal disorder, orgasm disorder, or simply sexual dysfunction. Physical causes of a low

libido may include pain, adverse effects of hundreds of common pharmacological medications (especially antidepressants), drug abuse, smoking,
hormone imbalances, numerous chronic medical conditions (especially nervous system disorders and blood-flow/circulation disorders), surgeries (particularly in the region of the genitals), radiation therapy, and chemotherapy.

Depending on underlying causes, modern medicine uses psychotherapy, pharmacological interventions, lifestyle changes, physical therapy, and
surgery to improve libido. Viagra, with worldwide annual sales exceeding
billions of dollars, is by far the best-selling pharmaceutical drug brought
to the market. This has held true since its introduction, despite reports of
Viagra's adverse effects, including death. However, men hoping to regain
youthful desires and long-lost intensities of romance, love, and courtship
soon realized this journey's limits. There is only so much that enhanced
blood flow to the penis can do to resolve emotional deficits. While prof-
its remain high, this realization may be responsible for the first reported
decline of sales on all erectile-dysfunction pharmaceuticals in 2010.

Cannabis and Libido Enhancement

Some of the neurochemistry associated with sexual arousal and cannabis
bears similarities. Both dilate pupils, elevate heart rates, alter endocrine
releases, affect brain signaling, induce euphoria, relax muscles, produce
changes in blood perfusion, and shift respiratory patterns.

Hindu Tantric scriptures and practices dating back more than a thou-
sand years reveal age-old uses of cannabis to enhance sexual pleasure and
bring about enlightenment. In fact, several ancient cultures that deified
sensuality and sexual practices in order to produce extraordinary states
of consciousness and facilitate enlightenment used cannabis to achieve
their goals.

Experiences from the latter two centuries present a picture of cannabis
producing both libido stimulation and depression. Scientific studies today
focus on this paradox of whether cannabis is a sexual stimulant or depres-
sant. Researchers have gained insights by comparing accounts from modern
users, historical records,[1] the world's therapeutic prescription manuals,[2] and
scientific studies on cannabinoids.[3]

The comparisons show that a properly dosed use of the plant may stimulate heightened sensations, increase stamina, deepen intensity of orgasms,

and produce a more profound sense of intimacy. Furthermore, some people who feel anxious before lovemaking have discovered that the plant's anti-anxiety properties can ease the tension and stress often associated with performance problems. Males have reported harder erections, while females described increases in lubrication and clitoral swelling during sex.

It is important to note that each of these properties depends on a very subjective therapeutic window. For instance, too high a dose can deepen anxieties and reduce sensations. While these effects fade as the body metabolizes the plant, user experience teaches to err on the side of caution and suggests beginning with low to medium doses gently and over time.

Study Summary

Drugs	Type of Study	Published Year, Place, and Key Results	CHI
Anandamide	Animal (rats)	2007—University of Michigan: Enhances pleasure experience.[3]	2

Total CHI Value 2

Strain-Specific Considerations

The body's own anandamide activates CB1 and CB2 receptors relatively equally.

Sativas and sativa-heavy hybrids present with a higher THC:CBD/CBN ratio, which, similar to anandamide, tends to activate both receptors relatively equally.

Mind-Body Medicine and Libido Enhancement

An ebb and flow of libido is normal and natural. Asexuality is not an illness but rather a naturally occurring condition. However, if a person experiences loss of libido and desires a return or increase in virility and sexual arousal capacity, it is helpful to explore underlying causes.

Observations have shown that men who suppress anger or hostility toward their partner or all women in general, and men who recycle and harbor their anger or hostility have lower testosterone profiles and a lower libido. The resulting sexual dysfunction may bring these emotional tendencies to the surface.

In summary, aggravating factors may include suppressed or harbored anger, especially at the gender one feels attracted to, and performance anxieties.

Consider working with the appropriate release of anger and hostility toward the gender one feels attracted to; changing belief(s) that create feelings of anger at the gender one feels attracted to; and reducing or ending performance-based anxieties.

Powerful Questions

Is there a part of me that wants to make my partner feel sexually unattractive? If so, why?

Where do I experience lack or loss of libido?

How do I feel about it?

How deep is that feeling?

How can I feel and release the feeling(s) appropriately and with harm to none?

What is at the bottom of the feeling(s)?

What belief do I find at the core of this feeling(s)?

Do I need to practice healing work regarding that belief?

Am I willing to replace this core belief(s)?

Suggested Blessings

May you lose yourself in long-lasting ecstasy.

May you experience the healing powers of a multitude of orgasmic pleasures.

May you feel your virility and creativity last beyond the points of no return.

May you find new depth of ecstatic union that fuels deeper levels of love and intimacy.

Suggested Affirmations

Sex is normal. Sex is fun. Safety is a great libido enhancer.

Love is the most exalted of all aphrodisiacs.

Anecdote

Bill had performance problems in bed, and much as he said he wanted intimacy, he was terrified of it. He described his past relationships as difficult, always leaving him feeling ambivalent toward his ex-girlfriends and women in general. Typical statements were "Women, you can't live with them, and you can't live without them." "First they love you, then they hurt you."

Eventually he realized that the only common denominator in all his relationships was himself. He pondered the thought as he inhaled. It wasn't long before a typical memory emerged; Gina had told him about an affair. And, while they had a relationship that made such events okay, he felt jealous and even envious but pretended not to be. After all, he had agreed to an open relationship. But now, examining his emotional reaction, he realized the fullness of his envy. He felt he could never have as much fun as women (Gina) had. However, instead of his usual knee-jerk reaction denying his envy, he relaxed. Bill looked deeper and longer until he unveiled his inability to create for himself what he thought Gina had. With that embrace of an otherwise intolerable emotion, he felt oddly empowered.

That night, he had a dream. He was watching a beautiful woman (not Gina) dancing sensuously. The dancer seemed to move to music only she could hear and feel—a music that moved her to orgasmic ecstasy that never seemed to end. After a while, she approached him and simply said, "Would you like me to teach you how to do this?" Bill responded with a single word, "Yes."

Since that fateful night, Bill explained, sexual intimacy had new and intriguing dimensions he never before imagined, and his troubles in bed vanished.

Let Food Be Thy Medicine

Anise ∾ Cacao ∾ Cinnamon ∾ Clove ∾ Ginger
Grains of Paradise ∾ Maca ∾ Nutmeg

Anise: Greek herbalists traditionally used anise to promote menstruation, increase breast milk production, facilitate birth, and enhance libido. University of Athens scientists have taken a closer look at anise in the context of finding a safe alternative to estrogen replacement therapies in the prevention of osteoporosis. Anise exhibits estrogen receptor modulator-like properties that produce bone-cell formation without causing breast and cervical cancer cell proliferation.[4]

Cacao: Neurologist Dr. Alan Hirsch, Director of Chicago's Smell and Taste Treatment and Research Foundation, discovered that people's sexual stimulation increases when exposed to the scent of chocolate. (See endnote 1.)

Cinnamon: Neurologist Dr. Alan Hirsch, Director of Chicago's Smell and Taste Treatment and Research Foundation, established that male sexual stimulation increases with exposure to the scent of cinnamon. Furthermore, researchers from Washington concluded that cinnamon might play a beneficial role in lowering high blood pressure, which can contribute to male sexual dysfunction.[5]

"Barefoot Doctors" in rural China use cinnamon sticks to prepare a decoction used in the treatment of male sexual dysfunction.

Clove: This spice has long held a standing reputation in the Unani traditions as an aphrodisiac for males. Now, an Aligarh Muslim University study may provide further clues as to why it works in the treatment of male sexual dysfunction. Researchers noted that normal male rats given a 50% alcoholic extract of clove (from 100 mg/kg to 500 mg/kg) registered significantly enhanced sexual appetites without any noticeable side effects.[6]

Ginger: Unani traditional medicine has long used ginger to enhance sexual function and fertility in males. Scientists from Riyadh, Saudi Arabia, used a rodent experiment to test the influence of ginger as part of their diet. The results showed that ginger significantly increased sperm motility (movement) and content without any toxic side effects.[7]

Grains of Paradise: Researchers from Yaoundé, Cameroon, using a rodent model, discovered that 115 mg/kg of a water-based extract of grains of paradise significantly increased male arousal and sexual function.[8]

Maca: Sexual dysfunction and loss of sexual interest are all too common side effects of selective-serotonin reuptake inhibitor (SSRI) pharmaceuticals, which are used in the treatment of depression. A study from Massachusetts General Hospital (2008) tested whether maca, a Peruvian high-altitude root vegetable, could mitigate SSRI-induced sexual dysfunction. The majority of study participants were women. Results showed a dose-dependent (3 gm daily) significant improvement with an increase in libido. Numerous other studies have confirmed the plant's libido-enhancing properties in males as well.[9]

Nutmeg: Unani traditions boast of nutmeg's long-standing reputation as a male aphrodisiac. An Aligarh Muslim University study found that when rats were given a 50% alcoholic extract of nutmeg as well as clove (500 mg/kg), male rats experienced an increased sexual appetite without any noticeable side effects.[10]

Lung Diseases
Asthma
Evidence-Based Confidence Level and Therapeutic Potential

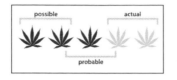

Total Number of Studies Reviewed: 7

CHI Value: 24

Asthma is typically a chronic medical problem, ranging from mild breathing problems similar to those associated with a head cold to severe and life-threatening emergencies that require rapid 911 interventions and transport to the nearest open emergency room.

Asthma does not discriminate. People from all walks of life suffer from asthma; however, children and senior citizens are the most vulnerable. Some children outgrow their asthma while others do not. The causes for asthma are poorly understood, and no pharmacological cure exists. Orthodox medicine focuses on diminishing occurrences and trying to control acute symptoms.

Physicians typically use oxygen and bronchodilators (such as Albuterol, Azmacourt, Ventolin, or Theo-Dur) to open constricted tubes leading to the lungs. However, there is evidence that regular use of inhalers contributes to making asthma worse over time. Other commonly used pharmaceuticals include steroids and drugs that stimulate beta-2 adrenergic receptor sites (receptors that enlist responses including the relaxation of the smooth muscles in the upper airways).

Some of the main triggers of an asthma attack include emotional distress, dust, dust mites, molds, smoking, strong smells, pollution (indoor and outdoor), industrial chemicals, food additives, colds, coughs, and strenuous exercise.

Common signs and symptoms include difficulty breathing, wheezing, pale skin, diaphoresis (sweating), fear and anxiety, tightness in the chest, coughing (clear sputum), or spasms of the upper airways.

If you have an asthma attack, follow your doctor's advice or call 911.

Cannabis and Asthma

It has long been known that the inhalation of burned materials contributes to diseases of the lung. This is especially true when smoking commercial cigarettes. It is almost counterintuitive to believe that inhaling cannabis can reduce symptoms or be otherwise therapeutically beneficial to people with a lung disease such as asthma. However, if smoking can be tolerated without the spasm of coughing, the therapeutic effects of relaxation and upper airway expansion—both important goals in treating asthma—may arrive relatively quickly.

Since 1974, studies have been conducted to document the effects of cannabinoids on human patients with asthma. In the first of such trials (1974) researchers developed a double-blind placebo-controlled cross-over study. Scientists enrolled ten patients with stable asthma to test and compare the efficacy of smoked cannabis, ingested THC, placebo, and a pharmaceutical (isoproterenol) commonly used in the '70s to treat asthma. Results showed that while the initial effect of isoproterenol was more pronounced, the effects of smoked cannabis and oral THC lasted longer. "These findings indicated that in the asthmatic subjects, both smoked marijuana and oral THC caused significant bronchodilation of at least 2 hours duration."[1]

By 1975, eight stable asthmatics were enrolled in another study to determine the effects of cannabis on asthma, both chemically and exercise-induced. Results showed that in both cases, smoked cannabis (THC 2%) produced a prompt correction of the bronchospasms and associated hyper-inflation, similar to isoproterenol.[2]

In 1976, another double-blind placebo-controlled study enlisted ten patients with asthma to learn more about the potential therapeutic properties of cannabinoids in controlling the disease. Results showed that: "Salbutamol and THC significantly improved ventilatory function. Maximal bronchodilation was achieved more rapidly with salbutamol, but at 1 hour both drugs were equally effective." The conducting scientist did not detect any variation in mood or heart rate during the application of THC and concluded that: "The mode of action of THC differs from that of sympathomimetic drugs (drugs which stimulate the sympathetic nervous system and increase heart rate and blood pressure), and it or a derivative may make a suitable adjuvant in the treatment of selected asthmatics."[3]

In the following year (1977), a study evaluated oral and smoked forms of THC compared to a placebo and isoproterenol in a random, double-blind trial conducted on eleven healthy people and five patients with asthma. Researchers measured airway dynamics and heart rates during the experiment. Results showed that aerolized THC was less pronounced than isoproterenol in producing bronchodilation in the short term (5 min.) but significantly better in the longer time ranges (1–3 hours). The authors wrote: "Aerosolized delta9-tetrahydrocannabinol caused significant bronchodilation in 3 of 5 asthmatic subjects, but caused moderate to severe bronchoconstriction associated with cough and chest discomfort in the other two.... These findings indicate that aerosolized delta9-tetrahydrocannabinol, although capable of causing significant bronchodilatation with minimal systemic side effects, has a local irritating effect on the airways, which may make it unsuitable for therapeutic use."[4]

These and the following study results have added more information about THC's ability to increase bronchodilation in asthma patients and highlight some of the differences in the available dosages, forms, and routes of administration of cannabinoids.

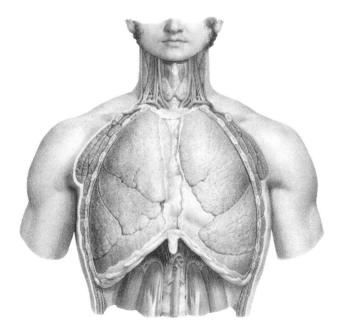

In 1978, researchers administered an aerosol containing THC to asthmatic patients in a steady state of dosage ranging from 50 to 200 mcg. Results showed that the treatment increased the peak expiratory flow rate and forced expiratory volume in one second, and that the onset, magnitude, and duration of the bronchodilator effect were dose-related.[5]

Comparing the synthetic cannabinoid Nabilone to the standard anti-asthmatic pharmaceutical Terbutaline, researchers discovered in 1983 that while Nabilone had some bronchodilation effects in healthy patients, it did not produce a therapeutic effect better than the placebo. The authors concluded that ". . . oral Nabilone (2 mg) does not result in significant acute bronchodilation in patients with asthma."[6]

Despite promising potential, for the next 20 years no studies on asthma and the therapeutics of cannabinoids appeared on the horizon of the usual publishing outlets.

However, by 2006 researchers from Boston had tested numerous novel molecules that exert their biological effects through the endocannabinoid system. The result of this exploration suggests the therapeutic potential of cannabinoids on inflammatory diseases such as asthma and allergic asthma.[7]

Strain-Specific Considerations

The primary cannabinoid used in these asthma studies was THC, which binds to both CB1 and CB2 receptors.

Sativas or sativa-dominant strains tend to contain a cannabinoid profile with a slightly higher THC:CBD/CBN ratio than that of indica or indica-dominant strains.

Mind-Body Medicine and Asthma

Grace and Graham examined the psychosomatic underpinnings of 19 patients and discovered that in the case of the participating subjects, asthma occurred when a patient was faced with a life situation they wished would just go away. They wished someone else would take responsibility for the situation and make it disappear, or wished to avoid it altogether. Typical statements were: "I wanted them to go away." "I didn't want anything to do with it." "I wanted to blot it all out, I wanted to build a wall between me and him." "I wanted to hole up for the winter." "I wanted to go to bed and pull the sheets over my head."

Study Summary

Drugs	Type of Study	Published Year, Place, and Key Results	CHI
Cannabinoids	Laboratory and animal	2006—Boston, Massachusetts: Potential reduction of inflammation in asthma and allergic asthma.[7]	1+2
Nabilone (2 mg) v. Terbutaline sulfate v. placebo	6 healthy people and 6 asthmatic patients	1983—Pulmonary Disease Division, Department of Medicine, University of California, Los Angeles, Calif.: Moderate bronchodilator action in healthy people but no difference compared to placebo in asthmatic patients.[6]	0
Aerosolized THC 50–200 mcg	Asthmatic patients in "steady state"	1978—Asthma Research Unit, Sully Hospital, Penarth, Welsh National School of Medicine, Heath Park, Cardiff, United Kingdom: THC produces bronchodilation in asthmatic patients[5]	3
Aerosolized THC, aerosolized placebo and isoproterenol, and 20 mg of oral and smoked THC	11 healthy people and 5 patients with asthma	1977—Bronchodilation lasts longer than with isoproterenol in healthy subjects. Among asthmatics 3 patients got better; 2 got worse.[4]	5
THC 200 mcg in ethanol (inhaler) v. salbutamol 100 mcg (Ventolin inhaler) v. placebo ethanol	10 asthmatic patients	1976—Asthma Research Unit and the Department of Pharmacology, Sully Hospital, Penarth, Welsh National School of Medicine, Heath Park, Cardiff, United Kingdom: THC significantly improved ventilatory function.[3]	5
Smoked cannabis 500 mg with 2% THC v. 500 mg of smoked placebo marijuana	8 asthmatic patients	1975—Division of Pulmonary Disease, Department of Medicine, UCLA School of Medicine, Los Angeles, Calif.: 2% cannabis and isoproterenol caused an immediate reversal of exercise-induced asthma and hyperinflation.[2]	3
2% natural marijuana (7 mg/kg) v. 15 mg of oral THC v. placebo v. isoproterenol	10 patients with stable bronchial asthma	1974—Smoked cannabis and oral THC caused significant bronchodilation for at least 2 hours.[1]	5

Total CHI Value 24

The authors concluded: "The reaction of the respiratory mucous membrane to a noxious agent is to exclude it by swelling of the membrane with consequent narrowing of the passageway, and to dilute it and wash it out by hypersecretion. When these changes are limited to the nose, the reaction is called vasomotor rhinitis (stuffy or runny nose from reasons other than allergies or infection); when they are sufficiently intense to include the bronchi, so that wheezing occurs, the name asthma is applied."[8]

Wheezing, a characteristic symptom of asthma, is an unmistakable sound. The tighter the airways, the higher the pitch. It appears akin to an internal smothering or a suppression of something that is felt should not be released. Asthma is a struggle to breathe in but especially to exhale.

Non-physical asthma triggers as well as non-physical asthma alleviators are well recognized and commonly noted in any emergency room setting. Most ER personnel know of cases in which a patient's respiratory distress was diminished or completely put to rest by "talking the patient down." Conversely, mental/emotional triggers of asthma have been studied. For instance, one such study published by the *American Journal of Psychiatry* (1987)[9] discovered that difficult or stressful dreams may contribute to asthma attacks while sleeping, and another experiment published by the American Psychological Association (1993)[10] discovered that asthmatic patients have up to three times the amount of nightmares compared to members of healthy control groups.

In summary, aggravating factors may include being faced with a life situation you wish would just go away, or wish that someone else would take responsibility for and make disappear; and a belief that avoidance would be the best course of (in)action.

Consider working toward deep relaxation; trust in the trustworthy; develop trust in self; and work with the paradox of relaxing in the presence of constricting emotions and experiences.

Powerful Questions

Which feelings produce stress responses and make me breathless?
Where do those feelings start?
What in life feels like it's smothering me?
Who smothers me but calls it love?
Are there tears I have not cried because I believe they must be kept inside at all cost?

Suggested Blessings

May you find a way to reduce your stress and ease the tight grip of fear and anxiety.
May you take refuge in the knowledge that all relaxation starts inside you.

May you find a way to let the beauty of life support you from your body's core to the distant horizons of your mind.

Suggested Affirmations

I am free to be me.

I am safe because "I am the master of my fate, I am the captain of my soul."[11]

Let Food Be Thy Medicine

Anise ∾ Bush Tea ∾ Cacao ∾ Garlic ∾ Nigella ∾ Turmeric

Anise: Iranian scientists discovered a possible mechanism that explains why many traditional healers have been using anise extracts and oils in the treatment of certain respiratory ailments. Anise extracts and essential oils possess bronchodilatory qualities (they open the upper airways).[12]

Bush Tea: A study from Karachi, Pakistan, determined why bush tea (rooibos or red tea) might be effective in cases of respiratory difficulties. Bush tea is a bronchodilator, antispasmodic, and contains blood pressure-lowering properties. It apparently achieves this by potassium (ATP) channel activation with a selective bronchodilatory effect.[13]

Cacao: A study from London, England, looked at a component of cacao, theobromine, in the context of treating a persistent cough and determined it to be effective as an anti-tussive (reduces coughing).[14]

Garlic: This versatile herb is used in Cuba for the treatment of asthma and to bring up phlegm during colds and flu.[15]

Nigella: Doctors from Mashhad University, Iran, evaluated the extracts from boiled nigella seeds on asthmatic adults and determined that patients using the extract reported a reduction in all asthma symptoms, including improved pulmonary function tests. Furthermore, patients experienced a reduced need for inhalers.[16]

Turmeric: Based on the evidence of numerous laboratory and animal trials, scientists from Vandoeuvre-Lès-Nancy, France, contend ". . . that curcumin plays a protective role in chronic obstructive pulmonary disease, acute lung injury, acute respiratory distress syndrome, and allergic asthma; its therapeutic action being on the prevention or modulation of inflammation and oxidative stress." Furthermore, and based on the substance of these studies, "these scientists suggest the beginning of clinical trials using turmeric to treat human patients with a variety of chronic and acute lung disorders."[17]

Chronic Obstructive Pulmonary Disease (COPD)
Evidence-Based Confidence Level and Therapeutic Potential

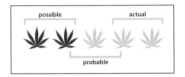

Total Number of Studies Reviewed: 2
CHI Value: 3

This type of lung disease is characterized by narrowing of the airways, which decreases the possible passage of gas exchange in and out of the lungs. In the paradigm of orthodox medicine, the major culprit of chronic obstructive pulmonary disease (COPD) is cigarette smoking. The constant presence of toxic gases produces an initial low-grade inflammation of the lung tissue. As the inflammation slowly progresses, the lungs develop chronic bronchitis, and symptoms such as chronic coughing occur. Burned carbon deposits deep inside the lung ultimately cause the slow destruction of alveoli (the lung structure that exchanges gases with the blood), leading to further deterioration and resulting in emphysema. At this stage of the disease, even the slightest exertion causes shortness of breath.

Cannabis and COPD

In 2005, researchers enrolled 18 patients with COPD, secondary weight loss, and limited exertion potential. To measure the potential therapeutic impacts of cannabinoids on these physical limitations, patients were given twice daily orally administered oil containing between 3.3 and 4.2 mg THC. After 16 days, results indicated an average weight gain of 1.5 kg and a 36% average increase in walking distance.[1] This is a significant achievement, especially when compared to orthodox treatment protocols.

Canadian scientists (2009) examined the effects of tobacco, tobacco with cannabis, and cannabis alone on COPD. Researchers interpret the resulting data: "Smoking both tobacco and marijuana synergistically increased the risk of respiratory symptoms and COPD. Smoking only marijuana was not associated with an increased risk of respiratory symptoms or COPD."[2]

Study Summary

Drugs	Type of Study	Published Year, Place, and Key Results	CHI
Smoking cannabis alone and smoking cannabis with tobacco	Population-based study	2009—Centre for Cardiovascular and Pulmonary Research, St. Paul's Hospital and the University of British Columbia, Vancouver, Canada: Tobacco with cannabis increases risk of COPD. Smoking cannabis alone does not increase risk of COPD.[2]	0
Cannabis oil	Human case study	2005—Presentation at the 2005 Conference of the German Society for Pneumology, Berlin, Karl-Christian Bergmann, Allergie- und Asthmaklinik, Bad Lippspringe, Germany: Increase in walking distance and significant weight gains.[1]	3

Total CHI Value 3

Strain- and Form-Specific Considerations

The human case study from Bad Lippspringe, Germany, used THC dissolved in oil. THC binds to CB1 and CB2 relatively equally.

Sativa and sativa-prominent strains contain higher THC:CBD ratios. Organic sativa oil extracts are made easily or may be purchased at your local dispensary.

Mind-Body Medicine and COPD

The barrel chest, a common symptom in patients with emphysema, merits interpretation. An impressive hyper-inflated, dominant body part mimics that of a person inflating his chest to look bigger and perhaps feel strong and in control. Vulnerability is generally interpreted as feared feelings (especially sadness, grief, hurt, love, or fear), which are often not expressed but rather held in. Un-exhaled feelings linger in the chest, pressing against the ribs and causing constant pressure that ultimately may contribute to a barrel chest. Difficulty exhaling is another common symptom for emphysema patients. Ironically, this strategy—to appear strong and in control all the time—ultimately produces very weak and actually physically vulnerable people who cannot leave the house without an oxygen tank or take a few steps without having to stop and catch their breath.

In summary, aggravating factors may include repressed emotions and a belief system that demands a denial of certain feelings and emotions.

Consider emotional release work, and challenge and change any belief that demands repression of emotions.

Powerful Questions

Are there tears that have never been shed?
What grief have I refused to release?
Which love has never been allowed to blossom?
What hurt still lingers after oh so many years?

Suggested Blessings

May you relax and release your fears.
May you find true strength and allow yourself to walk with ease.

Suggested Affirmations

It is safe to feel everything with strength and intensity.
My emotions are a gift and part of what it means to be human.
I can relax and release my breath fully and with ease.
I am safe and I am free.

Mental Disorders (in general)

Evidence-Based Confidence Level and Therapeutic Potential

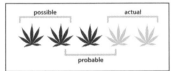

Total Number of Studies Reviewed: 30

Combined CHI Value: 83

The Diagnostic and Statistical Manual of Mental Disorders (DSM) published by the American Psychiatric Association stands as the primary system for mental illness diagnoses in the U.S. It contains about 400 different types of mental diseases and provides specific signs and symptoms to determine diagnoses, possible physiological and mental-emotional causes, and numerous treatment options.

What you will not find in the *DSM*, though, is a mystical, shamanic, or spiritual view of mental illness. And, while the symptoms may be exactly the same, the reason, means, and the resolution are framed in a much more positive light when a spiritual view is taken. Such a view brings hope, positive expectation, and a sense of wonder to the process of being or dealing with the "disturbed." One does not look at the situation as if "there is something wrong with the patient." In fact, an afflicted person may be seen as someone going through a deep transformation and a profound transcendence.

Christian spiritual traditions have referred to the onset of mental disturbances as the "Dark Night of the Soul." A Yoruba Shaman may look upon a mental patient and perceive a future healer. A Vipassana monk in Northern Thailand may look at the mental disturbance as the result of having met enlightenment's evil twin. While the *DSM* cites its reasons for a mental breakdown "dissociation," the monk may associate the disturbance with "staring into the abyss," "witnessing emptiness," or experiencing "no-self."

No matter which of these paradigms appeals to you, both suggest (at least in part) similar practical approaches that work on both sides of this perceptual divide to bring about the completion of the disturbance and give rise to the Phoenix and the emergence of the transformed and healed self. For example, a proper setting, a safe environment, and a good match between method or facilitator and "student" can enhance the healing process and minimize the risk of further debilitating effects.

If you work with a teacher, guide, physician, shaman, or therapist, make sure they are trustworthy, use evidence-based and/or time-proven methods, have the capacity to track your process, and can provide you with the best support possible.

And while a supportive and experienced teacher, therapist, or peer (group) can make a positive difference, consider that you are the most important member on your growth and healing team. During time of crisis employ forgiveness (for whatever part you may have played in it) and give yourself as much compassion, kindness, and love as possible.

While a conclusive understanding of ADHD and the endocannabinoid system (ECS) is still a work in progress, current research conducted primarily on rodents suggests that an ECS-based modulation of neurotransmitters such as dopamine, norepinephrine, GABA, and glutamate may be involved in reducing symptoms. Case studies and surveys conducted on patients with ADHD who successfully self-medicate with cannabis may support this hypothesis.

Researchers from Bordeaux, France (2009), suggest that "The balance between novelty-seeking and safety assessment is a key feature of adaptive behavior, and alterations in this equilibrium can lead to neuropsychiatric disorders."[4] Excessive novelty-seeking or poor impulse control are well-known and common features in ADHD. In the experiment conducted on rodents the researchers discovered that the endocannabinoid system influences the levels of impulse behavior and novelty seeking, and the balance between them. This balance was achieved via CB1 receptors using cortical glutamate (an excitatory neurotransmitter) for novelty-seeking and GABA (an inhibitory neurotransmitter) for controlling behavior. Thus, the dual capacity of the ECS to balance upper and downer effects simultaneously may present a new approach to treating ADHD.

Another experiment conducted on mice in Rome, Italy (2011), echoes the results from Bordeaux. Abnormal dopamine transmission in the striatum (the part of the forebrain that modulates the endocannabinoid system) plays a pivotal role in ADHD. Researchers point to CB1 receptors as novel molecular players in ADHD, and suggest that therapeutic strategies aimed at engaging the ECS might prove effective in this disorder.[5]

Researchers from Melbourne, Australia (2012), chemically induced ADHD-like symptoms in rats. After pre-treating one group of rodents with CBD (3 mg/kg) and another with clozapine (an anti-psychotic medication with off-label use for ADHD), the scientists measured and compared three symptoms: reduced investigative behavior, short attention span, and hyperactivity. Results demonstrated that CBD and clozapine treatment normalized social investigative behavior, reduced hyperactivity, but had no effects on the impairment to attention span.[6]

Consider a human case study from Heidelberg, Germany (2008), conducted on a 28-year-old male diagnosed with ADHD. Researchers describe their first meeting: "His attitude was pushy, demanding, and lacking distance. He expressed impatience, for example by drumming his fingers on the table. He also constantly shifted position, folded arms behind his head or leaned over the table in front of him." By the second meeting he had been taking Dronabinol (THC) as prescribed and "he appeared calm, but not sedated, organized and restrained." The researchers speculated, "There was evidence that the consumption of cannabis had a positive impact on performance, behavior and mental state of the subject." They went on to say that patients suffering from ADHD "... may—in some cases—benefit from cannabis treatment in that it appears to regulate activation to a level which may be considered optimum for performance."[7]

Data from a national U.S. survey of cannabis users (2,811 participants) was examined to determine possible associations between ADHD and cannabis use. Results suggest that daily cannabis-using patients self-medicated for hyperactive-impulsive symptoms of ADHD. The authors note: "These findings indirectly support research linking relevant cannabinoid receptors to regulatory control."[8]

Another survey conducted by the University of California, Irvine (2013), examined the results of self-treatment of ADHD symptoms and quality of sleep with cannabis. Researchers were surprised to find that males (56 participants) and females (20 participants) used cannabis for different reasons. Men used cannabis to treat inattention and females to improve the quality of sleep.[9]

Strain-Specific Considerations

The current status of scientific information suggests that both CB1- and CB2-based mechanisms are involved in modulating symptoms of ADHD. Thus both strains may offer therapeutic potential.

Mind-Body Medicine and ADD/ADHD

In a study conducted at the University of Oregon, researchers showed that that attention and self-regulation develop under the joint influence of genes and the environment, suggesting the possibility of epigenetic triggers and learned interventions.[10] Children who underwent a training method developed by NASA showed improvement in attention, intelligence, and conflict resolution skills when compared to untrained control groups. Additionally, investigations suggest that kids behave normal or more normally

Study Summary

Drugs	Type of Study	Published Year, Place, and Key Results	CHI
Cannabis	Data were collected in 2012 from a national U.S. survey of cannabis users	2014—Department of Psychology, University at Albany, New York, USA: These findings indirectly support research linking relevant cannabinoid receptors to regulatory control.[8]	3
Cannabis	76 cannabis-using patients with ADHD symptoms and poor quality of sleep.	2013—Department of Pediatrics, University of California, Irvine, USA: Men used cannabis to treat inattention, and females used it to improve the quality of sleep.[9]	3
CBD (3 mg/kg) and clozapine (1 and 3 mg/kg)	Animal study (rats)	2012—Monash Institute of Pharmaceutical Sciences, Monash University, Melbourne, VIC, Australia: Results demonstrated that CBD and clozapine treatment normalized social investigative behavior, reduced hyperactivity, but had no effects on the impairment to attention span.[6]	2
CB1 cannabinoids and antagonists	Animal study (mice)	2011—Clinica Neurologica, Dipartimento di Neuroscienze, Università Tor Vergata, Via Montpellier, Rome, Italy: Results point to CB1 receptors as novel molecular players in ADHD, suggesting that therapeutic strategies aimed at interfering with the ECS might prove effective in this disorder.[5]	2
Fatty acid amide hydro-lase (FAAH) inhibitor URB597 (increases anandamide), CB1 receptor inverse agonist AM251, HU210	Animal study (mice)	2009—NeuroCentre Magendie Université de Bordeaux, France: "These data show a tightly regulated influence of the ECS on impulsive behaviors and suggest the involvement of endocannabinoid signaling in the pathophysiological modulation of ADHD and related disorders."[4]	2
Cannabis (smoked), Dronabinol	Human case study (one patient)	2008—Institute of Legal and Traffic Medicine, Heidelberg University Medical Centre, Heidelberg, Germany: Cannabis improves symptoms of ADHD.[7]	3

Total CHI Value 15

when they are put in charge of the pace of their learning experience,[11] are in one-on-one relationships when learning, and are exposed to a learning environment that is rich in novelty and stimulation.

A form of meditation borrowed from Traditional Chinese Medicine was employed to see if short-term meditation could make a difference in attention-deficit conditions. Two groups of students were given five days of mindfulness training. A test was taken afterward by members of both groups. Those students with training showed greater improvement in conflict scores, as well as "lower anxiety, depression, anger, and fatigue, and higher vigor, a significant decrease in stress-related cortisol, and an increase in immunoreactivity."[12]

It is noteworthy that many children will outgrow ADHD, as suggested by the significantly smaller number of adults diagnosed with it. One possible explanation might be that adults have more freedom to choose a learning or work environment in which their liabilities can become assets. For instance, most adults (unlike many kids) can reject activities or jobs that require repetition or routine, and seek a work environment that is unpredictable, stimulating, and constantly changing.

Powerful Questions

What is going to happen if I just let myself feel bored?
What could happen if I infuse my energy into a boring moment?
How can I infuse a new perspective into the mundane?

Suggested Blessings

May your creativity spark novelty in every moment of your life.
May you discover that that every moment of daily rut and routine contains the seed of the unknown and unpredictable.
May you have the humility to see each moment as brand-new.
May your restlessness, impatience, and short attention span transform into an asset.

Suggested Affirmations

I have the capacity to produce novelty in every moment.
I have the humility to see every moment as brand-new.

Take Notice

Extended Attention Span Training (EAST), Self Mastery and Regulation Training (SMART)

Extended Attention Span Training (EAST) is a video game developed by NASA to ensure sustained attention, engagement, awareness, and a reduction of stress in individuals operating aircraft. The game is guided by a neurofeedback loop tied into the gaming activity that changes game elements in accordance with direct signals taken via electrodes attached to the pilot's skin.

Consider exploring the NASA spinoff called Self Mastery and Regulation Training (SMART), a video game available to the public that utilizes the same principles.

Anxiety
Evidence-Based Confidence Level and Therapeutic Potential

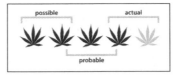

Total Number of Studies Reviewed: 4
CHI Value: 14

Generally speaking, anxiety is a normal reaction to the subjective experience of stress, such as in "performance anxiety." It can occur when anticipation of future events is associated in one's mind with thoughts and feelings not rooted in the present moment. While anxieties can be considered a normal part of life, chronic or constant anxiety can be debilitating to one's quality of life. In fact, such interference can produce very real physiological changes in the short and long term. It is estimated that almost two out of ten people in the U.S. suffer from some kind of anxiety disorder.[1]

Western medicine considers anxiety disorders mood disorders and defines five basic types: generalized anxiety disorder (GAD), obsessive-compulsive disorder (OCD), panic disorder, post-traumatic stress disorder (PTSD), and social anxiety disorder (social phobias).

Generalized Anxiety Disorder (GAD): GAD patients present with chronic worry about anticipated events constructed by their mind. Symptoms often include "feeling the other shoe is about to drop," unreasonable worry, tense and aching muscles (e.g., neck, shoulders), headaches, trembling and diaphoresis (sweating).

Obsessive-Compulsive Disorder (OCD): OCD patients are characterized by compulsive, often odd behavior that can be described as personal rituals, such as filling in all the letter O's when writing, not stepping on any cracks in the sidewalk, or constantly needing to wash their hands. Continuously occupying the mind with such trivial activities provides a sense of control for those who otherwise would focus on anticipated but unwanted thoughts or feelings.

Panic Disorder: Patients with panic disorder anxiety are prone to panic attacks. Acute short-term symptoms may begin as rapid heart rate, rapid breathing (hyperventilation), and a dry mouth, sometimes progressing to an anxiety attack with restlessness, chest tightness or pain, palpitations, shortness of breath, tingling, numbness (in the hands, feet, or lips), diaphoresis (sweating), feelings of impending doom or death, and inconsolability.

Post-Traumatic Stress Disorder (PTSD): PTSD develops after undergoing or witnessing a significant traumatic event. Patients frequently re-experience the trauma in their mind, either when dreaming or triggered by an external stimulus. They will often try to avoid all feelings and attempt to numb themselves against a constant dread of the return of the event. Some symptoms include "feeling on edge," flashbacks, constant fearful thoughts, sudden outbursts of anger, and an aversion to being close to anyone.

Social Anxiety Disorder: Social phobia patients are often defined by their anticipation of severely humiliating events. This type of anxiety disorder may be limited to a very narrow context, such as being extremely self-conscious about turning red (blushing) in public and then feeling judged by everybody in the room. Physical symptoms include a red face, trembling, sweating, nausea and/or difficulty forming words or sentences.

Doctors often prescribe pharmaceuticals (e.g., anti-anxiety drugs, antidepressants) or psychological intervention to treat anxiety, particularly when underlying physical causes are absent. Adverse effects of pharmaceutical anti-anxiety medication range from mild to fatal. A thorough risk versus benefit analysis is advisable before committing to such a regimen.

Cannabis and Anxiety (in general)

Various medical traditions use cannabis extracts because of their time-proven calming and sedative effects. Today numerous studies confirm that cannabinoids modulate mood states and can reduce anxiety. However, evidence has also shown that anxiety-reducing effects of cannabis are subjectively dose-specific. Too little can be sub-optimal, while too much can actually increase anxious feelings.

In 2005, teams from China, Canada, and the U.S. conducted a review of the available scientific literature on the topic of cannabinoids and anxiety and found that "Cannabis and its major psychoactive component (-)-trans-Delta-tetrahydrocannabinol, have profound effects on mood and can modulate anxiety and mood states."[2] In the same year, another international team of scientists examined a potent synthetic cannabinoid (HU210) in an experiment on rats. Most illegal substances have been reported to decrease the growth of new nerve cells in the hippocampus. However, chronic HU210 treatment promoted neurogenesis in the hippocampal regions of the rodents, which was likely to produce both an anxiolytic and antidepressant-like effect.[3]

In 2009, researchers from Boston collected data from 775 patients living with HIV/AIDS and suffering from six commonly associated symptoms: anxiety, depression, fatigue, diarrhea, nausea, and peripheral neuropathy. Study participants came from Kenya, South Africa, Puerto Rico, and ten different U.S. locations. Results showed that while the differences were relatively small, cannabis was considered somewhat more effective than standard prescription and over-the-counter medications in treating anxiety, depression, diarrhea, fatigue, and neuropathy. However, it proved less effective in cases of nausea.[4]

In 2010, researchers from São Paulo, Brazil, reviewed available studies on two cannabinoids, CBD and THC, and their impact on the psychiatric patient. Researchers considered CBD's therapeutic potential as an antipsychotic, anxiolytic, and antidepressant, while THC was considered as a potential adjuvant in the treatment of schizophrenia. The authors concluded: "Cannabinoids may be of great therapeutic interest to psychiatry; however, further controlled trials are necessary to confirm the existing findings and to establish the safety of such compounds."[5]

Strain-Specific Considerations

Cannabis, CBD, THC, and HU210 underwent testing in these trials in the context of anxiety. Cannabis contains the full spectrum of cannabinoids' and non-cannabinoids' biologically active ingredients that activate CB1 and

Study Summary

Drugs	Type of Study	Published Year, Place, and Key Results	CHI
Cannabidiol and THC	Meta-analysis	2010—Universidade de São Paulo, Brazil: Cannabidiol therapeutic potential: antipsychotic, anxiolytic, and antidepressant. THC: adjuvant in the treatment of schizophrenia.[5]	4
Cannabis	775 humans living with HIV/AIDS	2009—MGH Institute of Health Professions, School of Nursing, Boston: Cannabis considered effective in treating anxiety and depression and other symptoms in AIDS patients.[4]	3
HU210	Animal and laboratory study (rats)	2005—Multi-institutional and international study: Hippocampal cells are immunoreactive for CB1 receptors. Cannabinoids may induce hippocampal neurogenesis, which may explain their anxiolytic and antidepressant-like effects.[3]	2+1
Cannabis, cannabinoids	Literature review (meta-analysis)	2005—Psychiatric Drug Discovery, Lilly Research Laboratories, Eli Lilly and Company, Indianapolis, Indiana: Cannabis can modulate anxiety and mood states.[2]	4

Total CHI Value 14

CB2. CBD has greater affinity for CB2. THC binds relatively equally with both CB1 and CB2 receptors. HU210 possesses a higher affinity for CB1.

It appears that both signaling pathways (CB1 and CB2), individually as well as in combination, modulate anxiety. Indicas and indica-dominant hybrids, which tend to present with a lower THC:CBD/CBN ratio, are preferred. Many cannabis-using patients suffering from anxiety prefer the indicas' sedating, relaxing, and grounding effects.

Mind-Body Medicine and Anxiety

In the depths of anxiety reside the keys to our imagination and access to the power of our creativity. Thus, anxious people can imagine anything and everything that can go wrong. And most patients suffering from anxiety disorders know very well the power of their creativity, which when driven by anxiety can often produce the very thing so feared. The task here is to take back the power of your imagination from the part of the mind that has its sole focus on what could go wrong, and apply that mental power to what could go *right*.

Mild forms of anxiety occur when the mind anticipates challenging feelings. Anxieties progress to their debilitating forms when this anticipation interferes with normal daily functions and quality of life. Although most commonly associated with constricting feelings or emotions such as fear, anxiety can also be triggered by anticipation of expansive emotions such as an unprecedented love or joy or pride.

Powerful Questions

What was the "accident" or event that caused you to become a nervous wreck?

What trigger event(s) sets off your anxiety?

Who or what is getting on your nerves?

What can you learn about your anxiety?

Can you befriend your anxiety?

Can you have compassion for yourself when feeling anxious?

What belief(s) is locking your imagination on the object(s) of your anxiety?

What is the worst that could happen?

Can you come up with a plan B if the worst occurs?

When was the last time you felt relaxed, quiet, calm, secure, or confident?

Anecdote

Maria was a self-described worrywart. She worried excessively and needlessly until her constant anticipation of the worst possible scenario began to erode her health. She felt anxious, uncertain, uneasy, and irritable, which eventually produced a constant fatigue, insomnia, indigestion, and episodes of rapid heartbeats, hypertension, hyperventilation, and panic attacks. She sought a cannabis prescription for help with her disorder.

Maria describes her experience taking cannabis: "After a few minutes, I felt relaxed for what felt like the first time ever. I saw my worry like a dark cloud or mist right in front of me; but my reaction to it was noticeably different. I remained relaxed and curious where I normally would feel overwhelmed and panicky. Wherever I turned my mind's eye, my worry snapped into place in front me. I started to realize that I was the one pulling it with me at every turn of my imagination. I realized that I used my worry as a shield to protect myself from enemies sprung from my own imagination. I could see that my worry rose from the belief I held so dear that 'the world is a scary place' and that almost 'everybody is out to get me' in some way or another. I was a victim, thinking I had no power to do anything about it. Then I saw that I used my worry to separate myself from a memory I did not want to experience, an experience I pretended did not really exist.

"But what was it that I was so worried about? As I asked the question, I remembered an accident when I was little. I had run into traffic and was sideswiped by a car. I was okay but for a few abrasions. However, my parents were freaking out. 'I told you it is too dangerous to be out here by yourself!' 'People don't care and they will hurt you if you don't watch it.' I was kept inside for a long while and later strictly limited and supervised when outside. I saw how my parents used worry to excessively control my life. However, I also understood that that was then and this is now. I became aware that just because my parents did this does not mean I need to continue the behavior. I heard myself saying: I don't have to hide behind my worry any longer. I don't have to keep the world apart from me any longer."

This case demonstrated a relatively quick resolution engaging the underlying body-mind aspects of Maria's symptoms. Once Maria understood and answered the message of her chronic worry, the physical symptoms went away. Nowadays Maria hardly has any worries at all, and during those times when they do appear, she is confident that she'll get through it just fine. In those moments, Maria does not succumb to the feelings of stress and worry; she merely acknowledges the anxiety as part of the human experience that can be handled with a bit of mindfulness and attention. Maria considers herself cured.

See also "Ten Ways to Resolve Fear and Anxiety" on page 49.

Suggested Blessings

May you discover the natural confidence that comes from trusting yourself to be calm and quiet until action is required.

May you always find your natural balance between tension and relaxation.

Suggested Affirmations

I take back my imagination from the clutches of my anxieties and fears.

I imagine trusting myself.

I can relax, be calm, and feel safe.

I can imagine the good, the truth, and the beauty in this world.

I imagine what can go right.

Autism

Evidence-Based Confidence Level and Therapeutic Potential

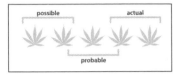

No Modern Cannabis Studies Available

Thirty years ago few people had ever heard the word "autism." Circa 1975, only one in 5,000 children was diagnosed with this condition.[1] Nowadays it is a household word, and almost everybody knows of someone suffering from the disease. The allopathic community considers autism a neurodevelopmental disorder that begins in very early childhood.

Among many psychological approaches to autism, applied behavioral analysis (ABA), developed by O. I. Lovaas, PhD,[2] appears to stand out in reported efficacy. Using ABA, improvements were seen in IQ, social skills, adaptive behavior, and academic progress.[3] However, while proven effective, ABA's one-on-one teaching conditions constitute a "full-time job" at about 40 hours a week, making it cost-prohibitive for many parents.

Pharmaceutical medications (such as Ritalin, an amphetamine-like drug) are given to millions of children every year to control symptoms. This leaves many parents little choice but to accept the risks of possible adverse effects, with reported deaths in the hundreds. No simple cure for autism exists, and there is a growing number of autistic patients. Government statistics suggest that the prevalence rate of autism is increasing 10–17% annually, doubling roughly every five years since 1980.[4] The facts are starkly clear: the pervasiveness of autism is growing exponentially. If current trends continue and no cure is found, we could be looking at a future reality where, by 2047, one in two people will be diagnosed as autistic.

Outwardly, autistic patients may look perfectly normal, but a closer look at their behavior reveals obvious differences from those unaffected. Autism is considered a spectrum disorder in which signs and symptoms range from mild to severe. Symptoms of autism include impaired social interaction and language skills, difficulty relating to others including peers, reduced or altered emotional or behavioral responses, difficulty making eye contact, no interest in sharing experiences, and repetitive focus and actions (ritualistic behavior such as lining up items is commonly noted). Depending on the condition's severity, autistic patients are often socially isolated and frequently considered social outcasts by others who do not know how to relate to them.

The reasons for autism's development and exponential growth remain a mystery within the modern medical system, which generally hypothesizes that genetic and environmental conditions are at play. More specific origination theories include biochemical causes, psychiatric causes, possible food components (e.g., gluten, casein, vitamin D deficiency), the overuse of pharmaceutical drugs (e.g., the use of antibiotics or oxytocin during birth), compromised immune system of one or both parents, vaccinations, neuro-inflammatory conditions, autoimmune conditions, imbalances of neurotransmitters, toxins (e.g., lead, mercury, pesticides), microbes (e.g., mold, viral load), or electromagnetic pollution.

"Autism is a very expensive disorder costing our society upwards of $35 billion in direct (both medical and non-medical) and indirect costs to care for all individuals diagnosed each year over their lifetimes."[5] As it stands, many autistic children will likely need lifelong care. Parents and caretakers need to make specific and practical long-term care plans that continue beyond their own lifetimes.

Cannabis and Autism

Scientists have learned a great deal from communicative autistic people. For one, autistic individuals process sensory information differently, thus producing an altered perception and, by extension, a different meaning given to reality.

Some cannabis users have reported similar experiences when using more than the therapeutically appropriate dose. For example, experiences of sensory disconnect between the eye and the ear, not unlike the disjointed soundtrack of a poorly dubbed foreign movie, have been noted to cause people to temporarily withdraw and display symptoms similar to those observed in autistic persons.

Based on these observations, it is hypothesized that dose-specific cannabinoids may somehow be involved in calibrating the connectivity among sensory input, perception, meaning, and the ability to respond and function.

Many parents have found themselves up against a wall. Feeling hopeless in the face of modern medicine's inability to understand the disease and its origin, perhaps lacking safe and effective assistance, many have turned to cannabis.[6] Based on anecdotal reports by some physicians, pediatricians, caretakers, and patients themselves that using cannabis had significant positive effects on patients suffering from autism, efforts are underway to learn more about if and how these reported therapeutic effects take place.

Positive results have been reported from ingestion of appropriate doses of cannabis or the pharmaceutical version of isolated cannabinoids, even in some extremely difficult cases where pharmaceutical treatment had proven ineffective or destructive. Reported results included reductions in tantrums, rage, self-injury, and property destruction, and improved happiness, an increased ability to learn, and flexibility in altering norms.

While it is known that the body's own endocannabinoid system is involved in mood regulation, no clinical study results exist to confirm or deny the anecdotally positive experiences of some autistics.

Cannabis and isolated cannabinoids can both have adverse effects, especially outside their appropriate therapeutic dosage; this must be cautiously considered, especially for children. However, parents faced with repeated ineffectiveness from prescribed pharmaceuticals may benefit in working with a qualified health care professional experienced in evaluating possible benefits of metered cannabis or prescription cannabinoids.

Mind-Body Medicine and Autism

Most differences between autistic and "normal" people are defined by the ability to function according to socially "normal" criteria. For most autistic people, their own symptoms are natural, and autism is nothing to be ashamed about. This is remarkable, and in contrast to many fully functioning "normal" people who often feel ashamed for something as simple as their face, height, or name. In this sense, it would seem that a majority of autistic people may have a more centered sense of their worth than a "normal" person.

Along the spectrum of ability to function, some autistics display extraordinary abilities in relatively narrow fields. Professor Treffert,[7] researcher at the University of Wisconsin Medical School, discovered in his research on savant syndrome that over half of all savants are autistics. Abilities include total musical recall,[8] total visual recall,[9] synesthesia,[10] and animal empathy.[11] A study by Patricia Howlin of King's College, London, suggests that as many as one-third of autistic people have some sort of savant-like capability in areas such as calculation or music.[12] Savant syndrome then is a case where the politically correct euphemism "differently abled" has real meaning. Autistic savants displaying super-natural ability alongside their sub-normal limitations demonstrate new possibilities for the human mind.

Since the senses of each autistic person seem in tune with realities different from those of non-autistic people, learning how these senses function may provide insights to better understand, communicate, and relate to a person with an autistic mind.

While the impact on parents, caretakers, and society at large is omnipresent and understood, we are left with questions about autism's alarming numbers and unknown possible environmental causes and psychosomatic influences. This mystery is still in need of much exploring.

Powerful Questions

How do the senses of this autistic person function?

What purpose does this extraordinary autistic state of mind serve?

What does this autistic person perceive that we do not?

Might there be a message inherent in autism?

Since autistics are usually oblivious to the music, motion, and symbology of neuro-typical or "normal" human-to-human communication using gesture, voice, body language, and facial muscles, answering the following questions may be useful.

How can I add voice and body to mere words?

How can I learn to understand facial expressions?

How can I make my facial expressions understood?

How can I add theatre to my message?

Suggested Blessings

May you find supportive teachers who can direct the autistic gaze and focus in fruitful directions.

May you be like a Hollywood star and learn easy and practical ways to add meaningful theatre to your expressions.

May you discover a way to add gesture, voice, body language, and facial expressions to linguistics, so as to be more fluent with others.

Depression
Evidence-Based Confidence Level and Therapeutic Potential

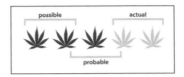

Total Number of Studies Reviewed: 8

CHI Value: 23

While brief episodes of "feeling depressed" are part of the human experience, prolonged, severe, or clinical depression can make it very difficult or even impossible to get out of bed in the morning and function normally. An estimated 350 million-plus people suffer from depression worldwide, according to a 2012 WHO estimate.[1] Symptoms vary but tend to include low energy or lack of interest in life, work, or pleasure.

Western medicine does not claim to know the causes for depression, but it hypothesizes that genetic predisposition, certain underlying medical conditions (e.g., hypothyroidism), toxins or nutritional deficiencies which alter normal neurochemistry, stressful life events (deep and sudden changes), or a combination of these and other factors are causal agents.

Treatment varies. Psychiatrists prescribe antidepressant medications, while psychologists employ psychotherapy. Some patients with milder forms of the disease find help in using the herb St. John's wort. Depression during longer nights in winter may also respond well to an exposure of full-spectrum light at home.

It is estimated that about 15% of clinically depressed patients will succeed in committing suicide. This morbidity combined with the other debilitating symptoms makes treatment of the disease and support of patients paramount.

Ironically, antidepressant drugs, marketed to treat depression and prevent suicides, are sold by the billions in the U.S. alone yet reportedly contribute to a significant rise in suicide rates. In fact, the FDA has commissioned major antidepressants like Paxil, Prozac, and Zoloft to post black-box warning labels regarding rise of suicidality.

Cannabis and Depression

Cannabinoids have proven effective in laboratory studies and rodent tests for antidepressant activity. These effects appear to share a similar mechanism of action as current antidepressant drugs such as the selective-serotonin reuptake inhibitors (SSRIs). Human trials have confirmed the antidepressant effects and mood-elevating properties of cannabis.

More specifically, in both a Tulsa study[2] (1995) and an experiment from Miami[3] (2002), researchers discovered that cannabinoids might play a therapeutic role in improving mood and reducing signs of depression. In 2005, an international team of scientists examined the impact of a potent synthetic cannabinoid (HU210) in an experiment on rats. Most illegal substances have been reported to decrease the growth of new nerve cells in the hippocampus. However, chronic HU210 treatment promoted neurogenesis in the hippocampal regions of the study rodents and appeared likely to produce both an anxiolytic and antidepressant-like effect.[4]

A Vancouver study (2007) confirmed the potential antidepressant effect of cannabinoids; specifically, enhanced CB1 activity in the hippocampus region of the brain produced an antidepressant-like effect in rats.[5] Scientists from Montreal, Canada (2007) lent further support for the hypothesis that cannabis modulates moods and possesses antidepressant-like properties via CB1 receptors.[6]

A Boston trial (2009) involved data collected from 775 patients living with HIV/AIDS and the manifestation of depression. Results revealed that cannabis was more effective in treating depression when compared with standard prescription and over-the-counter medications given for the same condition.[7]

Scientists from São Paulo, Brazil (2010), conducted a review of available studies on two cannabinoids (CBD and THC) and their impact on the psychiatric patient. Cannabidiol showed a therapeutic tendency as an antipsychotic, anxiolytic, and antidepressant, while THC emerged as a potential adjuvant in the treatment of schizophrenia.[8] In addition, an Oxford, Mississippi, experiment demonstrated that THC exerted antidepressant-like actions and "thus might contribute to the overall mood-elevating properties of cannabis."[9]

Study Summary

Drugs	Type of Study	Published Year, Place, and Key Results	CHI
Δ9-THC, Δ8-THC, CBG, CBN, CBC, CBD	Animal study (mice)	2010—University of Mississippi: THC and other cannabinoids exert antidepressant-like actions and mood elevation.[9]	2
CBD and THC	Meta-analysis	2010—Universidade de São Paulo, Brazil: Cannabidiol therapeutic potential: antipsychotic, anxiolytic, and antidepressant. THC: adjuvant in the treatment of schizrenia.[8]	4
Cannabis	775 humans living with HIV/AIDS	2009—MGH Institute of Health Professions, School of Nursing, Boston: Cannabis considered effective in treating anxiety and depression and other symptoms in AIDS patients.[7]	3
WIN55,212-2 (synthetic CB1 agonist)	Animal study (rats)	2007—Montreal, Canada: Central CB1 modulates mood and has antidepressant-like effects.[6]	2
HU210 (CB1 receptor agonist), URB597 (the fatty acid amide hydrolase inhibitor), AM251 (CB1 receptor antagonist)	Animal study (rats)	2007—Department of Psychology, University of British Columbia, Vancouver, Canada: Enhanced CB1 activity in the hippocampus region of the brain produces an antidepressant-like effect.[5]	2
HU210 (CB1 receptor agonist)	Animal and laboratory study (rats)	2005—Multi-institutional and international study: Hippocampal cells are immunoreactive for CB1 receptors. Cannabinoids may induce hippocampal neurogenesis, which may explain the anxiolytic and antidepressant-like effects.[4]	2
Oral doses of Delta-9-THC, 2.5 mg to 5 mg	Human clinical study (3 patients)	2002—Department of Medicine, University of Miami, Florida: Decrease in itching, improvement in sleep, and resolution of depression in patients with pruritus due to cholestatic liver disease.[3]	3
2.5 mg of Dronabinol twice daily or placebo	139 patients living with AIDS	1995—St. John's Hospital, Tulsa, Oklahoma: Improvement in mood (10% v. -2% for placebo).[2]	5

Total CHI Value 23

Strain-Specific Considerations

In these various studies, cannabinoids demonstrated the ability to modulate mood in depression via different pathways or mechanisms, chiefly among them THC and whole-spectrum cannabis. THC binds with both CB1 and CB2 relatively equally. It is hypothesized that cannabis, containing 70 cannabinoids and hundreds of non-cannabinoid ingredients, may work in concert to induce mood improvement via CB1 and CB2 activation as well as through the balancing influences of whole-plant constituents.

Delta-9-THC, Delta-8-THC, CBG, CBN, CBC, CBD, Cannabis, WIN55,212-2, HU210, and Dronabinol have been tested for treatment of depression. THC binds with both CB1 and CB2 relatively equally. Cannabigerol (CBG) binds with both CB1 and CB2. Cannabinol (CBN) has higher affinity for CB2. Cannabichromene's (CBC) underlying mechanism of action may not involve CB1 or CB2 receptors. Cannabidiol (CBD) has a greater affinity for CB2. WIN55,212-2 has a greater affinity for CB2. HU210 has a higher affinity for CB1 receptors. Dronabinol is an isomer (same molecular formula but different structural formula) of delta9-tetrahydrocannabinol.

Sativas and sativa-dominant strains tend to have a higher THC:CBD/CBN ratio and are generally sought after by cannabis-using patients suffering from depression for their stimulating, energizing, and uplifting potential.

Mind-Body Medicine and Depression

The emotional realities of a depressed person often include feeling weighed down by layers upon layers of unexpressed emotions such as hurt or anger. This accumulated emotional burden results in low energy and lack of interest in life, work, or pleasure. The prospect of expending energy to do some emotional house-cleaning when depressed can be depressing in and of itself. Healing depression requires patients to address and feel the layers of emotions that so depress the body, mind, and spirit. This is especially true when considering anger and hurt.

Anger is generally judged because of its direct association with violent expressions. Therefore, many consider it as something not okay to feel, or at least not for very long or with any real intensity. However, when discerning the complexities of anger, it is important to realize that as with any real feeling it can be liberating or imprisoning. For example, expressions of anger can be authentic or dramatic performances. Authentic anger is felt and released, while performing anger is harbored and stored. Anger can be used either to communicate or to manipulate others. Anger can be focused on the impact of an action which is easily correctable or it can be used to shame a person into thinking there is something wrong with them. Few role models exist that demonstrate how to express and release anger with intensity, focused appropriately for positive impact.

Consider adding a meditative approach when dealing with depression. This approach does not take any energy, only a bit of your imagination, and can be done in bed. Imagine whatever depresses you as a heavy weight (such as a duffelbag) lying on top of you (make it dirty, ugly, smelly). Now punch a tiny hole in the bottom of the bag. Slowly let the content flow out of the tiny hole and into the earth (she can handle it, probably turn it into fertilizer). Notice the weight becoming lighter (little by little). What does it feel like? Pay attention to the details. The more imaginative you can be, the more effective the technique can be. Remember that the autonomic nervous system does not know the difference between real and imagined events.

While numerous studies have shown that exercise (e.g., hiking, running) had a therapeutic effect on depression, an experiment conducted by a group of researchers from Germany and Canada demonstrated that type of gait (depressed vs. happy) had a direct impact on selective memory. Walking in a depressed fashion (e.g., slumped over, with hanging shoulders) made it easier to remember negative things. Conversely, walking in a happy fashion increased the tendency to remember positive things.[10] This gives the saying "put a bounce in your step" a new meaning.

Powerful Questions

Is it okay for you to feel angry?
How do you deal with your anger?
How intense do you allow your anger to get?
Does your anger leave a wave of destruction in its wake?

Similarly, for many people, it is not okay to feel hurt. Hurt is seen as a liability or vulnerability and considered a sign of weakness. Hurt diminishes trust and has the ability to destroy a healthy love of self, reduce the experience of one's worth, and otherwise negatively affect self-esteem and self-confidence.

Can you identify when your self-love suffers?
Do you notice when your self-esteem has taken a hit?
Do you see what reduces your self-confidence?
Is it okay for you to feel hurt?
How do you deal with your hurt?
Can you show hurt to others?
Can you show it to yourself?
Does hurt heal you?

Suggested Blessings

May you find a reason to get intricately involved with something that produces vibrant thoughts and juicy feelings.

May the process of thinking and feeling release the heaviness that so consumes your energy.

May you discover an omnipresent help to make this process easy or at least as easy as possible.

Suggested Affirmations

I have the capacity to feel and release what depresses me.

If I do not believe in this capacity I can ask for help in feeling and releasing all that is keeping me from living my life fully, substantially, and lightly.

It is okay to feel angry.

It is okay to feel hurt.

I can release my anger appropriately without hurting anyone.

I can heal my hurt and re-establish my sense of self-worth, rebuild my self-esteem, and regain confidence in myself.

Let Food Be Thy Medicine

Cacao ∾ Nutmeg

Cacao: Scientists from Tucson, Arizona, reported that chocolate is likely to be involved in increasing low levels of serotonin and dopamine (neurotransmitters involved in mood regulation).[11]

Nutmeg: An extract of nutmeg seeds (10 mg/kg) was found—in a mouse model—to have antidepressant properties similar to those of pharmacological antidepressants such as imipramine (15 mg/kg) and fluoxetine (20 mg/kg). The researchers from Guru Jambheshwar University in Hisar, India, stated: "The antidepressant-like effect of the extract seems to be mediated by interaction with the adrenergic, dopaminergic, and serotonergic systems."[12]

Manic-Depressive Disorder/Bipolar Affective Disorder (BAD)
Evidence-Based Confidence Level and Therapeutic Potential

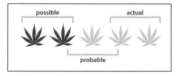

Total Number of Studies Reviewed: 5

CHI Value: 8

Psychiatry considers manic-depressive disorder to be a chronic mental illness characterized by dramatic and sudden mood swings ranging from manic to depressed and back. Onset of the illness is usually observed in late adolescence or early adulthood but has also been noted in younger people. While normal ups and downs in mood are part of being human, pathological mood swings severely reduce quality of life and the ability to function and maintain social relations. Subgroups of the illness are identified on a spectrum by severity of the disease and frequency of mood swings.

The scientific community believes that bipolar disorders have a variety of causes. Origins could be genetic, environmental (childhood trauma or abuse),[1] or physiological (e.g., brain, endocrine irregularities). Diagnosis is based on observation and clinical evaluation. Tests may be performed to rule out possible underlying causes or contributing diseases.

Western treatment consists of pharmacological interventions and talk therapy. The most commonly used pharmaceutical is an alkali metal—lithium—which functions as a potent mood stabilizer and has been proven to significantly prevent suicides in bipolar patients.[2]

Cannabis and Manic-Depressive Disorder

Scientists have conducted numerous studies to examine the effects of cannabis and cannabinoids on individuals with manic-depressive disorder. Results revealed that the body's own endocannabinoid system is involved in mood regulation. While some case studies reported possible beneficial effects vis-à-vis manic episodes, available evidence was too small and narrow to warrant using cannabis/cannabinoids for treatment. However, the plant and its products have been found to therapeutically influence the depressive aspect of the disease.

Study Summary

Drugs	Type of Study	Published Year, Place, and Key Results	CHI
Δ9-THC, Δ8-THC, CBG, CBN, CBC, and CBD	Animal study (mice)	2010—University of Mississippi: THC and other cannabinoids exert antidepressant-like actions and mood elevation.[3]	2
Cannabidiol (CBD)	Placebo-controlled human case study (2 patients with BAD)	2010—Department of Neuropsychiatry and Medical Psychology, Faculty of Medicine, University of São Paulo, Ribeirão Preto, São Paulo, Brazil: Ineffective for the manic episode of bipolar affective disorder.[4]	-5
Cannabis	Human case study, one patient diagnosed with BAD	2007—University of Louisville School of Medicine, Louisville, Kentucky: Cannabis reduced the number of depressed days and increased the number of hypomanic days.[5]	3
Cannabis and various other cannabinoids	Literature review	2005—Department of Psychiatry, University of Newcastle upon Tyne, Royal Victoria Infirmary, Newcastle upon Tyne, UK: Some patients claim that cannabis relieves symptoms of mania and/or depression.[6]	4
Cannabis	Human case studies	1998—Department of Psychiatry, Harvard Medical School, Boston, Massachusetts: Positive therapeutic impact based on individual case studies only.[7]	4

Total CHI Value 8

Strain-Specific Considerations

Only whole-plant cannabis and CBD (rather than other forms) have been tested for treatment of bipolar disorder. CBD was not proven effective, while whole-herb constituents could be supportive. CBD has a greater affinity for CB2. Whole cannabis contains cannabinoids activating CB1 and CB2.

Sativas and sativa-dominant strains tend to contain a higher THC:CBD ratio, which may slightly reduce CBD influence.

Some patients have reported on alternate strains of cannabis used during either the manic or depressive phase. During depressive phases, cannabis-using patients may benefit from sativas; while during manic phases, they might benefit more from an indica strain.

Mind-Body Medicine and Manic-Depressive Disorder

In a manic-depressive patient, the mind can swing relatively quickly between excessive excitement (mania) and feeling low in energy or spirit (depression). Both depression and mania can be a consequence of early childhood trauma or abuse. In that sense, the disease might work as a coping mechanism to separate the present state of mind from the encroachment of thoughts and feelings associated with a trigger event. A trigger can be anything the patient associates with the underlying trauma—weather, a certain song, a specific memory, a holiday, or a distinct smell.

It is well known that manic-depressive patients are more sensitive to stress than the normal person. External stress seems to draw the trigger event closer to the forefront of the mind and in so doing can become a source of stress itself. Together, external and internal stress can create a loop-like experience that can severely threaten the well-being of the patient and can give rise to manic-depressive episodes. The patient might believe that an episode of the disease is preferable to dealing with the trigger event that resides deep in the recesses of the unconscious.

Others have suggested that the rhythmic appearances of bipolar episodes may be an effort of the unconscious to bring the underlying trauma to conscious awareness in thin layers so that the conscious mind can process it. Thus, each episode may be one layer of an onion, only truly processed and transcended when the last layer is peeled away.

Suggested Blessings

May you have compassion for your manic-depressive responses.
May you be able to recognize your triggers.
May you embrace and befriend your triggers.
May you find a way to learn from your situation.
May you find a way to turn a liability into a present power or strength.

Suggested Affirmations

I can look and ask for practical assistance and support.
The more I learn about my triggers, the more I know about myself.
I will get to my truth and my truth shall set me free.

Post-Traumatic Stress Disorder (PTSD)
Evidence-Based Confidence Level and Therapeutic Potential

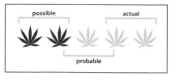

Total Number of Studies Reviewed: 3

CHI Value: 7

Post-traumatic stress disorder (PTSD) is a debilitating condition affecting the body, mind, and spirit. The condition results from direct or witnessed exposure to an extreme traumatic event such as war, police action, famine, earthquake, tsunami, assault, abuse, rape, kidnapping, torture, plane crash, explosions, life-threatening illness, or any situation involving the threat of death, extreme fear, dread, and helplessness. PTSD most often results from sudden trauma that happens without warning, was repeated over long periods of time, included intentional violence to body and psyche and/or involved grotesque injury and death, rape, or the loss of a close friend or relative.

While history brims with cases describing patients suffering from the symptoms of PTSD, the allopathic health care system, including hospitals charged with caring for veterans, has been very slow to acknowledge the disease. During WWI and WWII it was called "battle fatigue" or "shell shock," respectively. The British military placed more than 300 soldiers in front of a firing squad and shot them to death, ostensibly for cowardice before the enemy or desertion, when most of them were likely suffering from PTSD. The current term, PTSD, was formulated during the Vietnam War when thousands of soldiers came home suffering from a collection of common symptoms including guilt, depression, flashbacks, insomnia, or the inability to be close to loved ones. It was not until 1980 that PTSD was codified and included in the *Diagnostic and Statistical Manual of Mental Disorders (DSM)*.

With the advent of new imaging techniques, researchers discovered new insights pertinent to PTSD. A meta-analysis of available neuroimaging research suggests measurable physiological changes in the limbic system in patients with PTSD, namely changes in the amygdala, responsible for the processing of fear, the medial prefrontal cortex involved in decision making, and the hippocampus, needed for the formation of long-term memories. The analysis suggests that during episodes of activated PTSD, the hippocampus is diminished in size, neuronal integrity, and functional integrity. Furthermore, the medial prefrontal cortex appears to be volumetrically smaller and is hyporesponsive during symptomatic PTSD. Lastly, neuroimaging research reveals heightened amygdala responsivity in PTSD during symptomatic states.[1]

Not surprisingly, people exposed to the same traumatic events tend to respond differently. Some may experience only mild and passing symptoms, while others may feel numb, depressed, and suicidal or progress to developing full-blown PTSD. Symptoms often begin within three months after the traumatic event and may include profound lack of care for anything, emptiness, hopelessness, helplessness, worthlessness, shame, emotional numbness, distrust, paranoid behavior with hypervigilance, inexplicable fear, anxiety, lost memories, passivity, withdrawing, fits of anger with little or no provocation, irritability, impatience, lack of focus, insomnia, fitful sleep with sweating, nightmares, generalized weakness or fatigue, flashbacks, and avoidance of anything associated with the traumatic event.

Avoidance strategies themselves can become an additional problem for patients with PTSD. The compounding effects of detachment and unhealthy tension-reducing behaviors such as substance/food abuse, cutting, or promiscuous sex can make recovery more challenging.

The primary treatments within orthodox medicine are talk-therapy and pharmaceutical medications, primarily antidepressants and anxiolytics. However, misuse of prescription drugs and possible severe adverse effects with these classes of medication frame the clear and present limitations of pharmaceutical intervention. In addition, despite success from behavioral-cognitive therapies in the treatment of PTSD, patients often show vulnerability to reversal of progress by exposure to stress and stress triggers.

Cannabis and Post-Traumatic Stress Disorder

Recent discoveries (2009) from Haifa, Israel, show that the fear-processing center of the brain (amygdala) contains a significant number of endogenous cannabinoid receptors (CB1). Observation demonstrated that when the synthetic cannabinoid WIN55,212-2 was injected into the amygdala of rats, the cannabinoid modulated anxiety responses, especially extinction learning via regulation of the hypothalamic-pituitary-adrenal axis.[2] The Israeli study results further suggested that the cannabinoid supported inhibitory avoidance conditioning and extinction (the goal in PTSD therapies) by reducing the negative effects of stress.[3] Moreover, the same study from Haifa demonstrated that "microinjecting WIN55,212-2 into the basolateral amygdala (BLA) before exposing the rats to a stressor reversed the enhancing effects of the stressor on inhibitory avoidance (IA) conditioning and its impairing effects on IA extinction." This observation might explain why cannabinoids can modulate panic responses not just after extremely painful and traumatic events but also before.

An Ottawa study (2009) reported that cannabis could remove fear responses to stressors such as nightmares, poor sleep, night sweats, and flashbacks. Forty-seven PTSD patients suffering from nightmares that failed to adequately respond to standard pharmaceutical antidepressants and hypnotics received the synthetic cannabinoid Nabilone. Researchers wrote: "The majority of patients (72%) receiving Nabilone experienced either cessation of nightmares or a significant reduction in nightmare intensity. Subjective improvement in sleep time, the quality of sleep, and the reduction of daytime flashbacks and night sweats were also noted by some patients."[4]

Researchers (2008) from Richmond, Virginia, worked to determine the effect of the endocannabinoid system on learning and forgetting pleasant and unpleasant experiences. After analyzing the tests, the authors wrote: ". . . these results provide compelling support for the hypothesis that the endogenous cannabinoid system plays a necessary role in the extinction of aversively motivated behaviors but is expendable for appetitively motivated behaviors."[5]

Strain-Specific Considerations

WIN55,212-2, Nabilone, and Rimonabant have been tested for the treatment of PTSD. WIN55,212-2 binds with higher affinity to CB2. Nabilone is a synthetic cannabinoid similar to THC, which binds with both CB1 and CB2 relatively equally. Rimonabant is a CB1 antagonist known to reduce learned fear responses (extinction learning).

Study Summary

Drugs	Type of Study	Published Year, Place, and Key Results	CHI
WIN55,212-2	Animal study (rats)	2009—Haifa, Israel: WIN55,212-2 microinjected into the baso-lateral amygdala reduced stress-induced elevations in corticosterone levels.[2]	2
Nabilone	Human case study (47 patients diagnosed with PTSD)	2009—Ottawa, Canada: Reduction in nightmares, night sweats, daytime flashbacks, and improved sleep.[4]	3
Rimonabant (CB1 antagonist)	Animal study	2008—Richmond, Virginia, USA: Endogenous cannabinoid system is involved in forgetting painful events.[5]	2

Total CHI Value 7

While the human case study cited above relied on Nabilone, a synthetic cannabinoid similar to THC, many cannabis using-patients prefer indicas or indica-dominant hybrids with a relatively lower THC:CBD/CBN ratio, favoring the more relaxing and grounding properties of these strains.

Mind-Body Medicine and Post-Traumatic Stress Disorder

Psychosomatic researchers reported that WWII combat veterans who suffered from PTSD for decades possessed a chronically different thyroid hormone profile than normal men.[6] This was especially true for T3 concentrations, which were found to be higher than normal concentrations. T3 is a potent, fast-acting hormone that readily enters the brain and is involved in fight or flight. Scientists hypothesized that this constantly elevated hormone profile associated with stress and fear is involved in the mechanism of PTSD.

Scientists describe PTSD as a temporary breakdown of a natural and balanced response reaction between body and mind, between imagination and will, or between one's feeling and action.

Many of the symptoms or behaviors commonly seen in PTSD are coping mechanisms in the presence of an otherwise intolerable traumatic situation or memory of trauma. Irrational fears or anxieties, overly aggressive behaviors, substance abuse, pacing, rocking, and isolating or unsafe behaviors are set in motion to cope with the intolerable. However, while these coping mechanisms may be initially practical and useful in avoiding the key event, over time they become a liability.

In a way, PTSD symptoms physically manifest into a message that cannot be denied. Suppressed emotions can harm you. Appropriate emotional release can contribute to your healing.

Consider a study conducted at MIT (Massachusetts Institute of Technology) that has demonstrated a scientific basis for psychotherapy relevant to patients suffering from PTSD.[7] Researchers discovered the physiological underpinnings of a common mind-body therapy technique in which patients use a positive memory to diminish the impact of a traumatic one. This eventually leads to the inactivation of the traumatic emotional material and the toxic stress associated with it.

In summary, aggravating factors may include unresolved emotional trauma(s), beliefs that feeling and emotion are a weakness or liability, and the maintenance of negative coping strategies.

Consider the practice of forgiveness and acceptance, changing beliefs that devalue emotional experiences, and greater use of positive coping skills.

Anecdote

Jack talked his girlfriend Daniela into a bicycle ride through downtown San Francisco. While Jack was used to the traffic and pace of the city, Daniela was new to it. As they rode south on Market Street on their way to see the gold-plated roof of City Hall, a tractor-trailer slowly passed both of them. Jack saw Daniela wavering. Jack recalled, "She was getting really scared at the large wheels passing us. Daniela wobbled and flipped the bike. The large wheel rolled over the very top of her head and with a loud pop spilled its contents onto the street." Jack was still screaming uncontrollably when the paramedics arrived. He kept repeating, "I'll never forget that sound, I'll never forget that sound!"

Jack initially received treatment with pharmaceutical medication, but after a few days he discontinued them because he felt in a constant fog, with dizziness and blurred vision. He could not sleep, and when he did manage to get some sleep, he would wake up drenched in sweat. The nightmares came almost every night. Jack told his therapist that his heart would start racing and he'd break into a sweat and shake every time he saw a tractor-trailer passing by. Worse were the nightmares and terrifying sounds of himself screaming silently as if falling helplessly into an abyss. In contrast, during therapy sessions, Jack was unwilling to remember details of the event. He had difficulty expressing his feelings, and the symptoms persisted. One time at work when somebody opened a champagne bottle, the sudden sound triggered a fit. He was hard to console, and a co-worker took him home. Jack believed that safety and security were but an illusion.

After months of slow progress, a friend suggested that he obtain a cannabis prescription. He did, and for the first time in weeks, Jack relaxed into a deep and restful sleep, void of nightmares or night sweats. He felt more able to articulate and express the variety of his feelings about the event, especially his guilt. Over time he noticed that his guilt gave way to anger, which gave way to sorrow about Daniela's death, and slowly a sense of empathy and compassion became his new companions. Instead of "I'll never forget that sound," he now kept repeating, "As long as I hear the sound of my breath, I am safe."

Suggested Blessings

May you embrace yourself just as you are right now.

May you consider the possibility that all forgiveness benefits your health and aids in your healing.

Suggested Affirmations

I am okay just as I am right now.

I can feel and release even the most powerful emotions.

I am safe now, I feel safe now, and I know I am safe now.

It takes time to heal, but it will not take forever.

Hypervigilant behavior is but one way I can make myself feel safe.

Anger is a sign that my values have been violated.

I can use that anger constructively and without hurting anyone.

Schizophrenia
Evidence-Based Confidence Level and Therapeutic Potential

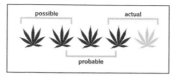

Total Number of Studies Reviewed: 4

CHI Value: 16

Schizophrenia remains one of the most common and serious yet least understood mental illnesses in the world today. Swiss psychiatrist Eugene Bleuler first used the word "schizophrenia" in 1911, which he derived from the Greek words *schizo* (to split) and *phren* (brain or mind). However, unlike common usage suggests, it does not necessarily refer to a split personality(-ies) but rather a split or disconnect between thinking and feeling. Symptoms often include hallucinations involving the senses, making it difficult for patients to communicate or connect to others and the world. These symptoms typically emerge in adolescence or early adulthood. Bleuler divided schizophrenic symptoms into positive and negative symptoms.

Positive symptoms (abnormal functions) may include hallucinations (involving one or several of the senses but most commonly hearing voices), misunderstanding or misinterpreting internal or sense-based experiences, difficulty expressing oneself verbally, lack of insight, social awkwardness (disorganization, inappropriate behavior), grandiosity, hostility, and feeling persecuted or suspicious.

Negative symptoms (reduction or absence of normal functions) may include amotivation, lack of affect, lack of eye contact, inappropriate emotional expressions, social isolation, poor hygiene, poor planning abilities, and poor follow-through.

The allopathic tradition considers this type of mental illness a chronic condition that requires lifelong treatment. In this paradigm, no cure exists and treatment consists of managing symptoms, employing antipsychotic pharmaceutical drugs with psychological or social support. While antipsychotic drugs can help with some symptoms, they also significantly increase the risks of developing a wide variety of adverse effects. This causes a majority of patients to discontinue use. Adverse effects, especially from long-term use, may include impotence, weight gain, and especially extrapyramidal[1] symptoms such as spasms of the neck, jaw, mouth, tongue, and face, restlessness, inability to hold still or maintain a posture, and rigidity. Serious adverse effects may include brain damage, low blood pressure, cardiac toxicity, diabetes, seizures, or death. However, considering the grave and often debilitating nature of this disease and in spite of considerable adverse effects, treatment enables many patients to live a relatively normal life.

Causes are not known but are considered to include a combination of environmental and genetic factors. Scientists have conducted tens of thousands of studies to better understand the reasons for this elusive disease. Modern science learned that prenatal stress could trigger subtle developmental changes, which might later develop into the disease. Prenatal stress,[2] family history,[3] social isolation,[4] inner city life,[5] sudden life-altering events such as migration,[6] or psychotic episodes are each commonly found in schizophrenia patients. Toxins, nutritional deficiencies, and other biological influences may also contribute and thus provide an opportunity for therapeutics such as detoxification and nutritional support.

Schizophrenic patients have excessive dopamine (a neurotransmitter) in their brain's mesolimbic system. Drugs such as methamphetamines or cocaine produce similar patient presentations in chemistry and behavior. Intense life-changing events can trigger the onset of the illness, especially in those who came from a schizophrenic family. Early child abuse has been identified with the development of certain mental disorders, and some mental health practitioners suggest a strong link to schizophrenia as well.[7]

Diagnosis involves observation and thorough history guided by the *Diagnostic and Statistical Manual of Mental Disorders (DSM)* to rule out underlying causes.

A variety of psychological traditions have taken their own views on schizophrenia. C. G. Jung, who believed that schizophrenia is related to unresolved early traumas, worked effectively with schizophrenic patients using non-authoritarian psychiatric work, free of drugs. Stanislav Grof's work on extraordinary states of consciousness and prenatal experiences describes schizophrenia as a type of spiritual crisis or emergency. Therapists associated with many disciplines around the world use numerous non-drug approaches to treat schizophrenia with varying degrees of success or cure rates. However, former schizophrenic patients who have healed their schizophrenic episode or spiritual emergency can be an invaluable help to people still stuck in the process.

Cannabis and Schizophrenia

While other studies on cannabis and schizophrenia exist, we selected two meta-analyses containing the majority of studies and two other relevant experiments for the purpose of providing a useful general overview.

In the year 2004, University of California–Irvine scientists discovered that the body's own cannabinoid anandamide levels in the cerebrospinal fluid (CSF) of untreated first-episode paranoid schizophrenics were eight times higher than that of healthy control subjects. Such an alteration remained absent in schizophrenics treated with "typical" antipsychotics. These results suggest that anandamide increases in acute paranoid schizophrenia patients and may be a compensatory adaptation to the disease state.[8] This might indicate a potential role of the endocannabinoid system in schizophrenia pathology and treatment.

Many schizophrenic patients have never been exposed to cannabis, and the vast majority of cannabis users do not develop psychotic events or subsequent schizophrenia. However, some observational studies present data demonstrating that cannabis use by still developing adolescents presents a statistical risk factor for developing schizophrenia. While cannabis is not a necessary or sufficient cause, in some cases it may be a co-factor.

To better understand why certain users may be vulnerable when the majority are not, it may be helpful to examine some studies. London researchers (2005) looked at specific genetic expressions among similar patients and discovered that those who carried a specific allele[9] (one of two or more versions of a gene) were most likely to exhibit psychotic symptoms.[10]

It is hypothesized that an experience with cannabis may combine with an existing genetic vulnerability to induce psychosis. "There are two ways to measure genetic liability to psychosis—directly and indirectly—and studies with both measures provide growing evidence that an underlying mechanism of gene-environment interaction explains the association between cannabis and psychosis."[11]

Based on the current evidence, it would be prudent for adolescents and young adults with a known family history of psychosis or schizophrenia to stay away from cannabis, or any other mind-altering substance, especially alcohol and speed-based drugs such as cocaine and methamphetamines.

Selected studies illuminate aspects of the interplay of genetic and environmental influences on developing schizophrenia. In 2009, German and U.S. researchers conducted a double-blind crossover clinical trial with 42 patients. Fulfilling *DSM-IV* criteria of acute paranoid schizophrenia, they compared the effectiveness of CBD with that of the antipsychotic Amisulpride for the treatment of acute schizophrenia. Results revealed that the CBD reduced symptoms similar to that of Amisulpride but with significantly lower incidence of side effects. The authors of the study concluded: "Cannabidiol revealed substantial antipsychotic properties in acute schizophrenia. This is in line with our suggestion of an adaptive role of the endocannabinoid system in paranoid schizophrenia, and raises further evidence that this adaptive mechanism may represent a valuable target for antipsychotic treatment strategies."[12]

Brazilian and Italian researchers conducted a meta-analysis of relevant literature in 2010 and suggested that THC was a potential adjuvant in the treatment of schizophrenia.[13] Additionally, CBD emerged with the most constant antipsychotic properties in dopamine- and glutamate-based models of schizophrenia.[14]

Study Summary

Drugs	Type of Study	Published Year, Place, and Key Results	CHI
Cannabidiol (CBD) and SR141716A (CB1 antagonist)	Meta-analysis	2010—University of Insubria, Italy: Potential novel approach for treating schizophrenia. CBD and THC meta-analysis. THC: adjuvant in the treatment of schizophrenia.[14]	4
CBD	Meta-analysis	2010—Universidade de São Paulo, Brazil: CBD therapeutic potential: antipsychotic, anxiolytic, and antidepressant.[13]	4
CBD vs Amisulpride	42 patients fulfilling DSM-IV criteria of acute paranoid schizophrenia	2009—Multinational research team, Cologne, Germany, and Irvine, California: Decrease in symptoms not different between both substances. CBD induced significantly less side effects.[12]	5
Anandamide	Antipsychotic-naive first-episode paranoid schizophrenics	2004—Department of Pharmacology, University of California–Irvine: Anandamide elevation in acute paranoid schizophrenia may be a compensatory mechanism.[8]	3

Total CHI Value 16

Strain-Specific Considerations

CBD, THC, and endogenous anandamide were examined in the context of schizophrenia. CBD has a greater affinity for CB2. THC and anandamide bind with CB1 and CB2 relatively equally.

Cannabis-using patients suffering from schizophrenia often choose a strain relative to their needs. If a generally more stimulating or uplifting effect is needed, patients tend to consider sativa or sativa-dominant strains. Those in need of a generally more relaxing or grounding effect tend to prefer indicas or indica-dominant strains with a relatively lower THC:CBD ratio, which likely favors CB2 activation.

Mind-Body Medicine and Schizophrenia

Schizophrenia is described by some patients as a loss of connection between thinking and feeling, with an accompanying sense of loss of soul. The latter suggests a need for a spiritual dimension in those patients' healing process.

Aggravating or contributing factors may include prenatal stress, family history of mental-health problems, toxins, nutritional deficiencies, other biological influences, social isolation, inner-city life, and sudden life-altering events such as migration.

Consider exploring nutritional support, detoxification, and support group(s) or therapy.

Powerful Questions

What was the trigger event?
What happened?
Has the negative loop ever been interrupted?
By what?
Is it possible to bring in other resources?

Suggested Blessing

May you recover from the sense of loss of soul.

Suggested Affirmation

I can discover peace and solitude, good friends, and practical help. I accept myself. I have compassion for myself.

Neurological Diseases (in general)

Evidence-Based Confidence Level and Therapeutic Potential

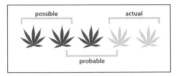

Total Number of Studies Reviewed: 69

Combined CHI Value: 215

To date, hundreds of different neurological disease classifications exist within orthodox medicine. While specific and unique in their presentation of signs, symptoms, and damages caused, the various conditions share

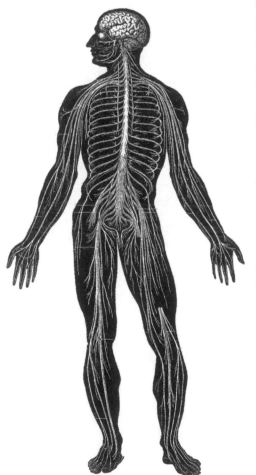

a common inability to properly transmit nerve impulses. This inability may be due to damage to the conduction network itself (nerve fibers) or difficulties in transmitting nerve impulses/signals at the energetic/electrical, molecular, or chemical levels. Specific disease manifestation largely depends on how and which aspect or part of the nervous system is affected.

Modern medicine basically divides the nervous system into the central nervous system (CNS), composed of the brain, spinal cord, and optic nerve, and the peripheral nervous system (PNS), consisting of nerve pathways from the spine extending outward toward the periphery of the body. The PNS is further divided into the autonomic nervous system and the enteric nervous system, the latter responsible for gastrointestinal or gut reactions. The autonomic nervous system also subdivides into the sympathetic and parasympathetic nervous systems, which up- or down-regulate automatic (involuntary) responses such as heartbeat, blood pressure, and hormonal release.

Orthodox medicine has identified a variety of possible culprits in the promotion of neurological diseases. They include toxins, lack of nutrition, infectious pathogens, radiation, accidents, as well as genetic and autoimmune causes. In many cases, though, both an exact causation and cure have so far escaped modern medicine. An arsenal of tests may provide insights into some of the specifics of disease development, and by extension manage progression. However, treatment is often limited to pharmaceutical medication or surgery. In addition, most neurological disorders are chronic, and the patient deteriorates over time.

Cannabis and Neuroprotection
Evidence-Based Confidence Level and Therapeutic Potential

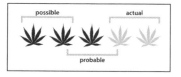

Total Number of Studies Reviewed: 4

CHI Value: 11

Cannabinoids assist in regulating functions associated with endocannabinoid receptor sites found in the human body. Endocannabinoid receptor sites (CB1 and CB2) are firmly embedded in all parts of the nervous system. More specifically, CB1 receptor sites are especially prominent in those parts of the brain (CNS) related to motor control, cognition, emotional responses, motivation, and homeostasis. CB2 receptor sites often sit outside the brain in the periphery, and they relate to the autonomic nervous system (ANS), immune system, cellular circulation, hormonal regulation, and gastrointestinal function. Scientists suspect that other undiscovered receptor sites exist in endothelial cells (cells that line the inside of blood vessels), which are referred to as non-CB1 or non-CB2.

By 2003, the U.S. federal government had issued itself a patent on a newly found property of cannabis making it "... useful in the treatment and prophylaxis of a wide variety of oxidation associated diseases such as ischemic, age-related, inflammatory and autoimmune diseases. The cannabinoids are found to have particular application as neuroprotectants; for example, in limiting neurological damage following ischemic insults such as stroke and trauma, or in the treatment of neurodegenerative diseases such as Alzheimer's disease, Parkinson's disease and HIV dementia."[1]

A multidisciplinary Bethesda, Maryland (2005), research team further examined the neuroprotective properties of cannabinoids by designing an experiment inducing rats to binge-drink alcohol. This activity causes substantial neurodegeneration in the brain, especially the hippocampus and the entorhinal cortex. Concurrently, the rats received CBD, a non-psychoactive cannabinoid. Results indicated that CBD could protect nerve cells from alcohol-induced toxicity in a dose-dependent manner.[2] Laboratory studies in Italy (2009)[3] and Spain (2010) echoed these results on the neuroprotective properties of cannabinoids. Researchers discovered that while the drug ecstasy (MDMA) produces hyperthermia, oxidative stress, and neuronal damage, especially at higher room temperatures, THC causes the opposite (namely hypothermic, anti-inflammatory, and antioxidant effects). Thus, researchers concluded that THC protects against MDMA neurotoxicity, at least in mice.[4]

Study Summary

Drugs	Type of Study	Published Year, Place, and Key Results	CHI
MDMA, THC	Animal study (mice)	2010—Departament de Ciències Experimentals i de la Salut, Grup de Recerca en Neurobiologia del Comportament, Universitat Pompeu Fabra, Barcelona, Spain: THC may have a neuroprotective effect against MDMA-induced neurotoxicity.[4]	2
JWH-015	Laboratory	2009—Santa Lucia Foundation Istituto di Ricovero e Cura a Carattere Scientifico, Rome, Italy: Endocannabinoids are neuroprotective.[3]	1
CBD	Animal study (rats)	2005—Multi-institutional, Bethesda, Maryland, USA: CBD was neuroprotective in a dose-dependent manner.[2]	2
Cannabinoids	In vitro and in vivo laboratory, animal, and human studies	2003—The United States of America as represented by the Department of Health and Human Services: Cannabinoids are neuroprotectants.[1]	1+2+3

Total CHI Value 11

Strain- and Form-Specific Considerations

Large cannabis leaves eaten in a salad or made into a juice may contain preventative properties in the context of neurological disorders. William L. Courtney, MD, a physician working with fresh cannabis, considers raw cannabis a dietary essential that provides potent preventative influences on several degenerative processes often involved with neurological diseases. These preventative features include neuroprotection and anti-inflammatory and antioxidant properties. These properties are echoed in the overall results of studies reviewed here and throughout this chapter.

Mind-Body Medicine and Neuroprotection in General

The breakdown of communication between command central (the brain) and the rest of the body may indicate a breakdown of non-physical dualities such as that of the mind and body, spirit and nature, dreams and reality, future and past, victimhood and responsibility, logic and intuition, or between will and imagination. Depending on one's perspective, this can be seen as an opportunity or as a mental illness—see Mental Disorders (in general).

Powerful Questions

What is getting on my nerves?
Who is getting on my nerves?
What hurts to communicate?
What is too dangerous to be communicated?
What must not be communicated?
Does it feel safer to withhold information?
Do I feel I cannot handle certain topics in my life?
What would happen if I talked about a taboo or charged topic?

Let Food Be Thy Medicine

Garlic ∽ Rosemary ∽ Turmeric

Garlic: Aged garlic extract may prevent the progression of Alzheimer's disease, according to the results of a rodent experiment that examined garlic in the treatment of Alzheimer's.[5]

Rosemary: At Hung-Kuang University, Taiwan, scientists concluded that " ... rosemary is an excellent multifunctional therapeutic herb; by looking at its potentially potent antiglycative bioactivity, it may become a good adjuvant medicine for the prevention and treatment of diabetic, cardiovascular, and other neurodegenerative diseases."[6]

Turmeric: In a meta-study, scientists provided an overview of decades of scientific studies on turmeric. Turmeric was noted as a therapeutic agent in Alzheimer's and Parkinson's diseases.[7]

Curcumin is a naturally occurring compound found in the rhizome of turmeric. Researchers from Nashville, Tennessee, examined the compound's ability to affect mice with multiple sclerosis (MS). Results of the study suggest that the amount of curcumin used to protect the mice from artificially induced MS corresponds to the amount found in the typical Indian diet. One author of the study reported that MS in India is very rare; and, while no human studies to date confirm the results, it certainly can't hurt to add some turmeric to your food.[8]

Alcohol Dependence/Abuse
Evidence-Based Confidence Level and Therapeutic Potential

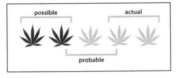

Total Number of Studies Reviewed: 4

CHI Value: 9

Alcohol abuse is one of the most common contributing factors to a great deal of pain and suffering. A neurological and mental illness, alcohol abuse causes or exacerbates a variety of serious social problems: domestic violence, child abuse, spousal abuse, homicide, suicide, purposeful injuries, falls, accidents, fatal overdose, loss of work, and increased poverty.

Alcohol abuse affects the entire body. Doctors name cardiovascular disease as the primary cause of death associated with alcohol abuse. Other health problems connected to alcohol abuse include poor absorption of food, cancer, cirrhosis of the liver, pancreatitis, gastritis, alcohol poisoning or overdose, aspiration of vomit, burns, drowning, damage to the nervous system, depression, dementia, and symptoms such as seizures, psychosis, and withdrawal delirium tremens (DTs).

A worldwide health problem, alcohol dependence impacts more males than females. However, women's bodies endure more rapid damage from the disease than do male bodies. In this author's experience as a paramedic, alcohol abuse-related health problems generate a majority of 911 emergencies, followed by nicotine-related health problems. Additionally, no antidote exists for the acute alcohol overdose common in binge drinking. In fact, orthodox medicine suggests no cure for chronic alcoholism. In this paradigm, patients remain alcoholics for life and must learn to manage the urge and maintain abstinence.

Long-term alcohol abuse induces neurochemical changes in brain physiology and structure, which serve to reinforce the psychological and physical need for alcohol and may lead to dependence. Therapy is basically two-fold. First, patients begin a process of detoxification and treatment through the initial withdrawal phases, followed by nutritional support consisting mainly of thiamine (vitamin B1). Second, doctors prescribe therapy, conducted usually in a peer-group setting.

Cannabis and Alcoholism

In 1970, Tod H. Mikuriya, MD, published a case involving an alcohol-dependent patient who significantly benefited from the ability of cannabis to reduce his alcohol consumption.[1] Thirty-four years later, Dr. Mikuriya followed up with a larger study incorporating 92 alcoholic patients. Forty-five patients found the treatment "very effective"; 38 found it "effective"; and nine patients reported that they had been able to give up alcohol altogether.[2]

Since then, studies conducted on mice in 2005[3] and 2008[4] suggest that blocking the CB1 receptor appears to effectively reduce the preference for alcohol and actual alcohol intake. Researchers speculate that medications targeting the CB1 receptors may be beneficial for the treatment of alcoholism.

While this research involved the body's own endocannabinoid receptor system (CB1), another experiment examined the neuroprotective properties of a specific cannabinoid (CBD) in the context of binge drinking. A multidisciplinary research team from Bethesda, Maryland, designed an experiment inducing rats to binge-drink alcohol—an activity causing substantial neurodegeneration in the brain, especially the hippocampus and the entorhinal cortex (2005). Concurrently, rats received CBD, a non-psychoactive cannabinoid, and results indicated that CBD could protect nerve cells from alcohol-induced toxicity in a dose-dependent manner.[5]

Study Summary

Drugs	Type of Study	Published Year, Place, and Key Results	CHI
CB1 antagonist	Animal study (mice)	2008—Division of Analytical Psychopharmacology, Orangeburg, New York: CB(1) antagonist receptor may reduce ethanol dependence.[4]	2
CBD	Animal study (rats)	2005—Multi-institutional, Bethesda, Maryland: CBD was able to protect nerve cells from alcohol-induced toxicity.[5]	2
CB1 antagonist	Animal study (rats)	2005—Behavioral Pharmacology Lab, Department of Medicine, Upton, New York: Blocking CB1 receptors may be beneficial for the treatment of alcoholism.[3]	2
Cannabis	Case study on 92 alcoholics	2004—California Cannabis Research Medical Group, Berkeley, CA: 45 patients found the treatment "very effective"; 38 found it "effective"; and 9 patients reported that they had been able to give up alcohol altogether.[2]	3

Total CHI Value 9

Strain-Specific Considerations

The drugs reviewed in these studies included cannabis (whole plant material), the isolated cannabinoid CBD, and CB1 antagonists. Cannabis contains cannabinoids that bind with both CB1 and CB2. CB1 antagonists block CB1 expression.

Indica strains and indica-dominant hybrids tend to have lower THC: CBD ratios favoring CB2 expression.

Mind-Body Medicine and Alcoholism

While not all stress-exposed children go on to develop alcoholism, severe childhood stressors have been associated with increased vulnerability to addiction. Researchers also suggest a genetic-environmental connection, which may contribute to one's vulnerability to later develop alcohol dependence.[6]

Consider exploring potential contributing or aggravating factors such as self-pity, hopelessness, shame, guilt, judgments, hard-heartedness, and blame. Perhaps work on replacing contributing factors with self-acceptance, forgiveness, gratitude, love, intimacy, a connection with something larger than oneself, finding what matters, passion, hope, and trust.

Powerful Questions

How or where have I lost the spirit I am trying to find in the bottle?
What is so intolerable in my life that I have to numb myself?
What is the crisis that always seems to loom at the edge of my reality?
What is too much for me to own?
Where am I convinced I cannot change?
What happened to my trust and my hope?
Who do I blame for my life?
Can I see what matters to me on the other side of blame?
Can I see my ability to forgive on the other side of blame?
Can I see my passion on the other side of blame?

Suggested Blessings

May you receive the vision needed to move through hopelessness and despair.
May you find the will and determination to manifest the vision to be found on the bottom of hopelessness and/or despair.

Suggested Affirmations

I accept myself right here, right now, just the way I am.
I can ask for help.
I can receive help.

Alzheimer's Disease

Evidence-Based Confidence Level and Therapeutic Potential

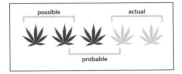

Total Number of Studies Reviewed: 4

CHI Value: 10

Alzheimer's disease (AD), a chronic degenerative illness that affects the mind and brain, is partially characterized by selective neuronal loss (AD kills brain cells) and cognitive deficits. Early symptoms include forgetfulness or a decrease in cognitive function, which eventually progresses to a gradual loss of communication abilities and significant behavioral changes. Eventually, the patient becomes completely dependent and bedridden. Death usually occurs from secondary sources such as trauma or chronic infections. The disease affects more women than men and usually begins between ages 50 and 60. AD is the main culprit for dementia. In 2007, it was the sixth leading cause of death in the U.S.[1]

Within the modern medical system, the causes of the disease remain unknown. In addition, the disease lacks a cure or effective treatment. Management of AD involves a multidisciplinary approach of supportive care, pharmaceutical medications, exercise, nutrition, and an assurance of the patient's safety through supervision. Depending on the progression of the disease, feeding tubes may be used to ensure adequate nutritional intake.

Generally speaking, scientists believe that AD originates in part from genetic, environmental, and lifestyle causes. Established risk factors include lack of exercise, obesity, hypertension, diabetes, depression, and smoking. More specifically, one hypothesis proposes beta-amyloid plaque as a factor, partially due to doctors observing higher concentrations in the brain cells of Alzheimer patients. Another discovery in AD involves a protein called tau, which in AD tangles and twists, preventing the delivery of nutrients to brain cells. Scientists believe that these plaques and tangles induce neurochemical and inflammatory changes responsible for the development of the disease.

No test exists, with the exception of an autopsy, to diagnose AD. However, the presence of dementia can be determined via a combination of cognitive and neurological examinations as well as various brain-imaging techniques.

While unable to explain the reason, observational studies reveal that higher levels of education, lifelong interests in learning, challenging activities, and social interactions can reduce the risk of the disease.[2]

Cannabis and Alzheimer's

Recent experiments suggest that the endocannabinoid system may play a significant role in the development of AD. One study (2005) from Madrid, Spain, discovered that ". . . cannabinoid receptors are important in the pathology of AD and that cannabinoids succeed in preventing the neuro-degenerative process occurring in the disease."[3] Another experiment from Madrid (2009) demonstrated that the CB2 agonist JWH-015 could induce the removal of native beta-amyloid from frozen human tissue.[4] Using available data from prior studies and experiments, scientists from Naples, Italy, conducted a meta-analysis (2008). Their results suggested that endocannabinoids likely produce a response that might counteract both the neurochemical and inflammatory consequences of beta-amyloid-induced tau protein hyperactivity. This might possibly be the most important underlying cause of AD.[5] While clinical trials are still lacking, researchers from British Columbia, Canada (2008), tested a patient with Alzheimer's-related behavioral symptoms, such as agitation and aggression, who failed to respond to such pharmaceuticals as neurontin, trazodone, quetiapine, and olanzapine. Scientists then gave the patient 0.5 mg of Nabilone, which significantly reduced his agitation levels. After doubling the dose, his symptoms were further reduced without any side effects.[6]

Study Summary

Drugs	Type of Study	Published Year, Place, and Key Results	CHI
CB2 agonist JWH-015	Laboratory	2009—Laboratorio de Apoyo a la Investigación, Hospital Universitario Fundación Alcorcón and Centro de Investigación Biomédica en Red sobre Enfermedades Neurodegenerativas, Madrid, Spain: Removal of native beta-amyloid.[4]	1
Cannabinoids in the context of AD, especially CBD.	Meta-analysis and literature review	2008—Endocannabinoid Research Group, Institute of Bio-molecular Chemistry, Consiglio Nazionale delle Ricerche, Naples, Italy: Results suggest a possible novel approach to AD. Might counteract neurochemical and inflammatory consequences of beta-amyloid-induced tau protein hyperactivity.[5]	4
Nabilone 0.5 mg X 1 pm and 0.5 mg X 2 daily	Human (1 patient)	2008—Division of Geriatric Psychiatry, Department of Psychiatry, University of British Columbia, Canada: Dramatic reduction in the severity of agitation and other behavioral symptoms.[6]	3
WIN55,212-2, HU210, and JWH-133	Rodent study	2005—Neurodegeneration Group, Cajal Institute, Consejo Superior de Investigaciones Científicas, Madrid, Spain: Neuro-protective in AD. Intracerebroventricular administration of the synthetic cannabinoid WIN55,212-2 to rats prevented beta-amyloid peptide-induced microglial activation, cognitive impairment, and loss of neuronal markers.[3]	2

Total CHI Value 10

Strain- and Form-Specific Considerations

The cannabinoids used in this study review include CBD, Nabilone, JWH-015, WIN55,212-2, HU210, and JWH-133.

CBD has a greater affinity for CB2. JWH-015 is a CB2 agonist. WIN55,212-2 has a greater affinity for CB2. JWH-133 is a potent CB2 agonist. Out of this group of cannabinoids, only HU210 has a higher affinity for CB1, and Nabilone is a synthetic cannabinoid similar to THC, which likely binds relatively equally to CB1 and CB2.

Indica and indica-dominant hybrids tend to present with a lower THC:CBD ratio, thus potentially favoring CB2 activation. Furthermore, raw fresh leaf or juice contains biologically active cannabinoids in the form of relatively non-psychoactive THC-acid and CBD-acid, which according to William L. Courtney, MD, a physician working with fresh cannabis as a dietary essential, can deliver a much higher concentration of CBD before any mind-altering effect may occur.

Mind-Body Medicine and Alzheimer's

The AD patient typically experiences a gradual loss of physical and mental abilities until s/he becomes completely dependent on others to care for basic bodily functions. Based on the image presented by the body, it would appear that AD is an attempt to return to the source of all life by way of the infant. Other options to return to the source of all life, such as the return through wisdom, appear nonexistent.

Physiologically, two parts of the brain are especially vulnerable to aggregation—the hippocampus (memory) and the amygdala (emotional reactions). This may suggest that clogged-up memories and related emotional reactions interfere with life. A part of the patient seems to have given up on conscious growing and learning and may attempt to seek a return, little by little, to a womb-like existence where all one's needs are met without conscious involvement or responsibility.

But, it doesn't have to be this way. In a case of mind over matter, numerous studies have demonstrated that the mind can continue to fully function even in the presence of Alzheimer's. In other words, even though the physical brain is affected by AD, people can maintain cognitive function. Via a review of epidemiological data and imaging evidence, researchers suggested possible reasons for this mismatch of a functioning mind in the presence of AD. Some researchers refer to it as "cognitive reserve," and others tend to use the term "neuroplasticity" (ability of a part of the brain to take over the function of another part). Scientists further suggested several qualities that could bring about and enhance cognitive reserve, even in old age. These included education, positive occupational experiences, high IQ, language skills, and participation in leisure activities.[7]

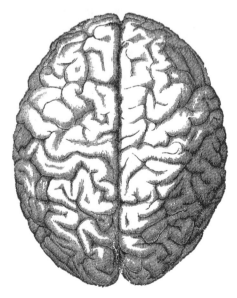

Aggravating factors may include social isolation, poor nutritional support, new skill or learning avoidance, and a belief that says "as the body ages the mind must fade away."

Mitigating factors may involve continuing education and learning opportunities, new activities or experiences, mental exercise and acquisition of new skills, new friendships and close relationships, and a belief in your ability to continue to grow even as your body grows older.

Powerful Questions

Where do I refuse to be responsible, even at the cost of freedom?
What do wise men have that children do not?
Where am I averse to learning new perspectives?
Where am I averse to learning new ways of being and doing?

Suggested Blessing

May you find a new and gentle way to return to the source of all life.

Suggested Affirmation

I will return the way of the wise wo/man.

Let Food Be Thy Medicine

Garlic ∾ Turmeric

Garlic: A rodent experiment to examine the impact of ingesting garlic on Alzheimer's disease concluded that aged garlic extract has a potential for preventing the progression of Alzheimer's disease.[8]

Turmeric: In a meta-study, scientists provide an overview of decades of scientific studies on turmeric. They summarized a long list of turmeric's potential therapeutic properties, including positive benefits for Alzheimer's patients.[9]

Take Notice

Infrared Light (670 nm)

A multi-institutional laboratory research project (2012) brought together scientists from nanotechnology, molecular medicine, and numerous other medical specialties. Using a laser-emitting infrared light at a frequency of 670 nm, scientists significantly reduced intracellular beta-amyloid aggregation with no ill-effects on cell proliferation. Researchers noted that infrared light at 670 nm can penetrate skull bone and underlying tissue beneath to a depth of several centimeters, making infrared light a potentially novel and non-invasive treatment for AD.[10]

Amyotrophic Lateral Sclerosis (ALS or Lou Gehrig's Disease)
Evidence-Based Confidence Level and Therapeutic Potential

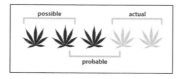

Total Number of Studies Reviewed: 7

CHI Value: 19

Lou Gehrig's disease or ALS is considered a chronic degenerative neurological illness associated with the selective loss of only those nerve cells needed for muscular motion located in the brain and spinal cord. *A-myo-trophic,* derived from ancient Greek, translates into no-muscle-nourishment, respectively. "Lateral" refers to muscles on either side of the affected nerve, and "sclerosis" means hardening. Without nourishment, a muscle wastes away and with it so does the ability to initiate movements.

The disease often begins spontaneously, and otherwise healthy adults suddenly show symptoms ranging from isolated muscle weakness, twitching, difficulty voicing speech, muscle cramps and spasms, and periods of uncontrollable laughter or crying, which progress to advanced-stage symptoms, namely difficulty swallowing. Breathing, while a mostly non-voluntary function, is also somewhat subject to will and, thus, is ultimately affected by ALS. Most ALS patients eventually die of respiratory failure. While late-stage ALS patients descend into total paralysis, their minds for the most part remain unaffected. One study estimated that, in the U.S. alone, about two people in 100,000 die of the disease.[1] While some patients survive for up to ten years, the majority of ALS patients die within three to five years after the onset of symptoms. However, one of the more famous ALS patients, Stephen Hawking, considered by many one of the most brilliant scientific minds to date, has shattered all life-expectancy statistics. He has not just survived ALS but has, in spite of his illness, produced a body of work earning him unprecedented international acclaim in both academia and the public domain.

Orthodox medicine does not know the exact causes of ALS and offers no cure. Although mostly observed in the elderly, ALS can affect anyone. While the vast majority of ALS patients have no family history of the disease, reports show two population groups with higher incidence of ALS. During the 1950s, ALS occurred at high rates in the U.S. territory of Guam.[2] More recently, military veterans, especially those who served in the Gulf War,[3] proved twice as likely to develop ALS than other population groups.[4] The last two observations have led to the hypothesis that ALS development may involve environmental components such as exposure to nerve toxins, present in both Guam in the '50s and during the Gulf War.

Doctors diagnose the disease by neurological examination, review of a patient's symptom progression, and results of nerve and muscle function tests. In the rare case of a possible hereditary link, genetic testing might be performed. Observing that ALS patients possess higher levels of glutamate in their spinal fluid, doctors have taken to one treatment currently available. The pharmaceutical drug riluzole is used to reduce glutamate levels, which may extend one's life span by up to two months. However, the drug does not reverse nerve damage, can be liver-toxic, and initiates a host of other adverse affects.

Cannabis and ALS

The number of studies examining the endocannabinoid system in the context of ALS continues to grow steadily. Researchers suggest that marijuana, with its pain-killing, muscle-relaxing, bronchodilating, saliva-reducing, appetite-stimulating, sleep-inducing, antioxidative and neuroprotective properties, may be a practical therapeutic agent in the management of ALS. Of all the studies reviewed in the summary below, the one that stands out in its potential practicality is the 2010 Seattle trial conducted on mice. It led scientists to suggest that an optimal treatment regimen for ALS would include "glutamate antagonists, antioxidants, a centrally acting anti-inflammatory agent, microglial cell modulators (including tumor necrosis factor alpha [TNF-alpha] inhibitors), an antiapoptotic agent, one or more neurotrophic growth factors, and a mitochondrial function-enhancing agent . . . to comprehensively address the known pathophysiology of ALS. Remarkably, cannabis appears to have activity in all of those areas."[5]

Study Summary

Drugs	Type of Study	Published Year, Place, and Key Results	CHI
Patients were randomly assigned to receive 5 mg THC twice daily followed by placebo or vice versa	27 ALS patients suffering from daily cramps	2010—Neuromuscular Diseases Unit, Kantonsspital St Gallen, Switzerland: No change in cramps.[6]	0
Cannabinoids	Mice	2010—Muscular Dystrophy Association/Amyotrophic Lateral Sclerosis Center, University of Washington Medical Center, Seattle, WA: Cannabinoids exhibited prolonged neuronal cell survival, delayed onset of ALS symptoms, and slower progression of the disease.[7]	2
Cannabinoids	Review	2010—Clinica Neurologica, Dipartimento di Neuroscienze, Università Tor Vergata, Rome, Italy: Cannabinoids regulate immune responses and protect nerve cell function and integrity.[8]	4
Cannabinoids	Review	2007—Department of Neurosciences, University of Rome Tor Vergata, Rome: The endocannabinoid system is involved in modulating neurodegeneration and neuroinflammation.[9]	4
CBN was delivered via subcutaneously implanted osmotic mini-pumps (5 mg/kg/day) over a period of up to 12 weeks	Mice	2005—Department of Neurology, University of Washington: Treatment significantly delays disease onset by more than two weeks while survival was not affected.[10]	2
Cannabis	131 ALS patients surveyed	2004—Department of Rehabilitation Medicine, University of Washington School of Medicine, Seattle, Washington: Cannabis may be moderately effective at reducing symptoms of appetite loss, depression, pain, spasticity, and drooling but not helpful with speech, swallowing, or sexual dysfunction.[11]	3
Cannabis	A review of preclinical and anecdotal data	2001—Muscular Dystrophy Association Neuromuscular Disease Clinic, University of Washington School of Medicine, Seattle, Washington: ALS patients may benefit from analgesia, muscle relaxation, bronchodilation, saliva reduction, appetite stimulation, and sleep induction effects of cannabis. In addition, marijuana's strong antioxidative and neuroprotective effects may prolong neuronal cell survival.[12]	4

Total CHI Value 19

Strain-Specific Considerations

The reviews, pre-clinical trials, and human case surveys analyzed in this section seem to generally suggest an employment of full-spectrum cannabinoids, which bind with both main endocannabinoid receptors. More specifically, CBN has proven effective in delaying the onset of symptoms in mice. To date, no human trial has been conducted to discover if these findings translate to the human experience.

Some cannabis-using patients suffering from ALS prefer to employ indicas or indica-dominant strains that tend to present with a higher CBD/CBN:THC profile than sativas or sativa-dominant hybrids.

Other cannabis-using ALS patients have reportedly benefited from prioritizing their symptoms and choosing a strain that addresses the top items.

Mind-Body Medicine and ALS

Many physicians and caregivers alike often assume that those with ALS must feel depressed and that this state of mind only increases as the disease takes its course. However, a recent study involving 56 ALS patients and many of their caregivers concluded that "clinical depression or significant depressive symptomatology is not an inevitable or common outcome of life-threatening illness, even in the presence of major disability."[13] In his 1939 farewell speech to fans, Lou Gehrig expressed nothing but gratitude for his life. He succumbed to ALS two years later. In a recent interview, Stephen Hawking responded to a question about fear of death: "I have lived with the prospect of an early death for the last 49 years. I'm not afraid of death, but I'm in no hurry to die. I have so much I want to do first. . . ."

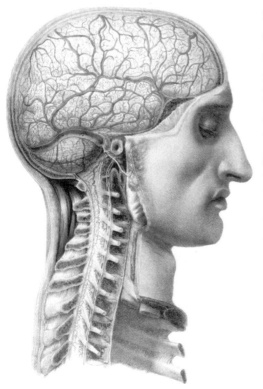

In ALS, the widening rift between the diminishing body and a fully functioning mind may offer some insight into its feedback or message. Worldly things fade away, leaving the inner world of mind fully functioning. Some neurologists refer to this unique condition as "locked-in syndrome." Research conducted on developing brainwave–computer interface technology hopes to enable "locked-in" minds to somewhat open the door to the world and interact.

Aggravating factors may include participation in the second Gulf War or other exposure to environmental toxins.

Consider working with gratitude, long-term projects, and passion for life.

Powerful Questions

Do I believe my body is keeping me from my mind's work or focus?
What does a separation between body and mind serve?
Do I consider my body a limitation or obstacle?
Why must I be locked in?
What would happen if the door stayed open?
What would happen if I came and went as I please?

Suggested Blessing

May you learn to enjoy the nature and beauty of body and mind.

Suggested Affirmation

I can complete my inner work and enjoy the gifts my body has to offer.

Epileptic Seizure (Status Epilepticus)
Evidence-Based Confidence Level and Therapeutic Potential

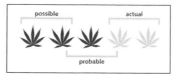

Total Number of Studies Reviewed: 5
CHI Value: 13

An emergency-room definition for status epilepticus (SE) is: continuous seizure activity lasting longer than five minutes or multiple seizures without regaining consciousness in between the seizures. This is a true emergency. SE, a potentially life-threatening condition, involves the brain and by extension the entire nervous system in a state of excessive nerve cell activity. Some people liken it to a short in the electrical system.

Several patients have reported an aura just prior to the onset of a seizure. This aura can be a smell, a visual shift in color, or a sense of psychic perceptions such as déjà vu or the sensation of shifting into "slow motion." It is a practical and useful sensation that helps the patient prepare for a coming event and allows her to reduce the risk of trauma and complications.

Other symptoms range from thrashing movements to loss of consciousness. They may include involuntary spasms of the body or parts of it, rapid heart rates, oral trauma from involuntarily biting cheek or tongue, incontinence, and confusion. Caution should be taken due to possible secondary trauma acquired from a fall.

Causes may include nerve toxins, hypoglycemia (low sugar), very high fevers (most common cause of SE in children), septic condition, trauma (especially to the head or spinal cord), tumors (especially brain and spinal cord), metabolic imbalances, acquired tolerance to anti-seizure medications, alcohol withdrawal, pharmaceutical drugs, street drugs, stroke (CVA), and hereditary or brain diseases.

Allopathic treatment consists of diagnosing and correcting, if possible, underlying causes. Diagnosed epileptic patients are given anti-seizure pharmaceuticals to reduce seizures and their intensity. Orthodox medicine currently has no cure for epilepsy.

Cannabis and Status Epilepticus

Researchers (2009) from the University of Reading, England, wrote, "Early studies suggested that cannabidiol (CBD) has anticonvulsant properties in animal models and reduced seizure frequency in limited human trials." Based on these early results, researchers conceived a study in which mice received a chemical substance (pentylentetrazol) known to produce generalized spasms similar to epileptic seizures. Cannabidiol (CBD), administered at a dose of 100 mg/kg, produced a significant reduction in the frequency of spasms and overall mortality,[1] thus confirming earlier findings.

The endocannabinoid system in the human body helps maintain an up/down (excitatory/inhibitory) balance within the central nervous system. With this understanding, neuroscientists (2009) from Rome, Italy, explored the relationship between epileptic activity and the amount of endocannabinoids present in cerebrospinal fluid. Doctors withdrew cerebrospinal fluid from patients suffering from diagnosed temporal lobe epilepsy and from healthy individuals. They measured the presence of two cannabinoids, anandamide and 2-arachidonoylglycerol (2-AG). Results revealed a significantly lower amount of anandamide in epilepsy patients when compared with the healthy controls, thus suggesting that the presence of anandamide, or lack thereof, may play a part in epilepsy.[2]

Based on prior research establishing the endocannabinoid system's involvement in hyperexcitability, particularly in the causation and control of seizures and status epilepticus (SE), scientists from the Commonwealth University in Virginia (2009) conducted an experiment to learn more about the endocannabinoid system during SE. They discovered that chemically induced SE caused a redistribution of cannabinoid receptor sites (CB1) in the hippocampus, suggesting a role for dysregulation of the endocannabinoid system during epileptogenesis.[3]

Pediatricians in Germany (2003) conducted the first human trial using pediatric patients suffering from a variety of neurological disorders including seizures. Doctors treated patients with Delta-9-THC with dosages ranging from 0.04 mg/kg body weight to 0.14 mg/kg body weight. The authors concluded: "In severely disabled children and adolescents, Delta-9-THC medication can have positive psychotropic effects, influences the degree of spasticity and dystonia, and occasionally seems to have an anticonvulsant action."[4]

In 2005, a group of international researchers from Leiden, Holland, and Rome, Italy, conducted a second and similar human trial on pediatric patients suffering from epileptic seizures who failed to respond to traditional pharmaceutical anti-seizure medications. Pediatric patients received an oil-based solution of cannabidiol (CBD). Each of the patients responded positively. The authors of the study concluded: "So far, obtained results in our open study appear encouraging for various reasons: 1) no side effects of such a severity were observed as to require CBD discontinuation; 2) in most of the treated children, an improvement of the crises was obtained equal to, or higher than, 25% in spite of the low CBD doses administered; 3) in all CBD-treated children, a clear improvement of consciousness and spasticity (whenever present) was observed."[5]

Study Summary

Drugs/Focus	Type of Study	Published Year, Place, and Key Results	CHI
Cannabidiol (CBD) 100 mg/kg	Animal study (mice)	2009—School of Pharmacy, University of Reading, Whiteknights, Reading, UK: Antispasmodic.[1]	2
Anandamide and 2-arachidonoyl-glycerol (2-AG)	Human patients with epilepsy	2009—Dipartimento di Neuroscienze, Università degli Studi di Roma Tor Vergata, Roma, Italy: Anandamide may prevent epilepsy.[2]	3
Cannabinoid receptor CB1 studied	Animal study (epileptic rats)	2009—Department of Neurology, Virginia Commonwealth University, Richmond, VA, USA: Authors suspect that redistribution of cannabinoid receptors CB1 in hippocampus may play a role in epilepsy.[3]	2
Cannabidiol (CBD)	18 children suffering from epileptic seizures who had no success with traditional pharmaceutical anti-seizure medications	2005—Multi-institutional research team from Holland and Italy: Safe and clear improvement of consciousness and spasticity.[5]	3
Delta-9-THC at dosages ranging from 0.04 mg/kg body weight to 0.14 mg/kg body weight	8 pediatric patients suffering from a variety of neurological disorders including seizures	2003—Pediatrician, Brunnenstrasse 54, Bad Wildungen, Germany: Positive psychotropic effects, influences the degree of spasticity and dystonia, and occasionally seems to have an anticonvulsant action.[4]	3

Total CHI Value 13

Strain-Specific Considerations

The relevant cannabinoids used in these trials against epilepsy include CBD, anandamide, and THC. Anandamide and THC bind relatively equally to CB1 and CB2. CBD has a greater affinity for CB2. The largest study to date (2005—see chart above) from Leiden, Holland, and Rome, Italy, used a CBD-infused oil on pediatric seizure patients.

Indicas or indica-dominant strains tend to have a higher CBD:THC ratio than sativas or sativa-heavy hybrids, thus favoring relative CB2 activation.

Mind-Body Medicine and Status Epilepticus

Julius Caesar suffered from epilepsy. In those days, people believed that epileptics were communing with the gods during a seizure event. Today some researchers echo this belief and past experience. The occurrences of temporal lobe seizure activity have been associated with religious vision and hyperreligiosity.[6]

The tonic-clonic jarring movements during an epileptic seizure simulate a short circuit without the circuit breaker present. The sparks simply continue to fly. Electrical energy keeps firing, overwhelming the nervous system, and the body responds in fits. The mental-emotional equivalent is overwhelming intense thoughts and feelings that the person refuses to consciously experience.

Studies exploring the significance of psychological tension in connection with seizure activity suggest that this tension, not immediately soluble in reality, can contribute to the occurrence of seizures. However, the resolution of such tension in a therapeutic setting could ameliorate seizure activities.[7]

Another researcher noted that seizure responses from relatively minor petit mal seizures to full-blown status epilepticus may appear as specific responses within the central nervous system, "... which abolishes consciousness when awareness of the discrepancy in the immediate situation between consciously acceptable responses and the true unconscious reactions threatens to disrupt the patient's existing pattern of integration."[8] This last finding suggests a conflict between the conscious and unconscious mind, a short due to crossed wires of conflicting beliefs, intentions, or experiences.

Another study examined the relationship between emotionally disturbed children and seizure activity. Researchers learned that sometimes the children would use the seizure activities as an unconscious defense mechanism—for instance, when witnessing the parents destroy each other psychologically. In such moments, the child would often succeed, temporarily ending the marital conflict. However, at other times, the child would display seizure activities to seek sympathy or attention and employ an avoidance mechanism such as procrastination when not wanting to do a certain task. This suggests that in some cases the frequency of seizure activity and the underlying psychodynamics were intertwined. "For example, greater passivity increased the frequency, and greater aggression decreased the frequency of petit mal attacks in two children; whereas increased anxiety probably caused more frequent psychomotor seizures in another child."[9]

A physician compiled the following examples. A patient never had seizures in college classes that he actively engaged in and liked when compared to classes he disliked. A trapeze artist had regular seizures except when he was working at the trapeze. A baseball player had seizures on the sidelines but never when playing ball. Another patient had regular seizures except when swimming. Based on these examples, this researcher suggested that mental activity that engages and appeals to the person might be employed in the treatment and prevention of seizure events.[10]

Given the rather elusive origin of seizures, those dealing with epilepsy might consider exploring the metaphysical underpinnings in order to better understand, cope, and ideally diminish seizures.

One particularly helpful mechanism includes increasing one's awareness of the trigger mechanisms involved in seizure development. Some epileptics have found success in this task by approaching it as a mindfulness exercise. Learning which signals from the environment such as sounds, music,[11] or lights can trigger a seizure is another way to be more aware of the complexities of this disease picture.

In summary, aggravating factors may include psychological tension from repressed memories and emotions, increased anxiety and passivity, negative affect, and lack of connection with the spiritual.

Consider working with integrating and healing childhood traumas, accepting and appropriately releasing repressed content, increasing assertiveness (appropriately expressed and without hurting anyone), engaging in profound spiritual connections or intensely enjoyed activities, and finding a positive perspective.

Powerful Questions

What thoughts or feelings overwhelm me?
What is too much for me to handle?
What is so intense that I want to throw in the towel?

Suggested Blessing

May you find a place in you where peace reigns supreme.

Suggested Affirmation

I release all fear.

Huntington's Disease

Evidence-Based Confidence Level and Therapeutic Potential

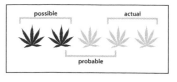

Number of Studies Reviewed: 5

CHI Value: 10

Huntington's disease (HD) or Huntington's chorea (abnormal twisting and writhing movements) is a degenerative genetic disease that affects the brain and nervous system, leading to loss of muscle control and dementia. A mutated form of the Huntington gene, found significantly more in Western Europeans, is thought to be responsible for disease development. The gene can be passed on to offspring. One parent with the mutation on one of the two DNA strand pairs is associated with a 50% chance that any offspring will develop the disease. If both parents have a single pair mutation, the risk for the offspring increases to 75%, and if both parents have dual pair mutation, development of Huntington's is a virtual certainty. Parents who may carry this gene may want to consider genetic testing.

Researchers currently ponder a variety of questions about Huntington's disease: How does the disease start? What causes or maintains the mutation? What activates the gene? Why does HD develop at a certain time after years of apparent dormancy? Why does HD begin earlier in some people and later in others?

Some scientists believe that the mutated gene codes for a protein that rather than forming and folding into functional protein molecules causes protein aggregation. These aggregated proteins clump together, collect, and eventually corrupt certain portions of the brain, causing the characteristic signs and symptoms of HD.

Once HD starts, the illness takes a predictable course for most patients. Symptoms usually begin with lack of coordination and ataxia (unsteady gait). They soon progress to chorea, dystonia (muscle contraction, twisting, and abnormal posturing), dementia, behavioral difficulties, and eventually death. No treatment exists within orthodox medicine for HD. However, to manage some of the disease complications, doctors may try certain treatments using a multidisciplinary approach composed of physical and speech therapies, neuroleptics (tranquilizing psychiatric pharmaceuticals), and other medication. If eating or drinking becomes too difficult, gastric tubes may be used. Huntington mortality statistics suggest that the leading causes of death are the development of pneumonia and heart disease followed by nutritional deficiencies, mental and cerebrovascular disorders, accidents, poisoning, and violence.[1]

Cannabis and Huntington's Disease

As early as 1986, researchers enrolled three patients suffering from HD whose disease progression continued to deteriorate and who did not respond to pharmaceuticals. Each received an oral form of the non-psychoactive cannabinoid CBD. After the first week of treatment, results revealed a mild improvement of 5 to 15% in objective and subjective tests. After week two, the improvement of 20 to 40% was observed using the same tests. The results remained stable for the following two weeks. The only adverse effect noted was a mild and transient hypotension.[2]

Five years later, researchers from the University of Arizona conducted a double-blind, randomized crossover trial testing the effects of oral CBD and placebo on 15 neuroleptic-free patients with HD. In this case, CBD proved only as effective as the placebo.[3]

In 2007, Spanish scientists examined the neuroprotective potential of CBD in the context of Huntington's disease. Results indicated that "... CBD provides neuroprotection against 3NP-induced striatal damage, which may be relevant for Huntington's disease, a disorder characterized by the preferential loss of striatal projection neurons.... This capability seems to be based exclusively on the antioxidant properties of CBD."[4]

Two more experiments published in 2011 examined the effects of cannabinoids on HD. In one study researchers from Madrid, Spain, examined whether Sativex (THC/CBD) was able to protect animals from HD progression and development. The authors observed, "In conclusion, this study provides pre-clinical evidence in support of a beneficial effect of the cannabis-based medicine Sativex as a neuroprotective agent capable of delaying disease progression in HD, a disorder that is currently poorly managed in the clinic, prompting an urgent need for clinical trials with agents showing positive results in pre-clinical studies."[5]

The other study from Madrid (also 2011) acknowledged cannabinoids as promising medicines for slowing the chronic degenerative progression of both Parkinson's disease and HD. Researchers examined in more detail the effects of CB1 and CB2 receptor activation on disease progression. Results demonstrated that "... activation of CB(2) receptors leads to a slower progression of neurodegeneration in both disorders." Furthermore, "... cannabinoids like $\Delta(9)$-tetrahydrocannabinol or cannabidiol protect nigral or striatal neurons in experimental models of both disorders in which oxidative injury is a prominent cytotoxic mechanism." Researchers concluded that "... the evidence reported so far supports that those cannabinoids having antioxidant properties and/or capability to activate CB(2) receptors may represent promising therapeutic agents in HD and PD, thus deserving a prompt clinical evaluation."[6]

Study Summary

Drugs/Focus	Type of Study	Published Year, Place, and Key Results	CHI
THC and CBD containing Sativex	Animal model (rats)	2011—Departamento de Bioquímica y Biología Molecular, Instituto Universitario de Investigación en Neuroquímica, Facultad de Medicina, Universidad Complutense, Madrid, Spain: Sativex is a neuroprotective agent capable of delaying disease progression in HD.[5]	1
Endocannabinoid system and cannabinoids, especially THC and CBD	Meta-analysis and review	2011—Departamento de Bioquímica y Biología Molecular III, Instituto Universitario de Investigación en Neuroquímica, Facultad de Medicina, Universidad Complutense, Madrid, Spain: The endocannabinoid system behaves as an endogenous neuroprotective system in both PD and HD.[6]	4
Arachidonyl-2-chloro-ethylamide (ACEA), a CB1 agonist; HU-308, a CB2 agonist; and cannabidiol (CBD)	Animal study (rats)	2007—Departamento de Bioquímica y Biología Molecular III, Universidad Complutense, Madrid, Spain: CBD provides neuroprotection, which may be relevant to Huntington's disease.[4]	2
Oral CBD (10 mg/kg/day for 6 weeks) and placebo (sesame oil for 6 weeks)	15 patients with Huntington's Disease	1991—Department of Pharmacology/Toxicology, University of Arizona, Tucson, USA: CBD was neither symptomatically effective nor toxic, relative to placebo.[3]	0
Orally administered CBD was initiated at 300 mg/d and increased 1 week later to 600 mg/d for the next 3 weeks	Three patients, 30 to 56, had HD for 7 to 12 ages years' duration	1986—Decreased choreic movements and severity.[2]	3

Total CHI Value 10

Strain-Specific Considerations

The relevant cannabinoids examined in this set of pre-clinical and human case studies include primarily CBD, THC, and Sativex. CBD has a greater affinity for CB2. THC binds relatively equally to CB1 and CB2. Sativex is a standardized plant cannabis extract containing THC and CBD in ratios similar to those in cannabis flowers.

Indica and indica-dominant strains or hybrids usually contain lower THC:CBD ratios, thus favoring CB2 activation when compared to sativas or sativa-leaning strains.

Mind-Body Medicine and Huntington's Disease

The threat of progression of HD and the relative certainty that the beginning of the end is near forces one's focus to be on living in the moment. The value of life is associated with youth, and the rest with pain and inevitable death. The archetype of youth rebelling against a predetermined destiny comes to mind. In a way, HD engages and sometimes challenges supernatural authorities such as destiny or the unconscious. It engages us in the intense choices ahead. Will I be choosing to look at life with gratitude for what I have now, or choosing to blame others and feel hopeless? Another strong component of HD is that of family burden and shared destiny in a movement toward less conscious control while uncontrollable unconscious dance-like movement increases. As consciousness retreats, it is apparently replaced by an unconscious release of energy.

To some people with HD, another choice may present itself: What if I were to embrace the inevitable unconscious dance of twisting, writhing energy exploding into my reality? What if I surrender consciously to the unconscious?

Powerful Questions

What comes up for me when looking at the past, present, and future?
What is my relationship to the conscious and the unconscious mind?
What is my relationship to the bridge between the conscious and the unconscious mind?
How do I feel about the unconscious?
What do I think of destiny?

Could I surrender to whatever emerges?

Could I embrace the emerging?

How do I feel about outside controlling forces?

How would I feel if I learned that those forces were set in motion by me for a good reason that I have purposefully forgotten?

Can I make peace with the coming unconscious dance?

Suggested Blessings

May all my blame turn to forgiveness.

May all my future fear become a present and creative love.

May all my hopelessness transcend into a creative vision carried by a determined will into the arms of loving possibilities.

Suggested Affirmation

I surrender to the loving hands of something larger than my unconscious or myself.

Multiple Sclerosis (MS)

Evidence-Based Confidence Level and Therapeutic Potential

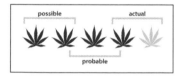

Total Number of Studies Reviewed: 26

CHI Value: 91

Orthodox medicine considers multiple sclerosis (MS) a chronic, inflammatory, and degenerative neurological illness with no cure and no exact cause. In fact, MS is one of the most common neurological diseases.

The meaning of the term "multiple sclerosis" provides a clue about the general picture of this illness. It derives from the Latin words *multi* and *plus,* which together translate into "manifold," and the Greek word *sclerosis* which translates as "hardness." Place the words together and we get "many folded hardness." Apply "manifold hardness" to the brain and spinal cord and we have a description of MS.

Multiple sclerosis is characterized by the breakdown of some of the thin sheets that cover the brain and spinal cord. These fat-based myelin sheets normally provide insulation and protection, but when lesions occur, nerve impulses misfire across the broken insulation, causing a variety of debilitating symptoms.

Scientists speculate that MS might be an autoimmune disease that inadvertently prompts adhesion molecules, which summon immune cells to fight an inflammation and thus contribute to the destruction of myelin sheets.[1] Other likely culprits include a combination of genetic factors, infections, and environmental influences such as decreased sun exposure and subsequent insufficient vitamin D.

Some pharmaceutical medications exist to manage symptoms as they develop or worsen, but they come with a steep price of significant side effects. MS may initially appear as acute attacks only, or it may progress to its chronic degenerative form in which symptoms accumulate and gradually worsen. Some of the most common symptoms include muscular spasms affecting the eyes, bladder, and bowels, numbness, increased weakness, ataxia, slurred speech and/or acute and chronic pain.

Due to limited success within the allopathic model, many MS patients have turned to other healing methodologies in the hope of finding help and relief.

Cannabis and MS

The earliest study listed in the National Library of Health took place in 1981 when researchers found motivation in anecdotal accounts of MS patients who reported that inhaling cannabis gave relief from spasticity. This, combined with the scientific discovery that THC is able to inhibit spasms in animal studies, opened the door to a multitude of scientific inquiries.

While initial studies merely focused on observing the effect of cannabis on the most common symptoms of MS, later studies worked to discover the mechanisms underlying the observed therapeutic effects.

The scientific community began to build on the data accumulated. The therapeutic frame of cannabis in the context of MS became more clear and defined. A reduction in spasticity was recognized as only the first of many benefits. Cannabis use also reduced pain, depression, anxiety, paresthesia, neuropathic pains, sleep disturbances, urge incontinence, and nocturnal polyuria.

Even the U.S. federal government issued itself a patent on the neuroprotective properties of cannabinoids employed in the treatment of several diseases involving inflammation and the nervous system, such as MS.

One of the latest animal studies on the cannabinoid receptor systems alludes to the involvement of cannabinoids in the inhibition of brain adhesion molecules, which in turn may be responsible for some therapeutic effects on MS. If clinical trials can confirm these results, scientists may be able to partly understand how to slow or even reverse the progression of MS.

While the 26 studies listed here differ in approach, scope, and methodology, the results share a common denominator. For patients suffering from MS, cannabis may be a potent ally in alleviating the disease's symptoms. Furthermore, cannabinoids may slow the progression of the illness itself and thus provide an improvement to long-term survival and quality of life.

Warning: Most clinical studies report adverse effects of cannabis use in addition to benefits dependent on dose and form. Adverse effects include reduced balance and posture, nausea, and dizziness; and at high dosages, negative psychological symptoms such as anxiety. These studies indicated that when used within the proper subjective therapeutic dose, cannabinoids' potential adverse effects are usually well tolerated and negligible, especially when compared to the beneficial effects.

To determine the best possible therapeutic window for you, seek advice from peers with MS who have used cannabis themselves, and consult a licensed health care professional familiar with cannabinoids.

See also "How to Establish Your Subjective Therapeutic Window" on page 20.

Strain-Specific Considerations

The majority of the studies reviewed in this section used whole-plant matter or the pharmaceutical plant derivative Sativex, a cannabinoid combination containing THC and CBD in similar proportions to the strain *Cannabis sativa.* Whole-flower cannabis and Sativex activate both CB1 and CB2 receptors.

Sativa or sativa-dominant hybrids usually contain a higher THC:CBD ratio, activating both CB1 and CB2 receptors, while indicas or indica-dominant strains usually contain lower THC:CBD ratios, favoring CB2 signaling.

Study Summary

Drugs/Focus	Type of Study	Published Year, Place, and Key Results	CHI
WIN55,212-2	Animal study (mice)	2009—Neuroimmunology Group, Functional and Systems Neurobiology Department, Cajal Institute (CSIC), Madrid, Spain: Inhibition of brain adhesion molecules may produce therapeutic effects in MS.[2]	2
Free-dose cannabis plant extract (Sativex)	17 patients with MS: double-blind, placebo-controlled, crossover study	2009—University of Rome "Sapienza," Rome, Italy: Within therapeutic doses, no impairment or negative psychological symptoms noted. However, at high dosages, negative psychological symptoms noted.[3]	5
THC:CBD as an oral spray	18 patients with MS: randomized, double-blind, placebo-controlled, crossover study	2009—Department of Neurological Sciences, University of Rome "Sapienza," Rome, Italy: RIII reflex threshold increased and RIII reflex area decreased plus pain reduction.[4]	5
Anandamide AEA, PEA, 2-AG, and OEA levels	50 patients with MS and 20 control subjects	2008—Centre for Study of Demyelinating Diseases, Department of Medical and Surgical Specialities and Public Health, Ospedale S Maria della Misericordia, University of Perugia, Perugia, Italy: "Significantly reduced levels of all the tested eCBs were found in the CSF of patients with MS compared to control subjects. . . ."[5]	3
Dronabinol	Case study of a 52-year-old woman with MS, paroxysmal dystonia, complex vocal tics, and marijuana dependence	2008—Mental Health Service Line, Department of Veterans Affairs Medical Center, Washington, DC, USA: Improvement in sleep, decreased anxiety, decreased reduction of craving and illicit use."[6]	3
Sativex (THC:CBD)	66 patients with MS	2007—Walton Centre for Neurology and Neuro-surgery, Liverpool, UK: THC/CBD was effective in reducing pains with no evidence of tolerance for the 2 years tested.[7]	5
THC:CBD daily	189 patients with MS	2007—Royal Berkshire and Battle NHS Trust, Reading, UK: Reduction in spasms.[8]	5
Endocannabinoids (AEA) & (2-AG) levels, metabolism, binding, and physiological activities	26 patients with MS, 25 healthy controls, and an animal study (mice)	2007—Multi-departmental study from Italy. Clinica Neurologica, Dipartimento di Neuroscienze, Università Tor Vergata, Rome, Italy: Targeting the endocannabinoid system might be useful for the treatment of MS.[9]	5
Endocannabinoid agonists	Animal study (mice)	2007—Department of Neuro-inflammation, Institute of Neurology, University College London, UK: CB(1) receptor is the main cannabinoid target for an antispastic effect.[10]	2

Drugs/Focus	Type of Study	Published Year, Place, and Key Results	CHI
Cannabinoids studied	Laboratory	2006—Center for Drug Discovery, Northeastern University, Boston, MA, USA: Results suggest a therapeutic potential of cannabinoids on inflammatory diseases such as MS.[11]	1
Cannabis extract, THC, or placebo	630 MS patients	2006—Urogynaecology Unit, Derriford Hospital, Plymouth, Devon, UK: Both cannabis extract and THC showed significant reductions in urge incontinence.[12]	5
Sativex as an oromucosal spray; each spray delivers 2.7 mg THC and 2.5 mg CBD. Average use in this study was 22–32 mg/day THC and 20–30 mg/day CBD.	Patients with MS	2006—Hunters Moor Regional Neurological Rehabilitation Centre, Newcastle upon Tyne, UK: Reduction in spasticity, neuropathic pain, and neuropathic pain of other etiologies.[13]	3
Cannabinoid HU210	Animal study (rats)	2006—Department of Physical Medicine and Rehabilitation, University of Saskatchewan, Saskatoon, Canada: "HU210 dramatically reduced peroxynitrite-induced axonal injury…."[14]	2
Cannabinoids	A meta-analysis of human, animal, and laboratory studies	2005—Neurologische Klinik mit Klinischer Neurophysiologie, Medizinische Hochschule Hannover, Germany: "…there is reasonable evidence for the therapeutic employment of cannabinoids in the treatment of MS-related symptoms."[15]	4
Whole-plant cannabis-based medicine, containing (THC:CBD) and delivered via an oromucosal spray	66 patients with MS	2005—Walton Centre for Neurology and Neurosurgery, University of Liverpool, UK: Reduction of pain and sleep disturbance in MS.[16]	5
Oromucosal spray, Sativex containing (THC:CBD)	Meta-analysis on 368 human patients with various neurological disorders including MS	2005—In some trials, THC:CBD spray significantly reduced neuropathic pain, spasticity, muscle spasms, and sleep disturbances.[17]	4
Whole-plant cannabis-based medicine, containing (THC:CBD) and delivered via an oromucosal spray, as adjunctive analgesic treatment. Each spray delivered 2.7 mg of THC and 2.5 of CBD, and patients could gradually self-titrate to a maximum of 48 spray in 24 hours.	66 patients with MS	2005—Walton Centre for Neurology and Neurosurgery, University of Liverpool, UK: "Cannabis-based medicine is effective in reducing pain and sleep disturbance in patients with multiple sclerosis-related central neuropathic pain and is mostly well tolerated."[18]	3

Drugs/Focus	Type of Study	Published Year, Place, and Key Results	CHI
Oromucosal spray (Sativex) 5containing a cannabis-based extract (THC:CBD) at 2.5–120 mg of each daily in divided doses	160 outpatients with MS	2004—Oxford Centre for Enablement, Windmill Road, Oxford, UK: Significant reduction of spasms.[19]	5
THC and CBD; 2.5 mg of each per spray for eight weeks followed by THC only (2.5 mg THC per spray)	15 MS patients with lower urinary tract symptoms	2004—Dept. of Uro-Neurology, Institute of Neurology and National Hospital for Neurology and Neurosurgery, London, UK: Urinary urgency, the number and volume of incontinence episodes, frequency and nocturia all decreased significantly. Pain, spasticity, and quality of sleep improved significantly.[20]	3
Cannabis, inhaled	420 patients with MS	2003—Office of Medical Bioethics, University of Calgary, Canada: Reduced anxiety, depression, spasticity, and chronic pain.[21]	3
Cannabis, inhaled	112 patients with MS	1997—University of Arizona Health Sciences Center, Tucson, AZ, USA: Reduced spasticity, pain, tremor, depression, anxiety, and paresthesia.[22]	3
Nabilone 1 mg every 2nd day	1 patient with MS	1995—Reduced muscle spasms and nocturia.[23]	3
One marijuana cigarette containing 1.54% THC	10 MS patients and 10 normal volunteers	1994—Department of Neurology, University of Michigan, Ann Arbor: Inhaled cannabis reduced balance in MS patients.[24]	3
One marijuana cigarette	1 MS patient	1989—Department of Clinical Neurophysiology, University of Göttingen, Germany: Chronic motor handicaps improved while smoking a marijuana cigarette.[25]	3
THC oral 2.5–15 mg once or twice daily	13 MS patients	1987—Department of Psychiatry, UCLA School of Medicine, Los Angeles, California: At doses greater than 7.5 mg, significant improvement in patient ratings of spasticity compared to placebo.[26]	3
Either 10 or 5 mg THC or placebo once daily	9 patients suffering from spasticity from various etiologies incl. MS	1981—10 mg THC significantly reduced spasticity.[27]	3

Total CHI Value 88

Mind-Body Medicine and MS

A cross-cultural study of patients with MS from the U.S. and Israel showed that both patient groups experienced similar concurrent psychological challenges at the time of the emergence of MS symptoms. These challenges were "characterized as a psychologically stressful situation involving difficulty in coping and feelings of helplessness."[28] Later studies revealed emotional stress as a potential trigger for the onset, exacerbation, and relapse of disease activity.[29]

Aggravating elements may include difficulty in coping, feelings of helplessness, and emotional stress.

Consider learning or adapting positive coping mechanisms to reduce trigger events.

Powerful Questions

How do I turn my energies on myself?

What do I try to control in my reality even though I know I can't?

How do I have impact in life when I don't want to participate?

Where and why am I so hardhearted with myself, others, and the whole world?

Where and why am I so rigid with what I perceive as right and wrong?

What other perspectives can help me melt my stubbornness away?

Where are my tears wanting and where are they wasted?

What keeps me from facing changes and unforeseen events?

What paralyzes my courage and substance?

How do I love myself so as to allow a world where I am free and where I am safe?

Why does it hurt to move or to show backbone?

How do I numb my senses or myself?

Why is life so exhausting?

Suggested Blessings

May our buds and leaves assist you in the calming of your fears.

May they elevate your mood and help dispel numbness, anxiety, and depression.

May we help relax the tension and spasms, and diminish the exhaustion. Relax; release the grip of your mental fists, release control, and surrender to a calming night of blissful sleep.

Suggested Affirmation

May I release the hard beliefs and toughness of thought to give way to the flexibility of gentle and strong internal borders.

Let Food Be Thy Medicine

Turmeric ∾ Vitamin D

Turmeric: Ayurvedic practitioners, herbalists, and naturopaths have long known about the multitude of potent therapeutic properties of *Curcuma longa* or turmeric. Curcumin is a naturally occurring compound found in the rhizome of the plant. Now researchers from Nashville, Tennessee, have examined the compound's ability to affect mice with MS. Results of the study revealed a similarity between the amount of curcumin used to protect the mice from artificially induced MS and that found in the typical Indian diet. One author of the study reported that MS in India is very rare, and while no human studies to date confirm the results, it certainly can't hurt to add some turmeric to your food.[39]

Vitamin D: Researchers in Stockholm, Sweden, suggest that vitamin D is important for MS patients. "One of the environmental factors that has been implicated in MS and autoimmune diseases, such as type I diabetes, is vitamin D deficiency."[31]

If applicable, see also Inflammatory Diseases and/or the section on Pain.

Parkinson's Disease

Evidence-Based Confidence Level and Therapeutic Potential

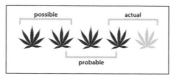

Total Number of Studies Reviewed: 4

CHI Value: 14

Western medicine considers Parkinson's disease a chronic degenerative brain/nervous system disorder. An estimated 50,000 new cases of Parkinson's arise in the U.S. every year. Scientists believe that this degenerative disease results from the loss of specific nerve cells that produce the chemical dopamine (a naturally occurring neurotransmitter), causing symptoms like shaking extremities, stiffness, loss of balance, shuffling steps, difficulty swallowing, insomnia, blank expressions, and emotional problems.

Cannabis and Parkinson's Disease

U.S. Department of Health and Human Services (2003) researchers received a patent on cannabinoids as antioxidants and neuroprotectants. Based on a multitude of earlier studies, these scientists noted in their U.S. patent abstract that ". . . cannabinoids are found to have particular application as neuroprotectants, for example in limiting neurological damage following ischemic insults, such as stroke and trauma, or in the treatment of neurodegenerative diseases, such as Alzheimer's disease, Parkinson's disease, and HIV dementia."[1]

A study (2004) from Hradec Kralove, Czech Republic, reports that almost half of all patients who used cannabis to treat symptoms associated with their Parkinson's noted a reduction in resting-state tremors, reduced bradykinesia (slowed ability to start and/or continue movements), less muscle rigidity, and decreased side effects from levodopa (a common Parkinson's medication)-induced dyskinesias (repetitive spastic motions). It took an average reported time of 1.7 months for these effects to take hold.[2]

In 2009 East Lansing, Michigan, researchers reported on the case of a 24-year-old woman suffering from hyperkinetic movement disorder presenting with tremors, generalized dystonia, unstable standing position, dysarthria (speech disorder), and mild anorexia. The patient reportedly tried the usual pharmacological medications such as benztropin, clonazepam, and tetrabenazin, but these failed to achieve the desired therapeutic impact. Doctors at the Department for Neurology, University of Michigan, then treated the woman with a cannabinoid during her pregnancy, after which her symptoms improved significantly.[3]

European scientists (2009) from Naples, Italy, know very well that neurodegenerative diseases remain one of the main causes of death in the industrialized world. They are also keenly aware that very few allopathic therapies currently exist for most neurodegenerative diseases. Thus in searching for novel approaches, they studied cannabinoids. Their research concluded that ". . . among Cannabis compounds, cannabidiol (CBD), which lacks any unwanted psychotropic effect, may represent a very promising agent with the highest prospect for therapeutic use."[4]

Study Summary

Drugs/Focus	Type of Study	Published Year, Place, and Key Results	CHI
Cannabidiol (CBD)	Meta-analysis	2009—Department of Experimental Pharmacology, Faculty of Pharmacy, University of Naples Federico II, Naples, Italy: Cannabidiol (CBD) may represent a very promising agent with the highest prospect for therapeutic use in the treatment of neurodegenerative illness.[4]	4
Dronabinol 5 mg 3x daily	Human case study	2009—Department for Neurology, University of Michigan: Reduction of hyperkinetic movement disorder.[3]	3
Cannabis, taken orally or inhaled	Patients with Parkinson's	2004—Department of Pharmacology and Toxicology, Faculty of Pharmacy, Charles University, Hradec Kralove, Czech Republic: Reduction in resting-state tremors, bradykinesia, muscle rigidity, and side effect of levodopa-induced dyskinesias.[2]	3
Cannabinoids, esp. cannabidiol (CBD)	Meta-analysis	2003—United States federal government: Useful in the treatment of neurodegenerative diseases such as Parkinson's disease.[1]	4

Total CHI Value 14

Strain-Specific Considerations

The cannabinoids reviewed in these studies focus especially on CBD but also include Dronabinol and whole cannabis (taken by mouth or inhaled). CBD has a higher affinity for CB2. Dronabinol, a synthetic cannabinoid prescription medication, is an isomer (same molecular formula but different structural formula) of Δ9-tetrahydrocannabinol. No information was given as to the strain used in the whole-cannabis case study. Both the prior meta-analysis conducted by U.S. government researchers from the Department of Health and Human Services (2003) and that of a team of Italian scientists (2009) highlight CBD as "... a very promising agent with the highest prospect for therapeutic use."

Indica and indica-dominant hybrids tend to contain lower THC:CBD ratios, thus favoring CB2 signaling.

Mind-Body Medicine and Parkinson's Disease

Emotions commonly associated with the body language expressed by Parkinson's disease may offer some insights into the underlying body-mind influences. For instance: shaking extremities (extreme fear); stiffness (fear of pain or movement); aphasia (frozen speech—too shocked to talk); loss of balance (paradoxical emotions pulling in different directions); shuffling steps (chronic exhaustion); difficulty swallowing (shock/fear, frozen expression); insomnia (inability to let go of the thought process); blank expressions (hiding behind a facade); and emotional problems (unresolved experiences).

Powerful Questions

Shaking extremities (extreme fear): What is the chronic and age-old fear my body is demonstrating to me? What fear or dread is shaking me to the core?

Stiffness (fear of pain or movement): What do I believe will happen to me when I move forward in life?

Aphasia (frozen speech; too shocked to talk): What has taken away my voice?

Loss of balance/ataxia (paradoxical emotions pulling in different directions): What emotions are pulling me in opposite directions? What keeps me off balance?

Shuffling steps (chronic exhaustion): What causes my internal exhaustion? What keeps me from walking through life with vitality?

Difficulty swallowing (shock/fear; frozen expression): What emotion sticks in my throat? What keeps me from easily swallowing nurturing food?

Insomnia (inability to let go of the thought process): Why can't I surrender my mind to the darkness of the night?

Blank expressions (hiding behind a facade): What shock has paralyzed my
facial expression? What is a numb face protecting me from?

Long-standing emotional problems (unresolved experiences): What emotional luggage demands release?

Suggested Blessings

May all fears fade away like dew in the morning sun.

May love replace all that is fear.

Suggested Affirmations

I trust myself. I trust those that are trustworthy.

I release all forms of control and doubt.

I can make room for any contradicting feelings until something completely new emerges.

Let Food Be Thy Medicine

Turmeric: In a large meta-study, scientists reviewed decades of scientific
studies on turmeric. They summarize a list of turmeric's potential therapeutic properties, including in cases of Parkinson's disease.[5]

Tourette Syndrome

Evidence-Based Confidence Level and Therapeutic Potential

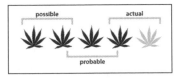

Total Number of Studies Reviewed: 10

CHI Value: 38

Gilles de la Tourette Syndrome (GTS), more commonly referred to as
Tourette syndrome (TS), is considered a developmental (most likely inherited) neurological and psychiatric disorder characterized by the presence
of chronic motor and phonic tics. Tics (uncontrollable, repetitive, and
non-rhythmic movements of select muscle groups including those needed

to speak) provoke involuntary sounds, phrases, taboo words, or oddly appearing jerking motions such as slapping or grimacing. Tics range from being a minor inconvenience to completely debilitating. Most people with tics perceive their onset as similar to sensing when one needs to sneeze or yawn. Some tics can be controlled while others cannot. Interestingly, even controllable tics appear irresistible, like an itch that demands scratching.

TS usually develops during childhood, though some kids do outgrow the syndrome later in life. Although orthodox medicine has not pinpointed a root cause for the syndrome, scientists suggest that genetic, environmental, and metabolic factors and/or the neurotransmitters dopamine and serotonin may play a leading role. In mild cases, reassurance and education can be enough to provide the practical resources for coping with and managing the condition. TS does not affect intelligence or life span and, unlike many other neurological disorders, TS is not degenerative. TS affects males significantly more often than females, but is relatively equally distributed across all ethnic groups. TS may disappear for periods of time and then reappear.

Physicians diagnose TS by conducting a thorough history and neurological examination, and using a process of elimination of other diseases with similar symptoms. If doctors suspect abnormalities of the central nervous system, they might perform an MRI to examine the patient's brain physiology. Pharmaceutical medications used in TS prove mostly ineffective with intolerable side effects.

Cannabis and Tourette Syndrome

Researchers from the University of Texas suggested as early as 1989 that cannabinoids could prove helpful in enhancing the effects of pharmaceuticals (neuroleptics) in relieving tics.[1] In addition, the authors of a study conducted at the Medical School Hanover, Germany (1998), wrote: "High densities of cannabinoid receptors were found in the basal ganglia and hippocampus, possibly indicating a functional role of cannabinoids in movement and behavior."[2]

Of all the studies listed in the summary below, four stand out in that they used the gold standard of randomized, double-blind, placebo-controlled methodology. Each of them showed cannabis to significantly reduce tics without the presence of serious adverse reactions.[3]

Study Summary

Drugs/Focus	Type of Study	Published Year, Place, and Key Results	CHI
THC	Case study (15-year-old boy with TS)	2010—Department of Psychiatry and Psychotherapy, Georg-August-University Göttingen, Germany: Administration of Delta-9-THC improved tics considerably without adverse effects.[4]	3
THC	A review of two double-blind trials on cannabinoids and TS	2009—Birmingham and Solihull Mental Health Trust, Birmingham, UK: Although both trials reported a positive effect from Delta-9-THC, the improvements in tic frequency and severity were small.[5]	0
Up to 10 mg/day of THC	Randomized, double-blind, placebo-controlled study of 24 patients with TS	2003—Department of Clinical Psychiatry and Psychotherapy, Medical School of Hanover, Germany: Results provide more evidence that THC is effective and safe in the treatment of tics.[6]	5
Up to 10 mg THC	Randomized, double-blind, placebo-controlled study on 24 patients suffering from TS	2003—Department of Clinical Psychiatry and Psychotherapy, Medical School of Hanover, Germany: Trends toward significant improvement during and after treatment.[7]	5
THC 5.0, 7.5, or 10.0 mg	Randomized, double-blind, placebo-controlled crossover single-dose trial of Delta-9-THC (5.0, 7.5, or 10.0 mg) used on 12 adult TS patients	2001—Department of Clinical Psychiatry and Psychotherapy, Medical School of Hanover, Germany: Significant improvement of tics when compared to placebo. No serious adverse reactions occurred.[8]	5
THC 5 to 10mg	12 patients with TS in a randomized, double-blind, placebo-controlled crossover trial	2001—Department of Clinical Psychiatry and Psychotherapy, Medical School of Hanover, Germany: A single-dose treatment with Delta-9-THC in patients suffering from TS does not cause cognitive impairment.[9]	5
Endogenous endocannabinoids system	Review	2000—Cannabis-Forschungs-Gruppe in der Medizinischen Hochschule, Abt. Klinische Psychiatrie und Psychotherapie: Dysregulation in the endogenous cannabinoid/anandamide system could possibly play an important role in the etiology of TS.[10]	4
Cannabinoids	Review	1999—Department of Clinical Psychiatry and Psychotherapy, Medical School of Hanover, Germany: Evidence that cannabinoid are of therapeutic value in the treatment of tics in Tourette syndrome.[11]	4
Cannabis	64 patients with TS	1998—Department of Clinical Psychiatry and Psychotherapy, Medical School of Hanover, Germany: Reduction or complete remission of motor and vocal tics and an amelioration of premonitory urges and obsessive-compulsive symptoms.[12]	3

Drugs/Focus	Type of Study	Published Year, Place, and Key Results	CHI
Cannabinoids	Review	1989—Laboratory of Psychobio-chemistry, University of Texas, El Paso, USA: May significantly enhance the therapeutic value of neuroleptics in motor disorders.[13]	4

Total CHI Value 38

Strain-Specific Considerations

The majority of the studies reviewed in this section on TS primarily used THC. However, whole-plant cannabis THC also binds relatively equally to both CB1 and CB2 receptor sites.

Sativa and sativa-dominant hybrids usually contain a higher THC:CBD ratio.

Mind-Body Medicine and Tourette Syndrome

TS begins during childhood. Like a self-fulfilling prophecy, the fear of public awkwardness often materializes. Fear of being seen with tics often precedes the awkward tics in movement or sudden outbursts of verbal shouts. Patients frequently describe the anticipation as similar to the sensation of a sneeze building up, followed by a release of the pre-sneeze tension.

Aggravating factors may include stress from chronic fears, anxiety, and negative expectations.

Consider working with positive stress-coping mechanisms and learning to replace negative expectations with positive ones.

Powerful Question

Are there other ways to deal with my fears of humiliation besides manifesting them?

Suggested Blessing

May you learn to shift dread to positive anticipation.

Suggested Affirmation

I have a powerful imagination and I get to choose the focus of my creativity moment by moment.

Obstetrical and Gynecological Difficulties and Concerns (OBGYN) (in general)

Combined Evidence-Based Confidence Level and Therapeutic Potential

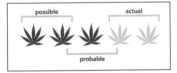

Total Number of Studies Reviewed: 5

Combined CHI Value: 11

Obstetricians specialize in the care of women during pregnancy, while gynecologists specialize in women's health. In practice, many physicians specialize in both obstetrics (OB) and gynecology (GYN), and OBGYN clinics are generally set up to examine, diagnose, and treat women in the areas of family planning (contraception), menstruation, chronic pelvic pain, fertility, pregnancy and prenatal care, sexually transmitted diseases, preventative care (pap smear, cancer screening), and menopausal concerns.

OBGYN and Cannabis

Plants used to assist women in managing their reproductive freedom and health have been around since Eve and the apple. Religious control mainly and sadly has prevented and destroyed much of this time-proven wisdom of the ages. However, many ideas still exist in the collective memory of the wise women and men who found means to carry on the natural ways of old.

Cannabis was once a plant consistently employed across a wide range of cultures to manage and treat gynecological issues by healers, midwives, herbalists, and doctors versed in the art of natural healing. Used by Sumerian physicians and later by their Egyptian counterparts, the plant has made its way into many other cultures to ease difficult childbirth, menstrual difficulties, threatened abortion, morning sickness, postpartum bleeding, eclampsia, urinary difficulties, gonorrhea, menopausal symptoms, and decreased libido; and it has also been used as a possible abortifacient.[1]

A physician's nineteenth-century Materia Medica describes one of the plant's efficacious properties as a stimulant for uterine muscle fibers. As such, it was used in the treatment of subinvolution (the uterus's inability to return to its normal size after delivery), menorrhagia (heavy menstrual bleeding), dysmenorrhea (painful menses), and to diminish uterine pain in general.[2]

Few modern studies exist, making OBGYN a field of medicine in which practitioners and women alike are left without scientifically grounded guidelines concerning the use of cannabis.

Abortion, Miscarriage, and Fertility

Certain plant cannabinoids bind to the same set of receptors as the body's own cannabinoid anandamide. They similarly exert influence on the earliest processes of conception and egg implantation in the uterine wall and thus play a significant role in fertility. While studies have shown that low levels of anandamide enhance egg implantation and higher levels diminish egg implantation,[1] few physicians are able to translate these discoveries into practical and therapeutic applications.

These dose-dependent and opposing properties of cannabis are not new to researchers and are commonly found in other therapeutic contexts such as pain or mental-states modulation. These opposing properties may also explain the historical medical references to cannabis in the prevention of miscarriage and at the same time its use as an early abortifacient.

Although reports exist about the adverse effects of cannabinoids on pregnancies, the discovery of endocannabinoids and their receptors in the female reproductive organs in rodents suggests the system's role in modulating pregnancy. In a trial conducted on mice, scientists from the Vanderbilt University Medical Center (2002) examined the role that the endocannabinoid system plays during normal pregnancy. Results revealed that levels of anandamide in the uterus and CB1 receptors on the fertilized egg work together toward a successful implantation in the uterine wall.[2] If these discoveries are confirmed in other mammals and in humans, the endocannabinoid system may well turn out to play a significant role in the success or failure of pregnancies.

Either way, historical observation and a review of medical records suggest caution with opportunity for those wishing to get pregnant or those wishing to avoid pregnancy altogether.

Once the fetus is implanted, it is most vulnerable to the impact of environmental substances during the first trimester.

Childbirth Pain

Nineteenth-century medical records describe the cannabis plant's effects on childbirth as being able to reduce pain, increase uterine contractions, modulate lactation, and reduce inflammation associated with vaginal pains or mastitis.

Anecdotal evidence[1] from observations and surveys of cannabis clinics, patients, and physicians supports historical records that describe the efficacy of cannabis in easing childbirth and childbirth pains.

Based on time-proven safety records and the discoveries of the body's own natural endocannabinoid system and its role in the modulation of spasms, pain, and inflammation, it is easy to see why historical obstetric and gynecological (OBGYN) treatments employed cannabis for cramps, pains, and inflammation. However, while some of these historical records are available, no modern data exist to better understand how the plant constituents specifically affect childbirth pains or other OBGYN-related problems.

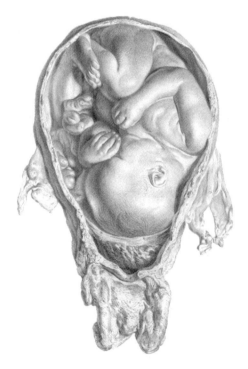

Endometriosis
Evidence-Based Confidence Level and Therapeutic Potential

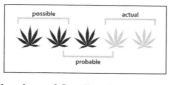

Number of Studies Reviewed: 2

CHI Value: 5

The endometrium, the interior lining of the uterus, is governed by hormonal changes. Endometriosis is a proliferation of interior cells outside the uterus. Displaced cells continue to respond to hormonal changes and behave as they would inside the uterus; however, without an easy exit they remain, causing growth and adhesions. This can be extremely painful. Growths and adhesions may spread throughout the pelvic cavity and form attachments on the ovaries, bowels, or any other surrounding tissue.

Primary symptoms often include generalized pelvic pains, difficult periods, painful sexual intercourse, and bleeding. Tests to determine endometriosis include a pelvic examination and ultrasound; however, the only way to be certain of endometrial tissue growth outside the uterus is via a laparoscopy. With the patient under full anesthesia, a physician inserts an instrument (laparoscope) into the woman's abdomen to visually check.

The exact causes of endometriosis remain unclear. Doctors hypothesize that a cause of endometriosis lies in unexpelled menstrual blood containing endometrial cells that returns via the fallopian tubes to the pelvic cavity. This process is called retrograde menstruation. Orthodox treatments include pain management, hormonal supplementation, and surgery.

Cannabis and Endometriosis

Researchers discovered that the endocannabinoid system plays a part in uterine function and dysfunction. This understanding combined with the historical application of phyto-cannabinoids to alleviate endometrial pain suggests that the endocannabinoid system may also be involved in alleviating pain and disease development.

Researchers from Florida State University (2010) discovered that CB1 receptors are present in nerve cells that innervate endometrial growths, and that CB1 activation reduces pain sensation. The authors wrote, "Together these findings suggest that the endocannabinoid system contributes to mechanisms underlying both the peripheral innervation of the abnormal growths and the pain associated with endometriosis, thereby providing a novel approach for the development of badly-needed new treatments."[1]

Another laboratory experiment (2010) in Paris, France, conducted on human endometriotic cell line confirmed in vivo (on rodents), reported several discoveries. Scientists noted that the synthetic cannabinoid WIN55,212-2 abrogated the growth of endometriotic tissue and exerted an anti-proliferative effect in mice implanted with endometrial tissue. This finding suggests a possible link between the endocannabinoid system and novel treatments.[2]

Study Summary

Drugs/Focus	Type of Study	Published Year, Place, and Key Results	CHI
CB1 agonists and antagonists	Animal study (rats)	2010—Florida State University: CB1 decreases endometriosis-associated hyperalgesia.[1]	2
WIN55,212-2	Animal study (mice)	2010—Université Paris Descartes, Paris, France: Abrogated the growth of endometriotic tissue and exerted an anti-proliferative effect.[2]	1+2

Total CHI Value 5

Strain-Specific Considerations

WIN55,212-2 binds with higher affinity to CB2 than CB1 receptors.

Indicas and indica-dominant strains generally present with a lower THC:CBD ratio, thus favoring CB2 expression.

Mind-Body Medicine and Endometriosis

Endometriosis is one of many underlying physical conditions that can cause chronic pelvic pain. Researchers have examined the psychological profiles of women with chronic pelvic pain. Results suggest a connection between changes in hormone profiles and exposure to chronic stress or post-traumatic stress disorders, especially in those patients who were victims of physical or sexual abuse.[3]

The disease picture of endometriosis may suggest a misplaced creativity. Cells leave the natural seat of biological creation and instead grow where they are not meant to grow, causing pain and damage. This may reflect the difference between creating life versus controlling life. Whenever we create life by making changes within, we create life from a natural and sustainable position. However, when we want to create life by trying to control others, we leave our natural domain and create, more often than not, very difficult circumstances that can harm us and the other people around us.

Aggravating factors may include chronic stress, guilt, and exposure to severe traumatic events such as sexual or physical abuse (PTSD).

Consider learning positive coping mechanisms and releasing guilt and its destructiveness.

Powerful Questions

Do you feel you have nothing to say about what happens in the bedroom?

If so, do you blame your partner for that situation?

Do you feel like you have to control others to get what you want?

Is there an aspect of your sexuality that you don't like, hate, resent, or feel guilty about?

Are you financially dependent on another, and how do you feel about it?

Do you feel the need to lie in the bedroom?

Suggested Blessing

May you realize that women who create change within are healers.

Suggested Affirmation

I decide what to think or feel! I create change without controlling anybody.

Menstrual Pain

Evidence-Based Confidence Level and Therapeutic Potential

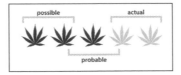

Number of Studies Reviewed: 1

CHI Value: 3

The Latin word for "month," *mensis,* is the basis for the term "menses" or "menstruation." The average duration of one complete cycle is about 28 days, coinciding with the approximate amount of time it takes for the moon to wax and wane. At the end of a cycle, a women's body regenerates a new lining inside the uterus. It discharges the old lining.

Many women have noticed that when the color of their menstrual blood is fairly dark, thick, and clotted, more cramps occur than when it is more liquid and bright red. Brighter blood is more oxygenated and generates an easy flow, while thick, clotted, and poorly oxygenated blood is more difficult to expel.

Typical allopathic treatments for menstrual cramps include non-steroidal anti-inflammatory drugs (NSAIDs) such as ibuprofen or Aleve.

Cannabis and Menstrual Pain

While the specifics of cannabis-based pain control are well established, little information exists to date to elucidate the impact of cannabinoids on menstrual pain. However, the proven antispasmodic effects of the plant alongside its analgesic and anti-inflammatory properties may form the historical basis for its use in the treatment of menstrual cramps. The single human case study published by researchers from Hürth, Germany, suggests that menstrual pain is among the many painful conditions for which cannabis is used as analgesia.[1]

Study Summary

Drugs/Focus	Type of Study	Published Year, Place, and Key Results	CHI
Cannabis	Case study	2003—Nova-Institute, Hürth, Germany: Cannabis is used to treat menstrual pain.[1]	3

Total CHI Value 3

Mind-Body Medicine and Menstrual Pain

Women who give life are mothers. The primordial cyclical rhythms of nature such as birth, death, and regeneration are part of the feminine power. Guided by subtle hormonal changes, the monthly flow of blood washes away the old mucosal lining of the uterus to prepare for its renewal.

Difficulties in embracing the power of the feminine may get expressed in difficult menstruations (dysmenorrhea). Women's blogs addressing dysmenorrhea report similar stories of "not being heard by my doctor" and "feeling disrespected" or "belittled" by health care providers when searching for relief from menstrual pain. These stories reveal an underlying theme of power and powerlessness.

This theme is further confirmed by women who empowered themselves through their own research or by joining other women with the same problems in their search for solutions to menstrual pain. These women discovered the importance of listening to subtle and not so subtle changes in their bodies. Some now view this monthly activity as a beautiful way of getting rid of toxins.

Aggravating factors may include dehydration, unhealthy food choices, and denial or judgments of feminine energy.

Consider drinking more water about seven days before the start of menstruation, limiting unhealthy foods, and embracing and cherishing the feminine in yourself.

Powerful Questions

Do I buy into the notion that my period is punishment for being female?
How do I feel about my menses and why?
Where do I reject my feminine energy?
Where do I judge my feminine?
Where are my male and female energy out of balance?

Suggested Blessing

I embrace the feminine power of creation in my body and my mind.

Suggested Affirmation

I listen to my body and respond in nurturing and loving ways.

Let Food Be Thy Medicine

Anise ∾ Fennel

Anise: Greek herbalists have long used anise and fennel to promote menstruation, increase breast milk production, facilitate birth, and enhance libido. University of Athens scientists have taken a closer look at anise in order to find a safe alternative to estrogen replacement therapies to prevent osteoporosis. In their study anise exhibited estrogen receptor modulator-like properties that produce bone cell formation without causing breast and cervical cancer cells to proliferate.[2]

Fennel: Fennel extract was found to be a more potent pain relief agent than mefenamic acid (such as Ponstel) in primary dysmenorrhea of high-school girls whose age averaged thirteen. In fact, it proved so effective that 80% of the fennel group no longer needed to rest in order to cope with the aches and pain.[3] Fennel is a safe plant to use, while mefenamic acid can produce serious side effects.

Morning Sickness

Evidence-Based Confidence Level and Therapeutic Potential

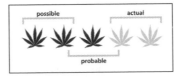

Number of Studies Reviewed: 1

CHI Value: 3

An estimated 50% of all pregnant women develop some kind of morning sickness, usually starting in the middle of the first trimester (at about six weeks). Normally, these episodes of nausea and vomiting are self-limiting and disappear toward the end of the first trimester (three months). While women can experience nausea and vomiting at any time of the day, these symptoms more commonly occur in the morning hours.

One hypothesis for morning sickness and the associated heightened senses of smell and taste is a fetal protection mechanism. Foods normally harmless to the mother may contain substances that could easily harm a developing fetus. When substances are detected by smell or taste that could harm the fetus, nausea develops to prevent the mother from ingestion or to produce vomiting after ingestion. Midwives often advise their clients to go with their desires for certain food items and avoid those that produce revulsion.

Cannabis and Morning Sickness

After an egg is fertilized, it stays in the fallopian tube for three days, then moves into the uterus for implantation. Morning sickness generally begins weeks after successful implantation. As mentioned earlier in the section on abortion, miscarriage, and fertility, levels of endogenous anandamide via CB1 and CB2 play a deciding role in the process of implanting the fertilized egg in the uterine wall. The cannabinoid THC binds to the same receptors and therefore may also play a significant role in egg implantation.

University researchers (2006) from Victoria, Canada, collected self-assessment data from 51 pregnant women who inhaled cannabis to alleviate their symptoms of morning sickness. Their analysis indicated that the 40 women who chose to treat morning sickness with inhaled cannabis found it to be either "extremely effective" or "effective."[1]

Study Summary

Drugs/Focus	Type of Study	Published Year, Place, and Key Results	CHI
Cannabis inhaled	51 pregnant women with morning sickness	2006—Michael Smith Foundation for Health Research Postdoctoral Fellow, Department of Sociology, University of Victoria, BC, Canada: "Effective" or "extremely effective."[1]	3

Total CHI Value 3

Mind-Body Medicine and Morning Sickness

Changes during pregnancy can be intense experiences caused by vastly different hormone profiles and other physiological and psychological changes. Women may feel disconcerted by the simple fact that generally liked foods now produce aversion, yet they develop cravings for items normally despised. Pondering these changes in lifestyles and identities combined with the necessary preparations for the newcomer may increase the impact of disruption to normal routines. A sense of overwhelm, fear, and being out of control may set in and contribute to the development of morning sickness.

The body produces the involuntary and rapid development of nausea and vomiting as a protective mechanism in the presence of a threat such as poison. The emotional underpinnings for nausea and vomiting, even when no physical threat is present, are very similar. When a perceived threat to the normal sense of self is detected or when the anticipation of mental-emotional upheaval is part of the experience, people often respond with fear and anxiety followed by symptoms of nausea. If intense enough, vomiting occurs.

See also the section on Vomiting.

Suggested Blessings

May you find delightful wonder as you ponder the unknown.
May you relax with ease and throw away the clinging blanket of fear.
May you walk through the web of anxiety as easy as one, two, three.

Suggested Affirmations

I am the author of my thoughts.
I am the architect of my perspectives.
I only choose beliefs that produce a feeling of safety.

Pregnancy

Much controversy surrounds the use of cannabis during pregnancy. Discoveries indicate that the presence of the brain's own cannabinoid, anandamide, triggers the endocannabinoid systems (CB1 and CB2). CB1 and CB2 receptors are present in reproductive glands and organs and, thus, may play a role in the modulation of conception, pregnancy, pain relief, and the birth experience itself.[1]

A study from 1983 enrolled 313 women who decided to home-deliver their children.[2] Of these, 41 women reported using marijuana. Researchers compared these two groups, and results showed that while both groups were generally similar, those women using marijuana made less money on average and were more likely to consume alcohol and cigarettes during pregnancy than non-users. Statistical evaluations revealed that the 41 women experienced slightly increased rates of difficulty at time of labor.

Osteoporosis

Evidence-Based Confidence Level and Therapeutic Potential

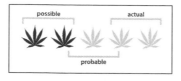

Total Number of Studies Reviewed: 3

CHI Value: 5

Osteoporosis directly translates from Greek as the disease of "porous bones" where the density of the bones diminishes over time. Cells that destroy aged bone cells are normally offset by cells that form new bones of proper strength and density. In osteoporosis, the balance shifts and more cells are destroyed than are created.

Once porous, the bones are vulnerable to stress fractures. The disease is most common in women, especially after hormone balances shift during menopause, and in patients who received steroids for chronic conditions.

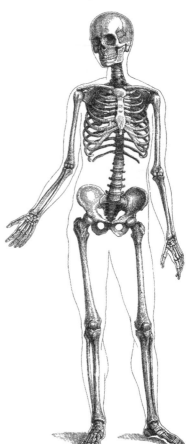

Although there are limited known symptoms, orthodox medicine identifies numerous preventable risk factors (e.g., smoking) and underlying diseases that may contribute to osteoporosis. Within this model of medicine, treatment consists mainly of pharmaceuticals, some nutritional modification (minerals, vitamin D), and exercise. Doctors diagnose the disease via dual energy x-ray absorptiometry, which measures bone mineral density. Other imaging options include quantitative CT scans and quantitative ultrasound. Unlike the other imaging machines, ultrasound provides the added benefits of no harmful ionizing radiation. Other tests may be included to rule out underlying contributing diseases.

Cannabis and Osteoporosis

A German study (2005) discovered that cannabinoids binding with CB1 and CB2 receptors regulate osteoclast (cells that remove bone tissue) activity and bone mineral density alike—thus partaking in the balance of removing old bone cells and sustaining bone density.[1] The same experiment revealed that the activation of CB2 receptors plays a role in the development of osteoporosis. The data from two Israeli studies (2006,[2] 2009[3]) confirmed that cannabinoids help maintain bone density and prevent age-related bone loss. All three studies provide the potential basis for new methods in prevention and treatment of age-related bone loss in both genders as well as postmenopausal osteoporosis.

Study Summary

Drugs/Focus	Type of Study	Published Year, Place, and Key Results	CHI
THC	Pre-clinical study	2009—Bone Laboratory, the Hebrew University of Jerusalem, Israel: THC maintains bone remodeling and protects against age-related bone loss.[3]	1
Endogenous cannabinoid system	Animal study (mice)	2006—Bone Laboratory, the Hebrew University of Jerusalem, Israel: Diminished endocannabinoid receptors increase bone loss.[2]	2
Endogenous cannabinoid receptors CB1 and CB2	Animal study (mice)	2005—Department of Psychiatry, Life and Brain Center, University of Bonn, Germany: CB1 and CB2 can regulate osteoclast activity and bone mineral density, and CB2 receptors play a role in the development of osteoporosis.[1]	2

Total CHI Value 5

Strain-Specific Considerations

The pre-clinical trials in this section suggest potential involvement of both receptor sites in modulating osteoporosis. Scientists focused their research on the cannabinoid THC, which binds with both CB1 and CB2.

Sativa or sativa-dominant strains generally contain a higher THC:CBD ratio.

Mind-Body Medicine and Osteoporosis

The skeleton functions to protect vital organs and produce a rigid support system. This enables the attached flexible counter system of muscles to exert force and allows the body to contract and expand, thus producing movement and enabling physical tasks.

The hollowness of bones provides strength despite their relatively light weight. An exterior of collagen and minerals protects the interior contents of soft and spongy yellow and red bone marrow. The red marrow produces blood cells while the yellow marrow stores fat cells as energy reserves.

In the disease picture of osteoporosis, the structure of life has become porous or brittle. At any time, a simple misstep can result in serious bone fractures. Hip and backbone fractures are most common, followed by broken ribs or wrists. In the internal architecture of patients with the disease, life may appear to offer no support; or if some support is still present, it appears transient and temporary. The patient is left dreading the inevitable end, and resignation and hopelessness may ensue. Giving up on life may suck the marrow of the bone until the remaining hollow house of cards collapses.

Osteoporosis often becomes a concern during menopause when we have the opportunity to shift more of our attention from the body to the inner workings of our spiritual nature and design.

Suggested Blessings

May you find strength and support in the wisdom of your mind, spirit, and soul.

May you find the juice of life in places you never thought to look.

Suggested Affirmation

I can choose to think of life as supporting me as gracefully as the air supports the flight of the eagle.

Let Food Be Thy Medicine

Anise: Greek herbalists use anise and fennel to promote menstruation, increase breast milk production, facilitate birth, and enhance libido. University of Athens scientists took a closer look at anise hoping to find a safe alternative to estrogen replacement therapy to prevent osteoporosis. Anise exhibited estrogen receptor modulator-like properties that produced bone-cell formation without causing breast and cervical cancer cells to proliferate.[4]

Pain (in general)

Evidence-Based Confidence Level and Therapeutic Potential

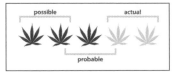

Total Number of Studies Reviewed: 19

Combined CHI Value: 62

For more information on specific cannabinoid and pain studies, see the following "Pain" subsections.

Pain affects the body, mind, one's quality of life, and overall well-being. It is a highly subjective experience, and people have significantly different thresholds for pain, an aspect influenced by many cultural factors. Pain produces unpleasant sensory and emotional experiences due to injury or even threat of injury. Tiny sensory organs called nociceptors present throughout the skin, blood vessels, muscle tissue, organs, and other strategic parts of the body stand ready to immediately signal the threat or presence of pain. Once the nociceptors are stimulated by the threat or presence of tissue damage from heat, pressure, or chemicals, rapid signals produce complex changes to the affected tissue and central nervous system. In turn, this increases respiration, heartbeat, and blood pressure. The whole organism, body and mind, quickly responds to stop or minimize pain and ensure survival.

Pain is the main reason people seek medical attention. While many describe pain with terms like sharp, dull, burning, or radiating, physicians specializing in pain distinguish between two basic types: neuropathic pain (usually chronic) and nociceptive pains (usually time-limited). Further differentiation includes referred pain, visceral pain, and parietal pain. Referred pain is present at a distance from the point of origin. Sometimes a person with a heart attack experiences pains radiating down the left arm or up into the neck. Visceral pains are associated with specific organs such as the liver or bowels but are usually not specifically localized. Parietal pains normally present at a precise location and claim association with inflammation at the lining of organs.

Traditional allopathic treatment begins with a search for underlying causes. Depending on the results of diagnostic tests, care consists of pharmaceutical medications addressing the underlying cause and then targeting the pain itself (analgesics). Major analgesic groups include acetaminophen, non-steroidal anti-inflammatory drugs (NSAIDs), and opioids.

Doctors believe that acetaminophen acts on the brain to reduce pain. Sold in the form of many brand names such as Tylenol, the drug breaks down in the liver, which is also the reason for its more serious adverse effects—liver toxicity. "Acetaminophen overdose is the leading cause for calls to Poison Control Centers (>100,000/year) and accounts for more than 56,000 emergency room visits, 2,600 hospitalizations, and an estimated 458 deaths due to acute liver failure each year."[1]

Besides the pain-killing properties of NSAIDs, they reduce fever and inflammation. Over a hundred million NSAIDs with brand names like Bayer Aspirin or the various forms of ibuprofen (Advil, Midol, Motrin, etc.) are sold every year in the U.S. alone.[2] Scientists hypothesize that NSAIDs inhibit enzymes (COX) involved in the neurochemical reaction needed for pain to occur. Major adverse affects include internal bleeding from gastrointestinal ulcers, heart attacks, strokes, and renal failure. "Each year 41,000 older adults are hospitalized, and 3,300 of them die from ulcers caused by NSAIDs. Thousands of younger adults are hospitalized."[3]

Opioids are effective painkillers because they bind to the body's opioid receptors in the nervous system and thus reduce or eliminate pain. Derived from the poppy plant, opioids are one of the oldest analgesics known to mankind. Patients report simultaneous experiences of mood-altering sedation, constipation, constricted pupils, and a reduction in respiratory rates. While short-term use of opioids can be an effective means of controlling pain, long-term use can lead to addiction. Two of the deadliest prescription drugs for pain in the U.S. are the opioids oxycodone and fentanyl, responsible for nearly 10,000 fatalities within seven years.[4]

Cannabis and Pain

For the last 5,000 years, cannabis has been used as an analgesic in nearly all ancient cultures from Sumeria to China, Babylon, the Indus Valley, and Judean, Greek, Roman, and Islamic civilizations.[5] The plant's prominent role and presence in the healing arts continued in early Western medicine. In addition to pain relief, cannabis serves as an anti-inflammatory and relaxing agent to body and mind to the present day. Recent discoveries confirm that cannabis is safe and effective when used properly to treat both neuropathic pain and in some cases nociceptive pain.[6]

While hundreds of studies and modern scientific data confirm the time-proven analgesic properties of the plant, they also elucidate some of the complex neurochemical workings of cannabinoids on pain within the human nervous system.

Foremost, scientists point to a relatively recent discovery that the human body contains its own naturally occurring endocannabinoid system. Naturally occurring cannabinoids or external cannabinoids, like those found in marijuana, signal cannabinoid receptors to regulate a wide variety of physiological processes including that of the sensation of pain. Two types of receptors, Cannabinoid Receptor I and II (CB1 and CB2), employ specific regulatory functions.

Broadly speaking, CB1 receptors are located in the central nervous system (brain and spinal cord), which controls information received by the senses and enables response reactions and behaviors. These receptors are located in parts of the brain that regulate motor control, attention, emotion, thinking (cerebellum), habits (basal ganglia and limbic system), and memory functions (hippocampus), and they are also found in both the male and female reproductive systems.

Here it is perhaps important to note that CB1 receptors are absent in the part of the brain that regulates heart and respiratory function (the medulla oblongata). This makes using cannabinoids as pain management safer than opiates, which can cause damage and death from respiratory deficiencies or arrests. Cannabinoids cannot replace opiates' strong analgesic properties, especially in cases of new trauma or injuries. However, in conjunction with a reduced amount of opiates, cannabinoids can produce a synergy of effective pain control while reducing the risk of adverse effects and the habit-forming potential of opiates. "Pre-clinical studies indicate that Delta(9)-THC and morphine can be useful in low dose combination as an analgesic."[7]

CB2 receptors cluster in the periphery of the body, especially in tissue involved in proper immune responses. The spleen houses a high concentration of CB2 receptors, for example. CB2 receptor engagement thus becomes important for treatment of chronic pain associated with autoimmune diseases in which the body's own immune system turns on itself.

Numerous plant-based cannabinoids, other plant-based (non-cannabinoid) constituents, synthetic cannabinoids, and those produced naturally by the human body engage significantly in reducing inflammation, which often goes hand-in-hand with autoimmune disease. An overview of existing studies (2004–2009) determined that cannabinoids effectively relieve pain involving inflammation such as in post-surgery patients, rheumatism, rheumatoid arthritis, chronic neuropathic pain, and fibromyalgia.[8]

Acetaminophen, non-steroidal anti-inflammatory drugs (NSAIDs), and opioids possess numerous therapeutic applications. However, patients in need of pain control, particularly those concerned about habit-forming substances and adverse effects, may benefit from a broader risk-benefit analysis, especially in cases of pain for which cannabinoids have proven efficacy.

Cannabis too can induce unwanted results. It is important to remember that using cannabis in excess of the subjective therapeutic dosage window (See "Is Cannabis Safe?," page 18) can induce adverse effects including an increase in pain,[9] anxiety, paranoia, or irritability. However, when compared to other options, "cannabis has a unique distinction of safety over four millennia of analgesic usage: no deaths due to direct toxicity of cannabis have ever been documented in the medical literature."[10]

Beyond the anti-inflammatory properties, analgesia, and potential to reduce the use of opiates, cannabis reduces painful spasms, diminishes anxieties associated with the anticipation of pain, induces rest and sleep, and can gently elevate mood—all essential elements to healing.

We list only three of many studies on the effects of cannabis and pain sensations to illustrate some interesting results and their implication for treatment.

A Worcester, Massachusetts, study (2009) cast a wide net for relevant studies on cannabinoids used for pain management "... published in the last 5 years on the activities of all classes of cannabinoids, including the endogenous cannabinoids such as anandamide, related compounds such as the elmiric acids (EMAs), and non-cannabinoid components (200–250 constituents) of Cannabis that show anti-inflammatory action."[11] Results indicated that all types of cannabinoids as well as non-cannabinoid parts of the plant effectively reduce pain from inflammation such as in post-surgery patients and cases of rheumatism, rheumatoid arthritis, chronic neuropathic pain, and fibromyalgia.

Multiple studies reveal that cannabinoids reduce neuropathic pains. A randomized, double-blind, placebo-controlled, crossover study from Rome, Italy (2009), on humans with multiple sclerosis (MS) was the first to examine the impact of cannabinoids on nociceptive pains using noxious stimulation via reflex tests. The authors observed ". . . that cannabinoids modulate the nociceptive system in patients with MS."[12]

San Diego-based scientists demonstrated the importance of dose in relation to therapeutic efficacy (2009). In a randomized, double-blind, placebo-controlled, crossover human trial, 15 healthy volunteers received capsaicin (the ingredient in cayenne pepper that makes it hot) injections in opposite forearms. The injections were spaced at 5- and 45-minute intervals after smoking cannabis of three different concentrations (2%, 4%, and 8% THC by weight). Scientists measured participants' pain levels and pain thresholds. The results supported the importance of dose dependency in pain reduction. "Five minutes after cannabis exposure, there was no effect on capsaicin-induced pain at any dose. By 45 min after cannabis exposure, however, there was a significant decrease in capsaicin-induced pain with the medium dose and a significant increase in capsaicin-induced pain with the high dose."[13]

WARNING/DISCUSSION

While the analgesic effects of cannabis are time-proven and empirically established, the study from San Diego adds a unique perspective to this common knowledge base. As a result, for those wishing to use cannabis to reduce pain, it is advisable to start out at a low dose and work up slowly to determine the most effective and appropriate therapeutic window. (See page 20.)

Mind-Body Medicine and Pain

Pain gets our attention. It can save lives and prevent or minimize damage. Beyond the positive attributes of pain as feedback and protective device, man-made belief(s) in punishment demands pain, as does guilt with its constant insistence on using pain as a means of making amends.

Pain can motivate new choices and inspire us to avoid choices that lead to pain in the first place. Pain lets you know where attention is immediately needed. The worse the pain, the more acute the demand for attention. This is true for acute or sudden pain as well as chronic pain. Pain demands change.

Normally, once pain receives attention, new choices are quickly implemented. The hand that nears fire is removed and the pain stops. The individual creates a strong memory to be more careful with fire in the future. The dentist drills into a nerve, motivating healthier choices about sugar and flossing habits. A relationship ends and may break the proverbial heart, leading to reflections on learning more about loving and intimacy.

While each person's experience with pain is unique, a common thread is simultaneous separation from and longing for someone or something. We experience pain in the physical, emotional, mental, and spiritual realms. A child falls and scrapes her knees. Separated from her sense of well-being while crying innocent tears, she yearns to return to it. A young man loses his first love and longs to hold her again. An author inadvertently pushes the wrong button on her computer and loses her entire manuscript; she feels a part of her has died with it. A Rabbi finds himself in a pit of despair, wondering about his normally unshakable faith.

Everybody has pain at one point or another in his or her life's journey. It is a part of the human experience. Pain can be a terribly destructive emotion, a terrifying state of being that produces isolation and exhaustion. It is for these and other reasons that many people want to numb themselves to pain by ignoring it, denying it, or masking it. However, these perhaps understandable reactions to pain do not produce healing but sadly ensure its continuation, re-emergence, and eventual amplification. Pain will continue to exist somewhere in the complexity of being until it is healed.

Pain begins as an emotional reality. If addressed and healed in the non-physical theatre, its existence will dissolve. If, however, pain is ignored, denied, masked, or otherwise avoided, the emotion will seek healing through more forceful and solidified means. For instance, avoided pain born of betrayal and humiliation may develop into an autoimmune disease where the body's own defense mechanism turns on itself. Thus the drama of pain that previously played on an emotional stage is moved to the more dense physical form in a renewed effort to draw more conscious understanding of where internal change, forgiveness, and healing are needed.

Aggravating factors may involve guilt and belief(s) in punishment.

Consider working with releasing guilt, grief, pain, and hurt in the emotional realm and employing forgiveness.

For pain due to inflammation, see also Inflammatory Diseases. For cancer pain, see the subsection below entitled "Pain Due to Advanced Cancer."

Powerful Questions

What is my pain keeping me from doing?

How do I feel about it?

What am I separated from and what am I longing for?

Is this pain pointing to some unfinished loss or grief?

Am I masking pain with punishing guilt?

Am I avoiding pain with numbing judgments or prejudices?

Am I denying pain by numbing it with self-pity?

Am I constantly avoiding pain with numbing medications?

Am I avoiding pain with imprisoning depression?

Am I running from pain by becoming addicted or obsessed?

Am I avoiding pain through focusing on blame and betrayal?

Suggested Blessing

May you forgive yourself or another for the pain.

Suggested Affirmation

I have healed pain before and I can do it again.

Let Food Be Thy Medicine

Cacao ∞ Cayenne ∞ Clove ∞ Fennel ∞ Garlic ∞ Ginger
Grains of Paradise ∞ Myrrh ∞ Nigella ∞ Rosemary

Cacao: German scientists at the University Witten-Herdecke concluded that the long-term ingestion of cacao with a high content of flavanols provides several markers of healthy skin. This might affect pain sensation near the skin, provide photo protection, improve blood circulation, increase skin density and hydration, and decrease skin roughness and scaling.[14]

Cayenne: In a meta-analysis of studies, University of Toronto doctors determined that cayenne cream used as a topical ointment treated the symptoms of chronic back pain better than a placebo.[15]

Cayenne stimulates peripheral circulation. In Cuba, a topical tincture and cream are used to produce circulatory benefits and treat aches and pains of lumbago, arthritis, and rheumatism.[16]

Cayenne is approved by the German Commission E as an external application for painful muscle spasms. Do not use it for longer than two days on the same region of tissue in order to avoid local skin inflammation.[17]

The FDA approved a cream, under the brand name Zostrix, which contains concentrated capsaicin. The company markets the cream mostly to arthritis sufferers to reduce pain, but also to reduce the pain that often lingers after an attack of shingles (a herpes-caused skin infection). A tube of Zostrix cream usually sells for about US$15–20. A homemade cayenne pepper cream costs pennies in comparison.[18]

Clove: In a study conducted in Mansoura, Egypt, patients suffering from chronic anal fissures received a preparation of clove oil 1% cream. Healing occurred in five times as many patients as in the control group. The 1% clove cream patients also experienced a greater reduction in resting anal pressure than those in the control group.[19]

A Tunisian study reported in the National Library of Medicine determined that essential oil of clove extract possessed analgesic, anti-inflammatory, antioxidant, antimicrobial, antifungal, antiviral (*Herpes simplex*—HSV and hepatitis C), antibacterial (including several of the multi-drug-resistant *Staphylococcus epidermidis*), and insect-repellant properties.[20]

Fennel: The German Commission E approved fennel seeds and oil in the treatment of pain associated with: "Dyspepsia such as mild, spastic gastrointestinal afflictions, fullness, flatulence. Catarrh of the upper respiratory tract."[22]

A Kerman, Iran, study discovered that fennel extract possessed a more potent pain relief agent than mefenamic acid (such as Ponstel) in primary dysmenorrhea of high-school girls whose age averaged 13. In fact, it proved so effective that 80% of the fennel group no longer needed to rest in order to cope with aches and pains.[23] Fennel is a safe plant to use, while mefenamic acid can produce serious side effects.

Garlic: Cubans use garlic for the treatment of inflammation, muscular pains, back pains, synovitis (inflammation of a membrane in the knee joint), and painful varicose veins.[24]

Ginger: A researcher from Durban, South Africa, supports the time-proven use of ginger by traditional African healers for its effective treatment of painful and chronic arthritic inflammatory conditions and its ability to achieve better metabolic control in patients with type II adult-onset diabetes.[25]

Grains of Paradise: Scientists from the University of Ibadan, Nigeria, explored this spice used in wound-healing practices throughout the ages. The spice's ability to stabilize the cell membrane[26] of injured tissue sites appears to reduce the need for reconstruction and to speed healing. Furthermore, scientists laud the spice's strong antioxidant properties, which enable the body to more effectively scavenge free radicals common in injuries.

Another study from the same Nigerian university suggests that the analgesic (pain-reducing) properties of the spice are specific to sites with inflamed tissue only. They do not reduce the pain perceptions of non-inflamed tissue sites.[27]

Myrrh: The German Commission E approved myrrh for the topical treatment of mucous membrane inflammation, such as in sore throats.[28]

Based on traditional practice and evidence-based medicine, a researcher from Bethesda, Maryland, reported on myrrh's significant antiseptic, anesthetic, and anti-tumor properties, which are most likely due to a specific alkene called furanosesquiterpene, present in essential oil of myrrh.[29]

Nigella: Doctors use ionizing radiation to treat many cancer patients. However, the radiation does not discriminate between cancer cells and healthy cells, resulting in massive tissue damage across the board. A study from Afyon, Turkey, using a rodent model, found that *Nigella sativa* oil ingestion (1 ml/kg body weight) and injections of glutathione might minimize radiation damage to healthy tissue. The study reports: "These results clearly show that NS and GSH treatment significantly antagonize the effects of radiation. Therefore, NS and GSH may be a beneficial agent in protection against ionizing radiation-related tissue injury."[30]

Rosemary: Cubans use an infusion of rosemary leaves to treat liver and gallbladder complaints, and to reduce painful abdominal spasms due to gas and flatulence.[31] The herb has been approved by the German Commission E for "Internal: Dyspeptic complaints. External: Supportive therapy for rheumatic diseases, circulatory problems."

Chronic Non-Malignant Pain

Evidence-Based Confidence Level and Therapeutic Potential

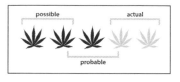

Total Number of Studies Reviewed: 2

CHI Value: 5

Chronic non-malignant pains (CNMPs) are defined as non-cancerous pains lasting longer than three months yet significantly impairing quality of life. A study conducted in Germany surveying available data from 1995 to 2009 discovered that about 17% of all pain falls into this category. The most common forms of CNMP non-responsive to pharmaceutical and non-drug treatment include musculoskeletal pains of the neck, shoulder, and back.[1]

Cannabis and CNMP

Researchers from Warsaw, Poland, conducted an animal study (2008) and discovered that cannabinoid agonists activate both endocannabinoid receptors CB1 and CB2. Cannabinoids reduced sensitivity to pain in a dose-dependent fashion. Furthermore, it was discovered that the COX-1 inhibitors such as indomethacin (a non-steroidal anti- inflammatory drug commonly used to reduce fever, pain, and stiffness) might increase these cannabinoid properties at low dosages.[2]

A human case study (2008) from Jerusalem, Israel, examined Dronabinol, the synthetic version of THC, in the context of CNMP. Researchers observed: "Cannabinoids have been used for pain relief for centuries, and recent studies have investigated their analgesic and anti-inflammatory mechanisms, as well as clinical efficacy, in treating chronic pain." In this study scientists wanted to examine the effects of THC on patients with CNMP unresponsive to conventional pharmacotherapy. Out of 13 participating patients, five reported an adequate response while eight patients reported an inadequate or no response to Dronabinol. The authors concluded that "... oral THC may be a valuable therapeutic option for selected patients with CNMP that are unresponsive to previous treatments, though further research is warranted to characterize those patients."[3]

Study Summary

Drugs	Type of Study	Published Year, Place, and Key Results	CHI
Dronabinol (synthetic isomer of THC)	Case study (13 patients)	2008—Department of Anesthesiology, Hadassah-Hebrew University Medical Center, Jerusalem, Israel: Dronabinol is a possible therapeutic option in the treatment of chronic non-malignant pain not responsive to other analgesics.[3]	3
CB1 and CB2 agonists	Animal study	2008—Department of Pharmacodynamics, Medical University of Warsaw, Poland: May reduce pain sensitivity and may work synergistically with NSAIDs.[2]	2

Total CHI Value 5

Strain-Specific Considerations

The relevant cannabinoid used in this section was Dronabinol, a synthetic prescription medication, which is an isomer (same molecular formula but different structural formula) of Δ9-tetrahydrocannabinol. THC binds relatively equally with both CB1 and CB2.

Sativa and sativa-dominant strains usually contain higher THC:CBD ratios.

Mind-Body Medicine and CNMP Medicine

See Pain (in general), the section immediately preceding this.

Migraine
Evidence-Based Confidence Level and Therapeutic Potential

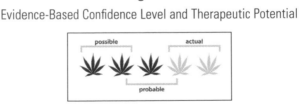

Total Number of Studies Reviewed: 3
CHI Value: 10

Migraines are recurring headaches that range from moderate to severe. Severe migraines lasting for hours or days can be debilitating to the point where all you want to do is draw the curtains and curl up into the fetal position. One patient described it this way: "The pulse of my own heartbeat becomes a drum of pain pounding against the walls of my skull with no end in sight." The pain can induce nausea and vomiting. Other symptoms often include severe sensitivity to light and sounds.

A number of people see paranormal flashes of light (called auras) signaling the migraine's arrival, while other early indications (prodromes) might consist of a craving for chocolate, aversion to noise, or sudden mood shifts to depression, anxiety, or elation. Additional prodromes include sluggishness, stiff neck, gastrointestinal problems, or very subjective oddities such as the sensation of a hot face yet feeling chilly, or the flare-up of hemorrhoids.

Within the allopathic tradition, the cause and cure for migraines remain unknown. Physical causes considered include abnormalities in blood vessels of the scalp or brain. While scientists also hypothesize that hormonal change, stressors, weather changes,[1] and food sources may play roles as triggers in migraine attacks, evidence remains inconclusive. "Menstruation had the most prominent effect, increasing the hazard of occurrence or persistence of headache and migraine by up to 96%."[2] Management of triggers through individual observations, diaries, consequent implementation of trigger avoidance, and prophylaxis through supportive lifestyle choices such as nutrition and exercise has given back some sense of control to many patients.

In interview form, doctors diagnose patients by determining the specific pain history and examining frequency of attacks, duration, specific location, presence of aura, nausea, or vomiting, and impact on daily routines. Treatment consists of numerous oral and injectable pharmaceuticals. Depending on underlying physiology, sometimes blood vessel surgery provides relief. However, the overuse of pharmaceuticals (especially tricyclics and opiates) and the number of adverse effects have posed problems in their own right.

Epidemiologically, about 75% of all adult migraine sufferers in the United States are women. Estrogen is considered as one culprit to explain the gender discrepancy.[3] Additionally, studies suggest that migraine sufferers might be at an increased risk for stroke.[4]

Cannabis and Migraine

Ethan Russo's in-depth historical and scientific review and meta-analysis of cannabis in migraine treatment (Missoula, U.S., 2004) demonstrates the plant's effectiveness recorded throughout ancient medical literature and provides modern scientific rationale for its age-old reputation as an effective balm for headaches. Russo justifies potential use and further study of cannabinoids in the treatment of migraine based on modern biochemical discoveries that the plant constituents work through "... anti-inflammatory, serotonergic and dopaminergic mechanisms, as well as by interaction with NMDA and endogenous opioid systems."[5] He further suggests that certain conditions including migraines "... display common clinical, biochemical and pathophysiological patterns that suggest an underlying clinical endocannabinoid deficiency that may be suitably treated with cannabinoid medicines."[6]

In a single patient case study from New York (2006), researchers discovered that the patient's chronic frontal headaches (produced by increased intracranial pressure) as well as her other related symptoms of photophobia (sensitivity to light), transient blindness, enlarged blind spots, and tinnitus improved after smoking marijuana. Further experiments revealed that non-psychoactive oral Dronabinol administered at 5 mg twice a day relieved all of her symptoms without any reported weight gain.[7]

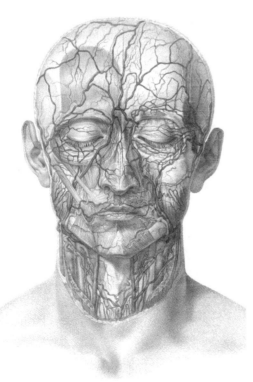

Researchers from Negev, Israel, (1985) obtained blood samples from patients diagnosed with migraines during an episode of migraine pain. They exposed the blood to the cannabinoids THC and CBD. Results indicated that THC, but not CBD, inhibited serotonin release from platelets (a blood component) in patients during migraine pains.[8] While the authors' discovery of THC's involvement in serotonin modulation in migraine blood plasma provided another possible clue about the exact mechanism by which cannabinoids reduce migraine pain, they acknowledged that other effects such as analgesia,[9] vasoconstriction,[10] and possible migraine preventative properties[11] might all play a role.

Study Summary

Drugs	Type of Study	Published Year, Place, and Key Results	CHI
Cannabis and Dronabinol	One human patient	2006—New York: Reduced all symptoms of pain, photophobia, transient blindness, enlarged blind spots, and tinnitus with both cannabis and Dronabinol.[7]	3
Cannabinoids	Meta-analysis of available studies	2004—GW Pharmaceuticals, Missoula, Montana: Endocannabinoid deficiency may underlie migraines.[5]	4
THC and CBD	Human patients diagnosed with migraines	1985—Negev, Israel: THC, but not CBD, inhibited serotonin release in blood samples during migraine pains.[8]	3

Total CHI Value 10

Strain-Specific Considerations

Russo's review suggests the possibility of an endocannabinoid deficiency in migraine pathology. The endogenous cannabinoid anandamide binds with both CB1 and CB2 relatively equally.

THC binds relatively equally with CB1 and CB2. Sativas and sativa-dominant strains generally contain a higher THC:CBD ratio.

Mind-Body Medicine and Migraine

The physicians Grace and Graham examined the psychosomatic underpinnings of migraines in 14 patients participating in their landmark study and wrote: "Migraine headaches occurred when an individual had been making an intense effort to carry out a definite planned program, or to achieve some definite objective. The headache occurred when the effort had ceased, no matter whether the activity had been associated with success or failure. The essential features were striving and subsequent relaxation." Typical statements were: "I had to get this done. . . . I had to meet the deadline. . . . I had a million things to do before lunch. . . . I was trying to get all these things accomplished."[12]

Consider the following statement from the PAMINA study: "The two days before menstruation and muscle tension in the neck, psychic tension, tiredness, noise, and odors on days before headache onset increased the hazard of headache or migraine, whereas days off, a divorced marriage, relaxation after stress, and consumption of beer decreased the hazard."[13]

The significant impact of state of mind was further explored in studies revealing that sex and orgasmic release altered migraine pains.[14] A group of 83 women suffering from migraines participated; 28 reported no relief, 27 reported some relief, 10 noted complete relief, and 3 women reported that the pain worsened.[15] While researchers do not know the mechanism by which sex and the orgasmic experience modulate migraine pains, they speculate that it may somehow alter the genesis of migraines.

In summary, aggravating factors may include perception of being forced, pushed, or pressured by others or one's own internal slave driver; two days before menstruation; muscle tension in the neck; and psychic tension, tiredness, and noise and odors on days before headache.

Benefits may be noticed from days off, a divorce, relaxation after stress, and consumption of beer.

Powerful Questions

I there something or someone it hurts to think about?

Anecdote

Martha was proud to be able to cram more appointments into a single day than anybody else. She worked out and took care of her family, friends, and associates. Martha maintained a tight ship at her two jobs, which she said she loved, and still found time to take self-improvement classes. She began having debilitating migraines in her forties. Her symptoms included photophobia, phonophobia, visual hallucinations, and nausea with intense vomiting that seemed to amplify her pain. Her physician tried pharmaceutical analgesia but Martha could not handle the adverse effects; it was adding to her nausea and was "too depressing in general." Confronted with the terrible choice of either living with her pain or the adverse effects, she went back to her doctor and asked for a cannabis prescription. Martha lowered the curtains, turned off the telephone and doorbell, and inhaled. She used an inhaler that delivered the cannabinoids without smoke, which she felt might make her cough and she dreaded the pain that would cause her. After a couple of inhalations, she noticed a pleasant relaxation, and within half an hour she fell into a blissful sleep. Martha awoke from her slumber without pain. For the first time, a medicine had really worked.

Suggested Blessing

May you find that state of mind that gives you peace.

Suggested Affirmations

I can slow down, listen to my body, relax my mind, and trust in life.
I can relax and bend like a blade of grass in the wind, and thus can
weather any storm and pressure with ease and fun, harming no one.

Neuropathies (in general)
Evidence-Based Confidence Level and Therapeutic Potential

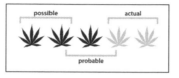

Total Number of Studies Reviewed: 5
CHI Value: 15

Neuropathies are pains generally caused over time by nerve damage from
past traumatic events (pressure, heat, cold, chemicals, radiation) or a progression of certain diseases, toxins, pathogens, or lack of nutrients. Deformities, scar tissue, impaired tissue metabolism, impairment of nerve fiber
insulation (demyelination), and inflammation all individually or together
contribute to neuropathies.

Neuropathies' classifications depend on the type of nerve(s) involved.
Pains from isolated nerve(s) (mononeuropathy or mononeuritis multiplex)
may result from the compression of a disc in the spinal column and can produce nerve pain extending to outward-lying tissue. Polyneuropathy affects
larger network nerve fibers and is often seen in diabetes or amyotrophic lateral sclerosis (ALS/Lou Gehrig's disease). Autonomic neuropathies are pains
involving nerves controlled by the involuntary nervous system, which can
debilitate all organs, systems, and functions governed by it such as the bladder, heart, and blood pressure. Another type of neuropathic pain, neuritis,
is an inflammation of nerve fiber(s) and is named for its underlying cause.

Symptoms correspond to the affected nerve fibers and the origin of the
neuropathy. Sensory symptoms can range from mild tingling and numbness

419

to debilitating pains shooting or burning down the path of the nerve. Motor symptoms range from mild weakness, cramps, or spasms to severe tremors with loss of function. Difficulty walking, using one's hands, and talking may be accompanied by severe pain. Impairment of autonomic functions can lead to incontinence, heart irregularities, postural hypotension, or difficulty in temperature regulation.

Allopathic treatments include analgesics, antidepressants, anti-seizure drugs, and synthetic cannabinoids such as Nabilone. Common underlying non-traumatic causes are iatrogenic, i.e., caused by allopathic treatments such as pharmaceutical drugs, surgery, chemotherapy, or radiation therapy. Other common causes include diabetes, multiple sclerosis, AIDS, and shingles *(Herpes zoster).*

With the exception of vitamin deficiency-induced neuropathies, patients typically find modern medicine's treatment of neuropathies ineffective. This often derives from the inability to cure many of the underlying illnesses. Treatment caution must also be exercised, as some of the medications used can be potentially habit-forming or result in dangerous adverse effects.

Cannabis and Neuropathies (in general)

The majority of randomized, placebo-controlled, crossover trials of the effects of cannabis on neuropathic pain discovered a marked therapeutic impact with few and manageable side effects. An overview of the existing studies on the subject of cannabinoids and neuropathies published between 2004 and 2009 mostly confirmed cannabinoids' effectiveness in relieving neuropathic pain.[1]

Strain-Specific Considerations

The cannabinoids reviewed here include the oromucosal spray Sativex, cannabis, and THC (oral spray). Those suggesting positive results included Sativex.

Sativex, a pharmaceutical plant derivative, is a cannabinoid combination containing THC and CBD in similar proportions as the strain *Cannabis sativa*. Cannabis contains THC and CBD in different ratios depending on the strain.

Sativa or sativa-dominant strains generally contain a higher THC:CBD ratio.

Study Summary

Drugs	Type of Study	Published Year, Place, and Key Results	CHI
Smoked cannabis placebo-controlled, crossover study	Human double-blind	2008—VA Northern California Health Care System, Department of Anesthesiology and Pain Medicine, University of California, Davis Medical Center, Davis, California, USA: Positive analgesic effects with peripheral neuropathic pain.[2]	5
Oral THC at an average dose of 16.6 mg	Open label prospective study on 8 patients with chronic refractory neuropathic pain	2004—Centre d'Evaluation et de Traitement de la Douleur, Hôpital Ambroise Paré Boulogne-Billancourt, France: No benefits observed and adverse effects noted in some patients.[3]	-5
Sativex, containing THC:CBD in an approximate 1:1 ratio, and GW-2000-02, containing primarily THC and placebo, delivered as oral sprays	48 human patients with neuropathic pain in a randomized, double-blind, placebo-controlled, three-period crossover study	2004—Royal National Orthopaedic Hospital, Brockley Hill, Stanmore, Middlesex, UK: Mild reduction of neuropathic pain. Improved sleep, no major adverse effects.[4]	5
Whole-plant extracts containing CBD:THC in a sublingual spray 2.5–120 mg/24 hours	A consecutive series of double-blind, randomized, placebo-controlled single-patient crossover trials of 24 patients with MS, spinal cord injuries	2003—Oxford Centre for Enablement, Windmill Road, Oxford, UK: Significant pain relief.[5]	5
Synthetic cannabinoid CT-3, a potent analog of THC-11-oic acid.	21 patients with chronic neuropathic pain, in a randomized, placebo-controlled, double-blind crossover trial	2003—Department of Anesthesiology, Pain Clinic, Hanover Medical School, Germany: Effective in reducing chronic neuropathic pain compared with placebo. No major adverse effects observed.[6]	5

Total CHI Value 15

Mind-Body Medicine and Neuropathies

Nerves communicate and connect each cell with the brain and nervous system, allowing trillions of different cells to efficiently work together and in balance for the benefit of the whole organism. Each cell listens and speaks. Each receives and transmits signals perceived by the seven common senses (sight, sound, touch, smell, taste, equilibrium, and imagination).

The disease picture of neuropathies suggests an element of communication about one's general experience of pain. For more information, see Pain (in general), Inflammatory Diseases, and Neurological Diseases.

Neuropathies—AIDS-Related

Evidence-Based Confidence Level and Therapeutic Potential

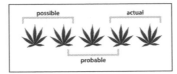

Number of Studies Reviewed: 2

CHI Value: 10

Cannabis and Neuropathies (AIDS-Related)

In 2007, researchers at San Francisco General Hospital conducted a randomized, placebo-controlled human trial on cannabis and AIDS-related neuropathies. Scientists discovered that HIV patients suffering from sensory neuropathies benefited equally from smoked cannabis as compared to oral pharmaceuticals used for chronic neuropathic pain. The authors concluded: "Smoked cannabis was well tolerated and effectively relieved chronic neuropathic pain from HIV-associated sensory neuropathy."[1]

The San Francisco results were confirmed two years later by an experiment in San Diego in which researchers conducted a double-blind, placebo-controlled, crossover trial of analgesia with smoked cannabis. Results showed that a majority of enrolled HIV patients with neuropathies experienced a 30% reduction in pains when compared to the placebo.[2]

Study Summary

Drugs	Type of Study	Published Year, Place, and Key Results	CHI
Cannabis (smoked)	Patients with chronic neuropathic pain from HIV-associated sensory neuropathy	2007—Community Consortium, Positive Health Program, San Francisco General Hospital, San Francisco, California: Smoked cannabis reduced daily pain by 34%.[1]	5
Smoked cannabis	HIV patients with neuropathies	2009—Department of Neurosciences, University of California, San Diego, California: 30% reduction in pains when compared to the placebo.[2]	5

Total CHI Value 10

Mind-Body Medicine and Neuropathies (AIDS-Related)

See sections on Bacterial and Viral Infections/HIV/AIDS and Neurological Diseases (in general).

Pain Due to Advanced Cancer

Evidence-Based Confidence Level and Therapeutic Potential

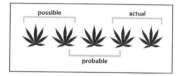

Number of Studies Reviewed: 2

CHI Value: 10

Cannabis and Pain Due to Advanced Cancer

In a double-blind, placebo-controlled study (2010) from Shrewsbury, UK, scientists enrolled 177 patients with advanced cancers who did not fully respond to the typical opiate-based painkillers. They administered a THC:CBD extract to determine its efficacy in treating pain. The results revealed that twice as many patients taking THC:CBD experienced a reduction of more than 30% from their normal pains when compared to the placebo group. The authors noted: "This study shows that THC:CBD extract is efficacious for relief of pain in patients with advanced cancer pain not fully relieved by strong opioids."[1]

Interestingly, in a San Diego double-blind, placebo-controlled, crossover trial of analgesia with smoked cannabis, HIV patients with neuropathies reported similar percentage results to the Shrewsbury study.[2]

Study Summary

Drugs	Type of Study	Published Year, Place, and Key Results	CHI
Sativex, THC:CBD	Double-blind, placebo-controlled human study	2010—Severn Hospice, Shrewsbury, Shropshire, UK: Relief for patients not fully responding to the typical opiate-based analgesics.[1]	5
Smoked cannabis	Double-blind, placebo-controlled, crossover human study	2009—Department of Neurosciences, University of California, San Diego, USA: Reduction of nerve pains.[2]	5

Total CHI Value 10

Strain-Specific Considerations

The cannabinoids examined in both double-blind, placebo-controlled human trials included Sativex and smoked cannabis. Sativex, a pharmaceutical plant derivative, is a cannabinoid combination containing THC and CBD in similar proportions as in the strain *Cannabis sativa*. Cannabis contains cannabinoids binding with CB1 and CB2, depending on the strain.

Sativas and sativa-dominant hybrids generally contain higher THC:CBD ratios.

Mind-Body Medicine and Pain Due to Advanced Cancer

See relevant sections on Cancer and Pain (in general).

Prion Diseases (Transmissible Spongiform Encephalopathies)

Evidence-Based Confidence Level and Therapeutic Potential

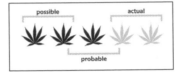

Number of Studies Reviewed: 1

CHI Value: 3

Scientists consider prions to be infectious proteins responsible for Creutzfeldt-Jacob disease in humans, bovine spongiform encephalopathy (mad cow disease) in cows, and scrapie in sheep. Currently, all prion diseases are fatal. Prion diseases primarily affect the brain and central nervous system. For clarification purposes, all types of prion diseases are also known as transmissible spongiform encephalopathies.

The exact cause or mechanism by which patients acquire prion diseases remains the subject of ongoing debate and analysis. Some current findings focus on ingestion of prion-contaminated meat. Past feeding practices in factory farms included grinding up dead cattle and feeding the protein back to live animals, thus providing a specific route of transmission. Kuru, another prion disease similar to Creutzfeldt-Jacob disease, was found mainly among members of a cannibalistic tribe in Papua New Guinea. Kuru has been in decline since the practice of cannibalism ended.[1]

Some orthodox medical treatments have accidentally transmittted Creutzfeldt-Jacob disease: older types of growth hormones extracted from pituitary glands of cadavers, blood transfusions,[2] and certain types of surgeries (brain, eye, or organ transplants). In addition, hospitals find prions extremely difficult to destroy once attached to hospital instruments and environments. Prions' resistance to normal methods of sterilization requires that hospitals take extra measures to reduce the possibility of transmission.

Possible causes of prion diseases include hereditary genes or mutations, accumulated toxins, viral influences, fungal influences, or a combination of these factors.

It is thought that when a prion enters the organism it is able to alter the signals that produce newly formed proteins. The newly generated proteins fold into unhealthy shapes. While normally the body's own enzyme, protease, can digest old or diseased proteins, prions are resistant to the enzyme. These protease-resistant prion protein accumulations in the central nervous system claim direct responsibility for neuropathogenesis and prion infectivity.[3] Once symptoms appear, degeneration is exponential. Most patients die within a year after the onset of symptoms.

Creutzfeldt-Jacob disease symptoms are very similar to other neurodegenerative diseases such as Alzheimer's and include confusion, forgetfulness, senility, apathy, irritability, seizures, muscle twitching, ataxia (wobbly gait), and loss of coordination. This list of common and varied indicators often leads to misdiagnoses. There is no test that can diagnose Creutzfeldt-Jacob disease. A brain biopsy can reveal the presence of the disease. However, drilling a hole into a patient's head just to confirm Creutzfeldt-Jacob disease is useless since no orthodox treatment exists.

Cannabis and Prions

Two recent factors necessitate finding a cure for the disease. First, variant forms have been transmitted through blood transfusions. Second, several countries have reported outbreaks of the disease due to contaminated beef consumption. Medical personnel urgently seek to determine a therapeutic agent that can slow the disease process or, preferably, effectively cure it.

Cannabinoids have known neuroprotective properties. In 2003, the U.S. federal government issued a patent on a newly found property of cannabis, declaring it "... useful in the treatment and prophylaxis of a wide variety of oxidation-associated diseases, such as ischemic, age-related, inflammatory and autoimmune diseases. The cannabinoids are found to have particular application as neuroprotectants; for example, in limiting neurological damage following ischemic insults, such as stroke and trauma, or in the treatment of neurodegenerative diseases, such as Alzheimer's disease, Parkinson's disease and HIV dementia."[4]

An experiment conducted in the laboratory and on animals (2007) showed that cannabidiol (CBD) not only inhibits accumulation of protease-resistant prion proteins but reduces their neurotoxic effects as well. CBD may be neuroprotective during prion infections.[5]

To date, no studies have examined the impact of cannabinoids in humans infected with prions. However, time-proven uses of CBD-rich cannabis for other neurological disorders suggest that CBD may offer hope as a treatment for Creutzfeldt-Jacob disease. Cannabinoids easily cross the blood-brain barrier and can reach affected tissue with relatively few side effects. No other treatment exists, and in light of the disease's dismal prognosis, any promising treatment approach warrants serious consideration.

Optimal dosage requirements and administration routes must still be determined. There are laboratory studies, however, that may prove instructive in this regard. For example, a 2007 study on mice established the neuroprotective value of CBD as follows: Mice were treated intraperitoneally three times per week for the indicated period of time, with 200 µl of 20 or 60 mg/kg CBD diluted 1:1:2 in an ethanol/cremophor/NaCl 0.9% mixture.[5]

Study Summary

Drugs	Type of Study	Published Year, Place, and Key Results	CHI
Injection of cannabidiol (CBD)[6]	Animal study (mice) and laboratory study	2007—International research institutions: CBD inhibited prion accumulation. CBD inhibited the neurotoxic effects of protease-resistant prion protein. CBD may be neuroprotective during prion infection.[5]	1+2

Total CHI Value 3

Strain- and Form-Specific Considerations

These laboratory and animal trials concluded that CBD may be the primary cannabinoid of interest in the context of prion accumulation and prion-related neuroprotection. No human trials have been conducted to date.

Indicas or indica-dominant hybrids tend to contain higher CBD:THC ratios when compared to sativa-based plants. Raw, fresh leaf or juice contains high concentrations of CBD in the form of CBD-acid.

Mind-Body Medicine and Prions

Prion diseases primarily affect the mind, the physical brain, and the central nervous system. It is said there comes a time in everybody's life when the prospect of returning to the source begins to be more in the forefront of the mind. There are two ways in which most people approach the inevitable. Either they return the way of the wise wo/man or they return the way of the infant. Prion disease bears similarity to those diseases that revert people to infancy, and this may be reflective of one side of this juncture.

However, in Creutzfeldt-Jacob disease, once symptoms appear, the disease progresses more rapidly than other such diseases, like Alzheimer's, where the degeneration occurs over the course of many years.

Powerful Questions

Where am I hopeless or despairing about my place in life?
Where am I helpless in my life?
Where am I refusing to let the world be as it is?
Is there a constructive way to channel my anger at life the way it is?
Why am I ready to throw in the towel?

Suggested Blessings

May you open to hitherto unseen wisdom and satisfying resources.
May we assist you in relaxing and finding a gentle place of forgiveness and well-being sourced within you.

Suggested Affirmations

I am always at the perfect place at the right time.
I can find a way to handle everything that comes my way.
It is okay to accept things as they are.

Sickle Cell Disease

Evidence-Based Confidence Level and Therapeutic Potential

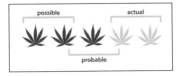

Number of Studies Reviewed: 2

CHI Value: 5

Sickle cell disease (SCD) is a genetic illness characterized by "flawed" red blood cells, which, instead of being round, mimic the shape of a sickle. Most likely, the body originally produced the mutation to protect itself from malaria parasites; now the disease claims responsibility for destroying one's quality of life or even shortening it. SCD is prevalent in people who descend from sub-Saharan Africa and other tropical regions where malaria runs rampant. Malaria is a cyclical disease and, in a real sense, SCD mirrors that cyclical nature. Carriers of one gene of sickle cell (sickle cell trait) may enjoy some protection from the malaria parasite and avoid SCD altogether. However, if both parents carry the sickle cell trait, the chance that their offspring will acquire sickle cell disease rises to one in four, and in this unlucky offspring, the disease turns chronic. The expression of the disease exists within a very wide range from relatively mild to moderate and severe. The frequency, intensity, and duration of a sickle cell crisis can also vary tremendously, but it usually lasts for about five to seven days.

The disease's symptoms derive from the misshapen red blood cells' inability to carry oxygen and nutrients to the body and from the clumping of cells, which causes occlusions. Resulting symptoms include anemia, low energy, pain, enlarged spleen, paleness of the skin, itching, infections with fever, rapid heartbeat, shortness of breath, stroke, autosplenectomy (destruction of the spleen), renal failure, and other organ damage. In addition, symptoms may progress to tissue death.

Orthodox treatments include pain medication, antidepressants, anti-anxiety medication, blood transfusions, surgery, other emergency care, and sometimes bone marrow transplants in children. Although presently orthodox medicine provides no cure, it can diagnose the trait and, thus, give potential future parents the information they need to make informed choices.

Cannabis and Sickle Cell Disease

A London-based experiment (2005) demonstrated that cannabis relieved pain, depression, and anxiety for sickle cell patients.[1] A research team from Minnesota (2010) came to similar conclusions in the course of an animal study. They genetically altered mice to produce human sickle cell hemoglobin while creating an internal environment similar to sickle cell crisis pain. Researchers then studied the effects of morphine and cannabinoids during objectively measurable experiences of pain. Results revealed that both morphine and cannabinoids reduced sickle cell-like pain in the animals.[2] Certainly more studies could provide a better understanding as to why and how cannabinoids reduce the symptoms of this disease.

Study Summary

Drugs	Type of Study	Published Year, Place, and Key Results	CHI
CP 55,940	Animal study (mice)	2010—University of Minnesota: Cannabinoids reduce sickle cell-like pain in mice.[2]	2
Cannabis inhalation	Human case study	2005—London, UK: Reduces pain, anxiety, and depression associated with sickle cell disease.[1]	3

Total CHI Value 5

Strain-Specific Considerations

The drugs tested against sickle cell disease in these trials included smoked cannabis and CP 55,940. The latter is 40 times more potent than Delta-9-THC and is extremely psychoactive. CP 55,940 is equally strong at CB1 and CB2 receptors.[3]

THC binds relatively equally to both CB1 and CB2. Sativas or sativa-dominant strains generally contain a higher THC:CBD profile.

Mind-Body Medicine and Sickle Cell Disease

Depression and anxiety among sickle cell patients are relatively common. A team of international researchers discovered that both psychological states were associated with an increased intensity and duration of pain on both crisis and non-crisis days when compared to sickle cell patients without anxiety or depression.[4]

The joy of life is connected to the flow of blood coursing through the veins. Just as blood nurtures and sustains cellular life, joy feeds and sustains a healthy mind. One's capacity for joy might be destroyed by holding on to beliefs such as "You are no good; you are flawed" or "There is something wrong with you." Sickle cells and malformed red blood cells are incapable of carrying sufficient nutrients to the body and, thus, cause much suffering.

When patients suffering from sickle cell disease are constantly faced with the threat of another crisis looming somewhere in the near future, anxiety and hopelessness further impact their mental and emotional lives.

Blood is also related to kin (blood bonds and blood relations with family, tribe, or group). Sickle cell disease is physically hereditary, but since the expression of the disease varies so greatly in duration and intensity, it is likely that non-physical signals such as the impact of deep-seated shame (perhaps passed down through the generations) may play a role in the severity of SCD.

Aggravating factors may include negative affect such as anxiety and depression.

Consider emotional release work, especially related to blood relatives; changing beliefs that produce anxiety or depression; and working toward positive affect.

Suggested Blessings

May you find a way to ease depression and diminish anxiety.

May our flowers soothe your pains and aches.

May they elevate your resonance and lighten your mood.

Suggested Affirmations

May the joy of life be my focus and my nourishment.

May it be a magnet for the miraculous and a lightning rod for the greatest joy of all.

Let Food Be Thy Medicine

Rosemary ∾ Vanilla

Rosemary: Approved by the German Commission E for: "Supportive therapy circulatory problems."

Vanilla: Researchers at the Children's Hospital of Philadelphia discovered that vanillin, a dietary compound in vanilla beans, was able to bind with sickle-shaped hemoglobin in rodents and, in doing so, improved oxygen transport—a key necessity for reducing symptoms in sickle cell patients. However, since vanillin is rapidly digested before it can reach the bloodstream, scientists are working to develop manmade intravenous compounds based on the spice.[5]

Skin Diseases (in general)

Evidence-Based Confidence Level and Therapeutic Potential

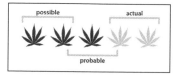

Total Number of Studies Reviewed: 4

CHI Value: 10

Diseases affecting the skin, hair, and nails are generally considered skin diseases. However, a majority of patients who seek treatment from a dermatologist also request cosmetic procedures such as hair removal, hair transplants, mole removal, wrinkle reduction, or liposuction. The dermatological treatment options include the three basic tools of Western medicine: pharmaceuticals, radiation (including laser and UVB), and surgery (cryosurgery, mole removal, hair transplants).

The Endocannabinoid System and Skin Diseases

A multi-institutional study (2009) with researchers from Germany, the United States, England, and Hungary identified the endocannabinoid system (ECS) in the skin for possible targeted approaches in the treatment of various skin diseases. It concluded that the main function of an endocannabinoid system in the skin is to control and balance growth, differentiation (the process of becoming a specific skin cell), and survival of skin cells as well as to produce proper immune responses. Researchers believe that the specific manipulation of the ECS might be beneficial in a multitude of human skin diseases including acne, dermatitis, dry skin, hair loss (alopecia, effluvium), hirsutism (excessive hair growth), itching, seborrhea, skin tumors, pain, and psoriasis.[1] The following chart gives an overview of key findings.

Condition	CB1	CB2
Skin cancer	Up-regulation of both ECS receptors CB1 and CB2 produces suppression of cancer cell growth, angiogenesis, and metastasis. Also induces apoptosis (cancer cell death).[2]	
Psoriasis	Up-regulation of both ECS receptors CB1 and CB2 will produce the suppression of keratinocyte proliferation and inflammation.[1]	
Hair loss	Down-regulation of CB1 stimulates hair growth.[1]	
Hirsutism (unwanted hair growth)	Up-regulation of CB1 produces the suppression of hair growth.[1]	
Seborrhea, acne		Down-regulation of CB2 produces an inhibition of sebum/lipid production.[1]
Dry skin		Up-regulation of CB2 increases sebum/lipid production and may remedy dry skin.[1]
Dermatitis (eczema)	Up-regulation of both CB1 and CB2 receptors produces a suppression of the immune/inflammatory process in cases of dermatitis.[1]	
Systemic sclerosis (scleroderma)		Up-regulation of CB2 induces a suppression of the immune/inflammatory process and fibrosis.[1]
Pain, itching	Up-regulation of CB1 and CB2 reduces pain and itching. Also inhibits transmission of signals in the nervous system.[1]	

A therapeutic up- or down-regulation could be achieved by using isolated specific cannabinoids (endo- and exo-), by utilizing agonists (drugs that selectively activate CB1 or CB2 receptors) or antagonists (drugs that selectively block one or the other of these receptor types), or by using specific strains known to increase activation of these receptors.

However, no isolated cannabinoid or whole plant constituents can perform such specific and isolated tasks (which also bring with them increases and severities in adverse effects that are not very well understood). In these specific cases no evidence-based rating was applicable and are noted as such.

Researchers (2007) from Debrecen, Hungary, discovered that human scalp hair follicles contain both endocannabinoid receptors and endocannabinoids, which were determined to be key players in hair growth regulation. Thus, type and dose-specific cannabinoids play a significant role in regulating unwanted hair growth and unwanted hair loss.[2]

Dermatologists are aware of the very limited and often ineffective allopathic options in the treatment of chronic itching. In a case study

(2006) from Münster, Germany, scientists learned that a cream containing N-palmitoyl ethanolamine, a fatty acid amide that enhances the action of anandamide, reduced the itching sensation in participating patients on an average of over 80%. The investigating neuro-dermatologists wrote: "Topical cannabinoid agonists represent a new, effective, and well-tolerated therapy for refractory itching of various origins. Creams with a higher concentration may be even more effective with broader indications."[3]

A study from Miami, Florida (2002), reported on the symptoms of itching from a different origin in three patients diagnosed with pruritus due to cholestatic liver disease that failed to respond to any other form of therapy. Researchers started them on a cannabis protocol and reported the following: "All patients were started on 5 mg of Delta-9-THC (Marinol) at bedtime. All three patients reported a decrease in pruritus, marked improvement in sleep, and eventually were able to return to work. Resolution of depression occurred in two of three. Side effects related to the drug included one patient experiencing a disturbance in coordination. Marinol dosage was decreased to 2.5 mg in this patient with resolution of symptoms. The duration of antipruritic effect was approximately 4–6 hrs in all three patients, suggesting the need for more frequent dosing. Delta-9-tetrahydrocannabinol may be an effective alternative in patients with intractable cholestatic pruritus."[4]

Study Summary

Drugs	Type of Study	Published Year, Place, and Key Results	CHI
ECS and various cannabinoids	Meta-analysis	2009—Multi-institutional/international study: "(T)argeted manipulation of the ECS (. . .) might be beneficial in a multitude of human skin diseases."[1]	3
ECS, anandamide, and THC	Laboratory	2007—Department of Physiology, University of Debrecen, Hungary: Endocannabinoids are present in human hair follicles. CB1 agonists may reduce unwanted hair growth, while CB1 antagonists might counteract hair loss.[2]	1
An emollient cream containing N-palmitoyl ethanolamine	Human case study	2006—Abteilung fur Klinische Neurodermatologie, Klinik und Poliklinik fur Hautkrankheiten, Universitatsklinikum Münster, Germany: Average of 80% reduction in itching during treatment of prurigo, lichen simplex, and pruritus.[3]	3
Oral doses of Delta-9-THC, 2.5 mg to 5 mg	Clinical study (3 patients)	2002—Department of Medicine, University of Miami, Florida, USA: Decrease in itching, improvement in sleep, and resolution of depression in patients with pruritus due to cholestatic liver disease.[4]	3

Total CHI Value 10

Strain-Specific Considerations

See sections on the individual skin diseases (below).

Mind-Body Medicine and Skin Disease

The skin is the largest organ of the body, sensing touch, vibration, and temperature. It is semi-permeable in that it prevents fluid loss and at the same time prevents water from washing out essential nutrients. The skin also absorbs some oxygen and small substances. Furthermore, the skin functions as a first line of defense and is involved in temperature regulation. It is at once border, boundary, and barrier, determining where one begins and ends. The skin is associated with self-image, identity, and individuality, which we present to the outside world.

The way a person feels about their skin (blemishes) often reveals the inner image they hold of themselves. Feeling ugly, feeling hideous, being embarrassed, or feeling ashamed or betrayed by one's own body are common emotional themes in the self-talk of patients with skin problems. Projecting these feelings onto others, thinking that everybody else feels the same way about their less-than-perfect skin, intensifies these emotional prisons. "If I feel ugly, I look ugly." It's no surprise that acne goes hand in hand with teenagers going through a change of life, body, image, and identity. Studies have confirmed that stress increases acne outbreaks.[5]

The emotional stress inflicted by a negative self-image constantly reinforced by negative self-talk and internal judgments shows up in body language, facial expressions, complexion, sense of well-being, and the way we carry ourselves. Stress reduces the ability of the body to heal itself[6] and worsens overall skin health in general by increasing hormone releases such as epinephrine and the steroid cortisol, which in turn over-stimulate sebaceous glands, producing skin eruptions.

Tracing these feelings back to the constricting pattern that comprises a person's self-image and replacing it with one that gives rise to a more positive sense of self-image can yield positive results in the emotional life and may also balance hormone levels. This increases the effectiveness of whatever healing regimen is engaged.

For more information, see the sections below on individual skin diseases. If applicable see also Cancer/Skin Cancer (Non-Melanoma), Cancer/

Melanoma (Malignant Skin Cancer), Bacterial and Viral Infections/Herpes, and Cancer/Kaposi's Sarcoma.

Let Food Be Thy Medicine

General Skin Health: Bush Tea ❧ Cacao ❧ Cajuput Cayenne ❧ Coconut ❧ Garlic ❧ Grains of Paradise ❧ Oregano Rosemary ❧ Turmeric

Bush Tea: This South African herb has been found to contain protective abilities against skin cell mutation.[7]

Cacao: German scientists at the University Witten-Herdecke (2006) concluded that the long-term ingestion of cacao with a high content of flavanols provides for several markers of healthy skin: photo protection, improved blood circulation, increased skin density and hydration, and a decrease in skin roughness and scaling.[8] Researchers from Tokyo, Japan, found that cacao bean extract, among other compounds, has protective properties against wrinkles caused by exposure to UV light.[9]

Cajuput: Various traditional practitioners use cajuput aka tea tree oil in the treatment of acne, eczema, psoriasis, dandruff, fungal infections, and bacterial infections.

Scientists at the Department of Infectious, Parasitic, and Immune-mediated Disease in Rome, Italy (2006), isolated a single compound found in tea tree oil believed to be the agent responsible in the destruction of *Candida albicans* fungus (a fungus implicated in vaginal yeast infections).[10]

Another Italian study (2006) found tea tree oil effective on superficial skin infestations, which had been caused by antibacterially resistant strains of staphylococcal bacteria. Tea tree oil is thus an important addition to the limited choices available to patients afflicted with these stubborn and possibly dangerous bacteria.[11]

U.S. doctors routinely prescribe Fluconazole, a pharmacological antifungal agent, to AIDS patients suffering from oral *Candida albicans* (fungal infection) inflammations. However, they found it often ineffective, leaving patients with no relief. In 2002, Detroit's Wayne State University School of Medicine scientists discovered that oral solutions of tea tree oil appeared to be effective when Fluconazole failed to work.[12]

Cayenne: Scientists from the "Big Easy" or New Orleans (2002), probably no strangers to wonderfully spicy foods, determined that an isolated compound made from cayenne is effective in the laboratory against a variety of fungi, including *Candida albicans.*[13]

Coconut: "In this study from Reykjavík, Iceland, researchers discovered in a laboratory experiment that medium-chain fatty acids, but especially capric acid ($C_{10}H_{20}O_2$), worked effectively in killing all strains of Neisseria gonorrhea."[14] Coconut is rich in medium-chain fatty acids.

Another laboratory study from the island determined how well medium-chain fatty acids destroy or inhibit the growth of other groups of bacteria. Both lauric acid and capric acid showed strong antibacterial abilities.[15]

Researchers demonstrated another aspect of lauric and capric acids' broad antimicrobial properties in the laboratory—this time against a fungus associated with yeast infections.[16]

Lauric acid and capric acid were also found to effectively inactivate chlamydia in the laboratory. This suggests that these two fatty acids found in relatively high concentrations in coconut milk and fat may play a role in the prevention of this particular bacterial infection as well.[17]

The authors of a study from Staten Island, New York, wrote: "Lipids can inactivate enveloped viruses, bacteria, fungi, and protozoa." By adding medium-chain fatty acids to HIV-infected blood products, the researchers learned that they could reduce the virus concentration by a very large number. Furthermore, the scientists expect that medium-chain fatty acids ". . . may potentially be used as combination spermicidal and virucidal agents."[18]

Garlic: Allicin (allylthiosulfinate, diallyl disulfide-S-monoxide), a potent, well-known, and well-researched antimicrobial and antifungal, is an active ingredient in garlic. A 2007 laboratory study from Ferrara, Italy, determined that concentrations of spray-dried garlic (1.5 gm per 10 mL) had the strongest fungicidal reaction of those tested.[19]

Grains of Paradise: Scientists from Ibadan, Nigeria (2008), explored this spice used in healing practices throughout the ages. The spice possesses the ability to stabilize the cell membrane[20] of injured tissue sites, thus reducing the need for reconstruction and speeding healing. Furthermore, scientists laud its strong antioxidant properties that enable the body to more effectively scavenge free radicals common in injuries.

Oregano: Veterinarians from Bologna, Italy (2005), studied the effects of several essential oils, including oil of oregano, against candida fungal infections. They found oregano to have "maximum inhibitory activity,"[21] of which the most active phenol component (acidic chemical compound) was carvacrol.

Rosemary: Scientists from Harbin, China (2007), confirmed the antimicrobial activity of the essential oil of rosemary against a variety of bacterial and fungal pathogens, including those of *Staphylococcus epidermidis, Escherichia coli,* and *Candida albicans.*[22]

An infusion of rosemary leaves is used in Cuba as a tonic for hair.[23]

Rosemary is approved by the German Commission E for external use as a supportive therapy for circulatory problems.

Turmeric: In a meta-study from Dallas, Texas (2007), scientists gave an overview of decades of scientific studies on turmeric. Among the long list of turmeric's potential therapeutic properties: promoter of wound-healing and effective in psoriasis.[24]

Acne

Evidence-Based Confidence Level and Therapeutic Potential

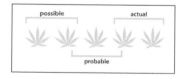

Total Number of Studies Reviewed: 1

Combined CHI Value: not applicable

Acne is a common skin disease affecting both genders during puberty. An increase in androgen hormones contributes to an increase in sebaceous gland activity, producing sebum (an oily/waxy substance), which when not properly discharged through the pores can cause back-ups, inflammation, and pimples. Allopathic treatment consists of topical pharmaceuticals, pills, laser therapy, phototherapy, and sometimes localized surgical procedures. No allopathic cure for acne exists.

The Endocannabinoid System and Acne

Condition	CB1	CB2
Acne		Down-regulation of CB2 will produce an inhibition of sebum/lipid production.[1]

Strain-Specific Considerations

Currently not applicable.

Mind-Body Medicine and Acne

The results of a large human study conducted on 94 teenagers concluded that stress-related inflammation played a significant role in breakouts.[2]

Becoming a grown-up is built in by nature. Adolescence is the process and the passage from childhood to a fully sexually capable body induced by gender-specific hormonal changes. These changes force an often-dramatic shift in physical image and intense internal mental and emotional landscapes, which are often difficult to embrace and own. The new and developing self-image is often disliked and rejected. For many, feeling ugly becomes a reality in the emerging pimples.

Powerful Questions

What are the symptoms keeping you from doing?

How do you feel about that?

Where do these feelings take you?

What scenarios or memories are associated with these feelings?

What is the meaning (messages, unhealthy beliefs/attitudes, etc.) that you have given to that scenario?

Can the answers to these questions direct your focus to support your capacity for self-healing?

Suggested Blessing

May you relax the stranglehold of "feeling ugly" for a moment so that you can fully accept yourself as a growing and maturing human being.

Suggested Affirmation

I have the capacity to define and find what is unique and beautiful inside of me.

Dermatitis (Eczema)

Evidence-Based Confidence Level and Therapeutic Potential

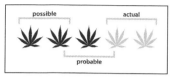

Total Number of Studies Reviewed: 1

CHI Value: 3

Dermatitis is an inflammation of the skin believed to be caused in part by coming in contact with irritants. It may also be due to effects from certain diseases or allergic sensitivities. Depending on the underlying cause, Western tradition uses topical and systemic pharmaceuticals such as steroids or antihistamines to reduce symptoms.

The Endocannabinoid System and Eczema

Condition	CB1 and CB2
Dermatitis (eczema)	Up-regulation of both ECS receptors CB1 and CB2 produces a suppression of the immune/inflammatory process in cases of dermatitis.[1]

Strain-Specific Considerations

THC binds with both CB1 and CB2 relatively equally. Sativas and sativa-dominant strains tend to present with a higher THC:CBD ratio.

Mind-Body Medicine and Dermatitis

Grace and Graham wrote: "Eczema occurred when an individual felt that he was being interfered with or prevented from doing something, and could in no way deal with the frustration.... His preoccupation was with the interference and the person or things thwarting him...." Typical statements (of 27 patients with eczema) were: "I want to make my mother understand but I can't.... I couldn't do what I wanted to but there wasn't anything I could do about it.... I was upset because it interfered with what I wanted to do.... I felt terribly frustrated." The researcher also noted themes of embarrassment and self-aggression in cases with eczema.[2]

Powerful Questions

What is the irritation that has gotten under the outer layer of your skin?
What is inflaming you?
What are you extra-sensitive about?
Where are you really thin-skinned?

Hair Growth—Unwanted (Hirsutism)
Evidence-Based Confidence Level and Therapeutic Potential

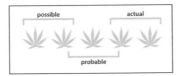

Number of Studies Reviewed: 1
CHI Value: not applicable

While male pattern hair growth in women is not an illness, it can be a great cosmetic and psychological concern. Western medicine considers an increased presence of male hormones or higher than normal levels of the hormone insulin to be causative agents. No allopathic cure is available, but suggested treatment includes pharmaceuticals and hair removal techniques.

The Endocannabinoid System and Hirsutism

Condition	CB1	CB2
Hirsutism	Up-regulation of CB1 will produce the suppression of hair growth.[1]	

Mind-Body Medicine and Hirsutism

A study comparing the emotional behavior of 30 patients dealing with hirsutism with an equal number of non-hirsute women discovered that hirsute women demonstrated greater tendency to exhibit severe and sudden shifts in mood as well as display significantly more hostile and irritable emotions.[2] The appearance of male pattern hair growth in women evokes intense emotional reactions in some, while others may find that displaying a more physically male image is to their liking. Hirsutism is often discovered paired with higher than normal levels of male hormones. While some women have dealt with hirsutism since puberty (hormonal changes), many discover hairs in new places during menopause (hormonal changes). Hirsutism is primarily a cosmetic issue unless it interferes with one's body image and identity.

Powerful Questions

What are the symptoms keeping you from doing?

How do you feel about that?

Where do these feelings take you?

What scenarios or memories are associated with these feelings?

What is the meaning (messages, unhealthy beliefs/attitudes, etc.) that you have given to that scenario?

Can the answers to these questions direct your focus to support your capacity for self-healing?

Suggested Blessing

May you realize the power, strength, and confidence of your animus (inner male energy) and let it inform your will and action in a balanced and harmonious way.

Suggested Affirmations

I can handle what life brings my way.

I protect myself by making sure my feelings are heard and respected.

Let Food Be Thy Medicine

Fennel: Fennel has been used as an estrogenic agent by traditional healers for centuries. Now scientists from Shiraz University, Iran, are looking at fennel's ability to help women who have developed hirsutism (growing hair like a male), even though they have normal menstrual cycles and normal levels of sex hormones. Researchers noted significant male type hair growth reduction when compared to the placebo. Of the two tested formulas (1% and 2%), 2% topical fennel extract proved most effective.[3]

Hair Loss (Baldness)

Evidence-Based Confidence Level and Therapeutic Potential

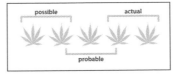

Number of Studies Reviewed: 1

CHI Value: not applicable

Until relatively recently, the allopathic tradition believed that male pattern baldness occurred in 3 out of 4 cases due to a gene passed down from the maternal father. Environmental signals, in addition to genetic influences, are thought to induce hormonal changes in the remainder. The role of a male sex hormone called dihydrotestosterone (DHT) is implicated but not fully understood. No allopathic cure is available. Some pharmaceutical and surgical procedures have been used with limited success.

The Endocannabinoid System and Baldness

Condition	CB1	CB2
Hair loss	Down-regulation of CB1 stimulates hair growth.[1]	

Strain-Specific Considerations

Currently not applicable.

Mind-Body Medicine and Hair Loss

Mythology associates hair with power, as in the biblical story of Samson and Delilah. Samson loses his supernatural strength after Delilah cuts off his hair while he sleeps. Hair is also connected to the body beautiful, virility, youthfulness, and sensuality. In the Western world, "long hair" has recently come to be associated with rebellion from values that are perceived to be old and outdated. Haircuts, hair colors, and styles can communicate and project a strong meaning, just as hair loss due to trauma, surgery, or chemotherapy may elicit intense feelings. While baldness is not a disease, it can have psychological consequences and can contribute to a negative self-image.

Powerful Questions

What are the symptoms keeping you from doing?

How do you feel about that?

Where do these feelings take you?

What scenarios or memories are associated with these feelings?

What is the meaning (messages, unhealthy beliefs/attitudes, etc.) that you have given to that scenario?

Can the answers to these questions direct your focus to support your capacity for self-healing?

Itching (Pruritis)
Evidence-Based Confidence Level and Therapeutic Potential

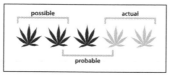

Number of Studies Reviewed: 3

Combined CHI Value: 10

The itch. While physiologically similar to the experience of pain, the response to an itch is not to withdraw but rather to scratch. Itching can be produced externally by temperature variations, slight electrical stimulation, parasites (lice, scabies), and contact with certain substances (natural or synthetic). Itching only occurs superficially on the outer layers of the skin.

Internal causes may include psychological origins (stress, hallucinations), brain tumors, multiple sclerosis, neuropathies, diabetes, certain hereditary causes, cholestatic liver disease, skin diseases (contagious or non-contagious), nerve damage, inflammation, wound-healing (skin trauma or burns), hives, allergic reactions, certain medication (pharmaceutical and holistic), fungus, parasites, eczema, or hormonal changes such as occur during menopause.

Orthodox dermatologists rely on internal and topical pharmaceuticals to reduce and suppress the itch. Common anti-itch medications include antihistamines and steroids. When these do not work, the itch continues affecting quality of life and contributing to frustration, hopelessness, and depression.

The Endocannabinoid System and Itching

Condition	CB1 and CB2
Pain, itching	Up-regulation of CB1 and CB2 produces a reduction of pain and itch by suppressing pain- and itch-producing substances as well as inhibiting transmission of signals in the nervous system.[1]

Strain-Specific Considerations

Both indica and sativa strains contain CB1- and CB2-activating cannabinoids. Future studies may confirm positive reports about the efficacy of cannabis from numerous cannabis-using pruritis sufferers who prefer a topical oil of their choice infused with whole-plant constituents to the use of inhaled cannabis.

Mind-Body Medicine and Pruritis

Similar to the indecision underlying some neck problems, chronic complaints of itching may also represent contradicting or conflicting desires. On one end of the spectrum, the sensation of an itch or tickling is a pleasurable and even sensual experience. On the other end, itching (especially the incessant type) can make someone want to jump out of his skin. In the latter case, scratching might produce temporary relief, but as soon as one stops scratching, the itch returns with a vengeance. Furthermore, the skin can only take so much scratching before it breaks and pain replaces the sensation. In some cases, patients prefer the pain to the itch and can scratch until bloody.

"Urticaria occurred when an individual saw himself as being mistreated. This mistreatment might take the form of something said to him or something done to him. He was preoccupied entirely with what was happening to him, and was not thinking of retaliation or of any solution of his problem." Typical statements were: "They did a lot of things to me and I couldn't do anything about it." "I was taking a beating." "My mother was hammering on me." "The boss cracked a whip on me." "My fiancée knocked me down and walked all over me but what could I do?"[2]

It is interesting to note that as with yawning, itching can be psychologically contagious, as evident by the observation that when one person in a group begins scratching others will soon follow their example.

Aggravating factors may include feeling mistreated or judged, indecisiveness, feeling victimized, and using pain to control an irritation or anxiety.

Consider working with gratitude and the employment of forgiveness; making a list of priorities; shedding any victim self-image and instead developing a sense of empowerment; or perhaps accepting or embracing a present irritation.

Powerful Questions

Where do I see myself as mistreated or judged?

In what ways do I feel like a victim?

What am I itching to get away from?

What has gotten under my skin?

What is driving me nuts?

Do I have paradoxical (conflicting) desires?

What am I itching to change?

Where am I indecisive?

Do I want to control an irritation even if it hurts?

Suggested Blessing

May you hold and respect contradictory desires until something completely new emerges to resolve the conflict.

Suggested Affirmation

I can find a place of peace and quiet in the midst of opposing energies and turmoil.

Psoriasis

Evidence-Based Confidence Level and Therapeutic Potential

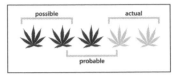

Number of Studies Reviewed: 1

CHI Value: 3

In the allopathic tradition, psoriasis is a chronic skin disease in which skin cells divide too rapidly; they build up and cause red and white, scaly-looking skin surfaces. While psoriasis can affect any area of the skin, it is often found on the elbows and knees. No allopathic cure is available. Management consists of topical medications, systemic pharmaceuticals, ultraviolet light therapy, and nutritional supplements.

The Endocannabinoid System and Psoriasis

Condition	CB1 and CB2
Psoriasis	Up-regulation of both ECS receptors CB1 and CB2 produces suppression of keratinocyte proliferation and inflammation.[1]

Strain-Specific Considerations

THC binds with both CB1 and CB2 relatively equally. Sativas and sativa-dominant strains tend to present with a higher THC:CBD ratio.

Mind-Body Medicine and Psoriasis

Constant anticipation of pain or hurt may play out on the physical stage. A cushiony build-up and thickening of the skin may occur. Areas of the body especially vulnerable are the knees and elbows, which during a fall are used to shield more vital body parts from damage. However, by becoming more thick-skinned, the affected area also loses sensitivity and becomes numb or itchy, painful, even inflamed.

Based on the chronic expectancy of pain, shame, and hurt, psoriasis patients might feel overly vulnerable. They may respond by being overly numb and aggressive in an attempt to compensate. Their projected fears may impact their relations with others and so become self-fulfilling prophecies.

By releasing chronic anxiety and accompanying anticipation of hurt, shame, and pain, and replacing underlying beliefs that constantly feed that anxiety, the patient can increase responsibility for his emotional reality. He may then more easily shift from the physical arena to a mental-emotional arena, informed by a positive self-image. This shift can remove stressors and allow whatever regimen the patient chooses to be more effective in achieving a lasting cure.

Powerful Questions

What are the symptoms keeping you from doing?

How do you feel about that?

Where do these feelings take you?

What scenarios or memories are associated with these feelings?

What is the meaning (messages, unhealthy beliefs/attitudes, etc.) that you have given to that scenario?

Can the answers to these questions direct your focus to support your capacity for self-healing?

Suggested Blessing

May our flowers help you to relax and discover a healthy and balanced response to the anxieties of life.

Suggested Affirmation

Anxiety is a part of life. I can learn to define and embrace anticipated feelings and emotions with confidence.

Let Food Be Thy Medicine

Turmeric: In a meta-study, scientists gave an overview of decades of scientific studies on turmeric. They summarized a long list of turmeric's potential therapeutic properties and noted that it is helpful in psoriasis.[2]

Seborrhea
Evidence-Based Confidence Level and Therapeutic Potential

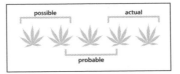

Number of Studies Reviewed: 1

CHI Value: not applicable

Seborrhea is an inflammation of the skin. It appears often in areas rich with sebaceous glands such as the face, chest, and the upper back or anywhere skin folds produce skin-to-skin contact. In the Western tradition, the causes are not currently known, but research has implicated stress as a possible contributing factor.[1] No allopathic cure is available. Treatment consists of using topical or systemic pharmaceuticals.

The Endocannabinoid System and Seborrhea

Condition	CB1	CB2
Seborrhea		Down-regulation of CB2 would produce an inhibition of sebum/lipid production.[2]

Strain-Specific Considerations

Currently not applicable.

Mind-Body Medicine and Seborrhea

The skin is inflamed similarly to that of dermatitis but in deeper layers. Stress is a likely contributing factor in the development of seborrhea.

Powerful Questions

What is the irritation that has gotten under the deeper layers of my skin? What is deeply irritating?

Systemic Sclerosis
Evidence-Based Confidence Level and Therapeutic Potential

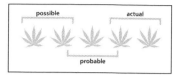

Number of Studies Reviewed: 1

CHI Value: not applicable

Orthodox medicine remains unclear as to the causes of this skin disease. Symptoms may include tough, tight, and hard skin, discolorations and/ or tight facial tone. Possible culprits include irritants, microbes, or an autoimmune response where the body considers certain skin cells foreign objects and attempts to eliminate them. For many patients, no allopathic cure is available. Managing treatments include topical and systemic pharmaceuticals.

The Endocannabinoid System and Systemic Sclerosis

Condition	CB1	CB2
Systemic sclerosis (Scleroderma)		Up-regulation of CB2 would induce a suppression of the immune/ inflammatory process and fibrosis.[1]

Strain-Specific Considerations

Not currently applicable.

Mind-Body Medicine and Systemic Sclerosis

The word *sclero-* in "sclerosis" or "scleroderma" is derived from the Greek word for "hard." Tough, thick skin and stone-faced or leathery facial expressions may reflect a belief system in which life is perceived as constantly dangerous and thus requiring a thick skin. Furthermore, emotional vulnerability displayed in facial expressions must be hidden behind a mask because it is seen as a liability.

Powerful Questions

What are the symptoms keeping you from doing?

How do you feel about that?

Where do these feelings take you?

What scenarios or memories are associated with these feelings?

What is the meaning (messages, unhealthy beliefs/attitudes, etc.) that you have given to that scenario?

Can the answers to these questions direct your focus to support your capacity for self-healing?

Suggested Blessing

May you find relaxation and peace.

Suggested Affirmation

I can find the internal resources needed to meet life's challenges, so I can now relax and trust in my known and yet-to-be-discovered powers, strengths, talents, and abilities.

Vomiting (in general)

Evidence-Based Confidence Level and Therapeutic Potential

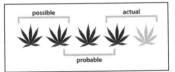

Total Number of Studies Reviewed: 27

Combined CHI Value (including Morning Sickness): 111

Vomiting involves involuntary but coordinated contractions of the stomach, respiratory, and esophageal muscles to forcefully eject the stomach's contents through the mouth or nose. Vomiting may occur as an autonomic response to the body's detection of poisons. Vomiting may also be induced voluntarily by stimulating the gag reflex through touch to the uvula or by taking an emetic (a substance that induces vomiting such as ipecac). Thus, vomiting can be a self-preservation mechanism; a self-induced evacuation of stomach content; or be brought on by disease or injury. *For Morning Sickness see OBGYN.*

Chemotherapy-Induced Nausea and Vomiting

Evidence-Based Confidence Level and Therapeutic Potential

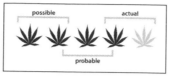

Total Number of Studies Reviewed: 24

CHI Value: 104

Nausea and vomiting are common occurrences following chemotherapy, as the toxic pharmacological agents do not differentiate between cancer cells and healthy cells. Retching and vomiting occur as a result of toxins detected by the brain. A signal travels from the vomiting center (area postrema), down cranial nerves, salivary glands, and diaphragmatic and gastrointestinal muscles, which initiates vomiting.

Anecdotal evidence from patients who smoked marijuana before chemotherapy and encountered significantly less nausea and vomiting ultimately led to clinical trials demonstrating the therapeutic properties of cannabinoids.

The following studies are part of the foundation on which physicians, patients, and advocacy groups base their recommendations that cannabinoids can greatly reduce chemotherapy-induced nausea and vomiting.

Cannabis and Chemotherapy-Induced Nausea and Vomiting

THC reduces nausea and vomiting via CB1.[1] The 24 studies reviewed here examined the effectiveness of cannabinoids in the treatment of chemotherapy-induced nausea and vomiting. They span a period of four decades. Studies conducted in the laboratory on animal, adult, and pediatric patients reached similar conclusions. Early studies focused on comparing the effectiveness of cannabinoids to the most common antiemetic pharmaceutical used at that time—prochlorperazine (generic of Compazine). Most studies reported cannabinoids as superior.

Later studies broadened their focus and reported that cannabinoids proved more effective than other antiemetics such as metoclopramide, chlorpromazine, thiethylperazine, haloperidol, domperidone, or alizapride. More recent studies examined the ability of cannabinoids, especially cannabidiol, to markedly reduce anticipated oxidative stress, inflammation, and cell death in the kidneys, therefore improving renal function in cancer pathologies.

Consideration: As in most cases where cannabinoids may be helpful, research suggests that a therapeutic window exists which may depend on individual tolerance. For instance, either a very high or low dose could offer a lack of antiemetic effects or adverse effects. To determine your optimal window, follow the advice of a licensed health care provider and your own subjective experience. See also "How to Find Your Subjective Therapeutic Window" on page 20.

Study Summary

Drugs	Type of Study	Published Year, Place, and Key Results	CHI
Cannabidiol	Animal study (mice)	2009—College of Medicine, Zhejiang University, Hangzhou, China: Cannabidiol markedly reduced the anticipated oxidative stress, inflammation, and cell death in the kidneys, and therefore improved renal function.[2]	2
Dronabinol orally starting at 2.5 mg the day before chemo and on day one. From day 2 and on, 10–20 mg daily.	64 cancer patients undergoing chemotherapy	2007—Bethesda Memorial Hospital, Comprehensive Cancer Care Center, Boynton Beach, Florida: Dronabinol proved as effective as ondansetron in reducing nausea and vomiting. Combination therapy was not more effective.[3]	3
Dronabinol and smoked cannabis	Review of selective studies	2003—The Cleveland Clinic Taussig Cancer Center, Cleveland, Ohio: Cannabinoids reduced chemotherapy-induced nausea and vomiting.[4]	4
Cannabinoids vs prochlorperazine, metoclopramide, chlorpromazine, thiethylperazine, haloperidol, domperidone, or alizapride	Review of selective studies	2001—Département Anesthésiologie, Genève, Department of Anaesthetics, Churchill, Pain Management Centre Nottingham, Department of Clinical Pharmacology, Radcliffe Infirmary, Oxford, UK: Cannabinoids were more effective anti-emetics than prochlorperazine, metoclopramide, chlorpromazine, thiethylperazine, haloperidol, domperidone, or alizapride.[5]	4
THC was administered orally (18 mg in an edible oil)	Children with cancer receiving chemotherapy	1995—Department of Pediatrics, Shaare Zedek Hospital, Jerusalem, Israel: Complete prevention of vomiting with negligible side effects.[6]	5
Oral THC (as Marinol) 10 mg every 6 hr v. pro-chlorperazine	67 cancer patients undergoing chemotherapy	1991—Prochlorperazine better than THC, but both drugs combined were better than either alone.[7]	4

Drugs	Type of Study	Published Year, Place, and Key Results	CHI
Nabilone and prochlorperazine v. metoclopramide and dexamethasone	Chemotherapy patients	1988—Department of Medical Oncology, Royal Infirmary, Glasgow: Better control of emesis with metoclopramide. Nabilone combination better tolerated.[8]	4
THC as oral Dronabinol 15 mg/m2 (m2=per body surface area) 1 hr before chemotherapy and every 4 hr thereafter for 24 hr v. prochlorperazine	36 cancer patients undergoing chemotherapy where pharmaceutical emetics were ineffective	1988—Division of Medical Oncology, Vincent T. Lombardi Cancer Research Center, Georgetown University, Washington, DC: THC was able to decrease nausea and vomiting in 23 of 36 patients compared to 1 of 36 receiving prochlorperazine.[9]	4
Cannabis (inhaled)	56 cancer patients undergoing chemotherapy unresponsive to standard anti-emetic drugs	1988—78% of treated patients demonstrated a positive response to marijuana.[10]	4
Nabilone and prochlorperazine	Pediatric chemotherapy patients	1987—Hospital for Sick Children and the University of Toronto: Nabilone more effective in reducing retching and vomiting.[11]	5
Nabilone and metoclopramide	Patients under-going radiation therapy	1987—Department of Radiotherapy, Queen Elizabeth Hospital, Birmingham, UK: No difference in effectiveness; more side effects noted with Nabilone.[12]	0
Nabilone 1 mg every 8 hours v. IV metoclopramide (1 mg kg – 1 to 3 hourly)	32 cancer patients undergoing chemotherapy	1986—Oncology, Charing Cross Hospital and University College Hospital, London: No difference between Nabilone and metoclopramide.[13]	5
Nabilone (oral)	18 pediatric patients	1986—Department of Haematology, The Children's Hospital, Sheffield, UK: Nabilone significantly reduced nausea and vomiting, and two-thirds of the kids expressed a preference for the drug.[14]	5
Nabilone (oral)	38 cancer patients receiving chemotherapy	1986—Nabilone is superior to domperidone for the control of chemotherapy-induced emesis.[15]	5
Oral Nabilone 2 mg x 2 daily v. prochlorperazine 15 mg	24 lung cancer patients receiving chemotherapy	1985—Nabilone was significantly superior to prochlorperazine in the reduction of vomiting episodes.[16]	5
Nabilone v. prochlorperazine	34 patients with lung cancer	1983—Symptom scores were significantly better for patients on Nabilone for nausea, retching, and vomiting.[17]	5

Drugs	Type of Study	Published Year, Place, and Key Results	CHI
Oral Nabilone 3 mg three times a day v. chlorpromazine administered at a dose of 12.5 mg IM	20 patients with advanced gynecological cancer	1983—Nabilone, when compared to chlorpromazine, did not significantly reduce vomiting, and most patients preferred Nabilone.[18]	5
Synthetic cannabinoid levonantradol (0.5, 0.75 or 1 mg) v. chlorpromazine (25 mg)	108 cancer patients	1983—0.5 mg levonantradol was a more effective anti-emetic than 25 mg chlorpromazine.[19]	5
THC v. prochlorperazine. THC was given by body surface area (BSA): BSA less than 1.4 m2 = 7.5 mg; BSA 1.4-1.8 m2 = 10 mg; and BSA greater than 1.8 m2 = 12.5 mg. Prochlorperazine was administered in a fixed dose of 10 mg.	212 cancer patients undergoing chemotherapies	1982—THC and prochlorperazine produced similar results but patients who felt THC in their system did better.[20]	5
Nabilone 2 mg x 2 daily v. prochlorperazine 10 mg x 2 daily	27 cancer patients undergoing chemotherapy who failed to respond to pharmacological anti-emetics	1982—Vomiting ejections and dry retching significantly reduced by Nabilone.[21]	5
Oral Nabilone 2 mg v. placebo chemotherapy	24 cancer patients undergoing	1982—"Nabilone is an effective anti-emetic agent for chemotherapy-induced nausea and vomiting."[22]	
Oral THC v. prochlorperazine v. placebo	55 chemotherapy patients	1981—Oral THC is far more effective than prochlorperazine and placebos.[23]	5
Nabilone v. prochlorperazine	113 cancer chemotherapy patients	1979—Nabilone is far more effective in reducing nausea and vomiting.[24]	5
Oral THC	20 cancer chemotherapy patients	1975—Sidney Farber Cancer Center, Peter Bent Brigham Hospital and Harvard Medical School, Boston: "No patient vomited while experiencing a subjective 'high'."[25]	5

Total CHI Value 104

Strain-Specific Considerations

The cannabinoids studied include Nabilone (or Nabilone-similar drugs such as Dronabinol, Marinol, Levonantradol) and to a lesser degree smoked cannabis, THC-infused oil, and lastly CBD. THC reduces nausea and vomiting via CB1.[2]

Nabilone is a synthetic cannabinoid similar to THC and binds with both CB1 and CB2 relatively equally. Smoked cannabis binds with CB1 and CB2 but at a different ratio depending on the strain. CBD has a greater affinity for CB2 expression than CB1.

Sativa and sativa-dominant strains tend to have higher THC:CBD ratios.

Mind-Body Medicine and Chemotherapy-Induced Nausea and Vomiting

The physical brain perceives a threat (a chemo-toxin) and instantly reacts to expel it. The mind's parallel might be the perception of an experience that brings great fear or even dread (such as a cancer diagnosis).

Powerful Questions

Do I express my emotions, especially those I do not like, appropriately and with intensity?

Can I release and forgive all hatred, pain, grief, and disapproval that I still carry from my past?

Can I love and approve of myself, right now, just as I am?

What is the ancient hatred I still carry with me?

What is that terrible secret that eats away at the substance of my soul?

Where does my hopelessness find fertile ground?

Suggested Blessing

May your changes strengthen your resolve to live a healthy life.

Suggested Affirmation

May all poisons and all fears leave you so all that remains is forgiveness and a world in which love reigns supreme.

Motion Sickness
Evidence-Based Confidence Level and Therapeutic Potential

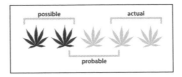

Total Number of Studies Reviewed: 2

CHI Value: 4

Seasickness, airsickness, and carsickness are associated with nausea, vomiting, dizziness, and vertigo. Motion sickness occurs due to discord between the movements perceived by the eyes versus those perceived by the inner ear. If this conflict finds no resolution, nausea may progress to vomiting. An estimated 7–28% of travelers experience acute motion sickness.[1]

Cannabis and Motion Sickness

While numerous studies elucidate the anti-emetic properties of cannabis, the Bradford study (2008) discovered that the cannabinoid THC prevented specific motion-induced nausea and vomiting in animals.[2]

A multi-institutional German study (2010) on human subjects further revealed that cannabinoid-receptor (CB1) expression was significantly lower in subjects who suffered from motion sickness compared to those who felt fine, indicating a relationship between reduced endocannabinoid activity and motion sickness. By extension, these discoveries represent a new possibility for treating aspects of motion sickness, mental stress, and physical nausea and vomiting.[3]

Strain-Specific Considerations

The cannabinoid studies on motion sickness employed anandamide, CBD, and THC. Anandamide and THC bind with CB1 and CB2 relatively equally. CBD tends to favor CB2 expression.

Sativa and sativa-dominant strains tend to contain a higher THC:CBD ratio.

Mind-Body Medicine and Motion Sickness

Grace and Graham wrote: "Nausea and vomiting occurred when an individual was thinking of something which he wished had never happened.

Study Summary

Drugs	Type of Study	Published Year, Place, and Key Results	CHI
ECS (CB1 and CB2), Anandamide	21 healthy male volunteers	2010—Multi-institutional German research group: CB1 expression in leucocytes 4 h after the experiment was significantly lower in volunteers with motion sickness than in participants without nausea and vomiting. Anandamide levels fell in subjects who got sick but rose in subjects who felt fine.[3]	3
Cannabidiol (CBD 0.5, 1, 2, 5, 10, 20, and 40 mg/kg), Delta(9)-tetrahydro-cannabinol (THC 0.5, 3, 5, and 10 mg/kg)	Animal study (Asian house shrew, S. urinus)	2008—The School of Pharmacy, University of Bradford, Bradford, West Yorkshire, UK: THC prevented motion-induced vomiting while CBD did not.[2]	1

Total CHI Value 4

He was preoccupied with the mistake he had made, rather than with what he should have done instead. Usually he felt responsible for what happened." Typical statements: "I wish it hadn't happened.... I was sorry I did it.... I wish things were the way they were before.... I made a mistake. ... I shouldn't have listened to him." The authors concluded: "Vomiting is a way of undoing something which has been done. It thus corresponds with the patients' wishes to restore things to their original situation, as if nothing has ever happened."[4]

The part of the human physiology responsible for producing motion-induced nausea and vomiting is an involuntary mechanism. This particular context may be indicative of fear as a response to mismatching or opposing experiences beyond one's control.

Suddenly the security that comes from feeling solid ground under one's feet disappears, replaced by the motion of the sea or by riding in a car down the serpentine roads of the Swiss Alps. Often the person at the helm of the sea vessel or behind the wheel of the car firmly in control of direction does not experience motion sickness to the same degree (or at all) as their passengers do.

NASA trains astronauts in parabolic flight maneuvers, in which temporary (about 30 sec.) weightlessness is achieved by flying an airplane following an elliptical flight pattern parallel to the Earth. This simulation is nicknamed "the vomit comet." Roughly two-thirds of all participants experience degrees of nausea or vomiting. Researchers blame anxiety or the anticipation of hitherto unknown sensations beyond one's control for this response.

Several factors point to the difference in participants' responses. Some found the sensation exciting while others experienced anxiety and fear. It is not unreasonable to make a connection between the blood levels of anandamide after parabolic maneuvers. In fact, levels dropped in subjects with motion sickness but rose in subjects who felt fine.[5] Those feeling fear may reject the change by ejecting the contents of their stomachs just as many warriors do before battle.

In summary, aggravating factors may include anxiety, a fearful anticipation, or reaction to unfamiliar sensations beyond one's control.

Consider the possibility of releasing anxiety by embracing excitement and feeding your curiosity rather than your anxiety.

Powerful Questions

What are the symptoms keeping you from doing?

How do you feel about that?

Where do these feelings take you?

What scenarios or memories are associated with these feelings?

What is the meaning (messages, unhealthy beliefs/attitudes, etc.) that you have given to that scenario?

Can the answers to these questions direct your focus to support your capacity for self-healing?

Suggested Blessings

May you relax and let go of fear.

May you find it as easy as 1-2-3 to let go of beliefs that produce unwarranted fear of change.

Suggested Affirmations

I have complete dominion over my mind.

I am the master of my belief.

I can choose thoughts that make me feel safe and secure.

Let Food Be Thy Medicine

Ginger: Researchers from Graz, Austria (2007), reported that while the abilities of ginger and cannabis to reduce nausea and vomiting are well established by a series of scientific studies, the focus on special receptor sites involved in nausea and vomiting remains unclear. They suggested more research.[6]

The German Commission E approved ginger for the prevention of motion sickness.[7]

Researchers from Zürich, Switzerland (1994), recruited thousands of volunteers to help determine how well seven different commonly used seasickness prophylactics worked. Researchers gathered data during whale-watching tours in Norway. In the control group (whose members did not receiving any prophylactics), 80% showed signs of seasickness, namely nausea with vomiting and malaise. In the group receiving a prophylactic, amongst seven agents, only about 4–10% of individuals experienced nausea with vomiting, and 16–23% experienced malaise independently of which prophylactic they took, thus indicating a similar effectiveness in preventing seasickness. The agents included ginger root, cinnarizine, cinnarizine with domperidone, cyclizine, dimenhydrinate with caffeine, meclozine with caffeine, and scopolamine, which seemed the least effective.[8]

In a double-blind, placebo-controlled study from Bangkok, Thailand (2006), ginger proved effective in preventing nausea and vomiting among patients receiving major gynecological surgery. The patients in the treatment group received two capsules of ginger taken one hour before the procedure (one capsule containing 0.5 gram of ginger powder).[9] Another study (2010) discovered that 650 mg of ginger given three times daily for a total of four days to pregnant women experiencing morning sickness worked even better than vitamin B-6 (another natural supplement commonly used for this purpose).[10]

Wound Care (in general)

Evidence-Based Confidence Level and Therapeutic Potential

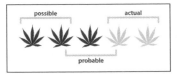

Total Number of Studies Reviewed: 10

Combined CHI Value: 32

Historically cannabis has been applied topically in the form of poultices, plasters, salves, tinctures, and oils to treat slow-healing wounds and skin ulcers (as in "diabetic foot" in turn-of-the-century American medicine). Cannabinoids have shown potent abilities to destroy and inhibit the growth of numerous microbes (see Bacterial and Viral Infections). Furthermore, the involvement of the endocannabinoid system in modulating inflammatory responses to both acute and chronic injuries may suggest a prominent and beneficial role in wound care. Anecdotes of modern-day users have reported successful treatments of slow-healing skin wounds with cannabis-infused honey and cannabis-infused oils.

Cannabis-Infused Honey

Modern medicine has rediscovered honey's ancient use in the care of infected wounds.[1] Applied to slow-healing skin wounds such as ulcerations, burns, or infected wounds, honey provides numerous therapeutic benefits. Honey is antibacterial, anti-inflammatory, improves circulation, reduces swelling, stimulates formation of new capillaries and connective tissue, and reduces pain. The Cuban Ministry of Health widely recommends honey as a skin-protective agent, as an antimicrobial for skin infections where it is prepared as a topical cream, as an alcohol tincture, and as oral drops.[2]

While no current studies examine the combined and possibly synergistic properties of honey and cannabis in infused form, it is interesting to note that many of the therapeutic properties of honey also exist in cannabis—most notably, anti-inflammatory and pain-reducing properties.

Cannabis-Infused Hempseed Oil

Oil made from hempseed is void of any mind-altering cannabinoids and has historically been used for the treatment of dry skin, as well as age-related skin blemishes and wounds. It is a rich and properly balanced source of omega-3 and omega-6 polyunsaturated fatty acids. Recent studies reveal that ingestion of hempseed oil positively changes fat profiles in the body and significantly reduces the symptoms of dryness, itching, and inflammation in atopic dermatitis.[3]

Some patients have combined the skin-healing and anti-inflammatory properties of hempseed oil by infusing it with cannabinoid-rich cannabis to create a topical ointment. The skin is the largest organ of the body and thus provides an ideal route for the gentle delivery of biologically active substances. Many cannabis-hemp oil users report a variety of benefits, including the shrinking of moles and age spots, localized and systemic pain relief, therapeutic relaxation of tight muscles and cramps, deeper and more restful sleep, the soothing of inflammation, and a subtle increase in libido, all with a gentle uplift in mood.

As with all natural, biologically active substances, effects are usually optimal within a specific therapeutic window, which may vary from person to person. Taking too much may aggravate symptoms. Taking too little may have a sub-optimal effect. As always, start slowly and increase application until you reach your therapeutic window. (See also page 20.)

Mind-Body Medicine and Wound Care

Few people wake up one morning and consciously choose to inflict injuries on themselves. However, within the paradigm that stipulates "you are the generator of all of your experiences," there are no exceptions. In cases of trauma, accidents, burns, wounds, and injuries, taking a step back and looking more carefully at the complex interplay of the conscious, subconscious, and unconscious often reveals free will at work.

While a person may never consciously decree "I am going to hurt myself today," he or she can become aware of consciously held beliefs concerning punishment. Nobody is perfect, everybody errs and makes mistakes; but with a belief in punishment, injuries will occur to meet a self-generated need. One might consider the use of guilt as motivation and its implicit demand for purification through punishment. This makes the choice for injury more clearly visible. An examination of self-hatred, inappropriately expressed anger, harbored anger, and underlying belief structures may reveal surprising aspects of the possible "why" and "how" of traumatic events.

Fractured Bones

Evidence-Based Confidence Level and Therapeutic Potential

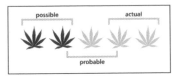

Total Number of Studies Reviewed: 4

Combined CHI Value: 9

Bone fractures are generally classified as closed or open (compound) fractures. The latter being fractures where bone segments are actually protruding through the surrounding tissue. Closed fractures can range in severity from mild hairline fractures, to partial fractures, or complete fractures but where the surrounding tissue is still intact.

A compound fracture is easy to spot. Bone is sticking out through the skin. There is severe pain, and localized swelling and bleeding is clearly present. Complete but closed fracture presents with dangling limbs, severe pain, and swelling, but without external blood loss. A closed but incomplete or partial fracture may only present with pain and swelling similar to a sprain or strain but most likely with increased intensities.

In the orthodox medical paradigm, a minor fracture such as a hairline fracture is merely immobilized and treated with pharmaceutical medication to reduce inflammation and pain. A completely fractured bone is set (realigned) manually, or surgically if necessary, and then placed into a semi-permanent cast for a period of 3 to 10 weeks (depending on location of fracture and age of patient), the idea being that the fracture must remain undisturbed to heal.

However, there is a downside to semi-permanent casts that was revealed by a study conducted on over 200 pediatric patients (average age of 8) by the University of Maryland School of Medicine (2014).[1] Researchers discovered that a whopping 93% of kids with fractures had iatrogenic complications (injuries caused by doctors or hospitals) arising from semi-permanent casts. Complications included swelling (edema), skin breakdown (ulceration), and poor healing due to inappropriate fracture immobilization.

Certain conditions such as osteoporosis, bone cancer, or brittle bone disease can make a person more vulnerable to fractures. Long-term smokers similarly are more vulnerable to fractures and once a fracture occurs smokers can take up to twice as long to heal as non-smoking patients with the same kind of injury.

Complications may occur when nerves are severed or impaired, producing loss of sensation or movement. In some cases a bone will not set in a condition called non-union or the bone will set but in the wrong spot causing a permanent misalignment which may require a manual fracturing and surgery to correct.

Cannabis and Fractured Bones

A study from Germany (2005) discovered that cannabinoids binding with CB1 and CB2 receptors regulate osteoclast (cells that remove bone tissue) activity and bone mineral density alike; thus, balancing the removal of old bone cells and sustaining bone density is a potential factor in fracture vulnerability and healing.[2] Similarly, data from two Israeli studies (2006,[3] 2009[4]) confirmed that cannabinoids help maintain bone density and prevent age-related bone loss, thus markedly reducing susceptibility to fractures in seniors.

And, more specifically, a new study conducted by a team of international researchers from Israel, Switzerland, and Sweden just published (2015) in the *Journal of Bone and Mineral Research* discovered that CBD, a primarily CB2 activating non-psychoactive cannabinoid, had the capacity to make fractured bones stronger while they heal ("enhancing the maturation of the collagenous matrix, which provides the basis for new mineralization of bone tissue") and thus not just strengthening fracture sites and making them harder to break in the future,[5] but also speeding the healing process itself.

Exploring Mind-Body Consciousness

The human body contains 206 bones. The skeleton protects vital organs and produces a rigid support system that enables the attached flexible counter system of muscles to exert force, allowing the body to contract and expand, thereby producing movement and enabling physical tasks.

Interestingly, a bone's hollowness provides its strength and light weight. The hard outer material is made from collagen and minerals, while the inside is filled with soft and spongy yellow and red bone marrow.

Study Summary

Drugs	Type of Study	Published Year, Place, and Key Results	CHI
CBD	Animal (rodents) study	2015—An international team of researchers from the Hebrew University of Jerusalem, Tel Aviv University, Institute for Biomechanics (Zürich), Lund University (Sweden), Hadassah-Hebrew University Faculty of Dental Medicine (Jerusalem). CBD leads to improvement in fracture healing.[5]	2
THC	Review study	2009 – Bone Laboratory, the Hebrew University of Jerusalem, Jerusalem, Israel. Maintains bone remodeling and protects against age-related bone-loss.[4]	3
Endogenous cannabinoids system	Animal study (mice).	2006 – Bone Laboratory, the Hebrew University of Jerusalem, Jerusalem, Israel. Diminished endocannabinoid receptors increase bone loss.[3]	2
Endogenous cannabinoids receptors (CB1) and (CB2).	Animal study (mice)	2005 – Department of Psychiatry, Life and Brain Center, University of Bonn, Germany. (CB1) and (CB2) can regulate osteoclast activity and bone mineral density and CB2 receptors play a role in the development of osteoporosis.[2]	2

Total CHI Value 9

Vulnerability to fractures may result from built-up pressure exerted by the growing resentments and accumulated guilt (with its demand for purification though punishment) for railing against outside authority, the fathers, the rulers, the gods, and their "shoulds" and "shouldn'ts." Fracture patients are unable to move about and are limited in their ability to complete daily tasks. This inability tends to bring up strong feelings, especially about what they can and cannot do anymore. It is in these feelings that significant meaning (relevant to the trauma) can be found.

Questions

Do you believe receiving support is weak or bad?

What support structure are you railing against?

What are the symptoms keeping you from doing?

How do you feel about it?

Where do these feelings take you?

What scenarios or memories are associated with these feelings?

What is the meaning (messages, unhealthy beliefs/attitudes, etc.) that you hold about that scenario?

Can the answer to these questions direct your focus to support your capacity for self-healing?

Suggested Blessing

May you find peace and balance within the structures and authorities in your life.

May you realize that you author your responses to the signals of your world.

Suggested Affirmation

Asking for help is a sign of strength.

I can find the right balance between asking for support and being self-reliant.

I am the author of my own experiences.

Take Notice

Consider this story: A few years back I had a chance to visit a traditional bone setter's clinic in Accra, Ghana. At the clinic called Aponchie, bone setters did what no western hospital would dare to do. Aponchie used basic field casts that could be undone daily to check, re-check, and topically treat and massage fracture sites and surrounding tissue. Daily checks without x-rays? Massaging a fracture site while the healing was in progress? Applying topical plant constituents that appeared to be a gooey mess of a mud-like substance to the damaged tissue as often as needed? My sterility-focused mindset had to take a break. Instead, I was invited to examine something new and very counterintuitive, something that challenged my modern medical training to the core.

I toured the clinic and was introduced to each patient, hearing each patient's story. One after another told me what had happened, how their bones, spine, arms, or legs were shattered by one or another horrific accident, harrowing tales of how they made it to the outskirts of town with dangling limbs before arriving at the clinic.

For instance, Michael, a fit young man in his early twenties had been playing soccer and sustained a kick to his shin so hard that it left his tibia and fibula (shin bones) protruding through his skin. He was taken and treated at the modern, western hospital, the VA in Accra.

After the cast came off, the skin above the fracture had healed but his bones had not set and his lower leg was left dangling (the nightmare of any fracture patient as well as their orthopedic surgeon).

Without much fanfare, his mother took him to Aponchie. The bone was set once more and placed in a temporary cast. He received daily treatments of touch, a topical poultice containing a combination of spices and local herbs that were placed on a single layer plastic bag (as a moisture barrier) that was finally wrapped with a common flexible bandage. And, twice a day, he was given the clinic's own herbal concoction for pain and healing. After about two weeks, the bones finally began to set. He was seeing the light at the end of a long tunnel.

And, while the bone setters at the clinic were willing to share some of the ingredients, the exact list was kept a secret. The elder of the bone setters solemnly pointed out that "too many times the white man has come and stolen medicinal knowledge, made billions, and shared none of it with those who discovered and generously shared it in the first place." Wow. After a long pause, I laughed to myself. I completely understood.

The few ingredients the bone setters were willing to discuss were local spices (rare in the western world), many of which are rich in a compound called beta-caryophyllene, chief among them black and white ashanti peppers (piper guineense) and alligator pepper (aframomum melegueta).

It wasn't until many years later when I was writing this book that I learned that beta-caryophyllene has the capacity to signal endocannabinoid receptors (CB2) and in doing so initiate a host of beneficial and therapeutic actions that speed the healing process.

For instance, once CB2 is activated, a number of biological changes take place in the human body that at once strengthen the immune system, reduce even severe inflammations and swelling, stimulate deep wound healing, and even produce some analgesic effects.

As you have noticed in the text above, the team of international researchers from Israel, Switzerland, and Sweden discovered that CBD and other primarily CB2 activating non-psychoactive cannabinoids have the capacity to make fractured bones stronger while they heal. Thus they not only strengthen fracture sites, but also speed the healing process itself, making it harder to break the bone in the future.

Post-Surgery Wounds
Evidence-Based Confidence Level and Therapeutic Potential

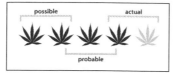

Number of Studies Reviewed: 1

CHI Value: 4

Wounds caused by surgical interventions require careful attention to possible complications signaled by an increase in pain, the presence of inflammation, swelling, discharge, discoloration and/or heat.

Cannabis and Post-Surgery Wounds

A 2009 Worcester, Massachusetts, study casts a wide net for meta-analysis, reviewing all cannabinoid studies "... published in the last 5 years on the activities of all classes of cannabinoids, including the endogenous cannabinoids such as anandamide, related compounds such as the elmiric acids

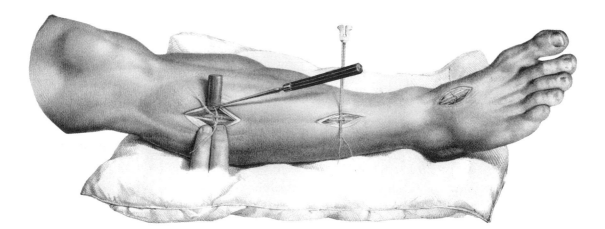

(EMAs), and non-cannabinoid components (200–250 constituents) of Cannabis that show anti-inflammatory action."[1] Results revealed that all types of cannabinoids as well as non-cannabinoid parts of the plant effectively reduce pain from inflammation associated with post-surgery patients, rheumatism, rheumatoid arthritis, chronic neuropathic pain, and fibromyalgia.

Study Summary

Drugs	Type of Study	Published Year, Place, and Key Results	CHI
All types of cannabi-noids (endogenous, plant-based, and synthetic)	Meta-analysis (2004–2009)	2009—University of Massachusetts Medical School, Worcester, Mass., USA: Cannabinoids effective in reducing pain for post-surgery patients.[1]	4

Total CHI Value 4

Mind-Body Medicine and Post-Surgery Wounds

See Wound Care (in general), immediately above and/or Spinal Cord Injuries, below.

Spinal Cord Injuries
Evidence-Based Confidence Level and Therapeutic Potential

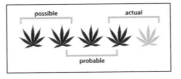

Total Number of Studies Reviewed: 5
CHI Value: 19

The spine is a marvel of the human body. It allows us to walk upright, bend, stretch, and reach. It is a solid load-carrying support system that is remarkably flexible while housing and protecting the spinal cord. Solid support is derived from vertebral bone rigidity, and flexibility is achieved by the placement of intervertebral discs (intervertebral fibrocartilage) between each of 26 spinal bones.[1] Seen from the side, the spine contains four curves that further allow for support, flexion, extension, and cushioning.

The brain and the spinal cord make up the central nervous system. The spinal cord is a relatively thick bundle of nerves descending from the medulla oblongata (the lowest part of the brain) through the center of the spine. Along its length, spinal cord nerves create junctions and exit the spine between each vertebra to ultimately connect all parts of the body in ever-smaller branching nerve fibers.

An injury to the spinal column most commonly results from external trauma (car crash, gunshot, etc.) but may also result from internal trauma (stroke, aneurysm) or via certain diseases (cancer). The location of damage in the spinal cord determines the degree of disability. For example, a paraplegic person is paralyzed from the waist down after sustained damage to the thoracic or lower spine. A quadriplegic person paralyzed from the neck down loses the ability to move his arms or legs after sustaining damage to the spinal cord in the neck or brain itself.

The management of spinal column injuries, where some sensation is still present, is often accompanied by chronic pain and uncontrollable muscle spasms of the back, arms, and legs.

Cannabis and Spinal Cord Injuries

The time-proven antispasmodic properties of cannabis have been confirmed by modern science in numerous human studies. Here we look at studies specifically related to spinal cord injuries and resulting spasms. As early as 1974, VA (U.S. Veterans Affairs) hospital-based researchers began looking at data suggesting a practical therapeutic antispasmodic benefit.[2] Later studies confirmed the efficacy of cannabinoids, especially THC. A study from Basel, Switzerland (2007), recommends a minimum dose of 15–20 mg daily to produce a therapeutic and measurable effect in reducing spinal cord injury-related spasmodic activity.[3]

Study Summary

Drugs	Type of Study	Published Year, Place, and Key Results	CHI
Oral THC, average daily dose 31 mg; rectal THC, average daily dose 43 mg	25 patients with spinal cord injuries and regular spasms	2007—REHAB Basel, Centre for Spinal Cord Injury and Severe Head Injury, Basel, Switzerland: THC is an effective antispasmotic. At least 15–20 mg per day required to achieve therapeutic effect.[3]	5
Dronabinol 2 x 5 mg increased gradually to 3 x 20 mg	5 patients with spinal cord injuries and regular spasms	1995—Medical College of Georgia, Augusta, GA, USA: Reduced spasms in 2 patients.[4]	3
Placebo v. 50 mg codeine p.o. (by mouth) v. 5 mg THC p.o.	A single patient with spinal cord injury and subsequent pains and spasms	1990—Psychologisches Institut für Beratung und Forschung, Zürich, Switzerland: THC produced significant reduction in spasticity.[5]	5
Inhaled cannabis	Data collected from 43 patients with spinal cord injury and related spasms	1982—Cannabis produced significant reduction significant reduction in spinal cord injury-related spasticity.[6]	3
Inhaled cannabis	10 patients with spinal cord injuries and resulting pain and spasms	1974—Spinal Cord Injury ward of the Miami, FL, VA Hospital: Decreased pain and spasms.[2]	3

Total CHI Value 19

Strain-Specific Considerations

Clinical trials employed cannabinoids from various sources: cannabis, THC, and Dronabinol (synthetic THC). Scientists tested them on patients with spinal cord injuries. Cannabis binds with both CB1 and CB2. THC and Dronabinol both bind with CB1 and CB2.

While both sativa and indica strains contain cannabinoids that activate CB1 and CB2, sativas or sativa-heavy strains tend to produce higher THC:CBD ratios.

Mind-Body Medicine and Spinal Cord Injuries

The spinal cord contains neural pathways connecting a trillion cells. It is analogous to a highway for electrical signals that control the entire body. Spinal cord injuries are like a sinkhole or collapsed bridge that blocks traffic in both directions, isolating previously connected communities. The most common causes of spinal cord injuries are car and motorcycle accidents followed by trauma from violence, falls, and sports accidents. These injuries usually present with some degree of paralysis, pain and/or spasms.

Paralysis patients often express an immobilizing terror or the feeling of being frozen with fear. Patients may say they are giving up external exploration of the world and focusing instead on their inner development. In that sense, spinal cord injuries provide an opportunity to (re) commit to a new direction. Paralysis may draw the patient's attention to a prior inability to relax the affected part(s) and spur him or her to consider what that part represents to them. Paralyzed legs may represent issues of progress or a shift in one's priorities in life. They may also relate to steadfastness or the ability to stand up for oneself. Paralysis below the belly button involves issues of sexuality and the release of stool and urine, and so love must be raised from the genitals to the heart. Stool relates to the element of earth and discerning that which matters. Paralysis reduces vertical height by half and challenges one to ask for help and to receive help. It may require a reassessment of the meaning of pride, humiliation, humility, and self-worth.

For pain considerations, see the opening section of Pain (in general).

Spasms (in forms ranging from minor twitching to serious cramps) may be reflective of a life force trying to shake up and wake up affected body parts. It may indicate a physical manifestation of contracting and fearful thoughts, emotions and/or underlying beliefs.

Powerful Questions

What was the last straw that broke?
What were the other straws that pushed me to the breaking point?
What broke my life in half?
What was the purpose of my life before?
What is the purpose of my life now?
How did I define my self-worth before?
How do I define my self-worth now?
What was I proud of before?
What am I proud of now?
Love before was . . . ?
Love now is . . . ?
Do I feel broken/humbled?
What is the affected body part a representation of?
What is the body function (lost) a representation of?

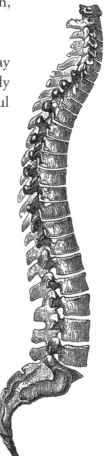

CHI = CANNABIS HEALTH INDEX

CHI ALSO = VITAL ENERGY = HEALTH

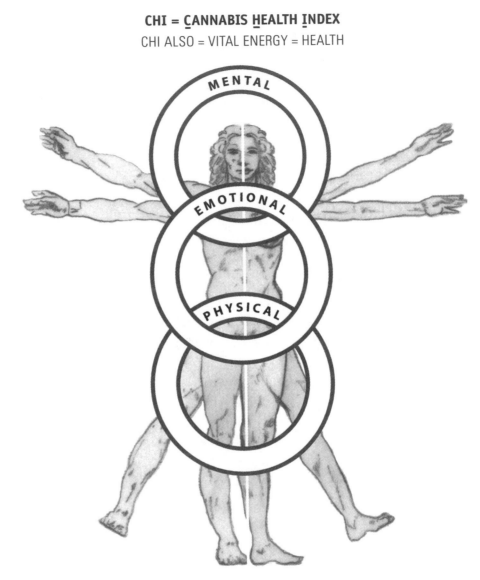

In ancient as well as modern perspectives, everything is energy and energy is called by many names:

"Chi" in Chinese Medicine

"Chi" = Prana in Yoga

"Chi" = The Great Spirit to Native Americans

"Chi" = "The Force" in *Star Wars*

"Chi" = The Psych in Psychology and Psychiatry

"Chi" = Vital Energy in nineteenth-century thinking

"Chi" = Quantum in the twenty-first-century thinking

Because chi is so vital, when it is impeded or out of balance, illness occurs.

The key to health is freeing and balancing chi through holistic mind-body medicine

Learn practical and easy ways to increase and revitalize your chi in the next chapter of *CHI*.

Chapter V
Integrating Mind-Body Medicine
for Deeper Healing

1. Applying the Healing Balm of Deep Relaxation

It is an easy intuitive leap to imagine the benefits of deep relaxation on the quality of mind as well as the physical body. However, beyond the common-sense need for rest, numerous recent studies have examined what specifically happens when we regularly enter a state of deep relaxation. And, the study results have been surprising.

But before we look at the health benefits of deep relaxation, let us have a brief look at what scientists are not talking about. Although going for a walk, taking a power-nap on the sofa, or sitting comfortably while watching a movie can be calming or relaxing, these activities are, generally speaking, not inducing what researchers have termed a "relaxation response" (RR). A "relaxation response" is defined as the opposite of the "stress response," also often referred to as fight, flight, or freeze.

During a RR the mind-body axis significantly changes hormonal and signal molecules in the brain, which in turn calms the sympathetic nervous system. It does so by reducing stress molecules (such as adrenalin or cortisol), calming heart rate, and reducing blood sugar, all of which are important to patients with cardiovascular illnesses and those suffering from adult-onset diabetes.

RR simultaneously produces an increase in the gas nitric oxide, which dilates (widens) major blood vessels, inducing a reduction in blood pressure. A double-blind, randomized trial conducted at the Body Medicine Center at Massachusetts General Hospital[1] demonstrated that this self-directed healing mechanism associated with RR is subject to conscious intervention and can easily be learned by almost anyone. Acquiring this skill could be especially helpful in patients with cardiovascular disease and hypertension, and those at risk of strokes.

Stress Response vs. Relaxation Response

Endocannabinoid receptors influence, modulate or regulate the function of each of the cells, tissues, glands, organs and systems in which they are contained. Cannabinoid receptors 1 (CB1) are present in the hypothalamus, the pituitary, and the adrenal glands.

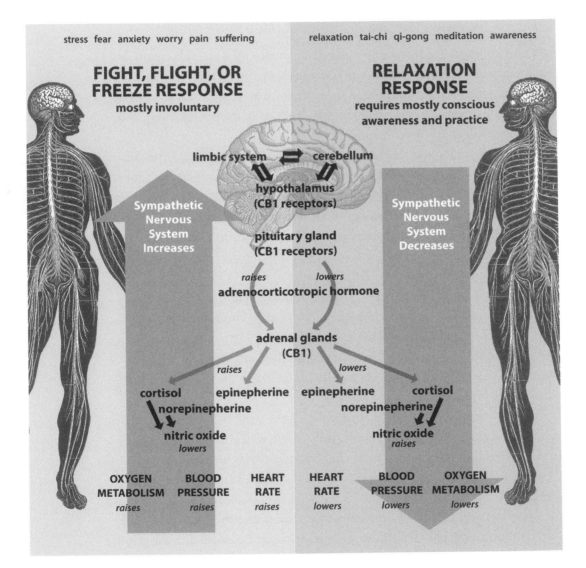

Furthermore, researchers are beginning to better understand how anandamide[2] (a cannabinoid made by nerve cells[3] in the human body) induces the widening of coronary arteries (which supply the heart), thus reducing hypertension and potentially benefiting numerous patient populations. If these findings can be confirmed in human trials it would suggest that we can learn to actively direct a RR by engaging the endocannabinoid system via physical signals (e.g., cannabis) or non-physical signals such as emotional states associated with certain meditation practices.

Researchers tested numerous mind-body techniques and discovered that people could learn to use ancient practices such as Tai Chi, Qi Gong, meditation,[4] repetitive prayer, and yoga as well as modern practices such as developing an awareness of emotional and behavioral stress responses or progressive muscle relaxation to induce a "relaxation response" and with it begin to consciously guide and support the healing process.

Using self-induced RR in hospital settings has already become popular due to its low-cost support in cases such as the treatment of potentially life-threatening illness such as hypertension and cardiac arrhythmias, but also in cases of chronic pain, psychological conditions such as autism,[5] anxiety and mild/moderate depression, as well as hormone-based premenstrual syndrome and infertility issues. Many physicians engage the patient's own capacity for self-healing by using the television set in the patient's room, where he or she can learn the techniques that produce a RR. As a result, patients spend less time recovering, prevent complications, and feel like an empowered member of their own healing team.

Patients (including those of advanced age) are encouraged to continue the practice of their choice at home as part of their health care regimen. The multiple positive results may include improved immune responses against tumors and microbes, and a healthier cardiovascular system, for example.

2. Using Your Emotional Intelligence for Deeper Healing

While we may never reach the ideal of being able to consciously direct all our emotional experiences, in working toward it we get better all the time.

For most of us it is easy to believe that we can create certain emotions. For instance, we are driving on the freeway and feel frustrated, bored, or even lonely. What do we do? We reach for the radio to find a tune that generates a "better" feeling. Another example might be feeling burdened with problems (real or imagined), worried, tense, and stressed. We book a massage and allow the bodyworker to help relax and soothe our tensions.

However, when it comes to certain other situations we believe we have nothing to do with how we are feeling in those moments. Let's say that you notice your boyfriend gets a message on his cell phone from an old lover. You might find yourself jealous. And rather than looking at the internal architecture of one's mind that gives rise to jealousy, many will focus on blaming him for this constricting emotion. Now, this is not to say that other people don't have impact. But we always have a choice about how we are going to look at the situation and therefore about how we are going to respond emotionally. We choose how we react.

Another example might be that you are home with family members for Thanksgiving dinner. You are a peace-loving liberal who has promised himself not to get upset when Uncle Henry starts his right-wing rant about the Second Amendment and the need for military empire. However, almost as soon as you sit down for dinner he begins, and all you can do is bite your lip and suppress your urge to lunge over the table and make him eat his words instead of his meal.

Learning to work with emotional authorship can offer other options. For instance, you could use this situation as feedback and accept yourself as a person who fuels your own expectation of conflict, demonstrating a potential lack of humility. After all, even Uncle Henry can have a change of heart. Or, you could explore your capacity for compassion or empathy for your own intense dislike of someone with different beliefs than yours. Or you could wonder and explore what the two of you have in common besides a capacity for passionate beliefs.

Each time we work toward emotional authorship we take an empowered position that does not rely on having to change someone else's mind—only our own.

Earlier in Chapter II we used the examples of fear and anxiety (cortisol, adrenalin) to illustrate the importance of understanding the two-way street between molecules and emotions and their influence on our health and well-being. At this point it is also important to point out that to equate a single emotion with a single molecule is a simplification, and in reality these connections are much more complex.

Complex emotional states may set into motion numerous cascading molecular reactions all at once. For instance, the relaxation response (as the opposite of "fight or flight") induces a set of changes in the human body and mind (see the Stress vs. Relaxation chart above) that involve the pituitary, hypothalamus, and adrenal glands as well as the endocannabinoid system.

However, the emerging observational patterns allow us to generalize and associate connective highlights. For example, in most chronically stressed people expansive emotions and their respective molecules have a health-supporting impact. On the other hand, most constricting emotions and their molecular counterparts, especially when they become chronic or highly concentrated, can make us more vulnerable to disease.

Being prone to constricting emotions (e.g., shame, defensiveness, guilt, anger, fear) diminishes our health and well-being. More specifically, studies have shown that persistent experiences of negative emotions and stress can worsen chronic degenerative diseases through an increase in the production of pro-inflammatory cytokines (cell-signaling protein molecules), which increase inflammation activity associated with aging, cardiovascular disease, osteoporosis, arthritis, type 2 diabetes, certain cancers, Alzheimer's disease, frailty, and functional decline, as well as periodontal disease, for example.[1]

A. Taking Ownership of Where You are Right Now

"We cannot change anything until we accept it."

—C. G. Jung

When we lack conscious ownership of thoughts and emotions that we have labeled intolerable or unacceptable, we spend a significant amount of energy engaged in avoidance mechanisms. For example, we may try to avoid unacknowledged emotions by bingeing on "comfort" foods that in fact make us ill, or reaching for any behavior or substance that acts like an emotional painkiller or numbing agent. This expenditure of energy on avoidance techniques often results in exhaustion, a constricting sensation in the physical body and in our emotional experience. And this misspent energy has real consequences for our health and vitality.

To reverse the damaging influence of our avoidance strategies and the loss of vital energy that comes with it, it is important to begin by accepting where we are, no matter where we find ourselves.[1] We need to find ways to accept and honor ourselves when we are wallowing in constricting emotions such as self-pity, hostility, grief, despair, or any thought or emotional state we have previously labeled intolerable or unacceptable, or simply do not want to acknowledge. We don't have to linger in this emotional state, but in order to shift our experience we must first accept where we are. Studies have shown that honest self-expression, alone or with a close and trusted friend(s), reduces both the frequency and the intensity of seemingly intolerable states of mind.

With time and a bit of practice, embracing our present condition can make it easier to tolerate even the most unwelcome situations. We may even begin to notice a shift in attitude from aversion to curiosity. It is this willingness to embrace the present moment rather than avoid it that, combined with a sense of wonder, allows us to change ourselves and so transcend our experience.

Cannabis, especially in combination with conscious intention and in the right setting for you, can bring to the surface otherwise hidden material which might seem intolerable in our normal frame of mind.[2]

> Robert, a man in his fifties, didn't remember ever feeling anything for his mother but intolerance, scorn, and impatience tempered by an occasional indulgence. In a state of relaxed and expanded awareness, he felt himself cry, child-like, "I want my mama, I want my mama." Once the previously unacceptable feelings of needing his mama when he was a child re-entered his awareness, Robert began to develop safer, deeper, and more meaningful relationships whereas previously his fear of intimacy led only to unsafe, shallow connections with women.

Consider the results from a study conducted at MIT (Massachusetts Institute of Technology). Researchers discovered the physiological underpinnings of a common mind-body therapy technique in which patients use a positive memory to diminish the impact of a traumatic one and thus inactivate the traumatic emotional material and the toxic stress that is associated with it.[3]

B. Releasing the Toxins of Suppressed/ Repressed Emotions

Humans are hard-wired to have thought and feeling. It is estimated that throughout the day we have tens of thousands of mental-emotional experiences. Both occur simultaneously, in a marriage immune to divorce, along with corresponding physiological changes that primarily depend on the intensity of each facet of the mental-emotional material.

Sigmund Freud, the Austrian physician and father of psychoanalysis, demonstrated the existence of the unconscious mind and provided a basic understanding of psychological problems and a therapeutic system with which to intervene. He also gave us the concepts of narcissism, infantile sexuality, and, of course, the Freudian slip—a slip of the tongue reflecting an unconscious emotion. (For example, in one of President John F. Kennedy's speeches he sculpted the air with his hand saying our country should encourage the "breast." He quickly corrected his "error" with the words "the best and the brightest.")

While the concept of an unconscious mind has played an important part in psychiatry and psychology since the nineteenth century, the idea of unconscious emotions is still difficult to accept for most of us who are accustomed to believing that we know what we are feeling: "I know when I'm angry." "I know fear." "Of course I know when I feel love." More importantly, for many of us it is difficult to accept the notion that suppressed, unconscious feeling could play a role in the development of illness and disease.[1]

For instance, in his book *The Pleasure Principle,* Freud describes the baby's blossoming sexuality and its clash and crash with reality. Based on his observational studies, Freud concluded that the infant's sexual impulses were incompatible with reality and the immature state of development of the child at that time. He associates this mismatch of desire and reality with the most painful feelings of failure and loss of love, leaving behind a permanent injury to self-regard. And, it is this damage to self-regard that Freud connects with the sense of inferiority commonly observed in neurotics and to varying degrees in the grown-up's psyche. Yet, while many adults may be aware of feelings of inferiority, not feeling good enough, or even that there is something wrong with them, few can remember this point of origin in the infant's psyche and the crash and burn of one's immature sexuality.

However, many people can access memories that reflect the same emotions, such as when they were told "what's wrong with you?" or "you are stupid" or "you will never amount to anything."

"Until you make the unconscious conscious, it will direct your life and you will call it fate."

—C. G. Jung

It may seem obvious that an infant can't be expected to process conflicting and intense emotions in a constructive way. So, we have an ally—the unconscious mind, which allows the baby to push aside and park the overwhelming emotions until the maturity and resources are available to work with them in a way that serves the individual's growth and evolution.

However, most often when the material and/or feelings re-emerge, we react with anxiety and fear and want to stuff them straight back out of our view, causing us to play ping-pong with the unconscious, which seems to continuously ask, "Are you ready to deal with this feeling yet?" And us saying, "No, no, not yet."

Reasons vary for suppressing emerging emotion. We may perceive danger, because to express anger in the wrong situation can be dangerous, even life-threatening. Often we may feel fear, including a fear that says if you examine the belief too closely that "you're a mistake" or "there is something wrong with you," you might find that it is true, so it is better not to look in the first place. We may believe that we are unable to cope. We may come across societal judgments or cultural taboos. (See the case study on page 212.)

The idea here is not that we need to discover every suppressed or repressed emotion, just enough of them for the pattern of hiding them to dissipate. As the pattern loses its stranglehold we will also notice that the reason for its existence in the first place will also lose its power. And perhaps for the first time, we can be truly free from past trauma and its often more debilitating meaning. We can then be empowered by the experiential knowledge of why we hid the emotions in the first place and perhaps even become grateful to the unconscious mind for its ability to take the trauma, hide it from our conscious mind, and patiently wait until such time when we are ready and willing to heal.

C. Identifying and Releasing Unhealthy Mental-Emotional Habits
BIAS, PREJUDICE, AND JUDGMENT

Generally speaking, biases, prejudices, and judgments are unhealthy, emotionally charged habits. More specifically, and for the purpose of this book, unhealthy habits are defined as those that are both physically and psychologically detrimental to our well-being. Biases can prevent us from thinking clearly, logically, and reasonably, and they may fuel chronic fear, anger, anxiety, or any other constricting emotional and stressful behavior such as defensiveness or power struggle.

The Merriam-Webster Dictionary defines bias as "a tendency to believe that some people, ideas, etc., are better than others that usually results in treating some people unfairly." Compare this to the same dictionary's definition of discernment: "the ability to see and understand people, things, or situations clearly and intelligently."

Multidisciplinary studies have established that it may be virtually impossible for a human being not to be biased. More than a hundred different types of biases have been described, and what they all have in common is that they automatically influence our judgments without the benefit of reason, logic, or critical thinking. What makes them dangerous to our health and well-being is that they often direct our choices and decisions in unhealthy ways for ourselves as well as others.

For instance, a study conducted at the University of Maryland (2000) examined hundreds of adolescents and adult smokers and discovered that the vast majority of them "agreed that smoking is addictive and causes death for 'most people' who smoke. However, for themselves personally, adolescent and adult smokers doubt that they would die from smoking even if they smoked for 30 or 40 years."[1] This disconnect in logic is commonly called "optimistic bias."

Consider another example. Have you noticed that it is easier to imagine things can go wrong than to imagine things will go right? The term for this is "negativity bias." It is perhaps easier to understand this concept in evolutionary terms, when the threat of dangerous animals lurking in the bushes was a daily reality, and more important to survival than, say, the discovery of tasty berries or learning a new skill. However, unchecked negativity bias can fuel chronic fear states, with detrimental impact on our physical and psychological health.

Similarly, scholars repeatedly demonstrated in numerous social studies that young black men are subject to widespread stereotyping and racism from both whites and African Americans alike. These findings were confirmed even in people who believed themselves aligned with the Civil Rights Movement or who would oppose racial inequality. Racial bias (especially if suppressed) contributes fears and anxieties, creating a constant brew of constricting emotions where blame, anger, and injustice are common responses, adding to social and personal ills and dysfunction.

If we want to diminish unhealthy habits, we need to recognize and reduce biases, prejudices, and judgments.

Overcoming Bias, Prejudice, and Judgment:

1. Recognize that you are human and as such have biases (don't feel guilty—take responsibility instead). By observing yourself and the circumstances that trigger a bias, you bring them to your consciousness (work with one at a time).
2. Own this bias by giving it emotional dimensions. (What is this emotion doing to you and others? What is this bias keeping you from doing and how do you feel about it?)
3. Don't not condemn yourself, just let it be okay.
4. Change by responding differently when you notice the trigger (learn, understand, evolve, and grow).

Recognizing negative patterns and letting oneself be with the emerging uncomfortable emotions, rather than using any of the available (and often addictive) avoidance mechanisms (smoking, judging, defensiveness, power struggle, shopping, etc.), discharges the old resistance. It also frees up the energy used to meet the age-old need for self-protection from an enemy long lost in a past event. A ghost of memory has been released. The old pattern and its meaning have fulfilled their purpose and can now be used to thrive and heal.

THREE DESTRUCTIVE HABITS: GUILT, MARTYRDOM, AND HARBORED ANGER

As mentioned before, it is important to remember that constricting emotions are not themselves harmful to our health provided they are expressed and let go of appropriately. However, three emotions—namely guilt, martyrdom, and harbored (righteous, fanatical) anger—tend to have only negative health consequences. And, while these three killers are responsible for much of human-caused pain and suffering in the world, and while they may appear stubborn to eradicate, they too can be seen for what they are, their ill-effects can be owned, they can be forgiven, and they certainly can be healed.

Guilt

A study conducted at the University of California suggests that when we engage in negative self-talk or self-blame we increase not just shame and guilt but also the number of pro-inflammatory cytokines in our body (which promote inflammation) and raise tumor necrosis factor–alpha receptor levels (involved in systemic inflammation).[2]

Guilt is often thought of as a feeling, but actually it functions more like a virus that infects our capacity to think and feel. For instance, when guilt infects anger it turns a normal human emotion into something we think we should not have. As such it forces us to live a lie, all-the-while hidden in the deep recesses of the mind where repressed anger boils, injecting toxic stress into body and mind. Without guilt, anger can flow freely, powerfully, and without hurting anyone.

When guilt shows up in the grieving process it can keep grief frozen and stuck in place. Once we direct guilt to give way to an underlying anger (for example), the experience of grief often shifts and puts us in touch with the love we feel for the missing.

Additionally, guilt is unhealthy motivation to behave a certain way. And sadly, many use guilt to blame, seek revenge, or punish. More specifically, guilt is used as a construct that seeks purification through punishment (of self or other).

Preventing guilt: A person guided by ideals (healthy motivations) and principles (specific behaviors that steer toward ideal), with the character to consistently apply said principles to inform all behavior, has no need for guilt.

Martyrdom

At its extreme, martyrdom can involve torture and horrific death. It is a form of fanatical anger that is at once arrogant, self-important, and destructive to anyone near. Martyrdom is a construct that emerges from the toxic emotional brew of feeling unappreciated, feeling as if one is treated wrongly, and feeling misunderstood by the whole world and everyone in it. Martyrdom describes people who use self-sacrifice and self-inflicted suffering as a front to punish and destroy others (e.g., suicide bombers, dying for one's beliefs). It can also apply to family members or partners who consistently work hard and/or suffer for another and consider this a form of self-sacrifice.

Preventing and ending martyrdom: It is impossible to feel martyrdom when we are in love, feel grateful and/or provide a gentle, caring intimacy to ourselves or another. Think about it—no martyr has ever been accused of having had too much fun, love, or enchantment in his or her life.

Also, you can avoid being mistreated or feeling overwhelmed by communicating when you have been giving too much or are given too much to do. Setting positive boundaries helps us to stay within our limits and capabilities.

Harbored Anger

Harbored anger is anger that is recycled as soon as it has been expressed, and as such is never released and continues to impact the body and the mind negatively. This anger is a never-ending and self-feeding loop of the same old emotional reaction to a specific trigger. It is often referred to as "ruminating."

Preventing fanatical anger: This requires a change of the underlying belief (e.g., "without this anger I am weak," "without this anger I lose my friends, family, or congregation"). Those examples are beliefs that need to be released and changed if the person is to move beyond his or her anger.

On Releasing Guilt, Martyrdom, and Harbored Anger

These three killer habits are all mental constructs that create a very destructive and unhealthy anger. Guilt creates repression, martyrdom creates destruction, and righteous anger makes anger a constant presence. The good news is that all three are in the domain of conscious intervention.

Each is based on a more or less conscious choice and as such can be easily changed or undone by another choice.

However, many times we do not let ourselves take the easy way (of choice) because we hold a judgment. If that is the case we can employ forgiveness. As we forgive guilt, martyrdom, and harbored anger we significantly strengthen our capacity to heal.

You might find one or more of the following techniques useful.

Forgiving judgments on feeling angry, guilty, or martyred: When you feel troubled by guilt, martyrdom, or fanatical anger you may want to ask your body for help. Focus on where in your body the trouble concentrates or collects. Ask yourself what am I judging here? See what comes up and release it by forgiving yourself. For instance, change "I am bad because I am angry" to "It is okay to be angry" or "I forgive myself for judging my anger." Similarly, you can change "There is something wrong with me because I am so hurtful" to "I forgive myself for being hurtful." Likewise: "I am so hateful" becomes "I forgive myself for judging my hate."

Once forgiveness is in place, the underlying anger in guilt can rise unrepressed to our consciousness and we can work to express it in appropriate, constructive, and safe ways. Once we forgive our martyrdom, we unlock its stranglehold and are able to make a new choice that sets us on a different course. And once we forgive our harbored anger we can get in touch with the source belief and replace it with one that begets different thoughts and emotions.

Releasing Anger: On a piece of paper write out your anger. Get descriptive and detailed. Use as many of your senses as possible. The idea here is not to show anyone but to get the anger out of your system. When you feel done, take the paper and safely destroy it. You will give your subconscious the message that this is how you want to deal with anger: honestly, in detail, and perhaps most importantly, without hurting anyone or getting yourself into some kind of trouble.

Releasing Harbored Anger: As above, write a description of your anger on a piece of paper. Again get your senses involved. When you feel done, take the paper but instead of safely destroying it, fold it and tuck it away for three days. After three days take it out and read it slowly. Write out your anger again. Fold and tuck it away for another three days. Take it out, read it slowly, and write out the anger again. But this time rip it up and destroy it safely. In this case you signal to your subconscious that you are going to change the way you are dealing with anger. It is like a dance move—you pace and lead beyond your past behavior and take a new direction. Your subconscious will get it and support the new way of safely expressing anger and being done with it, period.

The Way We Breathe Changes the Way We Feel:[3] Anger has a specific breath pattern of long and forced breaths (think of punching something away). The inhalation tends to be longer than the exhalation's phase, which may be accompanied by shouting or aggressive, rapid verbal expressions. By changing the way we breathe we can change the way we feel (also reducing heart rate and blood pressure).

Breathing consists of four phases: inhalation, top pause, exhalation, and bottom pause. In the case of an anxiety or panic attack, for instance, the breath is rapid and shallow, creating an unfavorable ratio of too much oxygen with too little CO_2. The body's reaction creates even more anxiety: a rapidly beating heart, increases in blood pressure, a dry mouth, and tingling or numbness in the hands, feet, or nose. Often the patient believes in an impending doom and imminent threat of non-being, despite reassurance.

In cases such as these, breathing into a brown paper bag can help return the ratio to a balanced state. However, a more powerful technique would be to teach the patient how to square their breath. By making each phase the same length of time, we superimpose an antidote for rapid breathing that induces a feeling of calm, being centered, and peaceful.

In case of a panic attack, consider the "square your breath" technique: Take a deep breath and count out how long it takes to complete your inhalation (start at the bottom and stop at the top). Now use the same number and hold your breath for the same length of time for all four phases. If you counted 4 seconds, it looks like this: Inhalation (1-2-3-4), Pause (1-2-3-4), Exhalation, (1-2-3-4), Pause (1-2-3-4). Continue to square your breath until you feel at peace.

D. Exploring and Building Healthy Mental-Emotional Habits
DISCERNMENT, CURIOSITY, AND TEMPERED POSITIVITY

There are many healthy emotional habits. Here we will highlight discernment because of the many healthy emotional qualities it often engenders.

Discernment is a healthy habit that according to the *Merriam-Webster Dictionary* produces "the ability to understand inner qualities or relationships." As opposed to biases, the habit of discernment allows us to intelligently explore, learn about, and understand the internal workings of what diminishes our health as well as what supports or restores our health and well-being.

Employing discernment enhances our capacity for curiosity or wonder. It is imbued with an inherent desire to understand an issue rather than to quickly judge it. Discernment creates a potent focus on possible solutions even when none currently seem to exist. It embraces complexities, which in turn make things easier rather than simple, as is the case with prejudice or bias. Discernment reduces false hope and nourishes real ones. It facilitates a solid foundation for being optimistic.

Additionally, when we look at the qualities that usually come with discernment (e.g., wonder, optimism, understanding), we notice that each and all of them tend to make us feel good. And while most of us, most of the time, welcome emotions that make us feel good, the idea that what feels good may be good for us warrants deeper investigation (and discernment).

Psychologist Barbara Fredrickson made an evolutionary argument in 2003 that positive feelings broaden minds and serve as valuable resources during times of hardship,[1] yet it wasn't until later that the mechanism by which positive emotions support physical health and contribute to healing was investigated. A study published in 2005 by researchers from London showed that positive emotions such as happiness can lower cortisol levels, reduce heart rate, and decrease fibrinogen stress responses.[2] The beneficial physiological results of positive emotions were further confirmed by a Harvard experiment (also published in 2005) demonstrating that curiosity and hope decrease the likelihood of developing hypertension.[3]

Positive emotional experiences have also been associated with longevity. One study reviewed autobiographical material of 180 Catholic nuns and compared this to the length of each nun's life. Researchers found that "positive emotional content reported in early-life autobiographies was strongly associated with longevity six decades later."[4] Study results were confirmed by another large population study from Texas, which concluded that "positive affect seems to protect individuals against physical declines in old age."[5]

Even single emotional words have impact on our mood and physiology. For example, research conducted at the University of Göttingen, Germany (2009), discovered that simply viewing single words such as *happy* or *brutal* reduced or increased anxiety, respectively.[6] The study suggests that thoughtfully selected and compassionate (kind, positive) words (or thought) alone can contribute to our ability to solve conflict, diminish stress, and enhance our coping mechanism. And while these scientists are not advocating the elimination of negativity (when there is a problem, there is a problem), they do suggest a focus on turning something negative into something positive.

For instance, observational studies conducted at the University of Washington (1998) have shown that couples who are working through a stressful conflict are much more likely to succeed if they manage a ratio of 5:1 positive feelings to negative ones during the process.[7] Similarly, research conducted at the University of Michigan found that for humans to flourish (to live within an optimal range of human functioning, one that connotes goodness, productivity, growth, and resilience), we need to employ positive affect to negative affect at a ratio of 3:1.[8]

If we apply this ratio to ourselves, especially during times of perceived stress or conflict, we may have a map to significantly enhance our capacity for self-healing and well-being.

Try to apply the 5:1 or 3:1 technique to yourself. For example, whenever you recognize hurtful or degrading self-talk such as "I am such an idiot," you can dispel the hurtful impact by simply acknowledging that "oh, look at that, I just judged myself" and "I can let that be okay," "I can forgive myself," "I can learn to let that go quickly and easily," "I can release the belief that a mistake must or should hurt me."

Applying discernment to positive thinking, we also get to look at the potential down-sides and important nuances. In what may seem counter-intuitive, studies have shown that positive thinking without action, or imagining a dream already realized, may rob us of the motivation needed to realize the goals.[9] A solution to this potential problem of untempered positivity comes to us from the University of Hamburg and the University of New York.[10] Researchers employed a method called "mental contrasting," where a desired future is imagined along with a focus on current reality or potential obstacles.

Mental contrasting produced motivational energy in alignment with a person's expectations of successfully attaining the desired future. Here is the caveat: the success of mental contrasting depends on the expectation of the person using it. In other words, if you believe it will work, it will. If you don't believe, however, the technique may significantly reduce your chance of success in achieving your goals. With that in mind, and for believers only:

Mental Contrasting Technique

1. Think about your goal. Invoke details using as many senses as you can. Let your mind wander and explore. Some people like to use a journal and write it out.
2. Focus on one big or numerous smaller positive aspects of your goal and flesh them out. Again, involve as many senses as you can to make it as real as you can.
3. Now, in the same fashion, look at what stands in your way of achieving your goal.
4. Focus on one big or numerous smaller positive aspects and flesh them out. Involve as many senses as you can to make it as real as you can. That is all there is to it.

THREE HEALING HABITS: GRATITUDE, COMPASSION, AND FORGIVENESS

Gratitude

Gratitude changes negative affect (e.g., guilt, hostility, anxiety), reduces the stress hormone cortisol, increases positive affect (e.g., caring, happiness, vigor), and produces a significant increase in DHEA (suspected anti-aging molecule).[1]

For instance, during a simple gratitude exercise patients at the University of California–Davis Medical Center Neuromuscular Disease Clinic were instructed to write down five things they were grateful for every day, using no more than one sentence to describe each item. After two months, researchers noted a heightened sense of well-being, more hours of sleep, and reduced pain compared to a control group whose members were asked to write one sentence about a grudge or a neutral emotional event on a daily basis.[2]

These findings from UC Davis are especially important when we look at the observation that negative affect (such as blame and sustained hostilities directed at others) has been shown in numerous studies to negatively impact mental and physical well-being. In one experimental study, 287 surviving heart-attack patients were followed and examined seven weeks after the attack and again after a period of eight years. Patients who reported that they had learned something from their experience were at significantly less risk for a second heart attack compared to patients who believed that others had caused their heart attack.[3] These results were confirmed by a meta-analysis of 45 independent studies that found hostility to be an independent risk factor for coronary heart disease.[4]

Experiencing and expressing gratitude enhances positive affect and leads to other measurable benefits, too. UC Davis study participants reported increases in optimism and happiness, fewer physical symptoms, positive states of alertness, greater attentiveness and determination, high energy, positive moods, feeling connected to others, increased empathy toward others, improved sleep, and more positive attitudes toward their family.

Kindness and Compassion

An experiment conducted at the University of North Carolina at Chapel Hill suggests a novel mechanism involving the vagus nerve by which kindness and compassion can make us happier and healthier.[5]

A key function of the vagus nerve is to communicate parasympathetic nerve impulses to the heart (reducing heart rate), arteries (lowering blood pressure), and digestive organs (optimizing digestion). The authors of the study report that the positive (expansive) emotions of kindness and compassion significantly increase vagal tone and thereby calm our heart and blood pressure, relax the mind, and create an optimal environment in which to absorb nutrients in the gut.

Participants of the study were instructed to meditate and to look at their own worries and concerns and then that of friends or family with kindness and compassion. While they were mentally observing the stressors in a meditative state, people were asked to repeat affirmations such as "may you live with ease," "may you feel safe," "may you feel healthy," and to keep returning to these thoughts when they noticed their minds wandering elsewhere. At the end of the study participants showed a higher vagal tone (lower heart rate and blood pressure) and an increase in overall expansive emotions such as joy, hope, or amusement. The authors of the study write, "Results suggest that positive emotions, positive social connections, and physical health influence one another in a self-sustaining upward-spiral dynamic."

Additionally, research has shown that every change we make produces a change in our chemistry as well as changes in our brain (new neurons and new connections). Learning a new skill produces new nerve clusters and connectivity in the part of the brain that becomes activated during the learning process. For instance, an international study centered at Harvard Medical School showed that using mindfulness meditation practices for eight weeks produced a significant increase in grey-matter density of the portions of the brain that are involved in learning and memory processes, emotion regulation, self-referential processing, and perspective-taking.[6]

In other words, what we have seen in the case of fear-based thinking (i.e., physical results such as increased stress, cortisol, epinephrine, low vagal tone) can be applied to compassion-based thinking (i.e., increased relaxation, oxytocin, and vagal tone). Showing kindness or compassion to yourself or to others changes your chemistry and your brain for the better. By working toward making kindness a habit rather than fear or aggression, we become nicer to ourselves as well as to others. We become empowered by transforming a host of constricting emotions and patterns into expansive ones. For example, we can turn self-indulgence into self-love, fear into curiosity, power struggle into open and compassionate communication—all of which in turn support our health and well-being.

> *"If you have fear of some pain or suffering, you should examine whether there is anything you can do about it. If you can, there is no need to worry about it; if you cannot do anything, then there is also no need to worry."*

—Dalai Lama

How to Strengthen Compassion Within?

Let us use a practical example. Bankruptcies or foreclosures are a serious crisis. The sustained mental and emotional stress commonly experienced during the months or years of a bankruptcy or foreclosure process is toxic stress.

This type of stress has been shown to increase the risk of developing chronic degenerative diseases such as hypertension, diabetes, heart disease, anxiety, and depression, as well as to increase drug abuse and domestic violence.

Considering compassion for yourself in dealing with a hostile bank or aggressive debt collectors can be a nurturing and supportive power in your corner. Ask yourself, is getting angry with the *banksters* helping you hold on to your home? Is anger helping you to think things through with attention to details? Is the constant presence of anger healthy for your body and your mind? Is losing your patience helping your sense of security and safety? Chances are the answers are no. This does not mean that you can't or shouldn't express yourself and employ strong counter measures in return.

Ask yourself, is it healthy to have compassion for yourself? Is it useful to step back and look at the bigger picture? Is it helpful to look at this crisis as a teacher from which you may learn something extraordinary? Chances are the answers could be yes.

The Dalai Lama teaches a technique called *Tong-Len* (meaning "giving and receiving") to strengthen the power of compassion within. *Tong-Len* reverses the habit of avoiding suffering and seeking pleasure. He instructs you to visualize, in the safety of your mind, a group of people on one side of the room. Now see these people suffering from turmoil and tragedy of all sorts such as homelessness, war, loss of health, or loss of loved ones. On the other side of the room imagine yourself as self-centered and indifferent to their suffering and pain. Now, in between that *selfish you* and the group of people in distress, place another representation of yourself as a neutral observer. Notice where you feel yourself naturally drawn. Looking objectively, chances are you will feel drawn to the group of people suffering. Now take in all the suffering of that group of despondent people and give love, joy, success, and any type of healing or soothing energy you can muster.

When we think we cannot do the meditation, it is because we come up against our own fears, anger, and despair. Now we can turn the practice on ourselves.

Take in any present or future suffering such as your fear, anger, or despair, and send compassion and forgiveness to yourself. This is the core of *Tong-Len*.

Forgiveness

Forgiveness is often mistaken for a weakness rather than seen as a strength. Some hold it as a shortcut or a cop-out. Others believe forgiveness is a cheap justification to just do whatever you want. It is often mistaken as giving up or admitting failure. Many people fear forgiveness: "If I do forgive I will reopen a wound, a hurt, a humiliation, and I don't want to ever deal with that 'awful' feeling again." Yet others think forgiveness is arrogant or that "only God forgives." With beliefs like these, it is no wonder that many don't want to engage the power contained in forgiveness. However, as you will see in the next paragraphs, to increase our capacity for self-healing it is imperative to make friends with forgiveness.

Psychoneuroendocrinology, the study of the interplay between emotions and hormones, has shown that hormone profiles respond to forgiveness.[7] In one study, merely imagining forgiving an offender produced measurable improvements in heart rate and blood pressure compared to study participants who were instructed to imagine not forgiving the offender.[8]

Beyond the physiological benefits of forgiving someone or oneself, studies have shown that forgiveness has other clear and measurable health benefits such as reduced hopelessness, defensiveness, blame, revenge, anxiety, and depression as well as increased optimism, self-efficacy, self-acceptance, and one's perceived level of social and emotional support. Forgiveness is also associated with the preservation of supportive and close relationships, greater satisfaction in life, transcendent consciousness, and spiritual connection.[9]

How do we access the power of forgiveness? One way to access the power in forgiveness is via engaging our capacity for thinking and feeling. This can be done by exploring and acknowledging whatever small or large part we may have played in the problem or issue we wish to forgive. Think of it this way: "you can't sell the car unless you own it." Always take the first step on the road to forgiveness by forgiving yourself. Perhaps it is for a bad choice you made. Perhaps you need to forgive yourself for an imprisoning fear or debilitating pain. Maybe your task is to forgive yourself for your ill-advised commitment to independence that refuses to let anybody help you. What can you learn from this situation? How do you feel about forgiving yourself? What resistances do you encounter? And, can you forgive that resistance?

To own the car so you can sell it (to continue the analogy), consider the following. In the privacy of a meditation, be with whatever feelings your responsibility engenders. Accept, embrace, and forgive that part of yourself. Now that you are forgiving yourself, consider what you don't have to do anymore. For instance, perhaps you can stop being so paranoid, stop being weak, stop being angry over and over again, or stop always being ready to argue or fight at the drop of a hat. Perhaps you now can see more of the love that was always here, but could not be seen for all the fear you held onto for dear life. Now, how does *that* feel?

E. Transforming Unhealthy Emotional Habits Into Positive Ones

As we have seen, bad habits can be detrimental to our health while good habits are powerful and easily accessed tools to support our health, healing, and well-being. In fact, healthy habits support us in our capacity to thrive without effort.

Addiction treatment research suggests that any habit can be broken down into three basic phases, namely a trigger event, the reaction, and finally the reward phase.

For instance, whenever Eric would feel anxious (the trigger), he would think about going shopping for something fun (the reaction). He went to a store and for a while he felt safe and in control (the reward). However, his insecurity was only intensified over time as his rising bills became an additional source for his anxiety, insecurity, and feeling of being out of control.

Whether we are talking about minor habits such as tapping one's foot incessantly when anxious or resorting to moderate or severe addiction habits, these three phases are operational. In response, there are numerous models that offer to break a negative habit. A look at any self-help section in a bookstore can yield abundant results. Those methods that tend to be more effective create awareness about the trigger phase, focus on replacing the choices of the reaction phase, and consciously examine the dimensions of the reward.

> For instance, Eric got help and learned to identify his trigger event (anxiety). He began to accept it without judgment and just allowed himself to be with his anxiety whenever it knocked at the door of his emotional reality. More specifically, he discovered that

simply focusing on automatic behavior such as his breath created the space to become aware of his other automatic behaviors, i.e., the shopping phase. Once he saw his emotional trigger and his habitual choices, he gained impulse awareness and with little effort replaced his expensive shopping habit while keeping his reward in place (feeling safe and secure). Eric consciously changed his unhealthy habit by configuring a list of optional behaviors that increased his sense of safety and security: he focused on his breath; allowed himself be with the anxiety without judgment; he would call an intimate friend and relish in the closeness of a warm and vulnerable conversation; or go for a relaxing walk in his favorite park behind his house.

TECHNIQUES TO TURN UNHEALTHY EMOTIONAL HABITS INTO POSITIVE ONES

Method 1: Choosing Words that Matter

The words we choose to communicate our thoughts and feelings about a stressful situation have a significant impact on how we experience it physiologically. For instance, in a study conducted by the University of Regensburg, Germany, researchers noted that during a stressful situation or crisis such as an emergency or a scheduled surgery, patients exhibit heightened and focused attention and increased susceptibility to suggestion.[1] This intensity-rich environment can be compared to a trance-like state where we are more vulnerable to negative words and suggestion. While on one hand hurtful or careless words can aggravate anxiety, stress, and pain, on the other hand carefully chosen and supportive words can offer an opportunity to benefit the patient. This mechanism is also true when applied to oneself.

In other words, we can choose to express ourselves using less intense or negative words. For example, "I am a bit anxious about the situation" is going to feel different to us than "I am terrified" or "I feel like I am going to die." You can try this yourself. Do you feel different when you hear yourself say: "I am a bit miffed about this" versus "I am pissed off" versus "I could f-ing kill you"? And while this may seem like just changing words, we in fact change the meaning of the constricting emotions and with it the emotional intensity.

Method 2: Inducing Relaxation Response

Scientists at the Benson-Henry Institute for Mind Body Medicine at Massachusetts General Hospital discovered that inducing a relaxation response (RR) resulted in specific gene expression for both short-term and long-term practitioners of RR. In other words, RR can change which genes are turned on and which genes are turned off. For instance, those human subjects who practiced RR initiated genes that significantly improved cellular metabolism, optimized oxygen consumption, and improved ability to respond to free radicals when compared to the control group of people who did not employ RR.[2]

Test the method when you feel stressed. We have the capacity to relax when we experience stress. Slow your mind and breathe, and focus on words that have positive meaning for you.

Both methods—careful choice of vocabulary and relaxation response (RR)—are part and parcel of our conscious intervention and can easily be learned and applied. In the beginning it may not feel like much, but over time, the effort to reduce negative affect and thus support your capacity for self-healing can yield significant results.

Method 3: Becoming a Cannabis Shaman

Here is an interesting observation and possibility. Using cannabis, like any behavior (such as shopping, sex, exercise, and using alcohol and drugs) can become an unhealthy psychological habit. However, within the proper therapeutic window and with conscious intention it can also function to transcend any unhealthy habit. Many cannabis-using patients have reported that the deep relaxation associated with cannabis made it easier to discover their own trigger without judgment, and to relax in the presence of otherwise intolerable emotions and become aware of the reward dimensions. By looking at these things we can gain impulse awareness and a better understanding of the value of our rewards, and thus open to the possibility of new choices and options that replace any negative behaviors in the reaction phase with those that support our health and well-being.

Method 4: Ending Negative Self-Talk

Ending the unhealthy habits of self-punishment, constricting rumination, and negative self-talk:

Step 1

Look specifically at how I self-punish and write it down. For instance:

If I humiliate, ridicule, or embarrass myself, I do it in this way (. . .).

When I engage in hostile self-talk, I say (. . .).

When I deny myself love, fun, or success, this is what it looks like (. . .).

When I stuff pain into my body, I usually put it into my (. . .).

Step 2

Now, that you know more clearly how you act as a self-punishing person, ask yourself what would a self-loving person do? Apply the new responses (of a self-loving person) in each and all of these specific scenarios and write those out as well.

Use the new script to make a different choice next time you see yourself about to act in a self-punishing way. Make that new choice until it becomes second nature.

You can use the same technique when you are dealing with your need to punish someone else.

With a little practice, the negative health impact of long-standing habits (e.g., binge drinking, arguing when upset) and entrenched ways of thinking (e.g., making catastrophic predictions, using prejudices) can be replaced with healthy habits of a positive nature (e.g., daily exercise, meditation, mindfulness) and positive ways of thought (e.g., seeing the best in people, discernment thinking). In doing so we nurture positive affect, reap the benefits of expansive emotions, improve the quality of our emotional life, and increase the generally healthy biological molecules associated with positive feelings.

3. Using the Power of Choice for Ongoing Healing

At the age of 37, Jill Bolte Taylor, a Harvard-educated brain scientist, suffered a serious stroke and simultaneously entered a state of extraordinary consciousness. Bleeding from a ruptured vessel in the left side of her brain caused her to lose numerous left-brain functions (the ability to "walk, talk, read, write, or recall any of my life"). After her stroke, she experienced cognitive shifts between the two sides of her brain. She lived two realities, as different as day and night. After a recovery process that took eight years, she wrote a book about her experience.[1]

Perhaps for the first time in medical history, a brain researcher was able to examine first-hand the right and left hemispheres of the brain and then explain the subjective experience of each. Taylor writes about the two halves of her brain as two minds with distinct personalities.

The left brain is all about logic, time, method, details, categorizing, and the internal voice of our individual self-perception as separate from others; it is always concerned about what happened in the past, and based on the past it is trying to connect and project what's going to happen in the future. During Jill Taylor's stroke, it was this part of her brain that was becoming more and more disabled.

Taylor describes her experience:

> My brain chatter went completely silent. [...] It was as if someone had taken a remote control and pushed the mute button. [...] I could not define where I began and where I ended. [...] I was captivated by the magnificence of the energy around me. [...] I felt enormous and expansive. [...] Any stress related to my job was gone. [...] I lost 37 years of emotional baggage. [...] In the wisdom of my dementia, I understood that this body was, by the magnificence of its design, a precious and fragile gift. It was clear to me that it functioned like a portal through which the energy of who I am can manifest here. I wondered how I could have spent so many years in this construct of life and never realize I was just visiting.[2]

In contrast with the left, the right brain is concerned with intuition, feeling, emotions, energy, oneness, and connection; it lives exclusively in the present moment, unconcerned about the past or the future. The right half "thinks" in pictures; the left, in words. The right perceives the input from our senses as a tapestry of energy (sounds, sights, smells, sensations, taste, and movement).

Taylor described her right-brain experience, now uninhibited by the left brain, in this way: "I am an energy being connected to the energy all around me through the consciousness of my right hemisphere. We are energy beings connected to one another through the consciousness of our right hemispheres as one human family. And right here, right now, we are all brothers and sisters on this planet, here to make the world a better place. And in this moment we are perfect. We are whole. And we are beautiful."[3]

Taylor called her cognitive shift to the right the "euphoric nirvana" of the right brain. When thinking with her right hemisphere, she experienced a complete sense of timeless well-being and peace. However, it was a switch back to the logical, sequential left that allowed her to recognize that she was having a stroke and ultimately enabled her to call for help.

Taylor's experience highlights the differences between the two sides of the brain and shows the capabilities of each.

She poses the question "Who are we?" and answers:

> We are the life force, power of the universe, with manual dexterity and two cognitive minds. And we have the power to choose, moment by moment, who and how we want to be in the world. Right here, right now, I can step into the consciousness of my right hemisphere where we are—I am—the life force power of the universe, and the life force power of the 50 trillion beautiful molecular geniuses that make up my form. At one with all that is. Or I can choose to step into the consciousness of my left hemisphere, where I become a single individual, a solid, separate from the flow, separate from you. I am Dr. Jill Bolte Taylor, intellectual, neuroanatomist. These are the "we" inside of me.[4]

Taylor's descriptions during her state of extraordinary consciousness may sound somewhat familiar to some cannabis patients. A similar cognitive shift to the right hemisphere occurs often during cannabis treatments, such as experiences of reduced stress or lack of stress, and intense sensations of peace and relaxation, even when aware of otherwise intolerable memories. Furthermore, increases in creativity, enhanced sensation of colors, sounds, taste, transcending life moments, feelings of connectedness to all of life, a sense of belonging where we are, gratitude, and an enhanced ability to empathically understand and forgive transgression may all be indicative of a shift in consciousness to the right brain.

Besides the potent choice of right-brain versus left-brain perspectives, neuroscientific research has demonstrated that even mundane-seeming choices like a word (and the way it is delivered) in a conversation or in one's thoughts (self-talk) have real and measurable impacts on health and well-being.

Magnetic resonance imaging (MRI) tests have shown that merely seeing the word "NO" for less than a second caused the instant release of stress molecules. When a negative word (anger, threat, danger) is perceived, the amygdala (the portion of our brain responsible for accessing and processing emotional memories) makes an association with a negative emotional memory and begins signaling the hypothalamus to activate the sympathetic nervous system. Epinephrine and norepinephrine are released into the bloodstream, readying us for an imagined foe or dangerous situation, even when there really is none.[5] The mind keeps busy exhausting itself trying to find solutions for mostly imaginary problems.

Unless we interrupt this mechanism consciously, the body responds with increased heart rate and blood pressure, along with changes in blood distribution; and the mind responds with fear-based projection, anger, defensiveness, or an avoidance mechanism instead of with empathy, logic, compassion, or reason (for example). Over time, this self-feeding loop takes its toll on our health and well-being.

However, while it is true that we seem hardwired to respond more strongly to negative situations, it is also true that we can pull our imagination away from the pattern of fear and begin to replace it with one based on positivity. Research has shown that to replace negative patterns (of thoughts and emotions) we must employ a ratio ranging between 3:1[6] to 5:1[7] positivity to negativity.

For most people this is a doable task. We know we can choose our words carefully and genuinely. We can choose to deliver these words in a relaxed and open fashion. We can choose to use our capacity to focus on positivity. In this way conscious choice can change our body and our mind in positive ways that support our health, well-being, and ability to thrive.

Suggested reading: This shift to the right can be learned and achieved without the traumatic experience of a stroke and without the use of cannabis. Several books have been written on the subject, examining the scientific understanding of left- and right-brain activity, and suggesting techniques and exercises to shift consciousness to the right. One of the more popular books is called *Drawing on the Right Side of the Brain* by Betty Edwards.

4. Reprogramming Unhealthy Beliefs and Building Beliefs that Heal

"A belief is not merely an idea the mind possesses; it is an idea that possesses the mind."

—Robert Bolt (*Lawrence of Arabia* and *Doctor Zhivago*)

Which came first, the chicken or the egg? When it comes to belief and experience, it seems that the same question may apply. Our thoughts and feelings shift in a new direction when specific underlying beliefs are challenged and changed.[1] It may help to think of life's experiences as the multidimensional manifestation of our beliefs, or, to put it differently, experiences can be considered our beliefs in motion. Experience tends to change when we make a fundamental shift in belief, choose a new path, or make a profound decision, which leads to a new way of seeing the world.

Belief is a subjective conviction in a so-called truth, or trust in the existence of something without rigorous proof.

Ayaan Hirsi Ali,[2] a Somali feminist, was raised as a Muslim fundamentalist. She describes her thoughts and feelings as a young woman, steeped in her family's culture, living on the Horn of Africa. Ali thought of Westerners and non-Muslims as infidels, and felt that their eternal punishment in the afterlife was just and right. She accepted the subservient roles of women, and she thought of female genital mutilation as normal and religiously justifiable.

It was not until she began to critically examine her religion, her socialization, her way of life, and its impact on women and men alike that her adopted beliefs began to erode and be replaced by new ones. She noticed that as her fundamental belief system shifted, so did her thoughts and feelings. She served a term as a Member of Parliament in Holland, and now she writes and talks about her change of heart and beliefs, and the new set of feelings and thoughts that were generated by them. Ali has continued to make appearances on television, talk shows, and panel discussions where she highlights her changes. Ali now defends equality between the sexes, advocates for human rights and access to education, and vehemently opposes the practice of genital mutilation. She argues with a palpable conviction against the views, beliefs, and practices of many traditional Muslims, clerics, and politicians. Ali not only challenges the tenets of Islam, she focuses particularly on its impact on girls and women in the Muslim world and Muslim families who have migrated to Europe or the U.S.

Ali is only one example of a public figure who demonstrates the connection between belief and experience. Examine any person who has had a change of heart, and you will likely discover an underlying belief that also changed. In health and in healing, it is important to realize that beliefs are not right or wrong. Beliefs are powerful, and they have real physiological consequences, such as female genital mutilations. It is with this in mind that we might want to shift toward beliefs that support life, and dismiss those that hurt life.

Researchers argue that, initially, beliefs are passed on by parents or significant caregivers and are readily received and accepted by the early developing psyche. Consider the work of Bruce Lipton, PhD, author of *The Biology of Belief,* who explores this connection with a puzzle: "Why do we need to teach children how to swim when practical experiences from water births have shown that all children, when born into water, have the innate ability to swim instinctively and without much effort, just like any other mammal?"[3] Lipton posits that children have been given a set of negative beliefs about water by their parents or caretakers, which in turn produces feelings of fear, trepidation, and ultimately the very real inability to swim safely and easily until it is relearned. During the process of learning how to swim, the kids will learn, little by little, to again believe that they can swim with ease and without harm, but it takes time to change their minds and reset their internal architecture.

The Power of Interpretation

While a traumatic or painful event may cause great stress to an organism, the chronic stress resulting from the meanings and negative interpretations of unhealthy beliefs that we often attach to the original event is potentially more debilitating than the original trauma.

Take the deep-seated and common belief that "the world is a scary place" which itself produces chronic fear, aggression, hostility, and a paranoid outlook on the world as a "dog eat dog," "might is right," "winner takes all" environment where competition and domination are forever on the horizon. People with significant fear-based beliefs will often try to control their environment and the people in it. One of several expressions of a fear-based belief structure is commonly referred to as a "type-A personality," which numerous studies have shown to be a potential precursor in the genesis of coronary artery disease.

Another example of real physiological changes stemming from belief-based negative affect comes from research conducted on patients suffering from post-traumatic stress disorder (PTSD). A meta-analysis of available neuroimaging research suggests real and measurable physiological changes in the limbic system in patients with PTSD. Changes occur in the amygdala, the part of the brain responsible for processing fear; the medial prefrontal cortex, involved in decision-making; and the hippocampus, the storage site of long-term memories. During episodes of activated PTSD the hippocampus is diminished in size, and reductions in neuronal integrity and functional integrity are evident. The medial prefrontal cortex also appears to shrink in size during symptomatic PTSD and is less responsive than usual. Finally, neuroimaging research reveals heightened amygdala responsivity during PTSD symptomatic states.[4]

Associated emotional symptoms of PTSD include profound lack of interest in anything, feelings of emptiness, hopelessness, helplessness, worthlessness, shame, emotional numbness, distrust, inexplicable fear, anxiety, impatience, irritability, and hostility. People with PTSD often exhibit paranoid behavior with hypervigilance, lost memories, a passive affect, withdrawal from regular activities, fits of anger with little or no provocation, lack of focus, insomnia, difficulties rising in the morning, fitful sleep with sweating, nightmares, generalized weakness or fatigue, flashbacks, and avoidance of anything associated with the traumatic event. Avoidance strategies can themselves become an additional problem for patients with PTSD. The compounding effect of detachment from actual or potential social supports and unhealthy attempts to reduce tension through substance abuse, overeating, cutting, or unsafe sexual practices can make recovery especially challenging.

The therapeutic benefits of leveraging a patient's belief system to support healing have been examined in recent years in many research studies. It seems that placebos (sugar pills) are just as therapeutic as standard pharmaceutical treatment for a wide variety of diseases.[5] While this may turn out to be bad news for pharmaceutical companies, it highlights the impact of belief on disease, health, and healing.

The Consequences of Belief

It does not matter if a belief is right or wrong. What matters is that they can have real consequences on our health and well-being.

Consciously engaging or increasing the body's own healing abilities may be accomplished by enlisting specific beliefs. In the case of placebos, this entails believing that the provided treatment will be effective. Though the placebo itself is not therapeutic, taking the placebo with the expectation of healing may enhance and focus the self-regenerating powers of the body, mind, and spirit. For the purpose of healing, it may or may not matter whether a belief is factually correct or not. The emotional state that results from one's belief determines the impact of the treatment on one's health. Beliefs can heal or hurt. Fortunately, we can choose to nourish or banish any beliefs we attach to a particular treatment. In this way, we are in control of the results. Some beliefs are more difficult to challenge and change, while others can yield easily.

> Jim used to like tofu. He had learned from his mother, an avid vegetarian, that soy was good for you and healthy. When Jim was finishing his last year at a pre-med college, he came across an in-depth research article written by a prominent scientist and expert in nutrition, published in a journal he had come to trust, that explained in compelling terms why soy is not good for you. Jim changed his mind and chose to avoid soy products. His thoughts and feelings were almost instantly different about tofu and other soy products.

Let's look at another example:

> Sarah grew up with her grandparents. When her grandfather was angry, he gave Sarah the silent treatment or left, slamming the door on his way out. Sarah was scared and felt terribly guilty after

such incidents. Sarah's grandfather instilled in her the belief that "anger is scary and that expressing anger is dangerous and unsafe." As a result, she avoided anger at all costs. While her suppression of anger may have been a useful survival mechanism in her childhood, later in life her anger aversion became a liability.

Sarah's anger aversion attracted abusive relationships, with anger appearing to come at her from seemingly everywhere but herself. Emotionally, she felt always on edge and drained of vitality, and her body felt tense, rigid, and sometimes numb. By the age of 35, she was taking prescription medications for chronic anxiety and high blood pressure.

After unpleasant adverse effects from pharmaceutical medications, Sarah obtained a prescription for cannabis. Her blood pressure dropped almost instantly. More important to her, for the first time in a long time, Sarah felt at ease. "It was like the plant put me in touch with a part of my mind that was fully capable of being relaxed and unencumbered by my normally anxious internal mode of being. I loved this unexpected and much-needed break. But the biggest kicker was that I noticed myself feeling angry as I was thinking of my boyfriend. I noticed a constricting sensation in my body, but I wasn't scared. Instead it was just sort of okay. One moment it was there, and I felt it; then it dissipated like smoke in the wind. I have since been able to repeat the same experience of feeling my anger even when I'm not using cannabis. Perhaps it's been a long time coming, but I do believe now that it is okay to feel angry."

Suggested Reading on the Topic of Changing Beliefs

Richard Bandler and John Grinder. *Neuro-linguistic Programming (NLP). The Structure of Magic, Vol. 1: A Book About Language and Therapy.* Science and Behavior Books, first edition (1975).

Richard Bandler and John Grinder. *Frogs into Princes: Neuro Linguistic Programming.* Real People Press (1989).

Stephen LaBerge, PhD. *Lucid Dreaming.* Ballantine Books (1991).

Sidney Rosen. *Ericksonian Hypnosis. My Voice Will Go with You: The Teaching Tales of Milton H. Erickson.* W. W. Norton & Company (1991).

5. Finding the Silver Lining and Wisdom in Your Illness

In the paradigm of "Disease is a Message," symptoms or diagnosed diseases are a request or demand for change. Here, the symptoms, or more specifically the feeling we have about our symptoms and what they keep us from doing, contain a message about the direction of change we need to take in order to heal.

Focused awareness, whether facilitated by cannabis or some other method, can provide a Rosetta Stone of sorts, that is, a guide for decoding the messages and feedback hidden in our illness.

For instance, psychotherapist Lawrence LeShan has worked with cancer patients for the past 50 years. Based on his extensive and numerous successful experiences with cancer patients (including those diagnosed as "end stage"), he published his findings in research papers and books highlighting a common denominator shared by those patients who went into and maintained remission: authenticity, or having learned to "sing their own song in life."[1] In other words, those patients who went into remission had answered their demand for change by learning to assertively communicate their needs and honestly express their emotions, even those hitherto considered taboo.

Another example comes to us from research conducted on heart disease. Numerous studies have shown that chronic negative affect (e.g., repressed anger, chronic hostilities, impatience) plays an important etiological (causative) role in developing cardiovascular illness.[2] However, when the invitation to change is answered by reducing the intensity and frequency of "hard-heartedness" (negative affect), the opposite is true. By developing qualities such as intimacy, kindness, and compassion within and with those around us, we support a healthy heart. Our ability to manage stress becomes more efficient and effective.[3]

As another example, a study published by the American Psychosomatic Society acknowledges prior reports of precipitating emotional or psychic trauma as a component in herpes breakouts. In particular, the study focused on a patient with repeated outbreaks of HSV-I who was ". . . able to consciously associate a relationship between the outbreak of the skin lesions and the existence of repressed hostility."[4]

Those patients who are able to prevent or abort an outbreak have learned to acknowledge and appropriately express their emotions, fostering a deeper intimacy with themselves and others. Those who have achieved freedom from recurring outbreaks have been able to change the beliefs that initially made suppression of "unacceptable" anger, especially around the area of affection, seem necessary. As a result, they no longer need to suppress anger, suppress what is true for them, or suppress their needs for affection through a kiss.

The interplay of the conscious mind and physiological feedback can serve as a sensitizing agent and reminder to pay attention to messages long before they manifest as highly undesirable symptoms. When initial messages are not acknowledged or responded to, the message may be repeated at a greater volume, that is, with a growing intensity. As the saying goes, an ounce of prevention is worth a pound of cure.

> Hilary was stressed and somewhat overwhelmed with the demands in her life. She had stepped on a nail and it hurt so badly that she had to really be careful about how she placed her foot. After ingesting a carefully dosed edible portion of cannabis, she began to relax, slow down, and just be with her discomforts, both physical and emotional. Hilary felt instantly better, her breathing became deep and calming, and she realized that she needed to slow down. Then she remembered that a week earlier she had gotten a speeding ticket on her way to run some errands. She smiled at herself for missing the initial feedback and message that cost her $156 and was strangely grateful to the ache in her foot. Hilary resolved to slow down.

The Benefits of Looking at Disease as a Message

Disease allows us to experience physically that which has previously been repressed psychologically.

Sometimes disease allows us to experience physically any unfinished psychological work. For instance, suppressed material such as emotions continuously wanders ghostlike between the body and the mind's conscious, subconscious, and unconscious realms. In this sense, suppressed emotions are similar to the elusive nature of most chronic diseases such as hypertension or cancer.

When we are finally ready to respond to the demand for change, it is paramount to interpret and understand the message correctly. If the message indicates that we must express emotions we have labeled "unacceptable" or face memories we have repressed, then this is the corrective action required to alter the internal landscape of our psyche. Traumatic memories may surface from the unconscious and be perceived in a cathartic, corrective, and therapeutic fashion. Through this process, unwanted, unwarranted, unhealthy, or conflicting beliefs—and their negative impact on vitality, aliveness, health, and well-being—may finally be seen and recognized as such by the conscious mind.

The insights resulting from these inner changes can reduce or end self-defeating tendencies and negative patterns that otherwise may lock disease in place. Deeper healing can then occur, healing that transcends a mere cessation of adverse symptoms and encompasses a spiritual dimension as well.

Self-respect grows as one's ability expands to face and deconstruct old emotional material. Self-esteem develops from the careful attention paid to the message and feedback of the disease. Connecting with the meaning of illness can lead to a greater appreciation and connection with our body and the life all around us.

For each disease covered by this book, the "disease as message" theme is probed in the sections related to "Mind-Body Consciousness."

6. Identifying and Dissolving Internal Barriers to Healing

"Condemnation does not liberate, it oppresses."

—C. G. Jung

When resistance to healing is present, a part of the self attributes something positive to the presence of the disease. Perhaps the most difficult thing to do in deep healing is to examine the reasons why you might not want to heal . . . or, if you're honest with yourself, why you aren't eager to be completely well this very minute. A reluctance to completely heal could be a reflection of your yearning for attention from others, a belief that you deserve punishment, misplaced family loyalties, fear of loss, or an idea like "as long as I am sick she will never leave me." Perhaps your illness has become an identity or a way of life, a way to get your needs met, or a means to feel special or in control, or to justify fanatical anger (that is, anger which is righteous, harbored, recycled, and punishing). Perhaps you see your illness as a way to avoid something such as unwanted responsibilities, difficult emotions, or the judgment of others.

"If someone wishes for good health, one must first ask oneself if he is ready to do away with the reasons for his illness. Only then is it possible to help him."

—Attributed to Hippocrates

If this reluctance to fully heal is not addressed and resolved, one will consciously or unconsciously nourish the disease rather than oneself.

> Emily was on vacation in Mexico with her sister Jane and her two nieces. As soon as they got to the beach resort Emily came down with a terrible cold and cough. She was unable to participate in any activities and became confined to her room. Emily was a body-mind therapist so she tried to understand the message of the cough. It did not take her long to determine that her cough was keeping Jane and her kids at a distance. She noticed that she felt angry when coughing. She realized that she did not want to be on vacation with kids, but out of misplaced family loyalties had allowed herself to agree to something she did not really want to do. Once she recognized that she had been using her cough to symbolically bark at her sister and her nieces, Emily also realized that her anger was misplaced. She allowed herself to gently feel her frustration and her anger at the situation and at herself for not respecting her preferences for the kind of vacation she really wanted. As her anger dissipated, she began to let it be okay that she'd messed up. She forgave herself, and within a day or two her symptoms diminished enough that she was able to make something of her remaining time with her family at the lovely tropical beach resort. She had, however, learned her lesson. Future vacations were planned and executed based on respecting what she really wanted, free of obligation.

While this chapter has examined some key elements of the internal mental-emotional architecture of mind, they are not the only possible scenarios. Sometimes the material that demands expression was never repressed. Some patients talk in terms of past-life influences or life-lessons. Others have discovered that, for them, the illness was related to the release of toxins that sometimes occurs when deep and profound internal changes are realized. Yet others have experienced transformations (e.g., a state of extraordinary consciousness) or rediscovered the potency of their attachment to a collective identity (e.g., an intense commitment to sharing a group's/tribe's/family's experience) as part of their very private and subjective healing experience.

Summary

- Suppressed or repressed emotions can make us sick and shorten our lives. They can be found and released, and this is part of the work of getting better.
- Constricting emotions are not themselves harmful to our health, provided they are expressed and let go of appropriately.
- Being prone to expressing expansive or positive emotions strengthens the immune system, improves quality of life, and contributes to longevity.
- To reverse the damaging influence of our avoidance strategies, and the loss of vital energy that comes with it, it is important to begin by accepting where we are, no matter where we find ourselves.
- "We have the power to choose, moment by moment, who and how we want to be in the world."—Jill Bolte Taylor, PhD
- Research has shown that experiencing and expressing gratitude enhances positive affect and results in measurable benefits.
- Merely imagining forgiving an offender produced measurable improvements in heart rate and blood pressure.
- Beliefs are not right or wrong, but in the area of health they have real and measurable physiological consequences. We get to choose.
- Disease is a message. Once the message is acknowledged, resistance to healing is dissolved.
- We approach every symptom or disease with resistance initially. Owning, forgiving, and releasing the resistance speeds recovery.
- Both cannabinoids and consciousness engage the body and the mind simultaneously. This facilitates shifts in awareness important to deep healing.

THE CANNABIS HEALTH INDEX

A Quick Guide to Evidence-Based Confidence Levels and Therapeutic Potentials

As new studies become available we continuously update them in the companion app @cannabishealthindex.com

Disease/Symptom	Number of Studies Reviewed	Combined CHI Value	Evidence-Based Confidence Level
Acid Reflux Disease	1	5	5.00
Age Related Macular Degeneration (ARMD)	1	1	1.00
Aging/Anti-aging	1	2	2.00
AIDS/HIV (in General)	1	3	3.00
Alcohol Dependence/Abuse	4	9	2.25
Alzheimer's Disease	4	10	2.50
Amyotrophic Lateral Sclerosis (ALS)	7	19	2.71
Anorexia & Cachexia	11	28	2.54
Antipyretic (see Fever)			
Antitussive (see Cough)			
Anxieties	4	14	3.50
Arthritis	3	6	2.00
Asthma	7	24	3.43
Atherosclerosis	3	6	2.00
Autism	0	0	0.00
Bacterial Infections (in General)	1	1	1.00
Total Number of Bacterial Studies Included			
Gonorrhea	0	0	0
Methicillin-Resistant Staphylococcus Aureus (MRSA)	1	1	1.00
Bipolar Affective Disorder (BAD)	5	8	1.60
Blood Pressure	2	5	2.50
Bone Cancer	3	8	2.67
Brain Cancer/Glioma/Glioblastoma	9	26	2.88
Brain Attack (CVA/Stroke)	3	8	2.66
Breast Cancer	6	11	1.83
Broken Bones	4	7	2.25

Disease/Symptom	Number of Studies Reviewed	Combined CHI Value	Evidence-Based Confidence Level
Cancer (in General) Total Number of Cancer Studies (not incl. CINV, CINS, or CCC)	50	100	2.00
Bone Cancer	3	8	2.67
Brain Cancer/Glioma/Glioblastoma	9	26	2.88
Breast Cancer	6	11	1.83
Cancer Caused by Cannabis (CCC)	6	-7	-1.17
Cancer Induced Night Sweats (CINS)	1	3	3.00
Cervical Cancer	2	2	1.00
Chemotherapy Induced Nausea & Vomiting (CINV)	24	104	4.33
Colon Cancer (Colorectal)	3	4	1.33
Kaposi's Sarcoma	2	1	0.50
Leukemia and Lymphoma (combined)	7	9	1.29
Liver Cancer	2	4	2.00
Lung Cancer	4	7	1.75
Melanoma (Malignant Skin Cancer)	1	1	1.00
Pains Due to Advanced Cancer	2	10	5.00
Pancreatic Cancer	2	4	2.00
Prostate Cancer	3	3	1.00
Rhabdomyosarcoma	2	1	0.50
Skin Cancer (Non-melanoma)	2	8	4.00
Thyroids Cancer	2	3	1.50
Cardiovascular Diseases (in General) Total Number of Cardiovascular Disease Studies Included	12	29	2.42
Cerebrovascular Accident (CVA)	3	8	2.66
Heart Disease	7	16	2.28
Hypertension	2	5	2.50
Stroke	3	8	2.66
Cerebrovascular Accident (CVA)	3	8	2.66
Cervical Cancer	2	2	1.00
Chemotherapy Induced Nausea & Vomiting (CINV)	24	104	4.33
Childbirth Pain	0	0	0

Disease/Symptom	Number of Studies Reviewed	Combined CHI Value	Evidence-Based Confidence Level
Chronic Obstructive Pulmonary Disease (COPD)	2	3	1.50
Cold & Flu	0	0	0
Colon Cancer (Colorectal)	3	4	1.33
Creutzfeld-Jacob's Disease	1	3	3.00
Cough	4	11	2.75
Cystitis (Interstitial)	1	3	3.00
Delirium tremens (DT's) (see Alcoholism or Seizures)			
Depression	8	23	2.88
Dermatitis	1	4	N/A
Diabetes Mellitus/Diabetes	6	11	1.83
Diabetic Ulcers (see Wound Care, Diabetes)			
Dystonia (see Huntington's Disease)			
Encephalitis	1	2	2.00
Endometriosis	2	5	2.50
Epilepsy	5	13	2.60
Epileptic Seizures	5	13	2.60
Eye Disease & Eye Function (in General) Total Number of Eye Studies Included	14	29	2.07
Age Related Macular Degeneration (ARMD)	1	1	1.00
Glaucoma	9	19	2.11
Improved Night Vision	1	3	3.00
Uveitis	3	6	2.00
Febrile Seizure (see Epileptic seizures and Fever)			
Fever	2	4	2.00
Fibromyalgia	3	14	4.66
Fractured Bones	4	7	2.25
Gastro-Esophageal Reflux Disease (GERD)	1	5	5.00
Glaucoma	9	19	2.11
Glioma/Glioblastoma	9	26	2.88
Gonorrhea	0	0	0

The Cannabis Health Index

Disease/Symptom	Number of Studies Reviewed	Combined CHI Value	Evidence-Based Confidence Level
Hair Growth (Unwanted)	1	4	N/A
Hair Loss/Baldness	1	4	N/A
Heartburn	1	5	5.00
Heart Disease	7	16	2.28
Hemorrhoids	0	0	0
Hepatitis	3	8	2.67
Herpes Virus	3	5	1.67
High Blood Pressure	2	5	2.50
Hirsutism	1	4	N/A
HIV/AIDS	1	3	3.00
Huntington's Disease	5	10	2.00
Hypertension	2	5	2.50
Improved Night Vision	1	3	3.00
Inflammatory Diseases	28	79	2.82
Total Number of Inflammatory Disease Studies Included (incl. Asthma, Dermatitis, Periodontitis, Hepatitis, IBS, GERD)			
Arthritis	3	6	2.00
Asthma	7	24	3.43
Atherosclerosis	3	6	2.00
Cystitis (Interstitial)	1	3	3.00
Dermatitis/Eczema	1	4	4.00
Periodontitis	1	2	2.00
Rheumatoid Arthritis	3	10	3.33
Inflammatory Diseases of the GI Tract	9	24	2.66
Total Number of GI-Based Inflammatory Disease Studies Included (incl. Hepatitis)			
Crohn's Disease (see IBS/IBD)			
Inflammatory Bowel Disease (IBD/IBS)	3	8	2.66
Gastro-Esophageal Reflux Disease (GERD)	1	5	5.00
Hepatitis	3	8	2.66
Pancreatitis	2	3	1.50
Ulcerative Colitis (see IBS/IBD)			

The Cannabis Health Index

Disease/Symptom	Number of Studies Reviewed	Combined CHI Value	Evidence-Based Confidence Level
Injuries (see Wound Care)			
Insomnia	1	5	5.00
Itching	3	10	3.33
Joint Pain (see Arthritis)			
Kaposi's Sarcoma	2	1	0.50
Lack of Appetite (see Anorexia/Cachexia)			
Lack of Female Libido (see Libido)			
Lack of Male Libido (see Libido)			
Libido	1	2	2.00
Liver Cancer	2	4	2.00
Leukemia	5	7	1.40
Lou Gehrig's Disease (ALS)	7	19	2.71
Lung Cancer	4	7	1.75
Lung Diseases	13	38	2.92
Number of Lung Disease Studies Reviewed (incl. Cough)			
Asthma	7	24	3.43
Chronic Obstructive Pulmonary Disease (COPD)	2	3	1.50
Cough	4	11	2.75
Lymphoma	2	2	1.00
Macular Degeneration	1	1	1.00
Mad Cow Disease	1	3	3.00
Manic Depressive Disorder	5	8	1.60
Melanoma	1	1	1.00
Menstrual Pain	1	3	3.00
Mental Disorders (in General)	30	83	2.77
Total Number of Mental Disorder Studies Reviewed			
Attention Deficit Disorder (ADD/ADHD)	6	15	2.50
Anxieties	4	14	3.50
Autism	0	0	0
Depression	8	23	2.88
Manic-Depressive Disorder/Bipolar Affective Disorder (BAD)	5	8	1.60

Disease/Symptom	Number of Studies Reviewed	Combined CHI Value	Evidence-Based Confidence Level
Mental Disorders (in General) *(continued)*			
Post-Traumatic Stress Disorder (PTSD)	3	7	2.33
Schizophrenia	4	16	4.00
Methicillin-Resistant Staphylococcus Aureus (MRSA)	1	1	1.00
Migraines	3	10	3.33
Miscarriage	0	0	0
Morning Sickness	1	3	3.00
Motion Sickness	2	4	2.00
Multiple Sclerosis (MS)	26	91	3.50
Nausea (see Vomiting)			
Neuropathies (in General)	5	15	3.00
Neurological Diseases (in General) Total Number of Neurological Disease Studies Included (exclud. Neuropathies)	69	215	3.12
Alcohol Dependence/Abuse	4	9	2.25
Alzheimer's Disease	4	10	2.50
Amyotrophic Lateral Sclerosis (ALS)	7	19	2.71
Delirium Tremens (see Alcoholism or Seizures)			
Dystonia (see Huntington's Disease)			
Epileptic Seizure	5	13	2.60
Huntington's Disease	5	10	2.00
Multiple Sclerosis	26	91	3.50
Parkinson's Disease	4	14	3.50
Tics (see Tourette's)			
Tourette's Syndrome	10	38	3.80
Neuro-Protective Properties of Cannabis in General Total Number of Studies Included	4	11	2.75
Obstetrical and Gynecological (OBGYN) (in General) Total Number of Gynecological Studies Included	4	11	2.75
Abortion, Miscarriage and Fertility	0	0	0
Childbirth Pain	0	0	0
Endometriosis	2	5	2.50

Disease/Symptom	Number of Studies Reviewed	Combined CHI Value	Evidence-Based Confidence Level
Menstrual Pain	1	3	3.00
Morning Sickness	1	3	3.00
Pregnancy	0	0	0
Osteoporosis	3	5	1.66
Obsessive-Compulsive Disorder (OCD) (see Anxiety)			
Pain (in General) Number of Pain Studies Reviewed (incl. Arthritis and Cystitis Pain)	19	62	3.26
Arthritic Pains	3	6	2.00
Cancer (Pain Due to Advanced)	2	10	5.00
Childbirth Pains	0	0	0
Chronic Non-malignant Pain	2	5	2.50
Cystitis Pains	1	3	3.00
Menstrual Pain	1	3	3.00
Migraines	3	10	3.33
Neuropathies (in General)	5	15	3.00
Neuropathies (AIDS Related)	2	10	5.00
Pancreatic Cancer	2	4	2.00
Parkinson's Disease	4	14	3.50
Periodontitis	1	2	2.00
Post Surgery Wounds	1	4	4.00
Post Traumatic Stress Disorder (PTSD)	3	7	2.33
Prion Diseases	1	3	3.00
Prostate Cancer	3	3	1.00
Pruritis (Itching)	3	10	3.33
Psoriasis	1	4	N/A
Rhabdomyosarcoma	2	1	0.50
Receding Gum Lines (see Periodontitis)			
Rheumatoid Arthritis	3	10	3.33
Schizophrenia	4	16	4.00
Seborrhea	1	4	N/A
Seizures (Epileptic)	5	13	2.60

Disease/Symptom	Number of Studies Reviewed	Combined CHI Value	Evidence-Based Confidence Level
Senile Dementia (see Alzheimer's)			
Sickle Cell Disease	2	5	3.00
Skin Cancer (Non-melanoma)	2	8	4.00
Skin Disease (in General) Number of Skin Disease Studies Reviewed	4	10	2.50
Acne	1	3	N/A
Dermatitis/Eczema	1	3	N/A
Hair Growth (Unwanted) Hirsutism	1	3	N/A
Hair Loss/Baldness	1	3	N/A
Pruritus (Itching)	3	10	3.33
Psoriasis	1	3	N/A
Seborrhea	1	3	N/A
Systemic Sclerosis	1	3	N/A
Spinal Cord Injuries	5	19	3.80
Stroke	3	8	2.66
Systemic Sclerosis	1	3	N/A
Thyroid Cancer	2	3	1.50
Tourette's Syndrome	10	38	3.80
Urethritis (see Interstitial Cystitis or Gonorrhea)			
Ulcerative Colitis (se IBD/IBS)			
Uveitis	3	6	2.00
Venereal Diseases (see Gonorrhea)			
Visual Impairment (see Eye diseases)			
Viral infections Total Number of Viral Studies Included (incl. KS)	14	30	2.14
Colds & Flu	0	0	0
Cough	4	11	2.75
Encephalitis (viral)	1	2	2.00
Hepatitis	3	8	2.67
Herpes	3	5	1.67
HIV/AIDS (in General)	1	3	3.00
Kaposi's Sarcoma	2	1	0.50

Disease/Symptom	Number of Studies Reviewed	Combined CHI Value	Evidence-Based Confidence Level
Vomiting (in General) Total Number of Nausea/Vomiting Studies Included	27	111	4.11
Chemotherapy Induced Nausea and Vomiting (CINV)	24	104	4.33
Morning Sickness	1	3	3.00
Motion Sickness	2	4	2.00
Withdrawal Syndrome (see Alcoholism, Epilepsy)			
Wounds (Post-Surgery)	1	4	4.00
Fractured Bones	4	7	2.25
Spinal Cord Injuries	5	19	3.80
Zoster (Herpes Zoster Virus/Shingles) (See Viral Infection, Herpes Simplex)			

NOTES

Introduction

1. Smith, R. 1991. "Where is the Wisdom...? The poverty of medical evidence." *BMJ* 303:798–99.

2. Sackett, David L., William M.C. Rosenberg, J.A. Muir Gray, R. Brian Haynes, W. Scott Richardson. 1996. "Evidence-based medicine: what it is and what it isn't." *BMJ* 312:7.

3. As of March 2015, the current Evidence-Based Practice Centers are located at:

   - Brown University
   - Duke University
   - ECRI Institute—Penn Medicine
   - Johns Hopkins University
   - Kaiser Permanente Research Affiliates
   - Mayo Clinic
   - Minnesota Evidence-based Practice Center
   - Pacific Northwest Evidence-Based Practice Center—Oregon Health and Science University
   - RTI International—University of North Carolina
   - University of Southern California
   - University of Alberta
   - University of Connecticut
   - Vanderbilt University

For more information visit the website of the U.S. Department for Health and Human Services: Agency for Healthcare Research and Quality, www.ahrq.gov /research/findings/evidence-based-reports/overview/index.html.

Chapter I: The Evidenced-Based Science of Medical Cannabis

1. Matsuda, L.A., Lolait, S.J., Brownstein, M.J., Young, A.C., and Bonner, T.I. 1990. "Structure of a cannabinoid receptor and functional expression of the cloned cDNA." *Nature* 346:561–64.

2. June 2, 2012, PubMed Search for the keyword "Endocannabinoid system" yielded 2,393 published scientific experiments.

3. Wolf, Susanne A., Anika Bick-Sander, Klaus Fabel, Perla Leal-Galicia, Svantje

Tauber, Gerardo Ramirez-Rodriguez, Anke Müller, Andre Melnik, Tim P. Waltinger, Oliver Ullrich, and Gerd Kempermann. 2010. "Cannabinoid receptor CB1 mediates baseline and activity-induced survival of new neurons in adult hippocampal neurogenesis." *Cell Communication and Signaling* 8:12.

4. Dickerson, Sally S., MA, Margaret E. Kemeny, PhD, Najib Aziz, MD, Kevin H. Kim, PhD, and John L. Fahey, MD. 2004. "Immunological Effects of Induced Shame and Guilt." *Psychosomatic Medicine* 66:124–31.

5. June 2, 2012, PubMed Search for the keyword "Cannabinoid" yielded 15,015 published scientific studies.

6. Radwan, ElSohly, El-Alfy, Ahmed, Slade, Husni, Manly, Wilson, Seale, Cutler, Ross. 2015 (May 22). "Isolation and Pharmacological Evaluation of Minor Cannabinoids from High-Potency Cannabis sativa." *J Nat Prod.*

7. Mechoulam, R., Ben-Shabat, S., Hanus, L., Ligumsky, M., Kaminski, N.E., Schatz A.R. et al. 1995. "Identification of an endogenous 2-monoglyceride, present in canine gut, that binds to cannabinoid receptors." *Biochem Pharmacol* 50:83–90.

8. Felder, C.C., Joyce, K.E., Briley, E.M., Mansouri, J., Mackie, K., Blond, O., Lai, Y., Ma, A.L., and Mitchell, R.L. 1995 (Sep). "Comparison of the pharmacology and signal transduction of the human cannabinoid CB1 and CB2 receptors." *Mol Pharmacol* 48(3):443–50.

9. Osei-Hyiaman, D., M. DePetrillo, P. Pacher, J. Liu, S. Radaeva, S. Bátkai, J. Harvey-White, K. Mackie, L. Offertáler, L. Wang, G. Kunos. 2005 (May). "Endocannabinoid activation at hepatic CB1 receptors stimulates fatty acid synthesis and contributes to diet-induced obesity." *J Clin Invest.* 115(5):1298–305.

10. Giuffrida, A., Leweke, F.M., Gerth, C.W., Schreiber, D., Koethe, D., Faulhaber, J. Klosterkotter J., Piomelli, D. 2004 (Nov). "Cerebrospinal anandamide levels are elevated in acute schizophrenia and are inversely correlated with psychotic symptoms." *Neuropsychopharmacology* 29(11):2108–24.

11. Maccarrone, Mauro, Tatiana Lorenzon, Monica Bari, Gerry Melino, and Alessandro Finazzi-Agrò. 2000 (Oct 13). "Anandamide Induces Apoptosis in Human Cells via Vanilloid Receptors: Evidence for a Role of Cannabinoid Receptors." *The Journal of Biological Chemistry* 275:31938–45.

Cozzolino R., Calì, G., Bifulco, M., and Laccetti, P. 2010 (Apr). "A metabolically stable analogue of anandamide, Met-F-AEA, inhibits human thyroid carcinoma cell lines by activation of apoptosis." *Invest New Drugs* 28(2):115–23.

Melck, Dominique, Luciano De Petrocellis, Pierangelo Orlando, Tiziana Bisogno, Chiara Laezza, Maurizio Bifulco, and Vincenzo Di Marzo. 2000. "Suppression of nerve growth factor Trk receptors and prolactin receptors by endocannabinoids leads to inhibition of human breast and prostate cancer cell proliferation." *Endocrinology* 141(1):118–26.

12. United States Patent Application 20060013777. Kind Code A1. Piomelli, Daniele. January 19, 2006. Assignee: The Regents of the University of California. Filed September 12, 2005.

13. Gaoni, Y., and Mechoulam, R. 1964. "Isolation, Structure, and Partial Synthesis of an Active Constituent of Hashish." *J. Am. Chem. Soc.* 86(8):1646–47.

14. Roth, Michael D. 2005 (Apr 7). "Pharmacology: Marijuana and your heart." *Nature* 434:708–09.

15. Hayakawa, K., Mishima, K., Abe, K., Hasebe, N., Takamatsu, F., Yasuda, H., Ikeda, T., Inui, K., Egashira, N., Iwasaki, K., and Fujiwara, M. 2004 (Oct 25). "Cannabidiol prevents infarction via the non-CB1 cannabinoid receptor mechanism." *Neuroreport* 15(15):2381–85.

16. Shmist, Y.A., Goncharov, I., Eichler, M., Shneyvays, V., Isaac, A., Vogel, Z., Shainberg, A. 2006 (Feb). "Delta-9-tetrahydrocannabinol protects cardiac cells from hypoxia via CB2 receptor activation and nitric oxide production." *Mol Cell Biochem* 283(1-2):75–83.

17. Hayakawa, K., Mishima, K., Abe, K., Hasebe, N., Takamatsu, F., Yasuda, H., Ikeda, T., Inui, K., Egashira, N., Iwasaki, K., Fujiwara, M. 2004 (Oct 25). "Cannabidiol prevents infarction via the non-CB1 cannabinoid receptor mechanism." *Neuroreport* 15(15):2381–85.

18. Tashkin, D.P., Shapiro, B.J., and Frank, I.M. 1974 (Apr). "Acute effects of smoked marijuana and oral delta9-tetrahydrocannabinol on specific airway conductance in asthmatic subjects." *Am Rev Respir Dis.* 109(4):420–28.

    Tashkin, D.P., Shapiro, B.J., Lee, Y.E., and Harper, C.E. 1975 (Sep). "Effects of smoked marijuana in experimentally induced asthma." *Am Rev Respir Dis.* 112(3):377–86.

    Williams, S.J., Hartley, J.P., and Graham, J.D. 1976. "Bronchodilator effect of delta1-tetrahydrocannabinol administered by aerosol of asthmatic patients." *Thorax* 31(6):720–23.

    Tashkin, D.P., Reiss, S., Shapiro, B.J., Calvarese, B., Olsen, J.L., and Lodge, J.W. 1977 (Jan). "Bronchial effects of aerosolized delta 9-tetrahydrocannabinol in healthy and asthmatic subjects." *Am Rev Respir Dis.* 115(1):57–65.

    Hartley, J.P., Nogrady, S.G., and Seaton, A. 1978 (Jun). "Bronchodilator effect of delta1-tetrahydrocannabinol." *Br J Clin Pharmacol.* 5(6):523–25.

    Gong, H. Jr., Tashkin, D.P., and Calvarese, B. 1983. "Comparison of bronchial effects of nabilone and terbutaline in healthy and asthmatic subjects." *Journal of Clinical Pharmacology* 23(4):127–33.

19. Karl-Christian Bergmann. "Dronabinol—eine mögliche neue Therapieoption bei COPD-Patienten mit pulmonaler Kachexie." Paper presented at the 2005 Conference of the German Society for Pneumology, Berlin, 17 March 2005. Karl-Christian Bergmann, Allergie- und Asthmaklinik, Bad Lippspringe, Germany.

20. Mechoulam, R., Peters, M., Murillo-Rodriguez, E., and Hanuš, L.O. 2007 (Aug). "Cannabidiol—recent advances." *Chemistry & Biodiversity* 4(8):1678–92.

21. Iuvone, T., Esposito, G., De Filippis, D., Scuderi, C., and Steardo, L. 2009 (Winter). "Cannabidiol: a promising drug for neurodegenerative disorders?" *CNS Neurosci Ther.* 15(1):65–75.

    Sagredo, O., Ramos, J.A., Decio, A., Mechoulam, R., Fernández-Ruiz, J. 2007 (Aug). "Cannabidiol reduced the striatal atrophy caused 3-nitropropionic acid in vivo by mechanisms independent of the activation of cannabinoid, vanilloid TRPV1 and adenosine A2A receptors." *Eur J Neurosci.* 26(4):843–51.

    Fernández-Ruiz, J., Moreno-Martet, M., Rodríguez-Cueto, C., Palomo-Garo, C., Gómez-Cañas, M., Valdeolivas, S., Guaza, C., Romero, J., Guzmán, M., Mechoulam, R., and Ramos, J.A. 2011 (Aug). "Prospects for cannabinoid therapies in basal ganglia disorders." *Br J Pharmacol.* 163(7):1365–78.

    Sandyk, Reuven, Consroe, Paul, Stern, Lawrence Z., and Snider, Stuart R. Tucson, AZ. 1986 (Apr). "Effects of cannabidiol in Huntington's Disease." *Neurology* 36 (Suppl 1):342.

22. Pelliccia, A., Grassi, G., Romano, A., and Crocchialo, P. "Treatment with CBD in oily solution of drug-resistant paediatric epilepsies." Paper presented on 9-10 September, 2005, Congress on Cannabis and the Cannabinoids, Leiden, The Netherlands.

23. Hamelink, Carol, Aidan Hampson, David A. Wink, Lee E. Eiden, and Robert L. Eskay. 2005 (Aug). "Comparison of cannabidiol, antioxidants, and diuretics in reversing binge ethanol-induced neurotoxicity." *JPET* 314(2):780–88.

24. Resstel, L.B., Tavares, R.F., Lisboa, S.F., Joca, S.R., Corrêa, F.M., and Guimarães, F.S. 2009 (Jan). "5-HT receptors are involved in the cannabidiol-induced attenuation of behavioural and cardiovascular responses to acute restraint stress in rats." *Br J Pharmacol.* 156(1):181–88.

25. Parolaro, D., Realini, N., Vigano, D., Guidali, C., and Rubino, T. 2010 (Jul). "The endocannabinoid system and psychiatric disorders." *Exp Neurol.* 224(1):3–14.

26. Crippa, J.A., Zuardi, A.W., and Hallak, J.E. 2010 (May). "Therapeutical use of the cannabinoids in psychiatry." *Rev Bras Psiquiatr.* 32, Suppl 1:S56–66.

27. Lewekel, F.M., Koethe, D., Pahlisch, F., Schreiber, D., Gerth, C.W., Nolden, B.M., Klosterkötter, J., Hellmich, M., and Piomelli, D. 2009. "S39-02

Antipsychotic effects of cannabidiol." *European Psychiatry* 24, Supplement 1:S207.

28. Weiss, L., Zeira, M., Reich, S., Slavin, S., Raz, I., Mechoulam, R., and Gallily, R. 2008 (Jan). "Cannabidiol arrests onset of autoimmune diabetes in NOD mice." *Neuropharmacology* 54(1):244–49.

29. Capasso, R., Borrelli, F., Aviello, G., Romano, B., Scalisi, C., Capasso, F., and Izzo, A. 2008 (July). "Cannabidiol, extracted from Cannabis sativa, selectively inhibits inflammatory hypermotility in mice." *Br J Pharmacol.* 154(5):1001–08.

30. Malfait, A.M., Gallily, R., Sumariwalla, P.F., Malik, A.S., Andreakos, E., Mechoulam, R., and Feldmann, M. 2000 (Aug 15). "The nonpsychoactive cannabis constituent cannabidiol is an oral anti-arthritic therapeutic in murine collagen-induced arthritis." *Proc Natl Acad Sci USA* 97(17):9561–66.

31. Napimoga, M.H., Benatti, B.B., Lima, F.O., Alves, P.M., Campos, A.C., Pena-Dos-Santos, D.R., Severino, F.P., Cunha, F.Q., and Guimarães, F.S. 2009 (Feb)."Cannabidiol decreases bone resorption by inhibiting RANK/RANKL expression and pro-inflammatory cytokines during experimental periodontitis in rats." *Int Immunopharmacol.* 9(2):216–22.

32. Takeda, S., Usami, N., Yamamoto, I., and Watanabe, K. 2009 (Aug). "Cannabidiol-2',6'-dimethyl ether, a cannabidiol derivative, is a highly potent and selective 15 lipoxygenase inhibitor." *Drug Metab Dispos.* 37(8):1733–37.

33. Massi, Paola, Angelo Vaccani, Stefania Ceruti, Arianna Colombo, Maria P. Abbracchio, and Daniela Parolaro. 2004 (Mar). "Antitumor effects of cannabidiol, a nonpsychoactive cannabinoid, on human glioma cell lines." *JPET* 308(3):838–45.

34. Massi, P., Vaccani, A., Bianchessi, S., Costa, B., Macchi, P., Parolaro, D. 2006 (Sep). "The non-psychoactive cannabidiol triggers caspase activation and oxidative stress in human glioma cells." *Cell Mol Life Sci.* 63(17):2057–66. Marcu, J.P., Christian, R.T., Lau, D., Zielinski, A.J., Horowitz, M.P., Lee, J., Pakdel, A., Allison, J., Limbad, C., Moore, D.H., Yount, G.L., Desprez, P.Y., McAllister, S.D. 2010 (Jan). "Cannabidiol enhances the inhibitory effects of {Delta}9-tetrahydrocannabinol on human glioblastoma cell proliferation and survival." *Mol Cancer Ther* 6.

35. Gertsch, J., Leonti, M., Raduner, S., Racz, I., Chen, J.Z., Xie, X.Q., Altmann, K.H., Karsak, M., Zimmer, A. 2008 (Jul 1). "Beta-caryophyllene is a dietary cannabinoid." *Proc Natl Acad Sci USA* 105(26):9099–104.

Horváth, Béla, Partha Mukhopadhyay, Malek Kechrid, Vivek Patel, Gali Tanchian, David A. Wink, Jürg Gertsch, and Pál Pacher. 2012 (Apr 15). "β-Caryophyllene ameliorates cisplatin-induced nephrotoxicity in a cannabinoid 2 receptor-dependent manner." *Free Radical Biology and Medicine* 52(8):1325–33.

36. Legault J., and Pichette, A. 2007 (Dec). "Potentiating effect of beta-caryophellene on anticancer activity of alpha-humulene isocaryophellene and palitaxel." *J Pharm Pharmacol* 59(12):1643–47.

37. Jirovetz, L., Buchbauer, G., Ngassoum, M.B., Geissler, M. 2002 (Nov 8). "Aroma compound analysis of Piper nigrum and Piper guineense essential oils from Cameroon using solid-phase microextraction-gas chromatography, solid-phase microextraction-gas chromatography-mass spectrometry and olfactometry." *J Chromatogr A.* 976(1-2):265–75.

38. Gertsch, J., Leonti, M., Raduner, S., Racz, I., Chen, J.Z., Xie, X.Q., Altmann, K.H., Karsak, M., Zimmer A. 2008 (Jul 1). "Beta-caryophyllene is a dietary cannabinoid." *Proc Natl Acad Sci USA.* 105(26):9099–104.

39. Ahmed, Aftab, M. Iqbal Choudhary, Afgan Farooq, Betül Demirci, Fatih Demirci, K. Hüsnü Can Başer. 2000 (Nov/Dec). "Essential oil constituents of the spice Cinnamomum tamala (Ham.)." *Flavour and Fragrance Journal* 15(6):388–90.

40. Singh, Vineeta, Atul Kumar Gupta, S. P. Singh, and Anil Kumar. 2012. "Direct analysis in real time by mass spectrometric technique for determining the variation in metabolite profiles of Cinnamomum tamala Nees and Eberm genotypes." *The Scientific World Journal.* Article ID 549265, 6 pages.

41. Ajaiyeoba, E.O., and Ekundayo, O. 1999 (Mar/Apr). "Essential oil constituents of Aframomum melegueta (Roscoe) K. Schum. seeds (alligator pepper) from Nigeria." *Flavour and Fragrance Journal* 14(2):109–11.

42. Umukoro, S., and Ashorobi, R.B. 2008 (Feb 12). "Further pharmacological studies on aqueous seed extract of Aframomum melegueta in rats." *J Ethnopharmacol.* 115(3):489–93.

43. Ibid.

44. Umukoro, S., and Ashorobi, R.B. 2007 (Feb 12). "Further studies on the antinociceptive action of aqueous seed extract of Aframomum melegueta." *J Ethnopharmacol.* 109(3):501–04.

45. Ibid.

46. Ndamukong, K.J., Ntonifor, N.N., Mbuh, J., Atemnkeng, A.F., Akam, M.T. 2006 (Mar). "Molluscicidal activity of some Cameroonian plants on Bulinus species." *East Afr Med J.* 83(3):102–09.

47. Umukoro, S., and Ashorobi, R.B. 2004. "Pharmacological evaluation of the antidiarrhoeal activity of Aframomum melegueta seed extract." *West African Journal of Pharmacology and Drug Research* 19.

Umukoro, S., and Ashorobi, R.B. 2005. "Effect of Aframomum melegueta seed extract on castor oil-induced diarrhea." *Pharmaceutical Biology* 43(4): 330–33.

48. Konning, G.H., Agyare, C., and Ennison, B. 2004 (Jan). "Antimicrobial activity of some medicinal plants from Ghana." *Fitoterapia* 75(1):65–67.

49. Kamtchouing, P., Mbongue, G.Y., Dimo, T., Watcho, P., Jatsa, H.B., Sokeng, S.D. 2002 (May). "Effects of Aframomum melegueta and Piper guineense on sexual behaviour of male rats." *Behav Pharmacol.* 13(3):243–47.

50. Jirovetz, L., Buchbauer, G., Ngassoum, M.B., Geissler, M. 2002 (Nov 8). "Aroma compound analysis of Piper nigrum and Piper guineense essential oils from Cameroon using solid-phase microextraction-gas chromatography, solid-phase microextraction-gas chromatography-mass spectrometry and olfactometry." *J Chromatogr A.* 976(1-2):265–75.

51. Chaudhry, N.M., and Tariq, P. 2006 (Jul). "Bactericidal activity of black pepper, bay leaf, aniseed and coriander against oral isolates." *J Pharm Sci.* 19(3):214–18.

52. Nalini, N., Manju, V., and Menon, V.P. 2006 (Summer). "Effect of spices on lipid metabolism in 1,2-dimethylhydrazine-induced rat colon carcinogenesis." *J Med Food.* 9(2):237–45.

53. Gülçin, I. 2005 (Nov). "The antioxidant and radical scavenging activities of black pepper (Piper nigrum) seeds." *Int J Food Sci Nutr.* 56(7):491–99.

54. Silva, Matos, Lopes, F. Silva, Holanda. 2004. "Composition of essential oils from three Ocimum species obtained by steam and microwave distillation and supercritical CO2 extraction." *ARKIVOC.* 4:66–71.

55. Blesching, U., PhD. *Spicy Healing: A Global Guide to Growing and Using Spices for Food and Medicine,* second edition (Berkeley, CA: Logos Publishing, 2009).

56. Pran N. Kaul, Arun K. Bhattacharya, Bhaskaruni R. Rajeswara Rao, Kodakandla V. Syamasundar, Srinivasaiyer Ramesh. 2003 (Jan 1). "Volatile constituents of essential oils isolated from different parts of cinnamon (Cinnamomum zeylanicum Blume)." *IndiaJournal of the Science of Food and Agriculture* 83(1):53–55.

57. Blesching, U., PhD. *Spicy Healing.* See note 55 above.

58. Jamshidi, R., Afzali, Z., and Afzali, D. 2009. "Chemical composition of hydro-distillation essential oil of rosemary in different origins in Iran and comparison with other countries." *American-Eurasian J. Agric. & Environ. Sci.* 5(1):78–81.

59. Blesching, U., PhD. *Spicy Healing.* See note 55 above.

60. Singh, G., Marimuthu, P., de Heluani, C.S., Catalan, C.A. 2006 (Jan 11). "Antioxidant and biocidal activities of Carum nigrum (seed) essential oil, oleoresin, and their selected components." *J Agric Food Chem.* 54(1):174–81.

61. Ibid.

62. Silva, Matos, Lopes, F. Silva, Holanda. 2004. "Composition of essential oils from three Ocimum species obtained by steam and microwave distillation and supercritical CO2 extraction." *ARKIVOC.* 4:66–71.

63. Akah, P.A., John-Africa, Lucy, and Nworu, C.S. 2007. "Gastro-protective properties of the leaf extracts of Ocimum gratissimum L. against experimental ulcers in rat." *International Journal of Pharmacology* 3:461–67.

64. Nwinyi, Obinna C., Chinedu, Nwodo S., Ajani, Olayinka O., Ikpo Chinwe, and Ogunniran, Kehinde O. 2009 (March). "Antibacterial effects of extracts of Ocimum gratissimum and Piper guineense on Escherichia coli and Staphylococcus aureus." *African Journal of Food Science* 3(3):077–081.

65. Calvo-Irabien, L.M., Yam-Puc, J.A., Dzib, G., Escalante-Erosa, F., Peña-Rodriguez, L.M. 2009. "Effect of postharvest drying on the composition of Mexican oregano (Lippia graveolens) essential oil." *Journal of Herbs, Spices & Medicinal Plants* 15(3).

66. Marciele Ribas Pilau, Sydney Hartz Alves, Rudi Weiblen, Sandra Arenhart, Ana Paula Cueto, Luciane Teresinha Lovato. 2011. "Antiviral activity of the Lippia graveolens (Mexican oregano) essential oil and its main compound carvacrol against human and animal viruses." *Brazilian Journal of Microbiology* 42:1616–24.

67. Alma, M. Hakkı; Ertaş, Murat; Nitz, Siegfrie; Kollmannsberger, Hubert. 2007. "Chemical composition and content of essential oil from the bud of cultivated Turkish clove." *BioResources* 2(2):265–69.

68. Blesching, U., PhD. *Spicy Healing.* See note 55 above.

69. Leonard E. Barrett, Sr. *The Rastafarians* (Massachusetts: Beacon Press, 1988), p. 255.

70. Harmatta, J. 1996. "Scythians" in *UNESCO Collection of History of Humanity—Volume III: From the Seventh Century BC to the Seventh Century AD* (Routledge/UNESCO), p. 182.

71. Herodotus. *The Histories of Herodotus,* Book IV, 72 (A. Knopf/Everyman's Library, 1910).

72. *Exodus,* Chapter 30, 30:22–30, 33.

73. Kaplan, Aryeh. *The Living Torah* (Moznaim, 1981), p. 442.

74. The Ebers Papyrus was dated by a reference to the reign of Imhotep to circa 1530 BCE, but other references in the text suggest that it was copied from the original text dating to circa 3000 BCE.

75. *Ebers Papyrus 821* (96, 7–96, 8) SmSmt-Pflanze, zerreiben in Honig, eingießen in ihre Scheide. Das bedeutet eine Zusammenziehung (der Gebärmutter).

76. ProCon.org Medical Marijuana. "Deaths from Marijuana v. 17 FDA-Approved

Drugs" (Jan. 1, 1997 to June 30, 2005)." http://medicalmarijuana.procon.org /view.resource.php?resourceID=000145.

U.S. Department of Health and Human Services. "Substance Abuse and Mental Health Services Administration. Mortality Data from the Drug Abuse Warning Network, 2002." See p. 18, table H, and p. 24 where it states: ". . . *marijuana is rarely the only drug involved in a drug abuse death. Thus, in many MSA's, the proportion of marijuana involved cases labeled as 'one drug' (i.e., marijuana only) will be zero or nearly zero."*

77. CDC. 2008 (Nov 14). "Smoking-Attributable Mortality, Years of Potential Life Lost, and Productivity Losses — United States, 2000—2004." *MMWR* 57(45):1226–28.

78. CDC. 2004 (Sep 24). "Alcohol-Attributable Deaths and Years of Potential Life Lost —United States, 2001." *MMWR* 53(37):866–70.

79. ProCon.org Medical Marijuana. "Deaths from Marijuana v. 17 FDA-Approved Drugs" (Jan. 1, 1997 to June 30, 2005)." http://medicalmarijuana.procon.org /view.resource.php?resourceID=000145.

80. Meier, M.H., Caspi, A., Ambler, A., Harrington, H., Houts, R., Keefe, R.S., McDonald, K., Ward, A., Poulton, R., Moffitt, T.E., Meier, M.H., Caspi, A., Ambler, A., Harrington, H., Houts, R., Keefe, R.S., McDonald, K., Ward, A., Poulton, R., Moffitt, T.E. 2012 (Oct 2). "Persistent cannabis users show neuropsychological decline from childhood to midlife." *Proc Natl Acad Sci USA* 109(40):E2657–64.

81. Silva, P., and Stanton, W. *From Child to Adult: The Dunedin Multidisciplinary Health and Development Study* (Oxford University Press, 1996).

82. Hashibe, M., Morgenstern, H., Cui, Y., Tashkin, D.P., Zhang, Z.F., Cozen, W., Mack, T.M., and Greenland, S. 2006 (Oct). "Marijuana use and the risk of lung and upper aerodigestive tract cancers: Results of a population-based case-control study." *Cancer Epidemiol Biomarkers Prev.* 15(10):1829–34.

83. O'Connell, Thomas J., and Bou-Matar, Ché B. 2007. "Long-term marijuana users seeking medical cannabis in California (2001–2007): Demographics, social characteristics, patterns of cannabis and other drug use of 4,117 applicants." *Harm Reduction Journal* 4:16.

84. Thompson, G.R., Rosenkrantz, H., Schaeppi, U.H., and Braude, M.C. 1973. "Comparison of acute oral toxicity of cannabinoids in rats, dogs and monkeys." *Toxicol Appl Pharmacol* 25:363–72.

85. Gregory T. Carter, Patrick Weydt, Muraco Kyashna-Tocha, and Donald Abrams. 2004 (May). "Medicinal Cannabis: Rational guidelines for Dosing." *IDrugs* 7(5):464–70.

86. Kulshrestha, R., Gupta, C.P., Shukla, G., Kundu, M.G., Bhatnagar, S.P., and Katiyar, C.K. 2008 (Aug). "The effect of water activity and storage temperature on the growth of Aspergillus flavus in medicinal herbs." *Planta Med.* 74(10):1308–15.

Chapter II: The Art and Science of Mind-Body Medicine

1. Helen Flanders Dunbar, *Emotions and Bodily Changes: A Survey of Literature on Psychosomatic Interrelationships, 1910–1933* (New York: Columbia University Press, 1935).

2. Franz Alexander, MD. *Psychosomatic Medicine: Its Principles and Applications* (New York: W.W. Norton & Company Inc., 1950).

3. Dunbar, *Emotions and Bodily Changes*.

4. Alexander, *Psychosomatic Medicine*.

5. Bruce H. Lipton, PhD. *The Biology of Belief: Unleashing the Power of Consciousness, Matter, & Miracles* (Carlsbad, CA: Hay House, 2008).

6. Leremy A. Colf, Alexander J. Bankovich, Nicole A. Hanick, Natalie A. Bowerman, Lindsay L. Jones, David M. Kranz, and K. Christopher Garcia. 2007 (Apr 6). "How a single T cell receptor recognizes both self and foreign MHC." Cell 129(1):135–46.

7. Candace Pert, PhD. *Molecules of Emotions: The Science Behind Body-Mind Medicine* (New York: Simon & Schuster, 1999).

8. Shelley L. Berger, Tony Kouzarides, Ramin Shiekhattar, and Ali Shilatifard. 2009. "An operational definition of epigenetics." *Genes & Dev.* 23:781–83.

9. Brian G. Dias and Kerry J. Ressler. 2014. "Parental olfactory experience influences behavior and neural structure in subsequent generations." *Nature Neuroscience* 17:89–96.

10. Kellermann, N.P. 2013. "Epigenetic transmission of holocaust trauma: can nightmares be inherited?" *Isr J Psychiatry Relat Sci.* 50(1):33–39.

11. Kahn, H.A., Medalie, J.H., Neufeld, H.N., Riss, E., and Gouldbourt, U. 1972. "The incidence of hypertension and associated factors: the Israeli ischemic heart disease study." *Am Heart J* 84:171–82. Cottington, E.M., Mathews, K.A., Talbott, E., Kuller, L.H. 1986. "Occupational stress, suppressed anger, and hypertension." *Psychosom Med.* 48:249–60.

12. Kahn, H.A., Medalie, J.H., Neufeld, H.N., Riss, E., and Gouldbourt, U. 1972. "The incidence of hypertension and associated factors: the Israeli ischemic heart disease study." *Am Heart J* 84:171–82.

13. Pettingale, K.W., Greer, S., and Tee, D.E.H. 1977. "Serum IgA and emotional expression in breast cancer patients." *J Psychosom Med* 21:395–99.

14. Ernest Harburg, PhD, Mara Julius, ScD, Niko Kaciroti, PhD, Lillian Gleiberman, PhD, and M. Anthony Schork, PhD. 2003. "Expressive/suppressive anger-coping responses, gender, and types of mortality: a 17-year follow-up (Tecumseh, Michigan, 1971–1988)." *Psychosomatic Medicine* 65:588–97.

15. Dimidjian, S., and Hollon, S.D. 2010 (Jan). "How would we know if psychotherapy were harmful?" *Am Psychol.* 65(1):21–33.

16. U.S. Department of Health and Human Services. National Institutes of Health. National Center of Complementary and Alternative Medicine (NCCAM). Meditation: An Introduction. Accessed April 15, 2015, http://nccam.nih.gov/health/meditation/overview.htm#sideeffects.

Molecules, Emotions, and Conscious Interventions—Complex Connections in the Endocannabinoid System

ACETYLCHOLINE

1. Tripathi, H.L., Vocci, F.J., Brase, D.A., and Dewey, W.L. 1987. "Effects of cannabinoids on levels of acetylcholine and choline and on turnover rate of acetylcholine in various regions of the mouse brain." *Alcohol Drug Res.* 7(5-6):525–32. Acquas, E., Pisanu, A., Marrocu, P., and Di Chiara, G. 2000 (Aug 4). "Cannabinoid CB1 receptor agonists increase rat cortical and hippocampal acetylcholine release in vivo." *Eur. J. Pharmacol.* 401(2):179–85.

ANANDAMIDE

1. Trezza, Viviana, and Vanderschuren, Louk J.M.J. 2009 (Jan). "Divergent effects of anandamide transporter inhibitors with different target selectivity on social play behavior in adolescent rats." *JPET* 328(1):343–50.

2. Heyman, E., Gamelin, F.X., Goekint, M., Piscitelli, F., Roelands, B., Leclair, E., Di Marzo, V., and Meeusen, R. 2012 (Jun). "Intense exercise increases circulating endocannabinoid and BDNF levels in humans—possible implications for reward and depression." *Psychoneuroendocrinology* 37(6):844–51.

3. Houser, S.J., Eads, M., Embrey, J.P., and Welch, S.P. 2000 (Feb 28). "Dynorphin B and spinal analgesia: induction of antinociception by the cannabinoids CP55,940, Delta(9)-THC and anandamide." *Brain Res.* 857(1-2):337–42.

4. Joseph, J., Niggemann, B., Zaenker, K.S., and Entschladen, F. 2004 (Aug). "Anandamide is an endogenous inhibitor for the migration of tumor cells and T lymphocytes." *Cancer Immunol Immunother.* 53(8):723–28.

5. Raichlen, D.A., Foster, A.D., Gerdeman, G.L., Seillier, A., and Giuffrida, A. 2012 (Apr 15). "Wired to run: Exercise-induced endocannabinoid signaling in humans and cursorial mammals with implications for the 'runner's high'." *J Exp Biol.* 215(Pt 8):1331–36.

6. Pakdeechote, P., Dunn, W.R., and Ralevic, V. 2007. "Cannabinoids inhibit noradrenergic and puringeric sympathetic cotransmission in the rat isolated mesenteric arterial bed." *British Journal of Pharmacology* 152:725–33.

Endogenous Opioids

1. Palkovits, M. 2000 (Oct 8). "The brain and the pain: neurotransmitters and neuronal pathways of pain perception and response." *Orv Hetil.* 141(41):2231–39.
2. Houser, S.J., Eads, M., Embrey, J.P., and Welch, S.P. 2000 (Feb 28). "Dynorphin B and spinal analgesia: induction of antinociception by the cannabinoids CP55,940, Delta(9)-THC and anandamide." *Brain Res.* 857(1-2):337–42.

Gamma-Aminobutyric Acid (GABA)

1. Streeter, C.C., Jensen, J.E., Perlmutter, R.M., Cabral, H.J., Tian, H., Terhune, D.B., Ciraulo, D.A., and Renshaw, P.F. 2007 (May). "Yoga asana sessions increase brain GABA levels: a pilot study." *J Altern Complement Med.* 13(4):419–26.
2. Ehrlich, I., Humeau, Y., Grenier, F., Ciocchi, S., Herry, C., and Lüthi, A. 2009 (Jun 25). "Amygdala inhibitory circuits and the control of fear memory." *Neuron* 62(6):757–71.
3. Lafenêtre, P.I., Chaouloff, F., and Marsicano, G. 2009 (Dec). "Bidirectional regulation of novelty-induced behavioral inhibition by the endocannabinoid system." *Neuropharmacology* 57(7-8):715–21.
4. Streeter, C.C., et al. 2007. "Yoga asana sessions increase brain GABA levels" (see note 1).

Oxytocin

1. Light, K.C., Grewen, K.M., and Amico, J.A. 2005. "More frequent partner hugs and higher oxytocin levels are linked to lower blood pressure and heart rate in premenopausal women." *Biol Psychol* 69:5–21.
2. Grewen, Karen M., PhD, Susan S. Girdler, PhD, Janet Amico, MD, and Kathleen C. Light, PhD. 2005 (Jul 1). "Effects of partner support on resting oxytocin, cortisol, norepinephrine, and blood pressure before and after warm partner contact." *Psychosomatic Medicine* 67(4):531–38.
3. Magon, Navneet, and Kalra, Sanjay. 2011 (Sept). "The orgasmic history of oxytocin: Love, lust, and labor." *Indian J Endocrinol Metab.* 15(Suppl3):S156–S161.
4. Kosfeld, M., Heinrichs, M., Zak, P.J., Fischbacher, U., and Fehr, E. 2005 (Jun 2). "Oxytocin increases trust in humans." *Nature* 435(7042):673–76.
5. Zak, P.J., Stanton, A.A., and Ahmadi, S. 2007 (Nov 7). "Oxytocin increases generosity in humans." *PLoS One* 2(11):e1128.

6. Brody, S. 2006. "Blood pressure reactivity to stress is better for people who recently had penile-vaginal intercourse than for people who had other or no sexual activity." *Biol Psychol.* 71:214–22.

7. Kovács, G.L., Sarnyai, Z., and Szabó, G. 1998 (Nov). "Oxytocin and addiction: A review." *Psychoneuroendocrinology* 23(8):945–62.

8. Vitalo, A., Fricchione, J., Casali, M., Berdichevsky, Y., Hoge, E.A., Rauch, S.L., Berthiaume, F., Yarmush, M.L., Benson, H., Fricchione, G.L., and Levine, J.B. 2009. "Nest making and oxytocin comparably promote wound healing in isolation reared rats." *PLoS One* 4(5):e5523.

9. Yang, J., Yang, Y., Chen, J.M., Liu, W.Y., Wang, C.H., and Lin, B.C. 2007 (May). "Central oxytocin enhances antinociception in the rat." *Peptides* 28(5):1113–19.

10. Legros, J.J. 2001 (Oct). "Inhibitory effect of oxytocin on corticotrope function in humans: Are vasopressin and oxytocin ying-yang neurohormones?" *Psychoneuroendocrinology* 26(7):649–55.

    Ditzen, B., Hoppmann, C., and Klumb, P. 2008. "Positive couple interactions and daily cortisol: on the stress-protecting role of intimacy." *Psychosom Med.* 70:883–89.

11. Kosfeld, M., Heinrichs, M., Zak, P.J., Fischbacher, U., and Fehr, E. 2005 (Jun 2). "Oxytocin increases trust in humans." *Nature* 435(7042):673–76.

12. Gimpl, G., and Fahrenholz, F. 2001 (Apr). "The oxytocin receptor system: structure, function, and regulation." *Physiol Rev.* 81(2):629–83.

13. De Laurentiis, A., Fernández-Solari, J., Mohn, C., Zorrilla Zubilete, M., and Rettori, V. 2010. "Endocannabinoid system participates in neuroendocrine control of homeostasis." *Neuroimmunomodulation* 17(3):153–56.

14. De Laurentiis, A., Fernández-Solari, J., Mohn, C., Burdet, B., Zorrilla Zubilete, M.A., and Rettori, V. 2010 (Apr 15). "The hypothalamic endocannabinoid system participates in the secretion of oxytocin and tumor necrosis factor-alpha induced by lipopolysaccharide." *J Neuroimmunol.* 221(1-2):32–41.

15. Russo, R.I., D'Agostino, G., Mattace, Raso G., Avagliano, C., Cristiano, C., Meli, R., and Calignano, A. 2012 (Nov). "Central administration of oxytocin reduces hyperalgesia in mice: Implication for cannabinoid and opioid systems." *Peptides* 38(1):81–88.

SEROTONIN

1. Williams, E., Stewart-Knox, B., Helander, A., McConville, C., Bradbury, I., and Rowland, I. 2006 (Feb). "Associations between whole-blood serotonin and subjective mood in healthy male volunteers." *Biol Psychol.* 71(2):171–74.

Peirson, A.R., and Heuchert, J.W. 2000 (Dec). "Correlations for serotonin levels and measures of mood in a nonclinical sample." *Psychol Rep.* 87(3, Pt 1):707–16.

2. Perreau-Linck, E., Beauregard, M., Gravel, P., Paquette, V., Soucy, J.P., Diksic, M., and Benkelfat, C. 2007 (Nov). "In vivo measurements of brain trapping of C-labelled alpha-methyl-L-tryptophan during acute changes in mood states." *J Psychiatry Neurosci.* 32(6):430–34.

3. Haj-Dahmane, S., and Shen, R.Y. 2011 (Sep). "Modulation of the serotonin system by endocannabinoid signaling." *Neuropharmacology* 61(3):414–20.

Epinephrine

1. Mezzacappa, Elizabeth S., Katkin, E.S., and Palmer, S.N. 1999. "Epinephrine, arousal, and emotion: A new look at two-factor theory." *Cognition and Emotion* 13(2):181–99.

2. Lutz, B. 2014 (Mar). "An institutional case study: Emotion regulation with HeartMath at Santa Cruz County Children's Mental Health." *Glob Adv Health Med.* 3(2):68–71.

Dopamine

1. Matsumoto, M., and Hikosaka, O. 2009 (Jun 11). "Two types of dopamine neuron distinctly convey positive and negative motivational signals." *Nature* 459(7248):837–41.

2. Badgaiyan, Rajendra D. 2010 (Dec 29). "Dopamine is released in the striatum during human emotional processing." *Neuroreport* 21(18):1172–76.

3. Freestone, P.S., Guatteo, E., Piscitelli, F., di Marzo, V., Lipski, J., and Mercuri, N.B. 2014 (Apr). "Glutamate spillover drives endocannabinoid production and inhibits GABAergic transmission in the Substantia Nigra pars compacta." *Neuropharmacology* 79:467–75.

Castelli, M., Federici, M., Rossi, S., De Chiara, V., Napolitano, F., Studer, V., Motta, C., Sacchetti, L., Romano, R., Musella, A., Bernardi, G., Siracusano, A., Gu, H.H., Mercuri, N.B., Usiello, A., and Centonze, D. 2011 (Nov). "Loss of striatal cannabinoid CB1 receptor function in attention-deficit/hyperactivity disorder mice with point-mutation of the dopamine transporter." *Eur J Neurosci.* 34(9):1369–77.

4. Castelli et al., ibid.

5. Salimpoor, V.N., Benovoy, M., Larcher, K., Dagher, A., and Zatorre, R.J. 2011 (Feb). "Anatomically distinct dopamine release during anticipation and experience of peak emotion to music." *Nat Neurosci.* 14(2):257–62.

6. Kjaer, T.W., Bertelsen, C., Piccini, P., Brooks, D., Alving, J., and Lou, H.C. 2002 (Apr). "Increased dopamine tone during meditation-induced change of consciousness." *Brain Res Cogn Brain Res.* 13(2):255–59.

NOREPINEPHRINE

1. Fernandez-Solari, J., Prestifilippo, J.P., Vissio, P., Ehrhart-Bornstein, M., Bornstein, S.R., Rettori V., and Elverdin, J.C. 2009 (Jun). "Anandamide injected into the lateral ventricle of the brain inhibits submandibular salivary secretion by attenuating parasympathetic neurotransmission." *Braz J Med Biol Res.* 42(6):537–44.

 Kurihara, J., Nishigaki, M., Suzuki, S., Okubo, Y., Takata, Y., Nakane, S., Sugiura, T., Waku, K., and Kato, H. 2001 (Sep). "2-Arachidonoylglycerol and anandamide oppositely modulate norepinephrine release from the rat heart sympathetic nerves." *Jpn J Pharmacol.* 87(1):93–96.

CORTISOL

1. Heyman, E., Gamelin, F.X., Goekint, M., Piscitelli, F., Roelands, B., Leclair, E., Di Marzo, V., and Meeusen, R. 2012 (Jun). "Intense exercise increases circulating endocannabinoid and BDNF levels in humans—possible implications for reward and depression." *Psychoneuroendocrinology* 37(6):844–51.

2. Gruenewald, T.L., Kemeny, M.E., Aziz, N., and Fahey, J.L. 2004 (Nov-Dec). "Acute threat to the social self: Shame, social self-esteem, and cortisol activity." *Psychosom Med.* 66(6):915–24.

GLUTAMATE

1. Navarrete, M., Díez, A., and Araque, A. 2014 (Oct 19). "Astrocytes in endocannabinoid signalling." *Philos Trans R Soc Lond B Biol Sci.* 369(1654).

2. Lafenêtre, P., Chaouloff, F., and Marsicano, G. 2009 (Dec). "Bidirectional regulation of novelty-induced behavioral inhibition by the endocannabinoid system." *Neuropharmacology* 57(7-8):715–21.

3. Ramikie, T.S., Nyilas, R., Bluett, R.J., Gamble-George, J.C., Hartley, N.D., Mackie, K., Watanabe, M., Katona, I., and Patel, S. 2014 (Mar 5). "Multiple mechanistically distinct modes of endocannabinoid mobilization at central amygdala glutamatergic synapses." *Neuron* 81(5):1111–25.

VASOPRESSIN

1. Guastella, A.J., Kenyon, A.R., Alvares, G.A., Carson, D.S., and Hickie, I.B. 2010 (Jun 15). "Intranasal arginine vasopressin enhances the encoding of happy and angry faces in humans." *Biol Psychiatry* 67(12):1220–22.

2. Moons, W.G., Way, B.M., and Taylor, S.E. 2014 (Jun). "Oxytocin and vasopressin receptor polymorphisms interact with circulating neuropeptides to predict human emotional reactions to stress." *Emotion* 14(3):562–72.

3. Marshall, A.D. 2013 (May). "Posttraumatic stress disorder and partner-specific social cognition: A pilot study of sex differences in the impact of arginine vasopressin." *Biol Psychol.* 93(2):296–303.

4. De Laurentiis, A., Fernández-Solari, J., Mohn, C., Zorrilla Zubilete, M., and Rettori, V. 2010. "Endocannabinoid system participates in neuroendocrine control of homeostasis." *Neuroimmunomodulation* 17(3):153–56.

5. Bachner-Melman, R., and Ebstein, R.P. 2014. "The role of oxytocin and vasopressin in emotional and social behaviors." *Handb Clin Neurol.* 124:53–68.

Chapter III: How to Use The Cannabis Health Index

1. Kitty C.M. Verhoeckxa, Henrie A.A.J. Korthout, A.P. van Meeteren-Kreikamp, Karl A. Ehlert, Mei Wang, Jan van der Greef, Richard J.T. Rodenburg, and Renger F. Witkamp. 2006 (Apr). "Unheated Cannabis sativa extracts and its major compound THC-acid have potential immuno-modulating properties not mediated by CB1 and CB2 receptor coupled pathways." *International Immunopharmacology* 6(4):656–65.

2. J. Bruce Moseley, MD, Kimberly O'Malley, PhD, Nancy J. Petersen, PhD, Terri J. Menke, PhD, Baruch A. Brody, PhD, David H. Kuykendall, PhD, John C. Hollingsworth, DrPH, Carol M. Ashton, MD, MPH, and Nelda P. Wray, MD, MPH. 2002. "A controlled trial of arthroscopic surgery for osteoarthritis of the knee." *N Engl J Med* 347:81–88.

3. Požgain I1, Požgain Z, and Degmečić D. 2014 (Jun). "Placebo and nocebo effect: A mini-review." *Psychiatr Danub.* 26(2):100–07.

4. Dean Radin, Leena Michel, Karla Galdamez, Paul Wendland, Robert Rickenbach, and Arnaud Delorme. 2012. "Consciousness and the double-slit interference pattern: Six experiments." *Physics Essays* 25(2).

5. Legault, J., and Pichette, A. 2007 (Dec). "Potentiating effect of beta-caryophellene on anticancer activity of alpha-humulene isocaryophellene and palitaxel." *J Pharm Pharmacol* 59(12):1643–47.

Chapter IV: Diseases and Symptoms A–Z

Aging/Anti-Aging

1. Schulz, T.J., Zarse, K., Voigt, A., Urban, N., Birringer, M., and Ristow, M. 2007 (Oct). "Glucose restriction extends Caenorhabditis elegans life span by

inducing mitochondrial respiration and increasing oxidative stress." *Cell Metab.* 6(4):280–93.

2. Aliev, G., Liu, J., Shenk, J.C., Fischbach, K., Pacheco, G.J., Chen, S.G., Obrenovich, M.E., Ward, W.F., Richardson, A.G., Smith, M.A., Gasimov, E., Perry, G., and Ames, B.N. 2009 (Feb). "Neuronal mitochondrial amelioration by feeding acetyl-L-carnitine and lipoic acid to aged rats." *J Cell Mol Med.* 13(2):320–33.

3. Baker, Darren J., Tobias Wijshake, Tamar Tchkonia, Nathan K. LeBrasseur, Bennett G. Childs, Bart van de Sluis, James L. Kirkland, and Jan M. van Deursen. 2011. "Clearance of p16Ink4a-positive senescent cells delays ageing-associated disorders." *Nature* 479:232–36.

4. Marchalant, Y., Brothers, H.M., Norman, G.J., Karelina, K., DeVries, A.C., and Wenk, G.L. 2009 (May). "Cannabinoids attenuate the effects of aging upon neuroinflammation and neurogenesis." *Neurobiol Dis.* 34(2):300–07.

5. Felder, C.C., Joyce, K.E., Briley, E.M., Mansouri, J., Mackie, K., Blond, O., Lai, Y., Ma, A.L., and Mitchell, R.L. 1995 (Sept). "Comparison of the pharmacology and signal transduction of the human cannabinoid CB1 and CB2 receptors." *Mol Pharmacol.* 48(3):443–50.

6. Ostir, G.V., Markides, K.S., Black, S.A., and Goodwin, J.S. 2000 (May). "Emotional well-being predicts subsequent functional independence and survival." *J Am Geriatr Soc.* 48(5):473–78.

7. Antonio Terracciano, PhD, Corinna E. Löckenhoff, PhD, Alan B. Zonderman, PhD, Luigi Ferrucci, MD, PhD, and Paul T. Costa, Jr., PhD. 2008. "Personality predictors of longevity: Activity, emotional stability, and conscientiousness." *Psychosomatic Medicine* 70:621–27.

8. Danner, D.D., Snowdon, D.A., and Friesen, W.V. 2001 (May). "Positive emotions in early life and longevity: Findings from the nun study." *Pers Soc Psychol.* 80(5):804–13.

9. Jacobs, T.L., Epel, E.S., Lin, J., Blackburn, E.H., Wolkowitz, O.M., Bridwell, D.A., Zanesco, A.P., Aichele, S.R., Sahdra, B.K., MacLean, K.A., King, B.G., Shaver, P.R., Rosenberg, E.L., Ferrer, E., Wallace, B.A., and Saron, C.D. 2011 (Jun). "Intensive meditation training, immune cell telomerase activity, and psychological mediators." *Psychoneuroendocrinology* 36(5):664–81.

10. Horváth, Béla, Partha Mukhopadhyay, Malek Kechrid, Vivek Patel, Gali Tanchian, David A. Wink, Jürg Gertsch, and Pál Pacher. 2012 (April 15). "β-Caryophyllene ameliorates cisplatin-induced nephrotoxicity in a cannabinoid 2 receptor-dependent manner." *Free Radical Biology and Medicine* 52(8):1325–33.

Gertsch, J., Leonti, M., Raduner, S., Racz, I., Chen, J.Z., Xie, X.Q., Altmann, K.H., Karsak, M., and Zimmer, A. 2008 (Jul 1). "Beta-caryophyllene is a dietary cannabinoid." *Proc Natl Acad Sci USA* 105(26):9099–104.

Anorexia and Cachexia

1. Strasser, F., Luftner, D., Possinger, K., Ernst, G., Ruhstaller, T., Meissner, W., Ko, Y.D., Schnelle, M., Reif, M., and Cerny, T. 2006. "Comparison of orally administered cannabis extract and delta-9 tetrahydrocannabinol in treating patients with cancer-related anorexia-cachexia syndrome: A multicenter, phase III, randomized, double-blind, placebo-controlled clinical trial from the Cannabis-in-Cachexia-Study-Group." *J Clin Oncol* 24(21):3394–3400.

2. Gómez, R., Navarro, M., Ferrer, B., Trigo, J.M., Bilbao, A., Del Arco, I., Cippitelli, A., Nava, F., Piomelli, D., and Rodríguez de Fonseca, F. 2002 (Nov 1). "A peripheral mechanism for CB1 cannabinoid receptor-dependent modulation of feeding." *J Neurosci.* 22(21):9612–17.

3. Wilson, M.M., Philpot, C., and Morley, J.E. 2007 (Mar-Apr). "Anorexia of aging in long-term care: Is Dronabinol an effective appetite stimulant?—a pilot study." *J Nutr Health Aging* 11(2):195–98.

4. Jo, Y.H., Chen, Y.J., Chua, S.C., Jr., Talmage, D.A., and Role, L.W. 2005 (Dec 22). "Integration of endocannabinoid and leptin signaling in an appetite-related neural circuit." *Neuron* 48(6):1055–66.

5. Dejesus, E., Rodwick, B.M., Bowers, D., Cohen, C.J., and Pearce, D. 2007. "Use of Dronabinol improves appetite and reverses weight loss in HIV/AIDS-infected patients." *J Int Assoc Physicians AIDS Care* 6(2):95–100.

6. Kirkham, T.C. 2005 (Sep). "Endocannabinoids in the regulation of appetite and body weight." *Behav Pharmacol.* 16(5-6):297–313.

7. Costiniuk, C.T., Mills, E., and Cooper, C.L. 2008 (Apr). "Evaluation of oral cannabinoid-containing medications for the management of interferon and ribavirin-induced anorexia, nausea and weight loss in patients treated for chronic hepatitis C virus." *Can J Gastroenterol.* 22(4):376–80.

8. Beal, J.E., Olson, R., Laubenstein, L., Morales, J.O., Bellman, P., Yangco, B., Lefkowitz, L., Plasse, T.F., and Shepard, K.V. 1995. "Dronabinol as a treatment for anorexia associated with weight loss in patients with AIDS." *Journal of Pain and Symptom Management* 10(2):89–97.

9. Maida, V. "The synthetic cannabinoid Nabilone improves pain and symptom management in cancer patients." Paper presented at the San Antonio Breast Cancer Symposium, December 2006.

10. Nelson, K., Walsh, D., Deeter, P., and Sheehan, F. 1994. "A phase II study

of delta-9-tetrahydrocannabinol for appetite stimulation in cancer-associated anorexia." *Journal of Palliative Care* 10(1):14–18.

11. Plasse, T.F., Gorter, R.W., Krasnow, S.H., Lane, M., Shepard, K.V., and Wadleigh, R.G. 1991 (Nov). "Recent clinical experience with Dronabinol." *Pharmacol Biochem Behav.* 40(3):695–700.

12. Mae Lynn Reyes-Rodríguez, PhD, Ann Von Holle, MS, Teresa Frances Ulman, PhD, Laura M. Thornton, PhD, Kelly L. Klump, PhD, Harry Brandt, MD, Steve Crawford, MD, Manfred M. Fichter, MD, Katherine A. Halmi, MD, Thomas Huber, MD, Craig Johnson, PhD, Ian Jones, MD, Allan S. Kaplan, MD, FRCP(C), James E. Mitchell, MD, Michael Strober, PhD, Janet Treasure, MD, D. Blake Woodside, MD, Wade H. Berrettini, MD, Walter H. Kaye, MD, and Cynthia M. Bulik, PhD. July 2011. "Posttraumatic stress disorder in anorexia nervosa." *Psychosomatic Medicine* 73(6):491–97.

13. Tracey D. Wade, PhD, Marika Tiggemann, PhD, Cynthia M. Bulik, PhD, Christopher G. Fairburn, FMedSci, Naomi R. Wray, PhD, and Nicholas G. Martin, PhD. 2008. "Shared temperament risk factors for anorexia nervosa: A twin study." *Psychosomatic Medicine* 70:239–44.

14. Olga Pollatos, MD, PhD, Beate M. Herbert, PhD, Rainer Schandry, PhD, and Klaus Gramann, PhD. 2008. "Impaired central processing of emotional faces in anorexia nervosa." *Psychosomatic Medicine* 70:701–08.

15. Tirapelli, C.R., de Andrade, C.R., Cassano, A.O., De Souza, F.A., Ambrosio, S.R., da Costa, F.B., and de Oliveira, A.M. 2007 (Mar 1). "Antispasmodic and relaxant effects of the hidroalcoholic extract of Pimpinella anisum (Apiaceae) on rat anococcygeus smooth muscle." *J Ethnopharmacol.* 110(1):23–29.

16. Cuban Ministry of Public Health, Havana. 1992. *Therapeutic Guide to Plant Pharmaceuticals and Honey Pharmaceuticals (Guia Terapeutica Dispensarial de Fitofarmacos y Apifarmacos).* Ministerio de Salud Publica, Ciudad de La Habana, Republica de Cuba.

17. Federal Republic of Germany. *Monographien der E-Kommission (Phyto-Therapie) (380 monographs). A therapeutic guide to herbal medicine evaluating the safety and efficacy of herbs for licensed medical prescribing in Germany.* Published between 1984 and 1994 in the Bundesanzeiger (official publication by the Federal Republic of Germany). Copies of the monographs are available at the Heilpflanzen-Welt Bibliothek: http://buecher.heilpflanzen-welt.de/BGA-Commission-E-Monographs/

18. Cuban Ministry of Public Health, Havana. *Therapeutic Guide to Plant Pharmaceuticals and Honey Pharmaceuticals.* 1992. See note 16 above.

19. Federal Republic of Germany. *Monographien der E-Kommission (Phyto-Therapie) (380 monographs).* See note 17 above.

20. Birdane, F.M., Cemek, M., Birdane, Y.O., Gülçin, I., and Büyükokurolu, M.E. 2007 (Jan 28). "Beneficial effects of Foeniculum vulgare on ethanol-induced acute gastric mucosal injury in rats." *World J Gastroenterol.* 13(4):607–11.

21. Ozbek, H., Ura, S., Dülger, H., Bayram, I., Tuncer, I., Oztürk, G., and Oztürk, A. 2003 (Apr). "Hepatoprotective effect of Foeniculum vulgare essential oil." *Fitoterapia* 74(3):317–19.

22. Cuban Ministry of Public Health, Havana. *Therapeutic Guide to Plant Pharmaceuticals and Honey Pharmaceuticals.* See note 16.

23. Blesching, Uwe, PhD. 2009. *Spicy Healing: A Global Guide to Growing and Using Spices for Food and Medicine* (Berkeley, California: Logos Publishing, 2nd Edition).

24. Cuban Ministry of Public Health, Havana. *Therapeutic Guide to Plant Pharmaceuticals and Honey Pharmaceuticals.* See note 16.

25. Goel, A., Kunnumakkara, A.B., and Aggarwal, B.B. 2008 (Feb 15). "Curcumin as 'Curecumin': From kitchen to clinic." *Biochem Pharmacol.* 75(4):787–809.

26. Federal Republic of Germany. *Monographien der E-Kommission (Phyto-Therapie) (380 monographs).* See note 17.

Bacterial Infections

Gonorrhea

1. Centers for Disease Control and Prevention. Page last updated: September 2, 2010. "Sexually Transmitted Diseases (STDs). Antibiotic-Resistant Gonorrhea. Only one remaining class of antibiotics is recommended for the treatment of gonorrhea." www.cdc.gov/std/gonorrhea/arg/default.htm

2. Giovanni Appendino, Simon Gibbons, Anna Giana, Alberto Pagani, Gianpaolo Grassi, Michael Stavri, Eileen Smith, and M. Mukhlesur Rahman. 2008. "Antibacterial cannabinoids from Cannabis sativa: A structure–activity study." *J. Nat. Prod.* 71(8):1427–30.

3. Touw, Mia. 1981 (Jan-Mar). "The religious and medicinal uses of cannabis in China, India and Tibet." *Journal of Psychoactive Drugs* 13(1).

4. Sam'l O.L. Potter, MA, MD, MRCP (Lond.) 1892. *A Compend of Materia Medica and Therapeutics and Prescription Writing; with especial references to the physiological actions of drugs.* (Philadelphia: U.S. Pharmacopeia. 5th Edition. P. Blakiston, Son & Co.), p. 124.

5. Advertised in the 1935 sales/price booklet, CANNABINE Comp. Mfg. By Chicago Pharmacal Co., 5547 E. Ravenswood Ave., Chicago, USA.

6. Takeda, S., Misawa, K., Yamamoto, I., and Watanabe, K. 2008 (Sep). "Cannabidiolic acid as a selective cyclooxygenase-2 inhibitory component in cannabis." *Drug Metab Dispos.* 36(9):1917–21.

7. Blesching, Uwe, PhD. 2009. *Spicy Healing: A Global Guide to Growing and Using Spices for Food and Medicine* (Berkeley, California: Logos Publishing, 2nd Edition).

8. Koutsky, L. 1997. "Epidemiology of genital human papillomavirus infection." *American Journal of Medicine* 102(5A):3–8.

9. Bergsson, G., Steingrímsson, O., and Thormar, H. 1999 (Nov). "In vitro susceptibilities of Neisseria gonorrhoeae to fatty acids and monoglycerides." *Antimicrob Agents Chemother.* 43(11):2790–92.

10. Bergsson, G., Arnfinnsson, J., Steingrímsson, O., and Thormar, H. 2001 (Oct). "Killing of Gram-positive cocci by fatty acids and monoglycerides." *APMIS.* 109(10):670–78.

11. Bergsson, G., Arnfinnsson, J., Steingrímsson, O., and Thormar, H. 2001 (Nov). "In vitro killing of Candida albicans by fatty acids and monoglycerides." *Antimicrob Agents Chemother.* 45(11):3209–12.

12. Bergsson, G., Arnfinnsson, J., Karlsson, S.M., Steingrímsson, O., and Thormar, H. 1998 (Sep). "In vitro inactivation of Chlamydia trachomatis by fatty acids and monoglycerides." *Antimicrob Agents Chemother.* 42(9):2290–94.

METHICILLIN-RESISTANT STAPHYLOCOCCUS AUREUS (MRSA)

1. Giovanni Appendino, Simon Gibbons, Anna Giana, Alberto Pagani, Gianpaolo Grassi, Michael Stavri, Eileen Smith, and M. Mukhlesur Rahman. 2008. "Antibacterial cannabinoids from Cannabis sativa: A structure–activity study." *J. Nat. Prod.* 71(8):1427–30.

2. Cutler, R.R., and Wilson, P. 2004. "Antibacterial activity of a new, stable, aqueous extract of allicin against methicillin-resistant Staphylococcus aureus." *Br J Biomed Sci.* 61(2):71–74.

3. Tsao, S.M., Hsu, C.C., and Yin, M.C. 2003 (Dec). "Garlic extract and two diallyl sulphides inhibit methicillin-resistant Staphylococcus aureus infection in BALB/cA mice." *J Antimicrob Chemother.* 52(6):974–80.

4. Edwards-Jones, V., Buck, R., Shawcross, S.G., Dawson, M.M., and Dunn, K. 2004 (Dec). "The effect of essential oils on methicillin-resistant Staphylococcus aureus using a dressing model." *Burns* 30(8):772–77.

5. Imai, H., Osawa, K., Yasuda, H., Hamashima, H., Arai, T., and Sasatsu, M. 2001. "Inhibition by the essential oils of peppermint and spearmint of the growth of pathogenic bacteria." *Microbios.* 106 Suppl 1:31–39.

6. Hada, T., Furuse, S., Matsumoto, Y., Hamashima, H., Masuda, K., Shiojima, K., Arai, T., and Sasatsu, M. 2001. "Comparison of the effects in vitro of tea tree oil and plaunotol on methicillin-susceptible and methicillin-resistant strains of Staphylococcus aureus." *Microbios*. 106 Suppl 2:133–41.

7. Bowling, F.L., Salgami, E.V., and Boulton, A.J. 2007 (Feb). "Larval therapy: a novel treatment in eliminating methicillin-resistant Staphylococcus aureus from diabetic foot ulcers." *Care* 30(2):370–71.

Viral Infections (in general)

1. Janice K. Kiecolt-Glaser, PhD, Lynanne McGuire, PhD, Theodore F. Robles, BS, and Ronald Glaser, PhD. 2002. "Psychoneuroimmunology and psychosomatic medicine: Back to the future." *Psychosomatic Medicine* 64:15–28.

   Kiecolt-Glaser, J.K., Loving, T.J., Stowell, J.R., Malarkey, W.B., Lemeshow, S., Dickinson, S.L., and Glaser, R. 2005 (Dec). "Hostile marital interactions, proinflammatory cytokine production, and wound healing." *Arch Gen Psychiatry* 62(12):1377–84.

2. Tabassum, A. Khan, Pratima A. Tatke, and Satish Y. Gabhe. 2006 (Nov 12-16). "Evaluation of aqueous extract of babool pods for in vitro anti-HIV activity." *Int Cong Drug Therapy HIV* 8: Abstract No. P399.

3. Chiang, L.C., Ng, L.T., Cheng, P.W., Chiang, W., and Lin, C.C. 2005 (Oct). "Antiviral activities of extracts and selected pure constituents of Ocimum basilicum." *Clin Exp Pharmacol Physiol*. 32(10):811–16.

4. Bourne, K.Z., Bourne, N., Reising, S.F., and Stanberry, L.R. 1999 (Jul). "Plant products as topical microbicide candidates: assessment of in vitro and in vivo activity against Herpes simplex virus type 2." *Antiviral Res*. 42(3):219–26.

5. Kurokawa, M., Hozumi, T., Basnet, P., Nakano, M., Kadota, S., Namba, T., Kawana, T., and Shiraki, K. 1998 (Feb). "Purification and characterization of eugenine as an anti-herpes virus compound from Geum japonicum and Syzygium aromaticum." *J Pharmacol Exp Ther*. 284(2):728–35.

6. Chaieb, K., Hajlaoui, H., Zmantar, T., Kahla-Nakbi, A.B., Rouabhia, M., Mahdouani, K., and Bakhrouf, A. 2007 (Jun). "The chemical composition and biological activity of clove essential oil, Eugenia caryophyllata (Syzigium aromaticum L. Myrtaceae): a short review." *Phytother Res*. 21(6):501–06.

7. Isaacs, C.E., Kim, K.S., and Thormar, H. 1994 (Jun 6). "Inactivation of enveloped viruses in human bodily fluids by purified lipids." *Ann N Y Acad Sci*. 724:457–64.

8. Esquenazi, D., Wigg, MD, Miranda, M.M., Rodrigues, H.M., Tostes, J.B., Rozental, S., da Silva, A.J., and Alviano, C.S. 2002 (Dec). "Antimicrobial and

antiviral activities of polyphenolics from Cocos nucifera Linn. (Palmae) husk fiber extract." *Res Microbiol.* 153(10):647–52.

9. Kutluay, S.B., Doroghazi, J., Roemer, M.E., and Triezenberg, S.J. 2008 (Apr 10). "Curcumin inhibits herpes simplex virus immediate-early gene expression by a mechanism independent of p300/CBP histone acetyltransferase activity." *Virology* 373(2):239–47.

COLDS AND FLU

1. World Health Organization (WHO). Media Center. "Influenza (seasonal)." Fact sheet No. 211. March 2014. www.who.int/mediacentre/factsheets/fs211/en/

2. Louis Sanford Goodman, Alfred Gilman, Laurence L. Brunton, and John S. Lazo. 2001. *Goodman & Gilman's The Pharmacological Basis of Therapeutics* (New York: McGraw-Hill, 10th Edition).

3. Toby L. Litovitz, MD, Wendy Klein-Schwartz, PharmD, MPH, K. Sophia Dyer, MD, Michael Shannon, MD, MPH, Shannon Lee, BSPharm, CSPI, and Meggan Power. 1998. *Annual Report of the American Association of Poison Control Centers Toxic Exposure Surveillance System 1997* (Elsevier Inc.).

4. The CDC website lists the following "possible side effects of antiviral drugs": "Some side effects have been associated with the use of flu antiviral drugs, including nausea, vomiting, dizziness, runny or stuffy nose, cough, diarrhea, headache and some behavioral side effects." Accessed April 16, 2015. www .cdc.gov/flu/antivirals/whatyoushould.htm

5. Nourjah, P., Ahmad, S.R., Karwoski, C., and Willy, M. 2006 (Jun). "Estimates of acetaminophen (Paracetomal)-associated overdoses in the United States." *Pharmacoepidemiol Drug Saf.* 15(6):398–405.

6. Wolfe, Sidney M., MD. 1989. "Antibiotics." Public Citizen's Health Research Group. Washington, DC. *Health Letter* 5(7):1–5.

7. A relatively unknown fact is that as of April 12, 2005, 11,302 (4,689 autism/ thimerosal and 6,613 non-autism/thimerosal) claims have been filed and compensation totaling more than $1.5 billion has been awarded to 1,910 families. Currently the program covers the following vaccines: diphtheria, tetanus, pertussis (DTP, DTaP, DT, TT, or Td), measles, mumps, rubella (MMR or any components), polio (OPV or IPV), hepatitis B, hepatitis A, Haemophilus influenzae type b (Hib), varicella (chicken pox), rotavirus, and pneumococcal conjugate. As of July 1, 2005, trivalent influenza vaccines have been covered under the VICP (Vaccine Injury Compensation Program). VAERS, P.O. Box 1100, Rockville, Maryland 20849-1100; Phone: 1-800-822-7967.

8. Grace, William J., MD, and Graham, David T., MD. Dept. of Medicine of the New York Hospital–Cornell Medical Center. 1952 (July 1). "Relationship of specific attitudes and emotions to certain bodily diseases." *Psychosomatic Medicine* 14(4):243–51.

9. Sheldon Cohen, PhD, William J. Doyle, PhD, Ronald B. Turner, MD, Cuneyt M. Alper, MD, and David P. Skoner, MD. 2003. *Emotional Style and Susceptibility to the Common Cold.* Department of Psychology (SC), Carnegie Mellon University, Pittsburgh; Departments of Otolaryngology (WJD, CMA) and Pediatrics (DPS), Children's Hospital of Pittsburgh, and the University of Pittsburgh School of Medicine, Pittsburgh, PA; and the Department of Pediatrics (RBT), Medical University of South Carolina, Charleston (now at the University of Virginia Health Sciences Center, Charlottesville, VA). *Psychosomatic Medicine* 65:652–57.

10. Cuban Ministry of Public Health, Havana. 1992. *Therapeutic Guide to Plant Pharmaceuticals and Honey Pharmaceuticals (Guia Terapeutica Dispensarial de Fitofarmacos y Apifarmacos).* Ministerio de Salud Publica, Ciudad de La Habana, Republica de Cuba.

11. Boskabady, M.H., and Ramazani-Assari, M. 2001 (Jan). "Relaxant effect of Pimpinella anisum on isolated guinea pig tracheal chains and its possible mechanism(s)." *J Ethnopharmacol.* 74(1):83–88.

12. Isaacs, C.E., Kim, K.S., and Thormar, H. 1994 (Jun 6). "Inactivation of enveloped viruses in human bodily fluids by purified lipids." *Ann N Y Acad Sci.* 724:457–64.

13. Federal Republic of Germany. *Monographien der E-Kommission (Phyto-Therapie) (380 monographs). A therapeutic guide to herbal medicine evaluating the safety and efficacy of herbs for licensed medical prescribing in Germany.* Published between 1984 and 1994 in the Bundesanzeiger (official publication by the Federal Republic of Germany). Copies of the monographs are available at the Heilpflanzen-Welt Bibliothek: http://buecher.heilpflanzen-welt.de/BGA -Commission-E-Monographs/

14. Cuban Ministry of Public Health, Havana. 1992. *Therapeutic Guide to Plant Pharmaceuticals and Honey Pharmaceuticals.* See note 10.

15. Federal Republic of Germany. *Monographien der E-Kommission (Phyto-Therapie) (380 monographs).* See note 13.

16. Ivanova, D., Gerova, D., Chervenkov, T., and Yankova, T. 2005 (Jan 4). "Polyphenols and antioxidant capacity of Bulgarian medicinal plants." *J Ethnopharmacol.* 96(1-2):145–50.

Cough

1. Gordon, R., Gordon, R.J., Sofia, D. 1976 (Feb). "Antitussive activity of some naturally occurring cannabinoids in anesthetized cats." *Eur J Pharmacol.* 35(2):309–13.

2. United States Patent Application 20060013777. Kind Code A1. Piomelli; Daniele. January 19, 2006. Assignee: The Regents of the University of California. Filed September 12, 2005.

3. Tan, W.C., Lo, C., Jong, A., Xing, L., Fitzgerald, M.J., Vollmer, W.M., Buist, S.A., and Sin, D.D. 2009 (Apr 14). "Marijuana and chronic obstructive lung disease: A population-based study." *CMAJ* 180(8):814–20.

4. United States Patent Application 20060013777; see note 2.

5. Jeanette M. Tetrault, MD; Kristina Crothers, MD; Brent A. Moore, PhD; Reena Mehra, MD, MS; John Concato, MD, MS, MPH; David A. Fiellin, MD. 2007. "Effects of marijuana smoking on pulmonary function and respiratory complications. A systematic review." *Arch Intern Med.* 167(3):221–28.

Encephalitis

1. Solbrig, M.V., Fan, Y., and Hazelton, P. 2013 (Nov 6). "Prospects for cannabinoid therapies in viral encephalitis." *Brain Res.* 1537:273–82.

Hepatitis

1. Venkatesh, L. Hegde, Shweta Hegde, Benjamin F. Cravatt, Lorne J. Hofseth, Mitzi Nagarkatti, and Prakash S. Nagarkatti. 2008 (Jul). "Attenuation of experimental autoimmune hepatitis by exogenous and endogenous cannabinoids: Involvement of regulatory T cells." *Molecular Pharmacology* 74(1):20–33.

2. Costiniuk, C.T., Mills, E., and Cooper, C.L. 2008 (Apr). "Evaluation of oral cannabinoid-containing medications for the management of interferon and ribavirin-induced anorexia, nausea and weight loss in patients treated for chronic hepatitis C virus." *Can J Gastroenterol.* 22(4):376–80.

3. Diana L. Sylvestre, Barry J. Clements, and Yvonne Malibu. 2006 (Oct). "Cannabis use improves retention and virological outcomes in patients treated for hepatitis C." *Eur J Gastroenterol Hepatol.* 18(10):1057–63.

4. Chiang, L.C., Ng, L.T., Cheng, P.W., Chiang, W., and Lin, C.C. 2005 (Oct). "Antiviral activities of extracts and selected pure constituents of Ocimum basilicum." *Clin Exp Pharmacol Physiol.* 32(10):811–16.

5. Chaieb, K., Hajlaoui, H., Zmantar, T., Kahla-Nakbi, A.B., Rouabhia, M., Mahdouani, K., and Bakhrouf, A. 2007 (Jun). "The chemical composition and biological activity of clove essential oil, Eugenia caryophyllata (Syzigium aromaticum L. Myrtaceae): A short review." *Phytother Res.* 21(6):501–06.

6. Deng, Y., Guo, Z.G., Zeng, Z.L., and Wang, Z. 2002 (Aug). "Studies on the pharmacological effects of saffron (Crocus sativus L.)—A review." *Zhongguo Zhong Yao Za Zhi.* 27(8):565–68.

HERPES VIRUS

1. Phan, N.Q., Siepmann, D., Gralow, I., and Ständer, S. 2010 (Feb). "Adjuvant topical therapy with a cannabinoid receptor agonist in facial post-herpetic neuralgia." *J Dtsch Dermatol Ges.* 8(2):88–91.

2. Medveczky, Maria M., Tracy A. Sherwood, Thomas W. Klein, Herman Friedman, and Peter G. Medveczky. 2004. "Delta-9 tetrahydrocannabinol (THC) inhibits lytic replication of gamma oncogenic herpes viruses in vitro." *BMC Med.* 2:34.

3. Blevins, R. Dean, and Dumic, Michael P. 1980. "The effect of Delta-9-tetrahydrocannabinol on Herpes simplex virus replication." *J Gen Virol.* 49:427–31.

4. Schneck, Jerome M. 1947. "The psychological component in a case of Herpes simplex." *Psychosomatic Medicine* 9:62–64.

5. Chiang, L.C., Ng, L.T., Cheng, P.W., Chiang, W., and Lin, C.C. 2005 (Oct). "Antiviral activities of extracts and selected pure constituents of Ocimum basilicum." *Clin Exp Pharmacol Physiol.* 32(10):811–16.

6. Bourne, K.Z., Bourne, N., Reising, S.F., and Stanberry, L.R. 1999 (Jul). "Plant products as topical microbicide candidates: assessment of in vitro and in vivo activity against Herpes simplex virus type 2." *Antiviral Res.* 42(3):219–26.

7. Kurokawa, M., Hozumi, T., Basnet, P., Nakano, M., Kadota, S., Namba, T., Kawana, T., and Shiraki, K. 1998 (Feb). "Purification and characterization of eugenine as an anti-herpes virus compound from Geum japonicum and Syzygium aromaticum." *J Pharmacol Exp Ther.* 284(2):728–35.

8. Chaieb, K., Hajlaoui, H., Zmantar, T., Kahla-Nakbi, A.B., Rouabhia, M., Mahdouani, K., and Bakhrouf, A. 2007 (Jun). "The chemical composition and biological activity of clove essential oil, Eugenia caryophyllata (Syzigium aromaticum L. Myrtaceae): A short review." *Phytother Res.* 21(6):501–06.

9. Esquenazi, D., Wigg, MD, Miranda, M.M., Rodrigues, H.M., Tostes, J.B., Rozental, S., da Silva, A.J., and Alviano, C.S. 2002 (Dec). "Antimicrobial and antiviral activities of polyphenolics from Cocos nucifera Linn. (Palmae) husk fiber extract." *Res Microbiol.* 153(10):647–52.

10. Kutluay, S.B., Doroghazi, J., Roemer, M.E., and Triezenberg, S.J. 2008 (Apr 10). "Curcumin inhibits Herpes simplex virus immediate-early gene expression by a mechanism independent of p300/CBP histone acetyltransferase activity." *Virology* 373(2):239–47.

Aggarwal, B.B., Sundaram, C., Malani, N., and Ichikawa, H. 2007. "Curcumin: the Indian solid gold." *Adv Exp Med Biol.* 595:1–75.

HIV/AIDS

1. Corless, I.B., Lindgren, T., Holzemer, W., Robinson, L., Moezzi, S., Kirksey, K., Coleman, C., Tsai, Y.F., Sanzero, Eller L., Hamilton, M.J., Sefcik, E.F., Canaval, G.E., Rivero Mendez, M., Kemppainen, J.K., Bunch, E.H., Nicholas, P.K., Nokes, K.M., Dole, P., and Reynolds, N. 2009 (May). "Marijuana effectiveness as an HIV self-care strategy." *Clin Nurs Res.* 18(2):172–93.
2. Tabassum, A. Khan, Pratima A. Tatke, and Satish Y. Gabhe. 2006 (Nov 12-16). "Evaluation of aqueous extract of babool pods for in vitro anti-HIV activity." *Int Cong Drug Therapy HIV* 8: Abstract No. P399.
3. Isaacs, C.E., Kim, K.S., and Thormar, H. 1994 (Jun 6). "Inactivation of enveloped viruses in human bodily fluids by purified lipids." *Ann N Y Acad Sci.* 724:457–64.

Cancer (in general)

1. World Health Organization. February 2009. *Fact sheet No 297. Cancer.*
2. Dr. John Gofman, Professor Emeritus in Molecular and Cell Biology at the University of California at Berkeley, demonstrated that past exposure to ionizing radiation partially caused by medical x-rays' procedures is responsible for more than 50% of all cancers, more than 50% of coronary heart disease cases, and about 75% of the breast-cancer problem in the United States:

   Gofman, John W. Radiation from Medical Procedures in the Pathogenesis of Cancer and Ischemic Heart Disease: Dose Response Studies with Physicians per 100,000 Population (San Francisco: Committee for Nuclear Responsibility, 1999).

   Gofman, John W. Preventing Breast Cancer: The Story of a Major, Proven, Preventable Cause of this Disease (San Francisco: Committee for Nuclear Responsibility, 2nd edition, February 1996).
3. Cohn, Victor. "Cancer curb is studied: Doctors eye drug found in marijuana." *Washington Post,* Aug 18, 1974.
4. Pan, H., Mukhopadhyay, P., Rajesh, M., Patel, V., Mukhopadhyay, B., Gao, B., Haskó, G., and Pacher, P. 2009 (Mar). "Cannabidiol attenuates cisplatin-induced nephrotoxicity by decreasing oxidative/nitrosative stress, inflammation, and cell death." *J Pharmacol Exp Ther.* 328(3):708–14.
5. Grossarth-Maticek, R., Siegrist, J., and Vetter, H. 1982. "Interpersonal repression as a predictor of cancer." *Soc Sci Med.* 16(4):493–98.

6. Shaffer, J.W., Graves, P.L., Swank, R.T., and Pearson, T.A. 1987 (Oct). "Clustering of personality traits in youth and the subsequent development of cancer among physicians." *J Behav Med.* 10(5):441–47.

7. LeShan, Lawrence, PhD. *Cancer as a Turning Point: A Handbook for People with Cancer, Their Families, and Health Professionals* (A Plume Book, 1989).

8. Fisher, Seymour, PhD, and Cleveland, Sidney E., PhD. "Relationship of body image to site of cancer." 1956. *Psychosomatic Medicine* 18:304–09.

9. Holland, Jimmie C., MD. 2002. "History of psycho-oncology: Overcoming attitudinal and conceptual barriers.*" Psychosomatic Medicine* 64:206–21.

10. Bacon, C., MD, Rennekerr, R., MD, and Cutler, Max, MD. 1952 (Nov 1). "A psychosomatic survey of cancer of the breast." *Psychosomatic Medicine* 14(6):453–60.

11. Everson, S.A., Goldberg, D.E., Kaplan, G.A., Cohen, R.D., Pukkala, E., Tuomilehto, J., and Salonen, J.T. "Hopelessness and risk of mortality and incidence of myocardial infarction and cancer." *Psychosomatic Medicine* 58(2): 113–21.

12. Meena, P.D., Kaushik, P., Shukla, S., Soni, A.K., Kumar, M., and Kumar, A. 2006 (Oct-Dec). "Anticancer and antimutagenic properties of Acacia nilotica (Linn.) on 7,12-dimethylbenz(a)anthracene-induced skin papillomagenesis in Swiss albino mice." *Asian Pac J Cancer Prev.* 7(4):627–32.

13. Dasgupta, T., Rao, A.R., and Yadava, P.K. 2004 (Feb). "Chemomodulatory efficacy of basil leaf (Ocimum basilicum) on drug metabolizing and antioxidant enzymes, and on carcinogen-induced skin and forestomach papillomagenesis." *Phytomedicine* 11(2-3):139–51.

14. Lee, E.J., and Jang, H.D. 2004. "Antioxidant activity and protective effect on DNA strand scission of rooibos tea (Aspalathus linearis)." *Biofactors* 21(1-4):285–92.

15. Marnewick, J., Joubert, E., Joseph, S., Swanevelder, S., Swart, P., and Gelderblom, W. 2005 (Jun 28). "Inhibition of tumour promotion in mouse skin by extracts of rooibos (Aspalathus linearis) and honeybush (Cyclopia intermedia), unique South African herbal teas." *Cancer Lett.* 224(2):193–202.

16. Kamaleeswari, M., and Nalini, N. 2006 (Aug). "Dose-response efficacy of caraway (Carum carvi L.) on tissue lipid peroxidation and antioxidant profile in rat colon carcinogenesis." *J Pharm Pharmacol.* 58(8):1121–30.

17. Mazaki, M., Kataoka, K., Kinouchi, T., Vinitketkumnuen, U., Yamada, M., Nohmi, T., Kuwahara, T., Akimoto, S., and Ohnishi, Y. 2006 (Feb). "Inhibitory effects of caraway (Carum carvi L.) and its component on N-methyl-N'-nitro-N-nitrosoguanidine-induced mutagenicity." *J Med Invest.* 53(1-2):123–33.

18. Sengupta, A., Ghosh, S., and Bhattacharjee, S. 2005 (Apr-Jun). "Dietary cardamom inhibits the formation of azoxymethane-induced aberrant crypt foci in mice and reduces COX-2 and iNOS expression in the colon." *Asian Pac J Cancer Prev.* 6(2):118–22.

19. Sánchez, A.M., Sánchez, M.G., Malagarie-Cazenave, S., Olea, N., and Díaz-Laviada, I. 2006 (Jan). "Induction of apoptosis in prostate tumor PC-3 cells and inhibition of xenograft prostate tumor growth by the vanilloid capsaicin." *Apoptosis* 11(1):89–99.

20. Beltran, J., Ghosh, A.K., and Basu, S. 2007 (Mar 1). "Immunotherapy of tumors with neuroimmune ligand capsaicin." *J Immunol.* 178(5):3260–64.

21. Banerjee, S., Panda, C.K., and Das, S. 2006 (Aug). "Clove (Syzygium aromaticum L.), a potential chemopreventive agent for lung cancer." *Carcinogenesis* 27(8):1645–54.

22. Banerjee, S., and Das, S. 2005 (Jul-Sep). "Anticarcinogenic effects of an aqueous infusion of cloves on skin carcinogenesis." *Asian Pac J Cancer Prev.* 6(3):304–08.

23. Ramljak, D., Romanczyk, L.J., Metheny-Barlow, L.J., Thompson, N., Knezevic, V., Galperin, M., Ramesh, A., and Dickson, R.B. 2005 (Apr). "Pentameric procyanidin from Theobroma cacao selectively inhibits growth of human breast cancer cells." *Mol Cancer Ther.* 4(4):537–46.

24. Howard, E.W., Ling, M.T., Chua, C.W., Cheung, H.W., Wang, X., and Wong, Y.C. 2007 (Mar 15). "Garlic-derived S-allylmercaptocysteine is a novel in vivo antimetastatic agent for androgen-independent prostate cancer." *Clin Cancer Res.* 13(6):1847–56.

25. Herman-Antosiewicz, A., Powolny, A.A., and Singh, S.V. 2007 (Sep). "Molecular targets of cancer chemoprevention by garlic-derived organosulfides." *Acta Pharmacol Sin.* 28(9):1355–64.

26. Lu, H.F., Yang, J.S., Lin, Y.T., Tan, T.W., Ip, S.W., Li, Y.C., Tsou, M.F., and Chung, J.G. 2007 (Mar-Apr). "Diallyl disulfide-induced signal transducer and activator of transcription 1 expression in human colon cancer colo 205 cells using differential display RT-PCRy." *Cancer Genomics Proteomics* 4(2):93–98.

27. Lee, H.S., Seo, E.Y., Kang, N.E., and Kim, W.K. 2008 (May). "[6]-Gingerol inhibits metastasis of MDA-MB-231 human breast cancer cells." *J Nutr Biochem.* 19(5):313-19.

28. Nomicos, E.Y. 2007 (Nov-Dec). "Myrrh: medical marvel or myth of the magi?" *Holist Nurs Pract.* 21(6):308–23.

29. Shishodia, S., Sethi, G., Ahn, K.S., and Aggarwal, B.B. 2007 (Jun 30). "Guggulsterone inhibits tumor cell proliferation, induces S-phase arrest, and

promotes apoptosis through activation of c-Jun N-terminal kinase, suppression of Akt pathway, and downregulation of antiapoptotic gene products." *Biochem Pharmacol.* 74(1):118–30.

30. Kaseb, A.O., Chinnakannu, K., Chen, D., Sivanandam, A., Tejwani, S., Menon, M., Dou, Q.P., and Reddy, G.P. 2007 (Aug 15). "Androgen receptor and E2F-1 targeted thymoquinone therapy for hormone-refractory prostate cancer." *Cancer Res.* 67(16):7782–88.

31. Ait Mbarek, L., Ait Mouse, H., Elabbadi, N., Bensalah, M., Gamouh, A., Aboufatima, R., Benharref, A., Chait, A., Kamal, M., Dalal, A., and Zyad, A. 2007 (Jun). "Anti-tumor properties of blackseed (Nigella sativa L.) extracts." *Braz J Med Biol Res.* 40(6):839–47.

32. Norwood, A.A., Tucci, M., and Benghuzzi, H. 2007. "A comparison of 5-fluorouracil and natural chemotherapeutic agents, EGCG and thymoquinone, delivered by sustained drug delivery on colon cancer cells." *Biomed Sci Instrum.* 43:272–77.

33. Goun, E., Cunningham, G., Solodnikov, S., Krasnykch, O., and Miles, H. 2002 (Dec). "Antithrombin activity of some constituents from Origanum vulgare." *Fitoterapia* 73(7-8):692–94.

34. Peng, C.H., Su, J.D., Chyau, C.C., Sung, T.Y., Ho, S.S., Peng, C.C., and Peng, R.Y. 2007 (Sep). "Supercritical fluid extracts of rosemary leaves exhibit potent anti-inflammation and anti-tumor effects." *Biosci Biotechnol Biochem.* 71(9):2223–32.

35. Goel, A., Kunnumakkara, A.B., and Aggarwal, B.B. 2008 (Feb 15). "Curcumin as 'Curecumin': From kitchen to clinic." *Biochem Pharmacol.* 75(4):787–809.
    Aggarwal, B.B., Kumar, A., and Bharti, A.C. 2003 (Jan-Feb). "Anticancer potential of curcumin: Preclinical and clinical studies." *Anticancer Research* 23(1A):363–98.

36. Lee, E.J., and Jang, H.D. 2004. "Antioxidant activity and protective effect on DNA strand scission of rooibos tea (Aspalathus linearis)." *Biofactors* 21(1-4):285–92.

37. Marnewick, J., Joubert, E., Joseph, S., Swanevelder, S., Swart, P., and Gelderblom, W. 2005 (Jun 28). "Inhibition of tumour promotion in mouse skin by extracts of rooibos (Aspalathus linearis) and honeybush (Cyclopia intermedia), unique South African herbal teas." *Cancer Lett.* 224(2):193–202.

38. Mitani, H., Ryu, A., Suzuki, T., Yamashita, M., Arakane, K., and Koide, C. 2007 (Apr-Jun). "Topical application of plant extracts containing xanthine derivatives can prevent UV-induced wrinkle formation in hairless mice." *Photodermatol Photoimmunol Photomed.* 23(2-3):86–94.

39. Singh, S.P., Abraham, S.K., and Kesavan, P.C. 1996 (Jul). "Radioprotection of mice following garlic pretreatment." *Br J Cancer Suppl.* 27:S102–104.

40. Cemek, M., Enginar, H., Karaca, T., and Unak, P. 2006 (Nov-Dec). "In vivo radioprotective effects of Nigella sativa L. oil and reduced glutathione against irradiation-induced oxidative injury and number of peripheral blood lymphocytes in rats." *Photochem Photobiol.* 82(6):1691–96.

41. Sharma, M., and Kumar, M. 2007 (Mar). "Radioprotection of Swiss albino mice by Myristica fragrans houtt." *J Radiat Res* (Tokyo) 48(2):135–41.

42. Soyal, D., Jindal, A., Singh, I., and Goyal, P.K. 2007 (Oct). "Modulation of radiation-induced biochemical alterations in mice by rosemary (Rosmarinus officinalis) extract." *Phytomedicine* 14(10):701–05.

43. Horváth, Béla, Partha Mukhopadhyay, Malek Kechrid, Vivek Patel, Gali Tanchian, David A. Wink, Jürg Gertsch, and Pál Pacher. 2012 (April 15). "β-Caryophyllene ameliorates cisplatin-induced nephrotoxicity in a cannabinoid 2 receptor-dependent manner." *Free Radical Biology and Medicine* 52(8):1325–33.

   Gertsch, J., Leonti, M., Raduner, S., Racz, I., Chen, J.Z., Xie, X.Q., Altmann, K.H., Karsak, M., and Zimmer, A. 2008 (Jul 1). "Beta-caryophyllene is a dietary cannabinoid." *Proc Natl Acad Sci USA* 105(26):9099–104.

Bone Cancer

1. Lozano-Ondoua, A.N., Wright, C., Vardanyan, A., King, T., Largent-Milnes, T.M., Nelson, M., Jimenez-Andrade, J.M., Mantyh, P.W., and Vanderah, T.W. 2010 (Apr 24). "A cannabinoid 2 receptor agonist attenuates bone cancer-induced pain and bone loss." *Life Sci.* 86(17-18):646–53.

2. Khasabova, I.A., Khasabov, S.G., Harding-Rose, C., Coicou, L.G., Seybold, B.A., Lindberg, A.E., Steevens, C.D., Simone, D.A., and Seybold, V.S. 2008 (Oct 29). "A decrease in anandamide signaling contributes to the maintenance of cutaneous mechanical hyperalgesia in a model of bone cancer pain." *J Neurosci.* 28(44):11141–52.

3. Idris, A.I. 2008 (Dec). "Role of cannabinoid receptors in bone disorders: Alternatives for treatment." *Drug News Perspect.* 21(10):533–40.

4. If the sternum is counted as 3 bones, the total number of bones is 208.

Brain Cancer

1. CT scans result in a relatively high exposure to cancer-causing ionizing radiation.

2. Surawicz, Tanya S., Faith Davis, Sally Freels, Edward R. Laws, and Herman R. Menck. 1998. "Brain tumor survival: Results from the National Cancer Data Base." *Journal of Neuro-Oncology* 40(2):151–60.

3. Sanchez, Cristina, Maria L. de Ceballos, Teresa Gomez del Pulgar, Daniel
    Rueda, Cesar Corbacho, Guillermo Velasco, Ismael Galve-Roperh, John W.
    Huffman, Santiago Ramon y Cajal, and Manuel Guzman. 2001 (Aug 1).
    "Inhibition of glioma growth in vivo by selective activation of the CB2 can-
    nabinoid receptor." *Cancer Research* 61:5784–89.

4. Massi, Paola, Angelo Vaccani, Stefania Ceruti, Arianna Colombo, Maria P.
    Abbracchio, and Daniela Parolaro. 2004 (March). "Antitumor effects of can-
    nabidiol, a nonpsychoactive cannabinoid, on human glioma cell lines." *JPET*
    308(3):838–45.

5. Massi, P., Vaccani, A., Bianchessi, S., Costa, B., Macchi, P., and Parolaro, D.
    2006 (Sep). "The non-psychoactive cannabidiol triggers caspase activation and
    oxidative stress in human glioma cells." *Cell Mol Life Sci.* 63(17):2057–66.

6. Blázquez, Cristina, Luis González-Feria, Luis Álvarez, Amador Haro, M. Llanos
    Casanova, and Manuel Guzmán. 2004 (Aug 15). "Cannabinoids inhibit the
    vascular endothelial growth factor pathway in gliomas." *Cancer Res.* 64:5617.

7. Guzman, M., Duarte, M.J., Blazquez, C., Ravina, J., Rosa, M.C., Galve-
    Roperh, I., Sanchez, C., Velasco, G., and Gonzalez-Feria, L. 2006. "A pilot
    clinical study of Delta(9)-tetrahydrocannabinol in patients with recurrent glio-
    blastoma multiforme." *Br J Cancer* 95(2):197–203.

8. Galanti, Gil, Tamar Fisher, Iris Kventsel, Jacob Shoham, Ruth Gallily, Raphael
    Mechoulam, Gad Lavie, Ninette Amariglio, Gideon Rechavi, and Amos Toren.
    2008. "*Δ9-Tetrahydrocannabinol inhibits cell cycle progression by down*-regulation
    of E2F1 in human glioblastoma multiforme cells." *Acta Oncologica* 47:1062.

9. Blázquez, C., Carracedo, A., Salazar, M., Lorente, M., Egia, A., González-
    Feria, L., Haro, A., Velasco, G., and Guzmán, M. 2008 (Jan). "Down-
    regulation of tissue inhibitor of metalloproteinases-1 in gliomas: A new marker
    of cannabinoid antitumoral activity?" *Neuropharmacology* 54(1):235–43.

10. Marcu, J.P., Christian, R.T., Lau, D., Zielinski, A.J., Horowitz, M.P., Lee, J.,
    Pakdel, A., Allison, J., Limbad, C., Moore, D.H., Yount, G.L., Desprez, P.Y.,
    and McAllister, S.D. 2010 (Jan). "Cannabidiol enhances the inhibitory effects
    of {Delta}9-tetrahydrocannabinol on human glioblastoma cell proliferation
    and survival." *Mol Cancer Ther* 6.

BREAST CANCER

1. World Health Organization. February 2009. *Fact sheet No 297. Cancer.*

2. U.S. National Institutes of Health. National Cancer Institute. July 23, 2010.
    "Breast Cancer Prevention. Factors Associated with Increased Risk of Breast
    Cancer. Ionizing radiation." www.cancer.gov/cancertopics/pdq/prevention
    /breast/healthprofessional#Section_178

3. Gofman, John W., MD, PhD. *Preventing Breast Cancer: The Story of a Major, Proven, Preventable Cause of This Disease* (San Francisco: Committee for Nuclear Responsibility, 2nd Edition, 1996).

4. Collaborative Group on Hormonal Factors in Breast Cancer. 2002. "Breast cancer and breastfeeding: collaborative reanalysis of individual data from 47 epidemiological studies in 30 countries, including 50,302 women with breast cancer and 96,973 women without the disease." *Lancet* 360(9328):187–95.

5. De Petrocellis, Luciano, Dominique Melck, Antonella Palmisano, Tiziana Bisogno, Chiara Laezza, Maurizio Bifulco, and Vincenzo Di Marzo. 1998 (Jul 7). "The endogenous cannabinoid anandamide inhibits human breast cancer cell proliferation." *PNAS* 95(14):8375–80.

6. Melck, Dominique, Luciano De Petrocellis, Pierangelo Orlando, Tiziana Bisogno, Chiara Laezza, Maurizio Bifulco, and Vincenzo Di Marzo. 2000. "Suppression of nerve growth factor Trk receptors and prolactin receptors by endocannabinoids leads to inhibition of human breast and prostate cancer cell proliferation." *Endocrinology* 141(1):118–26.

7. Ligresti, Alessia, Aniello Schiano Moriello, Katarzyna Starowicz, Isabel Matias, Simona Pisanti, Luciano De Petrocellis, Chiara Laezza, Giuseppe Portella, Maurizio Bifulco, and Vincenzo Di Marzo. 2006 (Sep). "Antitumor activity of plant cannabinoids with emphasis on the effect of cannabidiol on human breast carcinoma." *JPET* 318(3):1375–87.

8. Caffarel, María M., David Sarrió, José Palacios, Manuel Guzmán, and Cristina Sánchez. 2006 (Jul 1). "*Δ9-Tetrahydrocannabinol inhibits cell cycle progression in human breast cancer cells through Cdc2 regulation.*" *Cancer Res.* 66:6615.

9. McAllister, S.D., Christian, R.T., Horowitz, M.P., Garcia, A., and Desprez, P.Y. 2007 (Nov). "Cannabidiol as a novel inhibitor of Id-1 gene expression in aggressive breast cancer cells." *Mol Cancer Ther.* 6(11):2921–27.

10. Caffarel, M.M., Moreno-Bueno, G., Cerutti, C., Palacios, J., Guzmán, M., Mechta-Grigoriou, F., and Sanchez, C. 2008 (Aug 28). "JunD is involved in the antiproliferative effect of Delta9-tetrahydrocannabinol on human breast cancer cells." *Oncogene* 27(37):5033–44.

11. Bacon, C., MD, Rennekerr, R., MD, and Cutler, Max, MD. 1952 (Nov 1). "A psychosomatic survey of cancer of the breast." *Psychosomatic Medicine* 14(6):453–60.

12. Immunoglobulin A (IgA): antibodies made by the body's immune system in response to an invasion such as cancer.

13. Pettingale, K.W., Greer, S., and Tee, D.E.H. 1977. "Serum IgA and emotional expression in breast cancer patients." *J Psychosom Med* 21:395–99.

14. Weihs, Karen L., MD, Timothy M. Enright, PhD, and Samuel J. Simmens, PhD. 2008 (Jan 1). "Close relationships and emotional processing predict decreased mortality in women with breast cancer: Preliminary evidence." *Psychosomatic Medicine* 70(1):117–24.

15. Renneker, Richard E., MD, Robert Cutler, MD, Jerome Hora, MD, Catherine Bacon, MD, Garnet Bradley, MD, John Kearney, MD, and Max Cutler, MD. 1963. "Psychoanalytical explorations of emotional correlates of cancer of the breast." *Psychosomatic Medicine* 25:106–23.

16. White, Victoria M., PhD, Dallas R. English, PhD, Hamish Coates, PhD, Magdalena Lagerlund, PhD, Ron Borland, PhD, and Graham G. Giles, PhD. 2007. "Is cancer risk associated with anger control and negative affect? Findings from a prospective cohort study." *Psychosomatic Medicine* 69:667–74.

17. Chua, S., Arulkumaran, S., Lim, I., Selamat, N., and Ratnam, S.S. 1994. "Influence of breastfeeding and nipple stimulation on postpartum uterine activity." *Br J Obstet Gynaecol.* 101:804–05.

18. Newcomb, P.A., Storer, B.E., Longnecker, M.P. et al. 1994. "Lactation and a reduced risk of premenopausal breast cancer." *N Engl J Med.* 330:81–87.

    Collaborative Group on Hormonal Factors in Breast Cancer. 2002. "Breast cancer and breastfeeding: collaborative reanalysis of individual data from 47 epidemiological studies in 30 countries, including 50,302 women with breast cancer and 96,973 women without the disease." *Lancet* 360(9328):187–95.

    Tryggvadottir, L., Tulinius, H., Eyfjord, J.E., and Sigurvinsson, T. 2001. "Breastfeeding and reduced risk of breast cancer in an Icelandic cohort study." *Am J Epidemiol.* 154:37–42.

19. American Society of Plastic Surgeons (ASPS). 2000/2007/2008 "National Plastic Surgery Statistics." Accessed April 16, 2015. www.plasticsurgery.org /Documents/news-resources/statistics/2008-statistics/2008-top-5-cosmetic -surgery-procedures-graph.pdf

20. American Cancer Society. 2010. "Cancer Facts and Figures 2010." Atlanta, GA. Accessed April 16, 2015. www.cancer.org/acs/groups/content/@nho /documents/document/acspc-024113.pdf

21. Kassi, E., Papoutsi, Z., Fokialakis, N., Messari, I., Mitakou, S., and Moutsatsou, P. 2004 (Nov 17). "Greek plant extracts exhibit selective estrogen receptor modulator (SERM)-like properties." *J Agric Food Chem.* 52(23):6956–61.

22. Ramljak, D., Romanczyk, L.J., Metheny-Barlow, L.J., Thompson, N., Knezevic, V., Galperin, M., Ramesh, A., and Dickson, R.B. 2005 (Apr). "Pentameric procyanidin from Theobroma cacao selectively inhibits growth of human breast cancer cells." *Mol Cancer Ther.* 4(4):537–46.

23. Lee, H.S., Seo, E.Y., Kang, N.E., and Kim, W.K. 2008 (May). "[6]-Gingerol inhibits metastasis of MDA-MB-231 human breast cancer cells." *J Nutr Biochem.* 19(5):313-19.

24. Nomicos, E.Y. 2007 (Nov-Dec). "Myrrh: medical marvel or myth of the magi?" *Holist Nurs Pract.* 21(6):308–23.

25. Shishodia, S., Sethi, G., Ahn, K.S., and Aggarwal, B.B. 2007 (Jun 30). "Guggulsterone inhibits tumor cell proliferation, induces S-phase arrest, and promotes apoptosis through activation of c-Jun N-terminal kinase, suppression of Akt pathway, and downregulation of antiapoptotic gene products." *Biochem Pharmacol.* 74(1):118–30.

CANCER CAUSED BY CANNABIS?

1. Trabert, B., Sigurdson, A.J., Sweeney, A.M., Strom, S.S., and McGlynn, K.A. 2011 (Feb 15). "Marijuana use and testicular germ cell tumors." *Cancer* 117(4):848–53.

2. Singh, R., Sandhu, J., Kaur, B., Juren, T., Steward, W.P., Segerbäck, D., and Farmer, P.B. 2009 (Jun). "Evaluation of the DNA-damaging potential of cannabis cigarette smoke by the determination of acetaldehyde-derived N2-ethyl-2'-deoxyguanosine adducts." *Chem Res Toxicol.* 22(6):1181–88.

3. Berthiller, J., Straif, K., Boniol, M., Voirin, N., Benhaïm-Luzon, V., Ayoub, W.B., Dari, I., Laouamri, S., Hamdi-Cherif, M., Bartal, M., Ayed, F.B., and Sasco, A.J. 2008 (Dec). "Cannabis smoking and risk of lung cancer in men: A pooled analysis of three studies in Maghreb." *J Thorac Oncol.* 3(12): 1398–403.

4. Aldington, S., Harwood, M., Cox, B., Weatherall, M., Beckert, L., Hansell, A., Pritchard, A., Robinson, G., and Beasley, R. 2008 (Feb). "Cannabis use and risk of lung cancer: A case-control study." *Eur Respir J.* 31(2):280–86.

5. Hashibe, M., Morgenstern, H., Cui, Y., Tashkin, D.P., Zhang, Z.F., Cozen, W., Mack, T.M., and Greenland, S. 2006 (Oct). "Marijuana use and the risk of lung and upper aerodigestive tract cancers: Results of a population-based case-control study." *Cancer Epidemiol Biomarkers Prev.* 15(10):1829–34.

6. Hashibe, M., Straif, K., Tashkin, D.P., Morgenstern, H., Greenland, S., and Zhang, Z.F. 2005 (Apr). "Epidemiologic review of marijuana use and cancer risk." *Alcohol* 35(3):265–75.

CANCER-INDUCED NIGHT SWEATS

1. Hayakawa, K., Mishima, K., Nozako, M., Hazekawa, M., Ogata, A., Fujioka, M., Harada, K., Mishima, S., Orito, K., Egashira, N., Iwasaki, K., and Fujiwara, M. 2007 (Mar 27). "Delta9-tetrahydrocannabinol (Delta9-THC)

prevents cerebral infarction via hypothalamic-independent hypothermia." *Life Sci.* 80(16):1466–71.

2. Maida, V. 2008 (Jul). "Nabilone for the treatment of paraneoplastic night sweats: A report of four cases." *J Palliat Med.* 11(6):929–34.

CERVICAL CANCER

1. Sedjo, R.L., Roe, D.J., Abrahamsen, M., Harris, R.B., Craft, N., Baldwin, S., Giuliano, A.R. 2002 (Sep). "Vitamin A, carotenoids, and risk of persistent oncogenic human papillomavirus infection." *Cancer Epidemiol Biomarkers Prev.* 11(9):876–84.

2. Contassot, E., Tenan, M., Schnüriger, V., Pelte, M.F., and Dietrich, P.Y. 2004 (Apr). "Arachidonyl ethanolamide induces apoptosis of uterine cervix cancer cells via aberrantly expressed vanilloid receptor-1." *Gynecol Oncol.* 93(1):182–88.

3. Ramer, R., and Hinz, B. 2008 (Jan 2). "Inhibition of cancer cell invasion by cannabinoids via increased expression of tissue inhibitor of matrix metalloproteinases-1." *J Natl Cancer Inst.* 100(1):59–69.

4. Deng, Y., Guo, Z.G., Zeng, Z.L., and Wang, Z. 2002 (Aug). "Studies on the pharmacological effects of saffron (Crocus sativus L.)—A review." *Zhongguo Zhong Yao Za Zhi.* 27(8):565–68.

Colon Cancer

1. National Cancer Institute at the National Institutes for Health. "Colon and Rectal Cancer. Estimated new cases and deaths from colon and rectal cancer in the United States in 2010." www.cancer.gov/cancertopics/types/colon-and-rectal

2. Ruhaak, L.R., Felth, J., Karlsson, P.C., Rafter, J.J., Verpoorte, R., and Bohlin, L. 2011. "Evaluation of the cyclooxygenase-inhibiting effects of six major cannabinoids isolated from Cannabis sativa." *Biol Pharm Bull.* 34(5):774–78.

3. Patsos, H.A., Hicks, D.J., Dobson, R.R.H., Greenhough, A., Woodman, N., Lane, J.D., Williams, A.C., and Paraskeva, C. 2005. "The endogenous cannabinoid, anandamide, induces cell death in colorectal carcinoma cells: A possible role for cyclooxygenase 2." *Gut* 54:1741–50.

4. Wang, D., Wang, H. Ning, W., Backlund, M.G, Dey, S.K., and Dubois, R.N. 2008 (Aug 1). "Loss of cannabinoid receptor 1 accelerates intestinal tumor growth." *Cancer Res.* 68(15):6468–76.

5. Kune, Gabriel A., Susan Kune, Lyndsey F. Watson, and Claus Bahne Bahnson. 1991. "Personality as a risk factor in large bowel cancer: Data from the Melbourne Colorectal Cancer Study." *Psychological Medicine* 21:29–41.

6. Dasgupta, T., Rao, A.R., and Yadava, P.K. 2004 (Feb). "Chemomodulatory efficacy of basil leaf (Ocimum basilicum) on drug metabolizing and antioxi-

dant enzymes, and on carcinogen-induced skin and forestomach papilloma-genesis." *Phytomedicine* 11(2-3):139–51.

7. Kamaleeswari, M., and Nalini, N. 2006 (Aug). "Dose-response efficacy of caraway (Carum carvi L.) on tissue lipid peroxidation and antioxidant profile in rat colon carcinogenesis." *J Pharm Pharmacol.* 58(8):1121–30.

8. Deeptha, K., Kamaleeswari, M., Sengottuvelan, M., and Nalini, N. 2006 (Nov). "Dose-dependent inhibitory effect of dietary caraway on 1,2-dimethylhydrazine-induced colonic aberrant crypt foci and bacterial enzyme activity in rats." *Invest New Drugs.* 24(6):479–88.

9. Sengupta, A., Ghosh, S., and Bhattacharjee, S. 2005 (Apr-Jun). "Dietary cardamom inhibits the formation of azoxymethane-induced aberrant crypt foci in mice and reduces COX-2 and iNOS expression in the colon." *Asian Pac J Cancer Prev.* 6(2):118–22.

10. Nalini, N., Manju, V., and Menon, V.P. 2006 (Summer). "Effect of spices on lipid metabolism in 1,2-dimethylhydrazine-induced rat colon carcinogenesis." *J Med Food.* 9(2):237–45.

11. Gagandeep Dhanalakshmi S., Méndiz, E., Rao, A.R., and Kale, R.K. (2003). "Chemopreventive effects of Cuminum cyminum in chemically induced fore-stomach and uterine cervix tumors in murine model systems." *Nutr Cancer.* 47(2):171–80.

12. Norwood, A.A., Tucci, M., and Benghuzzi, H. 2007. "A comparison of 5-fluorouracil and natural chemotherapeutic agents, EGCG and thymoqui-none, delivered by sustained drug delivery on colon cancer cells." *Biomed Sci Instrum.* 43:272–77.

13. Deng, Y., Guo, Z.G., Zeng, Z.L., and Wang, Z. 2002 (Aug). "Studies on the pharmacological effects of saffron (Crocus sativus L.)—A review." *Zhongguo Zhong Yao Za Zhi.* 27(8):565–68.

14. Goel, A., Kunnumakkara, A.B., and Aggarwal, B.B. 2008 (Feb 15). "Curcumin as 'Curecumin': From kitchen to clinic." *Biochem Pharmacol.* 75(4):787–809.

Kaposi's Sarcoma (KS)

1. Luca, T., Di Benedetto, G., Scuderi, M.R., Palumbo, M., Clementi, S., Ber-nardini, R., and Cantarella, G. 2009 (Aug 15). "The CB(1)/CB(2) receptor agonist WIN-55,212-2 reduces viability of human Kaposi's sarcoma cells in vitro." *Eur J Pharmacol.* 616(1-3):16–21.

2. Chao, C., Jacobson, L.P., Jenkins, F.J., Tashkin, D., Martínez-Maza, O., Roth, M.D., Ng, L., Margolick, J.B., Chmiel, J.S., Zhang, Z.F., and Detels, R. 2009 (Feb). "Recreational drug use and risk of Kaposi's Sarcoma in HIV- and HHV-8-coinfected homosexual men." *AIDS Res Hum Retroviruses.* 25(2):149–56.

LEUKEMIA AND LYMPHOMA (IN GENERAL)

1. Howlader, N., Noone, A.M., Krapcho, M., Neyman, N., Aminou, R., Waldron, W., Altekruse, S.F., Kosary, C.L., Ruhl, J., Tatalovich, Z., Cho, H., Mariotto, A., Eisner, M.P., Lewis, D.R., Chen, H.S., Feuer, E.J., Cronin, K.A., and Edwards, B.K. (eds). "SEER Cancer Statistics Review, 1975-2008," National Cancer Institute, Bethesda, MD, http://seer.cancer.gov/csr /1975_2008/, based on November 2010 SEER data submission, posted to the SEER website, 2011.

2. World Health Organization (WHO). 2002. IARC Monographs on the Evaluation of Carcinogenic Risks to Humans. Non-Ionizing Radiation, Part 1: Static and Extremely Low-Frequency (ELF) Electric and Magnetic Fields. Volume 80." Accessed April 16, 2015. http://monographs.iarc.fr/ENG/Monographs/vol80/

LEUKEMIA

1. Thomas Powles, Robert te Poele, Jonathan Shamash, Tracy Chaplin, David Propper, Simon Joel, Tim Oliver, and Wai Man Liu. 2005 (Feb 1). "Cannabis-induced cytotoxicity in leukemic cell lines: The role of the cannabinoid receptors and the MAPK pathway." *Blood* 105(3):1214–21.

2. Liu, W.M., Scott, K.A., Shamash, J., Joel, S., and Powles, T.B. 2008 (Sep). "Enhancing the in vitro cytotoxic activity of Delta(9)-tetrahydrocannabinol in leukemic cells through a combinatorial approach." *Leuk Lymphoma.* 49(9):1800–09.

3. Robert J. McKallip, Wentao Jia, Jerome Schlomer, James W. Warren, Prakash S. Nagarkatti, and Mitzi Nagarkatti. 2006 (Sep). "Cannabidiol-induced apoptosis in human leukemia cells: A novel role of cannabidiol in the regulation of p22phox and Nox4 expression." *Mol Pharmacol.* 70(3):897–908.

4. Wentao Jia, Venkatesh L. Hegde, Narendra P. Singh, Daniel Sisco, Steven Grant, Mitzi Nagarkatti, and Prakash S. Nagarkatti. 2006. "*Δ9-Tetrahydrocannabinol-induced apoptosis in Jurkat leukemia T cells is regulated by translocation of Bad to mitochondria.*" *Mol Cancer Res* 4(8):549–62.

5. Gustafsson, K., Wang, X., Severa, D., Eriksson, M., Kimby, E., Merup, M., Christensson, B., Flygare, J., and Sander, B. 2008 (Sep 1). "Expression of cannabinoid receptors type 1 and type 2 in non-Hodgkin lymphoma: Growth inhibition by receptor activation." *Int J Cancer.* 123(5):1025–33.

6. Tan, K.L., Koh, S.B., Ee, R.P., Khan, M., and Go, M.L. 2012 (Sep). "Curcumin analogues with potent and selective anti-proliferative activity on acute promyelocytic leukemia: Involvement of accumulated misfolded nuclear receptor co-repressor (N-CoR) protein as a basis for selective activity." *ChemMedChem.* 7(9):1567–79.

Shan, Q.Q., Gong, Y.P., Guo, Y., Lin, J., Zhou, R.Q., and Yang, X. 2012 (May). "Anti-tumor effect of tanshinone II A, tetrandrine, honokiol, curcumin, oridonin and paeonol on leukemia cell lines." *Sichuan Da Xue Xue Bao Yi Xue Ban.* 43(3):362–66.

Kim, Y.S., Farrar, W., Colburn, N.H., and Milner, J.A. 2012 (Jul). "Cancer stem cells: Potential target for bioactive food components." *J Nutr Biochem.* 23(7):691–98.

7. Guenova, M.L., Michova, A., Balatzenko, G.N., Yosifov, D.Y., Stoyanov, N., Taskov, H., Berger, M.R., and Konstantinov, S.M. 2012 (May). "A particular expression pattern of CD13 epitope 7H5 in chronic lymphocytic leukaemia—a possible new therapeutic target." *Hematology* 17(3):132–39.

8. Deng, Y., Guo, Z.G., Zeng, Z.L., and Wang, Z. 2002 (Aug). "Studies on the pharmacological effects of saffron (Crocus sativus L.)—A review." *Zhongguo Zhong Yao Za Zhi.* 27(8):565–68.

LYMPHOMA

1. Gustafsson, K., Sander, B., Bielawski, J., Hannun, Y.A., and Flygare, J. (2009). "Potentiation of cannabinoid-induced cytotoxicity in mantle cell lymphoma through modulation of ceramide metabolism." *Mol Cancer Res* 7(7):1086–98.

2. Mauro Maccarrone, Tatiana Lorenzon, Monica Bari, Gerry Melino, and Alessandro Finazzi-Agrò. 2000. "Anandamide induces apoptosis in human cells via vanilloid receptors: Evidence for a protective role of cannabinoid receptors." *The Journal of Biological Chemistry* 275:31938–945.

3. Greene, William A., Jr., MD. 1954. "Psychological factors and reticuloendothelial disease." *Psychosomatic Medicine* 16:220–30.

4. Gouva, M., Damigos, D., Kaltsouda, A., Bouranta, P., Tsabouri, S., Mavreas, V., and Bourantas, K.L. 2009. "Psychological risk factors in acute leukemia." *Interscientific Health Care* 1:16–20.

5. Nomicos, E.Y. 2007 (Nov-Dec). "Myrrh: medical marvel or myth of the magi?" *Holist Nurs Pract.* 21(6):308–23.

6. Shishodia, S., Sethi, G., Ahn, K.S., and Aggarwal, B.B. 2007 (Jun 30). "Guggulsterone inhibits tumor cell proliferation, induces S-phase arrest, and promotes apoptosis through activation of c-Jun N-terminal kinase, suppression of Akt pathway, and downregulation of antiapoptotic gene products." *Biochem Pharmacol.* 74(1):118–30.

7. Goun, E., Cunningham, G., Solodnikov, S., Krasnykch, O., and Miles, H. 2002 (Dec). "Antithrombin activity of some constituents from Origanum vulgare." *Fitoterapia* 73(7-8):692–94.

Liver Cancer

1. Vara, D., Salazar, M., Olea-Herrero, N., Guzmán, M., Velasco, G., and Díaz-Laviada, I. 2011 (Jul). "Anti-tumoral action of cannabinoids on hepatocellular carcinoma: Role of AMPK-dependent activation of autophagy." *Cell Death Differ.* 18(7):1099–111.
2. Giuliano, M., Pellerito, O., Portanova, P., Calvaruso, G., Antulli, A., De Blasio, A., Vento, R., and Tesoriere, G. 2009 (Apr). "Apoptosis induced in HepG2 cells by the synthetic cannabinoid WIN: Involvement of the transcription factor PPARgamma." *Biochimie.* 91(4):457–65.
3. Ibid.
4. Felder, C.C., Joyce, K.E., Briley, E.M., Mansouri, J., Mackie, K., Blond, O., Lai, Y., Ma, A.L., and Mitchell, R.L. 1995 (Sep). "Comparison of the pharmacology and signal transduction of the human cannabinoid CB1 and CB2 receptors." *Mol Pharmacol* 48(3):443–50.

Lung Cancer

1. Gofman, John, MD, PhD. 1999. *Radiation from Medical Procedures in the Pathogenisis of Cancer and Ischemic Heart Disease* (San Francisco: Center for Nuclear Responsibility, 1st Edition).
2. Victor Cohn. 1974 (Aug 18). "Cancer curb is studied: Doctors eye drug found in marijuana." *Washington Post.*
   Munson, A.E., Harris, L.S., Friedman, M.A., Dewey, W.L., and Carchman, R.A. 1975 (Sep). "Antineoplastic activity of cannabinoids." *Journal of the National Cancer Institute* 55(3).
3. Hashibe, M., Morgenstern, H., Cui, Y., Tashkin, D.P., Zhang, Z.F., Cozen, W., Mack, T.M., and Greenland, S. 2006 (Oct). "Marijuana use and the risk of lung and upper aerodigestive tract cancers: Results of a population-based case-control study." *Cancer Epidemiol Biomarkers Prev.* 15(10):1829–34.
4. Ramer, R., and Hinz, B. 2008 (Jan 2). "Inhibition of cancer cell invasion by cannabinoids via increased expression of tissue inhibitor of matrix metalloproteinases-1." *J Natl Cancer Inst.* 100(1):59–69.
5. Preet, A., Ganju, R.K., and Groopman, J.E. 2008 (Jan 10). "Delta9-Tetrahydrocannabinol inhibits epithelial growth factor-induced lung cancer cell migration in vitro as well as its growth and metastasis in vivo." *Oncogene* 27(3):339–46.
6. Kissen, David M., and Eysenck, H.J. 1962 (Apr-June). "Personality in male lung cancer patients." *Journal of Psychosomatic Research* 6(2):123–27.
7. Grossarth-Maticek, Ronald, Kanazir, Dusan T., Schmidt, Peter, and Vetter, Hermann. 1985. "Psychosocial and organic variables as predictors of lung

cancer, cardiac infarct and apoplexy: Some differential predictors." *Personality and Individual Differences* 6(3):313–21.

8. Quander-Blaznik, Jutta. 1991. "Personality as a predictor of lung cancer: A replication." *Personality and Individual Differences* 12(2):125–30.

9. Banerjee, S., Panda, C.K., and Das, S. 2006 (Aug). "Clove (Syzygium aromaticum L.), a potential chemopreventive agent for lung cancer." *Carcinogenesis* 27(8):1645–54.

10. Nomicos, E.Y. 2007 (Nov-Dec). "Myrrh: medical marvel or myth of the magi?" *Holist Nurs Pract.* 21(6):308–23.

11. Shishodia, S., Sethi, G., Ahn, K.S., and Aggarwal, B.B. 2007 (Jun 30). "Guggulsterone inhibits tumor cell proliferation, induces S-phase arrest, and promotes apoptosis through activation of c-Jun N-terminal kinase, suppression of Akt pathway, and downregulation of antiapoptotic gene products." *Biochem Pharmacol.* 74(1):118–30.

Melanoma

1. Grant, W.B. 2002 (Mar 15). "An estimate of premature cancer mortality in the U.S. due to inadequate doses of solar ultraviolet-B radiation." *Cancer* 94(6):1867–75.

2. Gonzalez-Rosales, F., and Walsh, D. 1997. "Intractable nausea and vomiting due to gastrointestinal mucosal metastases relieved by tetrahydrocannabinol (Dronabinol)." *Journal of Pain and Symptom Management* 14(5):311–14.

3. Zutt, M., Hanssle, H., Emmert, S., Neumann, C., and Kretschmer, L. 2006. "Dronabinol for supportive therapy in patients with malignant melanoma and liver metastases." *Hautarzt* 57(5):423–27.

4. Cannabis Science, a U.S. biotech company, posted on their website the article entitled "Cannabis Science Updates Cancer Patient Progress As It Receives Verbal Confirmation By A Physician That Both Sites Of The Former Lesions Are Free Of Cancer Cells; Official Physician Documentation To Follow." Accessed April 6, 2015. www.cannabisscience.com/index.php/2011/497-cannabis-science-updates-cancer-patient-progress-as-it-receives-verbal-confirmation-by-a-physician-that-both-sites-of-the-former-lesions-are-free-of-cancer-cells-official-physician-documentation-to-follow

5. Jozsef Timar, Balazs Bani, Norbert Varga, and Istvan Kenessey. "Cannabinoid receptor-1 modulation induces apoptosis of human melanoma cells." Paper presented at the 99th American Association for Cancer Research (AACR) Annual Meeting, Apr 12-16, 2008; San Diego, CA.

6. A simple online search for "Phoenix Tears" or its advocate Rick Simpson will yield numerous results on any server or media site, such as YouTube. You can

also go directly to: Phoenix Tears Foundation (www.phoenixtearsfoundation.com), which was founded to pursue cannabinoid research and treatment, or visit Rick Simpson's home site (http://phoenixtears.ca/) or "Patients Out of Time," an all-volunteer non-profit 501(c)3 educational charity (www.medicalcannabis.com/).

7. Lee, E.J., and Jang, H.D. 2004. "Antioxidant activity and protective effect on DNA strand scission of rooibos tea (Aspalathus linearis)." *Biofactors* 21 (1-4):285–92.

8. Marnewick, J., Joubert, E., Joseph, S., Swanevelder, S., Swart, P., and Gelderblom, W. 2005 (Jun 28). "Inhibition of tumour promotion in mouse skin by extracts of rooibos (Aspalathus linearis) and honeybush (Cyclopia intermedia), unique South African herbal teas." *Cancer Lett.* 224(2):193–202.

9. Banerjee, S., and Das, S. 2005 (Jul-Sep). "Anticarcinogenic effects of an aqueous infusion of cloves on skin carcinogenesis." *Asian Pac J Cancer Prev.* 6(3):304–08.

10. Nomicos, E.Y. 2007 (Nov-Dec). "Myrrh: medical marvel or myth of the magi?" *Holist Nurs Pract.* 21(6):308–23.

11. Shishodia, S., Sethi, G., Ahn, K.S., and Aggarwal, B.B. 2007 (Jun 30). "Guggulsterone inhibits tumor cell proliferation, induces S-phase arrest, and promotes apoptosis through activation of c-Jun N-terminal kinase, suppression of Akt pathway, and downregulation of antiapoptotic gene products." *Biochem Pharmacol.* 74(1):118–30.

PANCREATIC CANCER

1. "World Health Organization (WHO) Tobacco-Free Initiative." Accessed April 16, 2015. www.who.int/tobacco/research/cancer/en/

2. Carracedo, A., Gironella, M., Lorente, M., Garcia, S., Guzmán, M., Velasco, G., and Iovanna, J.L. 2006 (Jul 1). "Cannabinoids induce apoptosis of pancreatic tumor cells via endoplasmic reticulum stress–related genes." *Cancer Res* 66:6748–55.

3. Fogli, S., Nieri, P., Chicca, A., Adinolfi, B., Mariotti, V., Iacopetti, P., Breschi, M.C., and Pellegrini, S. 2006 (Mar 20). "Cannabinoid derivatives induce cell death in pancreatic MIA PaCa-2 cells via a receptor-independent mechanism." *FEBS Lett.* 580(7):1733–39.

4. Bao, B., Ali, S., Banerjee, S., Wang, Z., Logna, F., Azmi, A.S., Kong, D., Ahmad, A., Li, Y., Padhye, S., and Sarkar, F.H. 2012 (Jan 1). "Curcumin analogue CDF inhibits pancreatic tumor growth by switching on suppressor microRNAs and attenuating EZH2 expression." *Cancer Res.* 72(1):335–45.

5. Wu, Z.H., Chen, Z., Shen, Y., Huang, L.L., and Jiang, P. 2011 (Aug).

"Anti-metastasis effect of thymoquinone on human pancreatic cancer." *Yao Xue Xue Bao*. 46(8):910–14.

PROSTATE CANCER

1. Leitzmann, M.F., Platz, E.A., Stampfer, M.J., Willett, W.C., and Giovannucci, E. 2004 (Apr 7). "Ejaculation frequency and subsequent risk of prostate cancer." *Journal of the American Medical Association*. 291(13):1578–86.

2. Melck, Dominique, Luciano De Petrocellis, Pierangelo Orlando, Tiziana Bisogno, Chiara Laezza, Maurizio Bifulco, and Vincenzo Di Marzo. 2000. "Suppression of nerve growth factor Trk receptors and prolactin receptors by endocannabinoids leads to inhibition of human breast and prostate cancer cell proliferation." *Endocrinology* 141(1):118–26.

3. Sami Sarfaraz, Farrukh Afaq, Vaqar M. Adhami, and Hasan Mukhtar. 2005 (Mar 1). "Cannabinoid receptor as a novel target for the treatment of prostate cancer." *Cancer Res* 65:1635.

4. Czifra, G., Varga, A., Nyeste, K., Marincsák, R., Tóth, B.I., Kovács, I., Kovács, L., and Bíró, T. 2009 (Apr). "Increased expressions of cannabinoid receptor-1 and transient receptor potential vanilloid-1 in human prostate carcinoma." *J Cancer Res Clin Oncol*. 135(4):507–14.

5. Ullrich, Philip M., PhD, Susan K. Lutgendorf, PhD, Jane Leserman, PhD, Derek G. Turesky, BA, and Karl J. Kreder, MD. 2005. "Stress, hostility, and disease parameters of benign prostatic hyperplasia." *Psychosomatic Medicine* 67:476–82.

6. White, Victoria M., PhD, Dallas R. English, PhD, Hamish Coates, PhD, Magdalena Lagerlund, PhD, Ron Borland, PhD, and Graham G. Giles, PhD. 2007. "Is cancer risk associated with anger control and negative affect? Findings from a prospective cohort study." *Psychosomatic Medicine* 69:667–74.

7. Sánchez, A.M., Sánchez, M.G., Malagarie-Cazenave, S., Olea, N., and Díaz-Laviada, I. 2006 (Jan). "Induction of apoptosis in prostate tumor PC-3 cells and inhibition of xenograft prostate tumor growth by the vanilloid capsaicin." *Apoptosis* 11(1):89–99.

8. Howard, E.W., Ling, M.T., Chua, C.W., Cheung, H.W., Wang, X., and Wong, Y.C. 2007 (Mar 15). "Garlic-derived S-allylmercaptocysteine is a novel in vivo antimetastatic agent for androgen-independent prostate cancer." *Clin Cancer Res*. 13(6):1847–56.

RHABDOMYOSARCOMA

1. Kaefer, M., and Rink, R.C. 2000 (Aug). "Genitourinary rhabdomyosarcoma." *Urologic Clinics of North America* 27(3):471–87.

2. Grufferman, S., Schwartz, A.G., Ruymann, F.B., and Maurer, H.M. 1993 (May). "Parents' use of cocaine and marijuana and increased risk of rhabdomyosarcoma in their children." *Cancer Causes Control.* 4(3):217–24.

3. Oesch, S., Walter, D., Wachtel, M., Pretre, K., Salazar, M., Guzmán, M., Velasco, G., and Schäfer, B.W. 2009 (Jun). "Cannabinoid receptor 1 is a potential drug target for treatment of translocation-positive rhabdomyosarcoma." *Mol Cancer Ther.* 9.

4. Deng, Y., Guo, Z.G., Zeng, Z.L., and Wang, Z. 2002 (Aug). "Studies on the pharmacological effects of saffron (Crocus sativus L.)—A review." *Zhongguo Zhong Yao Za Zhi.* 27(8):565–68.

Skin Cancer (Non-Melanoma)

1. Casanova, M. Llanos, Cristina Blázquez, Jesús Martínez-Palacio, Concepción Villanueva, M. Jesús Fernández-Aceñero, John W. Huffman, José L. Jorcano, and Manuel Guzmán. 2003. "Inhibition of skin tumor growth and angiogenesis in vivo by activation of cannabinoid receptors." *J Clin Invest.* 111(1):43–50.

2. Bíró, Tamás, Balázs I. Tóth, György Haskó, Ralf Paus, and Pál Pacher. 2009 (Aug). "The endocannabinoid system of the skin in health and disease: Novel perspectives and therapeutic opportunities." *Trends Pharmacol Sci.* 30(8):411–20.

3. Lee, E.J., and Jang, H.D. 2004. "Antioxidant activity and protective effect on DNA strand scission of rooibos tea (Aspalathus linearis)." *Biofactors* 21(1-4):285–92.

4. Marnewick, J., Joubert, E., Joseph, S., Swanevelder, S., Swart, P., and Gelderblom, W. 2005 (Jun 28). "Inhibition of tumour promotion in mouse skin by extracts of rooibos (Aspalathus linearis) and honeybush (Cyclopia intermedia), unique South African herbal teas." *Cancer Lett.* 224(2):193–202.

5. Banerjee, S., Panda, C.K., and Das, S. 2006 (Aug). "Clove (Syzygium aromaticum L.), a potential chemopreventive agent for lung cancer." *Carcinogenesis* 27(8):1645–54.

6. Banerjee, S., and Das, S. 2005 (Jul-Sep). "Anticarcinogenic effects of an aqueous infusion of cloves on skin carcinogenesis." *Asian Pac J Cancer Prev.* 6(3):304–08.

Thyroid Cancer

1. Alford, Erika Masuda, MD, Mimi I. Hu, MD, Peter Ahn, MD, and Jeffrey P. Lamont, MD. "Thyroid and parathyroid cancers." In *Cancer Management: A Multidisciplinary Approach.* 13th Edition (CMPMedica, 2011).

2. Ligresti, Alessia, Aniello Schiano Moriello, Katarzyna Starowicz, Isabel Matias, Simona Pisanti, Luciano De Petrocellis, Chiara Laezza, Giuseppe Portella,

Maurizio Bifulco, and Vincenzo Di Marzo. 2006 (Sep). "Antitumor activity of plant cannabinoids with emphasis on the effect of cannabidiol on human breast carcinoma." *JPET* 318(3):1375–87.

3. Cozzolino R., Calì, G., Bifulco, M., and Laccetti, P. 2010 (Apr). "A meta-bolically stable analogue of anandamide, Met-F-AEA, inhibits human thyroid carcinoma cell lines by activation of apoptosis." *Invest New Drugs* 28(2):115–23.

4. Harland, W.H. 1900. "Notes on two cases of exophthalmic goiter appearing suddenly in men who have been in action." *Brit. M. J.* 2:584.

5. Lidz, Theodore, MD. 1949 (Jan 1). "Emotional factors in the etiology of hyperthyroidism." *Psychosomatic Medicine* 11(1):28.

6. Mittelman, B. 1933. "Psychogenic factors and psychotherapy in hyperthyreosis and rapid heart imbalance." *J. Nerv. and Ment. Dis.* 77:465.

7. Agnes, Conrad. 1934. "A psychiatric study of hyperthyroid patients." *J. Nerv. & Ment. Dis.* 79:505.

Cardiovascular Health

Heart Disease

1. Xu, J.Q., Kochanek, K.D., Murphy, S.L., and Tejada-Vera, B. "Deaths: Final data for 2007. National vital statistics reports web release; vol. 58 no. 19." (Hyattsville, Maryland: National Center for Health Statistics. Released May 2010.)

2. Hayakawa, K., Mishima, K., Abe, K., Hasebe, N., Takamatsu, F., Yasuda, H., Ikeda, T., Inui, K., Egashira, N., Iwasaki, K., and Fujiwara, M. 2004 (Oct 25). "Cannabidiol prevents infarction via the non-CB1 cannabinoid receptor mechanism." *Neuroreport* 15(15):2381–85.

3. Shmist, Y.A., Goncharov, I., Eichler, M., Shneyvays, V., Isaac, A., Vogel, Z., and Shainberg, A. 2006 (Feb). "Delta-9-tetrahydrocannabinol protects cardiac cells from hypoxia via CB2 receptor activation and nitric oxide production." *Mol Cell Biochem* 283(1-2):75–83.

4. Lamontagne, D., Lépicier, P., Lagneux, C., and Bouchard, J.F. 2006 (Mar). "The endogenous cardiac cannabinoid system: A new protective mechanism against myocardial ischemia." *Arch Mal Coeur Vaiss.* 99(3):242–46.

5. Ronen Durst, Haim Danenberg, Ruth Gallily, Raphael Mechoulam, Keren Meir, Etty Grad, Ronen Beeri, Thea Pugatsch, Elizabet Tarsish, and Chaim Lotan. 2007. "Cannabidiol, a nonpsychoactive cannabis constituent, protects against myocardial ischemic reperfusion injury." *Am J Physiol Heart Circ Physiol* 293:H3602–H3607.

6. Ashton, J.C., and Smith, P.F. 2007 (Jul). "Cannabinoids and cardiovascular disease: The outlook for clinical treatments." *Curr Vasc Pharmacol.* 5(3):175–85.

7. Resstel, L.B., Tavares, R.F., Lisboa, S.F., Joca, S.R, Corrêa, F.M., and Guimarães, F.S. 2009 (Jan). "5-HT receptors are involved in the cannabidiol-induced attenuation of behavioural and cardiovascular responses to acute restraint stress in rats." *Br J Pharmacol.* 156(1):181–88.

8. Montecucco, F., Lenglet, S., Braunersreuther, V., Burger, F., Pelli, G., Bertolotto, M., Mach, F., and Steffens, S. 2009 (May). "CB(2) cannabinoid receptor activation is cardioprotective in a mouse model of ischemia/reperfusion." *J Mol Cell Cardiol.* 46(5):612–20.

9. Hayakawa, K., Mishima, K., Abe, K., Hasebe, N., Takamatsu, F., Yasuda, H., Ikeda, T., Inui, K., Egashira, N., Iwasaki, K., and Fujiwara, M. 2004 (Oct 25). "Cannabidiol prevents infarction via the non-CB1 cannabinoid receptor mechanism." *Neuroreport* 15(15):2381–85.

10. Barefoot, J.C., Dahlstrom, W.G., and Williams, R.B., Jr. 1983 (Mar). "Hostility, CHD incidence, and total mortality: A 25-year follow-up study of 255 physicians." *Psychosom Med.* 45(1):59–63.

11. Ibid.

12. Harburg, Ernest, PhD, Mara Julius, ScD, Niko Kaciroti, PhD, Lillian Gleiberman, PhD, and M. Anthony Schork, PhD. 2003. "Expressive/suppressive anger-coping responses, gender, and types of mortality: A 17-year follow-up (Tecumseh, Michigan, 1971–1988)." *Psychosomatic Medicine* 65:588–97.

13. Williams, Janice E., PhD, MPH; Catherine C. Paton, MSPH; Ilene C. Siegler, PhD, MPH; Marsha L. Eigenbrodt, MD, MPH; F. Javier Nieto, MD, PhD; and Herman A. Tyroler, MD. 2011. *Anger Proneness Predicts Coronary Heart Disease Risk* (American Heart Association, Inc.).

14. Harburg, Ernest, PhD, et al. 2003. "Expressive/suppressive anger-coping...." See note 12.

15. Everson, S.A., Goldberg, D.E., Kaplan, G.A., Cohen, R.D., Pukkala, E., Tuomilehto, J., and Salonen, J.T. "Hopelessness and risk of mortality and incidence of myocardial infarction and cancer." *Psychosomatic Medicine* 58(2):113–21.

16. Kubzansky, Laura D., PhD, David Sparrow, DSc, Pantel Vokonas, MD, and Ichiro Kawachi, MD. 2001. "Is the glass half empty or half full? A prospective study of optimism and coronary heart disease in the normative aging study." *Psychosomatic Medicine* 63:910–16.

17. Abd-Allah, A.R., Al-Majed, A.A., Mostafa, A.M., Al-Shabanah, O.A., Din, A.G., and Nagi, M.N. 2002. "Protective effect of Arabic gum against cardiotoxicity induced by doxorubicin in mice: A possible mechanism of protection." *J Biochem Mol Toxicol.* 16(5):254–59.

18. Rudkowska, I., and Jones, P.J. 2007 (May). "Functional foods for the preven-

tion and treatment of cardiovascular diseases: Cholesterol and beyond." *Expert Rev Cardiovasc Ther.* 5(3):477–90.

19. Suneetha, W.J., and Krishnakantha, T.P. 2005 (May). "Cardamom extract as inhibitor of human platelet aggregation." *Phytother Res.* 19(5):437–40.

20. Kaunitz, H. 1986 (Mar-Apr). "Medium-chain triglycerides (MCT) in aging and arteriosclerosis." *J Environ Pathol Toxicol Oncol.* 6(3-4):115–21.

21. Cuban Ministry of Public Health, Havana. 1992. *Therapeutic Guide to Plant Pharmaceuticals and Honey Pharmaceuticals (Guia Terapeutica Dispensarial de Fitofarmacos y Apifarmacos).* Ministerio de Salud Publica, Ciudad de La Habana, Republica de Cuba.

22. Federal Republic of Germany. *Monographien der E-Kommission (Phyto-Therapie) (380 monographs). A therapeutic guide to herbal medicine evaluating the safety and efficacy of herbs for licensed medical prescribing in Germany.* Published between 1984 and 1994 in the Bundesanzeiger (official publication by the Federal Republic of Germany). Copies of the monographs are available at the Heilpflanzen-Welt Bibliothek, last accessed April 16, 2015: http://buecher .heilpflanzen-welt.de/BGA-Commission-E-Monographs/

23. Okada, Y., Tanaka, K., Sato, E., and Okajima, H. 2006 (Nov 21). "Kinetic and mechanistic studies of allicin as an antioxidant." *Org Biomol Chem.* 4(22):4113–17.

24. Fukao, H., Yoshida, H., Tazawa, Y., and Hada, T. 2007 (Jan). "Antithrombotic effects of odorless garlic powder both in vitro and in vivo." *Biosci Biotechnol Biochem.* 71(1):84–90.

25. Chuah, S.C., Moore, P.K., and Zhu, Y.Z. 2007 (Nov). "S-allylcysteine mediates cardioprotection in an acute myocardial infarction rat model via a hydrogen sulphide mediated pathway." *Am J Physiol Heart Circ Physiol.* 293(5):H2693–701.

26. Wu, C.X., Wei, X.B., Ding, H., Sun, X., and Cheng, X.M. 2006 (Aug). "Protective effect of effective parts of Zingiber Officinale on vascular endothelium of the experimental hyperlipidemic rats." *Zhong Yao Cai.* 29(8):810–13.

27. El-Bahai, M.N., Al-Hariri, M.T., Yar, T., and Bamosa, A.O. 2009 (Jan 24). "Cardiac inotropic and hypertrophic effects of Nigella sativa supplementation in rats." *Int J Cardiol.* 131(3):e115–17.

28. Hsieh, C.L., Peng, C.H., Chyau, C.C., Lin, Y.C., Wang, H.E., and Peng, R.Y. 2007 (Apr 18). "Low-density lipoprotein, collagen, and thrombin models reveal that Rosmarinus officinalis L. exhibits potent antiglycative effects." *J Agric Food Chem.* 55(8):2884–91.

29. Deng, Y., Guo, Z.G., Zeng, Z.L., and Wang, Z. 2002 (Aug). "Studies on the

pharmacological effects of saffron (Crocus sativus L.)—A review." *Zhongguo Zhong Yao Za Zhi*. 27(8):565–68.

30. Goel, A., Kunnumakkara, A.B., and Aggarwal, B.B. 2008 (Feb 15). "Curcumin as 'Curecumin': From kitchen to clinic." *Biochem Pharmacol*. 75(4):787–809.

HYPERTENSION

1. He, J., and Whelton, P.K. 1997 (Sep). "Epidemiology and prevention of hypertension." *Med Clin North Am*. 81(5):1077–97.

2. Chobanian, A.V., Bakris, G.L., Black, H.R., Cushman, W.C., Green, L.A., Izzo, J.L., Jr., Jones, D.W., Materson, B.J., Oparil, S., Wright, J.T., Jr., and Roccella, E.J. 2003. "The Seventh Report of the Joint National Committee on Prevention, Detection, Evaluation, and Treatment of High Blood Pressure: The JNC 7 report." *Journal of the American Medical Association* 289:2560–72.

3. Crawford, W.J., and Merritt, J.C. 1979 (May). "Effects of tetrahydrocannabinol on arterial and intraocular hypertension." *Int J Clin Pharmacol Biopharm*. 17(5):191–96.

4. Ho, W.S., and Gardiner, S.M. 2009 (Jan). "Acute hypertension reveals depressor and vasodilator effects of cannabinoids in conscious rats." *Br J Pharmacol*. 156(1):94–104.

5. Ashton, J.C., and Smith, P.F. 2007 (Jul). "Cannabinoids and cardiovascular disease: The outlook for clinical treatments." *Curr Vasc Pharmacol*. 5(3):175–85.

6. Grace, William J., MD, and Graham, David T., MD. Dept. of Medicine of the New York Hospital–Cornell Medical Center. 1952 (July 1). "Relationship of specific attitudes and emotions to certain bodily diseases." *Psychosomatic Medicine* 14(4):243–51.

7. GWB-A & GWB-D taken from the General Well-being Schedule.

8. Jonas, Bruce S., ScM, PhD, and Lando, James F., MD, MPH. 2000. "Negative affect as a prospective risk factor for hypertension." *Psychosomatic Medicine* 62:188–96.

9. Jonas, Bruce S., PhD, Franks, Peter, MD, and Ingram, Deborah D., PhD. 1997. "Are symptoms of anxiety and depression risk factors for hypertension? Longitudinal evidence from the National Health and Nutrition Examination Survey I Epidemiologic Follow-up Study." *Arch Fam Med*. 6(1):43–49.

10. Lijing L. Yan, PhD, MPH; Kiang Liu, PhD; Karen A. Matthews, PhD; Martha L. Daviglus, MD, PhD; T. Freeman Ferguson, MPH, MSPH; Catarina I. Kiefe, MD, PhD. 2003. "Psychosocial factors and risk of hypertension: The Coronary Artery Risk Development in Young Adults (CARDIA) Study." *Journal of the American Medical Association* 290(16):2138–48.

11. Ostir, Glenn V., PhD, Ivonne M. Berges, PhD, Kyriakos S. Markides, PhD,

and Kenneth J. Ottenbacher, PhD. 2006. "Hypertension in older adults and the role of positive emotions." *Psychosomatic Medicine* 68:727–33.

12. Richman, L.S., Kubzansky, L., Maselko, J., Kawachi, I., Choo, P., and Bauer, M. 2005 (Jul). "Positive emotion and health: going beyond the negative." *Health Psychol.* 24(4):422–29.

13. Mann, S.J., and Delon, M. 1995 (Sep-Oct). "Improved hypertension control after disclosure of decades-old trauma." *Psychosomatic Medicine* 57(5):501–05.

14. Khan, A.U., and Gilani, A.H. 2006 (Dec). "Selective bronchodilatory effect of Rooibos tea (Aspalathus linearis) and its flavonoid, chrysoeriol." *Eur J Nutr.* 45(8):463–69.

15. Rudkowska, I., and Jones, P.J. 2007 (May). "Functional foods for the prevention and treatment of cardiovascular diseases: Cholesterol and beyond." *Expert Rev Cardiovasc Ther.* 5(3):477–90.

16. Taubert, D., Roesen, R., and Schomig, E. 2007 (Apr 9). "Effect of cocoa and tea intake on blood pressure: A meta-analysis." *Arch Intern Med.* 167(7):626–34.

17. Lahlou, S., Tahraoui, A., Israili, Z., and Lyoussi, B. 2007 (Apr 4). "Diuretic activity of the aqueous extracts of Carum carvi and Tanacetum vulgare in normal rats." *J Ethnopharmacol.* 110(3):458–63.

18. Cuban Ministry of Public Health, Havana. 1992. *Therapeutic Guide to Plant Pharmaceuticals and Honey Pharmaceuticals (Guia Terapeutica Dispensarial de Fitofarmacos y Apifarmacos).* Ministerio de Salud Publica, Ciudad de La Habana, Republica de Cuba.

19. Federal Republic of Germany. *Monographien der E-Kommission (Phyto-Therapie) (380 monographs). A therapeutic guide to herbal medicine evaluating the safety and efficacy of herbs for licensed medical prescribing in Germany.* Published between 1984 and 1994 in the Bundesanzeiger (official publication by the Federal Republic of Germany). Copies of the monographs are available at the Heilpflanzen-Welt Bibliothek: http://buecher.heilpflanzen-welt.de/BGA -Commission-E-Monographs/

20. Okada, Y., Tanaka, K., Sato, E., and Okajima, H. 2006 (Nov 21). "Kinetic and mechanistic studies of allicin as an antioxidant." *Org Biomol Chem.* 4(22): 4113–17.

21. Fukao, H., Yoshida, H., Tazawa, Y., and Hada, T. 2007 (Jan). "Antithrombotic effects of odorless garlic powder both in vitro and in vivo." *Biosci Biotechnol Biochem.* 71(1):84–90.

STROKE

1. The United States of America as represented by the Department of Health and Human Services. (Aidan J. Hampson, Julius Axelrod, and Maurizio Grimaldi)

Patent No. 09/674028 filed on 02/02/2001. Patent 6630507 issued on October 7, 2003. Estimated expiration date: 2021. Cannabinoids as antioxidants and neuroprotectants. www.patentstorm.us/patents/6630507.html

2. Hayakawa, K., Mishima, K., Nozako, M., Hazekawa, M., Irie, K., Fujioka, M., Orito, K., Abe, K., Hasebe, N., Egashira, N., Iwasaki, K., and Fujiwara, M. 2007 (Sep). "Delayed treatment with cannabidiol has a cerebroprotective action via a cannabinoid receptor-independent myeloperoxidase-inhibiting mechanism." *J Neurochem* 102(5):1488–96.

3. Hayakawa, K., Mishima, K., Nozako, M., Hazekawa, M., Ogata, A., Fujioka, M., Harada, K., Mishima, S., Orito, K., Egashira, N., Iwasaki, K., and Fujiwara, M. 2007 (Mar 27). "Delta9-tetrahydrocannabinol (Delta9-THC) prevents cerebral infarction via hypothalamic-independent hypothermia." *Life Sci* 80(16):1466–71.

4. CES-D = Center for Epidemiological Studies Depression Scale.

5. Ostir, Glenn V., PhD, Kyriakos S. Markides, PhD, M. Kristen Peek, PhD, and James S. Goodwin, MD. 2001. "The association between emotional well-being and the incidence of stroke in older adults." *Psychosomatic Medicine* 63:210–15.

6. Ibid.

7. Khan, A.U., and Gilani, A.H. 2006 (Dec). "Selective bronchodilatory effect of Rooibos tea (Aspalathus linearis) and its flavonoid, chrysoeriol." *Eur J Nutr.* 45(8):463–69.

8. Rudkowska, I., and Jones, P.J. 2007 (May). "Functional foods for the prevention and treatment of cardiovascular diseases: Cholesterol and beyond." *Expert Rev Cardiovasc Ther.* 5(3):477–90.

9. Cuban Ministry of Public Health, Havana. 1992. *Therapeutic Guide to Plant Pharmaceuticals and Honey Pharmaceuticals (Guia Terapeutica Dispensarial de Fitofarmacos y Apifarmacos).* Ministerio de Salud Publica, Ciudad de La Habana, Republica de Cuba.

10. Federal Republic of Germany. *Monographien der E-Kommission (Phyto-Therapie) (380 monographs). A therapeutic guide to herbal medicine evaluating the safety and efficacy of herbs for licensed medical prescribing in Germany.* Published between 1984 and 1994 in the Bundesanzeiger (official publication by the Federal Republic of Germany). Copies of the monographs are available at the Heilpflanzen-Welt Bibliothek: http://buecher.heilpflanzen-welt.de/BGA-Commission-E-Monographs/

11. Okada, Y., Tanaka, K., Sato, E., and Okajima, H. 2006 (Nov 21). "Kinetic and mechanistic studies of allicin as an antioxidant." *Org Biomol Chem.* 4(22): 4113–17.

12. Fukao, H., Yoshida, H., Tazawa, Y., and Hada, T. 2007 (Jan). "Antithrombotic effects of odorless garlic powder both in vitro and in vivo." *Biosci Biotechnol Biochem.* 71(1):84–90.

13. Wu, C.X., Wei, X.B., Ding, H., Sun, X., and Cheng, X.M. 2006 (Aug). "Protective effect of effective parts of Zingiber officinale on vascular endothelium of the experimental hyperlipidemic rats." *Zhong Yao Cai.* 29(8):810–13.

Diabetes Mellitus

1. Aubert, Ronald. 1995. *Diabetes in America* (2nd Edition, published by the National Institutes of Health, No. 95-1468), p. 3.

2. Ibid.

3. Weiss, L., Zeira, M., Reich, S., Slavin, S., Raz, I., Mechoulam, R., and Gallily, R. 2008 (Jan). "Cannabidiol arrests onset of autoimmune diabetes in NOD mice." *Neuropharmacology* 54(1):244-49.

   Also Weiss, L., Zeira, M., Reich, S., Har-Noy, M., Mechoulam, R., Slavin, S., and Gallily, R. 2006 (Mar). "Cannabidiol lowers incidence of diabetes in non-obese diabetic mice." *Autoimmunity* 39(2):143–51.

4. Zhang, F., Challapalli, S.C., and Smith, P.J. 2009 (Aug). "Cannabinoid CB(1) receptor activation stimulates neurite outgrowth and inhibits capsaicin-induced Ca(2+) influx in an in vitro model of diabetic neuropathy." *Neuropharmacology* 57(2):88–96.

5. El-Remessy, Azza B., Mohamed Al-Shabrawey, Yousuf Khalifa, Nai-Tse Tsai, Ruth B. Caldwell, and Gregory I. Liou. 2006. "Neuroprotective and blood-retinal barrier-preserving effects of cannabidiol in experimental diabetes." *American Journal of Pathology* 168:235–44.

6. Li, X., Kaminski, N.E., and Fischer, L.J. 2001 (Apr). "Examination of the immunosuppressive effect of delta9-tetrahydrocannabinol in streptozotocin-induced autoimmune diabetes." *Int Immunopharmacol.* 1(4):699–712.

7. Bujalska, M. 2008. "Effect of cannabinoid receptor agonists on Streptozotocin-induced hyperalgesia in diabetic neuropathy." *Pharmacology* 82(3):193–200.

8. Richman, L.S., Kubzansky, L., Maselko, J., Kawachi, I., Choo, P., and Bauer, M. 2005 (Jul). "Positive emotion and health: going beyond the negative." *Health Psychol.* 24(4):422–29.

9. Wales, J.K. 1995 (Feb). "Does psychological stress cause diabetes?" *Diabet Med.* 12(2):109–12.

10. Ingerski, L.M., Anderson, B.J., Dolan, L.M., and Hood, K.K. 2010 (Aug). "Blood glucose monitoring and glycemic control in adolescence: Contribution of diabetes-specific responsibility and family conflict." *J Adolesc Health.* 47(2):191–97.

11. Ruzaidi, A., Amin, I., Nawalyah, A.G., Hamid, M., and Faizul, H.A. 2005 (Apr 8). "The effect of Malaysian cocoa extract on glucose levels and lipid profiles in diabetic rats." *J Ethnopharmacol.* 98(1-2):55–60.

12. Eddouks, M., Lemhadri, A., and Michel, J.B. 2004 (Sep). "Caraway and caper: potential anti-hyperglycaemic plants in diabetic rats." *J Ethnopharmacol.* 94(1):143–48.

13. Rau, O., Wurglics, M., Dingermann, T., Abdel-Tawab, M., and Schubert-Zsilavecz, M. 2006 (Nov). "Screening of herbal extracts for activation of the human peroxisome proliferator-activated receptor." *Pharmazie.* 61(11):952–56.

14. Chaiyata, P., Puttadechakum, S., and Komindr, S. 2003 (Sep). "Effect of chili pepper (Capsicum frutescens) ingestion on plasma glucose response and metabolic rate in Thai women." *J Med Assoc Thai.* 86(9):854–60.

15. Kim, W., Khil, L.Y., Clark, R., Bok, S.H., Kim, E.E., Lee, S., Jun, H.S., and Yoon, J.W. 2006 (Oct). "Naphthalenemethyl ester derivative of dihydroxyhydrocinnamic acid, a component of cinnamon, increases glucose disposal by enhancing translocation of glucose transporter." *Diabetologia.* 49(10):2437–48.

16. Subash, Babu P., Prabuseenivasan, S., and Ignacimuthu, S. 2007 (Jan). "Cinnamaldehyde, a potential antidiabetic agent." *Phytomedicine* 14(1):15–22.

17. Kannappan, S., Jayaraman, T., Rajasekar, P., Ravichandran, M.K., and Anuradha, C.V. 2006 (Oct). "Cinnamon bark extract improves glucose metabolism and lipid profile in the fructose-fed rat." *Singapore Med J.* 47(10):858–63.

18. Prasad, R.C., Herzog, B., Boone, B., Sims, L., and Waltner-Law, M. 2005 (Jan 4). "An extract of Syzygium aromaticum represses genes encoding hepatic gluconeogenic enzymes." *J Ethnopharmacol.* 96(1-2):295–301.

19. Srinivasan, K. 2005 (Sep). "Plant foods in the management of diabetes mellitus: Spices as beneficial antidiabetic food adjuncts." *Int J Food Sci Nutr.* 56(6):399–414.

20. Sobenin, I.A., Nedosugova, L.V., Filatova, L.V., Balabolkin, M.I., Gorchakova, T.V., and Orekhov, A.N. 2008 (Mar). "Metabolic effects of time-released garlic powder tablets in type 2 diabetes mellitus: The results of double-blinded placebo-controlled study." *Acta Diabetol.* 45(1):1–6.

21. Al-Amin, Z.M., Thomson, M., Al-Qattan, K.K., Peltonen-Shalaby, R., and Ali, M. 2006 (Oct). "Anti-diabetic and hypolipidaemic properties of ginger (Zingiber officinale) in Streptozotocin-induced diabetic rats." *Br J Nutr.* 96(4):660–66.

22. Ojewole, J.A. 2006 (Sep). "Analgesic, antiinflammatory and hypoglycaemic effects of ethanol extract of Zingiber officinale (Roscoe) rhizomes (Zingiberaceae) in mice and rats." *Phytother Res.* 20(9):764–72.

23. Yang, S., Na, M.K., Jang, J.P., Kim, K.A., Kim, B.Y., Sung, N.J., Oh, W.K., and Ahn, J.S. 2006 (Aug). "Inhibition of protein tyrosine phosphatase 1B by lignans from Myristica fragrans." *Phytother Res.* 20(8):680–82.

24. Lemhadri, A. Zeggwagh, N.A., Maghrani, M., Jouad, H., and Eddouks, M. 2004 (Jun). "Anti-hyperglycaemic activity of the aqueous extract of Origanum vulgare growing wild in Tafilalet region." *J Ethnopharmacol.* 92(2-3):251–56.

25. Hsieh, C.L., Peng, C.H., Chyau, C.C., Lin, Y.C., Wang, H.E., and Peng, R.Y. 2007 (Apr 18). "Low-density lipoprotein, collagen, and thrombin models reveal that Rosmarinus officinalis L. exhibits potent antiglycative effects." *J Agric Food Chem.* 55(8):2884–91.

26. Goel, A., Kunnumakkara, A.B., and Aggarwal, B.B. 2008 (Feb 15). "Curcumin as 'Curecumin': From kitchen to clinic." *Biochem Pharmacol.* 75(4):787–809.

27. Gertsch, J., Leonti, M., Raduner, S., Racz, I., Chen, J.Z., Xie, X.Q., Altmann, K.H., Karsak, M., and Zimmer, A. 2008 (Jul 1). "Beta-caryophyllene is a dietary cannabinoid." *Proc Natl Acad Sci USA* 105(26):9099–104.

Horváth, Béla, Partha Mukhopadhyay, Malek Kechrid, Vivek Patel, Gali Tanchian, David A. Wink, Jürg Gertsch, and Pál Pacher. 2012 (Apr 15). "β-Caryophyllene ameliorates cisplatin-induced nephrotoxicity in a cannabinoid 2 receptor-dependent manner." *Free Radical Biology and Medicine* 52(8):1325–33.

Eye Disease and Eye Function
AGE-RELATED MACULAR DEGENERATION

1. Wei, Y., Wang, X., and Wang, L. 2009 (Jun 14). "Presence and regulation of cannabinoid receptors in human retinal pigment epithelial cells." *Mol Vis.* 15:1243–51.

2. Abd-Allah, A.R., Al-Majed, A.A., Mostafa, A.M., Al-Shabanah, O.A., Din, A.G., and Nagi, M.N. 2002. "Protective effect of Arabic gum against cardiotoxicity induced by doxorubicin in mice: A possible mechanism of protection." *J Biochem Mol Toxicol.* 16(5):254–59.

3. Hermann, F., Ruschitzka, F., Spieker, L., Sudano, I., Noll, G., and Corti, R. 2005 (Sep). "The sweet secret of dark chocolate." *Ther Umsch.* 62(9):635–37.

4. Jayaprakasha, G.K., Ohnishi-Kameyama, M., Ono, H., Yoshida, M., Jaganmohan, Rao L. 2006 (Mar 8). "Phenolic constituents in the fruits of Cinnamomum zeylanicum and their antioxidant activity." *J Agric Food Chem.* 54(5):1672–79.

5. Jirovetz, L., Buchbauer, G., Stoilova, I., Stoyanova, A., Krastanov, A., and Schmidt, E. "Chemical composition and antioxidant properties of clove leaf essential oil." 2006 (Aug 23). *J Agric Food Chem.* 54(17):6303–07.

6. Satyanarayana, S., Sushruta, K., Sarma, G.S., Srinivas, N., and Subba Raju, G.V. 2004. "Antioxidant activity of the aqueous extracts of spicy food additives—evaluation and comparison with ascorbic acid in in-vitro systems." *J Herb Pharmacother.* 4(2):1–10.

7. Birdane, F.M., Cemek, M., Birdane, Y.O., Gülçin, I., and Büyükokurolu, M.E. 2007 (Jan 28). "Beneficial effects of Foeniculum vulgare on ethanol-induced acute gastric mucosal injury in rats." *World J Gastroenterol.* 13(4):607–11.

8. Siddaraju, M.N., and Dharmesh, S.M. 2007 (Mar). "Inhibition of gastric H+, K+-ATPase and Helicobacter pylori growth by phenolic antioxidants of Zingiber officinale." *Mol Nutr Food Res.* 51(3):324–32.

9. Ivanova, D., Gerova, D., Chervenkov, T., and Yankova, T. 2005 (Jan 4). "Polyphenols and antioxidant capacity of Bulgarian medicinal plants." *J Ethnopharmacol.* 96(1-2):145–50.

10. Venkatesan, N., Punithavathi, D., and Babu M. 2007. "Protection from acute and chronic lung diseases by curcumin." *Adv Exp Med Biol.* 595:379–405.

11. Goel, A., Kunnumakkara, A.B., and Aggarwal, B.B. 2008 (Feb 15). "Curcumin as 'Curecumin': From kitchen to clinic." *Biochem Pharmacol.* 75(4):787–809.

GLAUCOMA

1. Hepler, R.S., and Frank, I.R. 1971. "Marihuana smoking and intraocular pressure." *Journal of the American Medical Association* 217(10):1392.

2. Crawford, W.J., and Merritt, J.C. 1979 (May). "Effects of tetrahydrocannabinol on arterial and intraocular hypertension." *Int J Clin Pharmacol Biopharm.* 17(5):191–96.

3. Song, Z.H., and Slowey, C.A. 2000 (Jan). "Involvement of cannabinoid receptors in the intraocular pressure-lowering effects of WIN55,212-2." *J Pharmacol Exp Ther.* 292(1):136–39.

4. Tomida, I., Azuara-Blanco, A., House, H., Flint, M., Pertwee, R.G., and Robson, P.J. 2006. "Effect of sublingual application of cannabinoids on intraocular pressure: A pilot study." *J Glaucoma* 15(5):349–53.

5. Plange, N., Arend, K.O., Kaup, M., Doehmen, B., Adams, H., Hendricks, S., Cordes, A., Huth, J., Sponsel, W.E., and Remky, A. 2007 (Jan). "Dronabinol and retinal hemodynamics in humans." *Am J Ophthalmol.* 143(1):173–74.

6. Green, K. 1998 (Nov). "Marijuana smoking vs cannabinoids for glaucoma therapy." *Arch Ophthalmol.* 116(11):1433–37.

7. Merritt, J.C., Perry, D.D., Russell, D.N., and Jones, B.F. 1981 (Aug-Sep). "Topical delta 9-tetrahydrocannabinol and aqueous dynamics in glaucoma." *J Clin Pharmacol.* 21(8-9 Suppl):467S–471S.

8. Merritt, J.C., Crawford, W.J., Alexander, P.C., Anduze, A.L., and Gelbart, S.S. 1980. "Effect of marihuana on intraocular and blood pressure in glaucoma." *Ophthalmology* 87(3):222–28.

9. Cooler, P., and Gregg, J.M. 1977 (Aug). "Effect of delta-9-tetrahydrocannabinol on intraocular pressure in humans." *South Med J.* 70(8):951–54.

10. Berger, Allan S., MD, and Simel, Paul J., MD. 1958. "Effect of hypnosis on intraocular pressure in normal and glaucomatous subjects." *Psychosomatic Medicine* 20:321–27.

IMPROVED NIGHT VISION

1. Russo, E.B., Merzoukib, A., Molero, J., Mesab, K., Freyd, A., and Bach, P.J. 2004 (Jul). "Cannabis improves night vision: A case study of dark adaptometry and scotopic sensitivity in kif smokers of the Rif mountains of northern Morocco." *J Ethnopharmacol.* 93(1):99–104.

UVEITIS

1. Toguri, J.T., Lehmann, C., Laprairie, R.B., Szczesniak, A.M., Zhou, J., Denovan-Wright, E.M., and Kelly, M.E. 2014 (Mar). "Anti-inflammatory effects of cannabinoid CB(2) receptor activation in endotoxin-induced uveitis." *Br J Pharmacol.* 171(6):1448–61.

2. El-Remessy, A.B., Tang, Y., Zhu, G., Matragoon, S., Khalifa, Y., Liu, E.K., Liu, J.Y., Hanson, E., Mian, S., Fatteh, N., and Liou, G.I. 2008. "Neuroprotective effects of cannabidiol in endotoxin-induced uveitis: Critical role of p38 MAPK activation." *Mol Vis.* 14:2190–203.

3. Xu, H., Cheng, C.L., Chen, M., Manivannan, A., Cabay, L., Pertwee, R.G., Coutts, A., and Forrester, J.V. 2007 (Sep). "Anti-inflammatory property of the cannabinoid receptor-2-selective agonist JWH-133 in a rodent model of autoimmune uveoretinitis." *J Leukoc Biol.* 82(3):532–41.

Fever/Temperature Regulation

1. Khalid Benamar, Menachem Yondorf, Joseph J. Meissler, Ellen B. Geller, Ronald J. Tallarida, Toby K. Eisenstein and Martin W. Adler. 2007 (Mar). "A novel role of cannabinoids: Implication in the fever induced by bacterial lipopolysaccharide." *JPET* 320(3):1127–33.

2. Hayakawa, K., Mishima, K., Nozako, M., Hazekawa, M., Ogata, A., Fujioka, M., Harada, K., Mishima, S., Orito, K., Egashira, N., Iwasaki, K., and Fujiwara, M. 2007 (Mar 27). "Delta9-tetrahydrocannabinol (Delta9-THC) prevents cerebral infarction via hypothalamic-independent hypothermia." *Life Sci.* 80(16):1466–71.

Fibromyalgia

1. Chakrabarty, S., and Zoorob, R. 2007 (Jul 15). "Fibromyalgia." *Am Fam Physician.* 76(2):247–54.

2. Skrabek, R.Q., Galimova, L., and Ethansand, Daryl K. 2008 (Feb). "Nabilone for the treatment of pain in fibromyalgia." *J Pain.* 9(2):164–73.

3. Ware, M.A., Fitzcharles, M.A., Joseph, L., and Shir, Y. 2010 (Feb 1). "The effects of Nabilone on sleep in fibromyalgia: Results of a randomized controlled trial." *Anesth Analg.* 110(2):604–10.

4. Burstein, Sumner H., and Zurier, Robert B. 2009 (Mar). "Cannabinoids, endocannabinoids, and related analogs in inflammation." *AAPS J.* 11(1):109–19.

5. Schweinhardt, P., Sauro, K.M., and Bushnell, M.C. 2008 (Oct). "Fibromyalgia: A disorder of the brain?" *Neuroscientist* 14(5):415–21.

6. Zautra, Alex J., PhD, Robert Fasman, MA, John W. Reich, PhD, Peter Harakas, MSc, Lisa M. Johnson, MA, Maureen E. Olmsted, PhD, and Mary C. Davis, PhD. 2005. "Fibromyalgia: Evidence for deficits in positive affect regulation." *Psychosomatic Medicine* 67:147–55.

7. Broderick, Joan E., PhD, Doerte U. Junghaenel, MA, and Joseph E. Schwartz, PhD. 2005. "Written emotional expression produces health benefits in fibromyalgia patients." *Psychosomatic Medicine* 67:326–34.

8. Walker, E.A., Keegan, D., Gardner, G., Sullivan, M., Bernstein, D., and Katon, W.J. 1997. "Psychosocial factors in fibromyalgia compared with rheumatoid arthritis: II. Sexual, physical, and emotional abuse and neglect." *Psychosomatic Medicine* 59(6):572–77.

9. Chenchen Wang, MD, MPH, Christopher H. Schmid, PhD, Ramel Rones, BS, Robert Kalish, MD, Janeth Yinh, MD, Don L. Goldenberg, MD, Yoojin Lee, MS, and Timothy McAlindon, MD, MPH. 2010. "A randomized trial of Tai Chi for fibromyalgia." *N Engl J Med* 363:743–75.

Hemorrhoids

1. Donovan, M. 1845 (Jan 1). "On the physical and medicinal qualities of Indian hemp (Cannabis indica); with observations on the best mode of administration, and cases illustrative of its powers." *Dublin Journal of Medical Science* (1836-1845) 26(3):368–402.

2. Shah, N.C., and Joshi, M.C. 1971. "An ethnobotanical study of the Kumaon region of India." *Economic Botany* 25(4):414–22.

3. Grace, William J., MD, and Graham, David T., MD. Dept. of Medicine of the New York Hospital–Cornell Medical Center. 1952 (July 1). "Relationship of specific attitudes and emotions to certain bodily diseases." *Psychosomatic Medicine* 14(4):243–51.

4. Bliss, D.Z., Jung, H.J., Savik, K., Lowry, A., LeMoine, M., Jensen, L., Werner, C., and Schaffer, K. 2001 (Jul-Aug). "Supplementation with dietary fiber improves fecal incontinence." *Nurs Res.* 50(4):203–13.

5. Elwakeel, H.A., Moneim, H.A., Farid, M., and Gohar, A.A. 2007 (Jul). "Clove oil cream: A new effective treatment for chronic anal fissure." *Colorectal Dis.* 9(6):549–52.

6. Cuban Ministry of Public Health, Havana. 1992. *Therapeutic Guide to Plant Pharmaceuticals and Honey Pharmaceuticals (Guia Terapeutica Dispensarial de Fitofarmacos y Apifarmacos).* Ministerio de Salud Publica, Ciudad de La Habana, Republica de Cuba.

Inflammation (in general)

1. Horváth, Béla, Partha Mukhopadhyay, Malek Kechrid, Vivek Patel, Gali Tanchian, David A. Wink, Jürg Gertsch, and Pál Pacher. 2012 (April 15). "β-Caryophyllene ameliorates cisplatin-induced nephrotoxicity in a cannabinoid 2 receptor-dependent manner." *Free Radical Biology and Medicine* 52(8):1325–33.

   Gertsch, J., Leonti, M., Raduner, S., Racz, I., Chen, J.Z., Xie, X.Q., Altmann, K.H., Karsak, M., and Zimmer, A. 2008 (Jul 1). "Beta-caryophyllene is a dietary cannabinoid." *Proc Natl Acad Sci USA* 105(26):9099–104.

2. Cuban Ministry of Public Health, Havana. 1992. Therapeutic Guide to Plant Pharmaceuticals and Honey Pharmaceuticals (Guia Terapeutica Dispensarial de Fitofarmacos y Apifarmacos). Ministerio de Salud Publica, Ciudad de La Habana, Republica de Cuba.

3. Ibid.

4. Khanna, D., Sethi, G., Ahn, K.S., Pandey, M.K., Kunnumakkara, A.B., Sung, B., Aggarwal, A., and Aggarwal, B.B. 2007 (Jun). "Natural products as a gold mine for arthritis treatment." *Curr Opin Pharmacol.* 7(3):344–51.

5. Tekeoglu, I., Dogan, A., Ediz, L., Budancamanak, M., and Demirel, A. 2007 (Sep). "Effects of thymoquinone (volatile oil of black cumin) on rheumatoid arthritis in rat models." *Phytother Res.* 21(9):895–97.

6. Goel, A., Kunnumakkara, A.B., and Aggarwal, B.B. 2008 (Feb 15). "Curcumin as 'Curecumin': From kitchen to clinic." *Biochem Pharmacol.* 75(4):787–809.

ARTHRITIS

1. Hootman, J., Bolen, J., Helmick, C., and Langmaid, G. 2006. "Prevalence of doctor-diagnosed arthritis and arthritis-attributable activity limitation—United States, 2003-2005." *MMWR* 55(40):1089–92.

2. Wolfe, Sidney M., MD, Larry D. Sasich, PharmD, MPH, Rose-Ellen Hope, RPh, and Public Citizen's Health Research Group. 1999. *Worst Pills, Best*

Pills—A Consumer's Guide to Avoiding Drug-Induced Death or Illness (New York: Pocket Books).

3. Malfait, A.M., Gallily, R., Sumariwalla, P.F., Malik, A.S., Andreakos, E., Mechoulam, R., and M. Feldmann. 2000 (Aug 15). "The nonpsychoactive cannabis constituent cannabidiol is an oral anti-arthritic therapeutic in murine collagen-induced arthritis." *Proc Natl Acad Sci* USA 97(17):9561–66.

4. Burstein, Sumner. 2005 (Mar). "Ajulemic acid (IP-751): Synthesis, proof of principle, toxicity studies, and clinical trials." *AAPS J.* 7(1):E143–E148.

5. Schuelert, N., Johnson, M.P., Oskins, J.L., Jassal, K., Chambers, M.G., and McDougall, J.J. 2011 (May). "Local application of the endocannabinoid hydrolysis inhibitor URB597 reduces nociception in spontaneous and chemically induced models of osteoarthritis." *Pain.* 152(5):975–81.

6. Schiel, K.A. 1999 (Oct). "A proposed psychosomatic etiologic model for rheumatoid arthritis." *Med Hypotheses.* 53(4):305–14.

7. Wise, B.L., Niu, J., Zhang, Y., Wang, N., Jordan, J.M., Choy, E., and Hunter, D.J. 2010 (Jul). "Psychological factors and their relation to osteoarthritis pain." Osteoarthritis Cartilage. 18(7):883–87.

8. Cuban Ministry of Public Health, Havana. 1992. *Therapeutic Guide to Plant Pharmaceuticals and Honey Pharmaceuticals (Guia Terapeutica Dispensarial de Fitofarmacos y Apifarmacos).* Ministerio de Salud Publica, Ciudad de La Habana, Republica de Cuba.

9. Khanna, D., Sethi, G., Ahn, K.S., Pandey, M.K., Kunnumakkara, A.B., Sung, B., Aggarwal, A., and Aggarwal, B.B. 2007 (Jun). "Natural products as a gold mine for arthritis treatment." *Curr Opin Pharmacol.* 7(3):344–51.

10. Haffor, A.S. 2010 (Mar). "Effect of myrrh (Commiphora molmol) on leukocyte levels before and during healing from gastric ulcer or skin injury." *J Immunotoxicol.* 7(1):68–75.

11. Tekeoglu, I., Dogan, A., Ediz, L., Budancamanak, M., and Demirel, A. 2007 (Sep). "Effects of thymoquinone (volatile oil of black cumin) on rheumatoid arthritis in rat models." *Phytother Res.* 21(9):895–97.

ATHEROSCLEROSIS

1. Lu, Dai, Kiran Vemuri, V., Duclos, Richard I., Jr., and Makriyannis, Alexandros. 2006 (Jul). "The cannabinergic system as a target for anti-inflammatory therapies." *Current Topics in Medicinal Chemistry* 6(13):1401–26. Bentham Science Publishers.

2. Takeda, S., Usami, N., Yamamoto, I., and Watanabe, K. 2009 (Aug). "Cannabidiol-2',6'-dimethyl ether, a cannabidiol derivative, is a highly potent and selective 15 lipoxygenase inhibitor." *Drug Metab Dispos.* 37(8):1733–37.

3. Zhao, Y., Yuan, Z., Liu, Y., Xue, J., Tian, Y., Liu, W., Zhang, W., Shen, Y., Xu, W., Liang, X., and Chen, T. 2010 (Jan). "Activation of cannabinoid CB2 receptor ameliorates atherosclerosis associated with suppression of adhesion molecules." *J Cardiovasc Pharmacol.* 9.

4. Miller, T.Q., Smith, T.W., Turner, C.W., Guijarro, M.L., and Hallet, A.J. 1996. "A meta-analytic review of research on hostility and physical health." *Psychol Bull.* 119:322–48.

5. Whiteman, Martha C., PhD, Ian J. Deary, and F. Gerald R. Fowkes. 2000 (Sep-Oct). "Personality and social predictors of atherosclerotic progression: Edinburgh Artery Study." *Psychosomatic Medicine* 62(5):703–14.

6. Roy, Brita, MD, MPH, MS, Ana V. Diez-Roux, MD, PhD, Teresa Seeman, PhD, Nalini Ranjit, PhD, Steven Shea, MD, and Mary Cushman, MD. 2010 (Feb/Mar). "Association of optimism and pessimism with inflammation and hemostasis in the Multi-Ethnic Study of Atherosclerosis (MESA)." *Psychosomatic Medicine* 72(2):134–40.

7. Rozanski, Alan, MD, Heidi Gransar, MS, Laura D. Kubzansky, PhD, Nathan Wong, MD, Leslee Shaw, PhD, Romalisa Miranda-Peats, MPH, Louise E. Thomson, MBChB, Sean W. Hayes, MD, John D. Friedman, MD, MPH, and Daniel S. Berman, MD. 2011 (Jan). "Do psychological risk factors predict the presence of coronary atherosclerosis?" *Psychosomatic Medicine* 73(1):7–15.

8. Rudkowska, I., and Jones, P.J. 2007 (May). "Functional foods for the prevention and treatment of cardiovascular diseases: Cholesterol and beyond." *Expert Rev Cardiovasc Ther.* 5(3):477–90.

9. Suneetha, W.J., and Krishnakantha, T.P. 2005 (May). "Cardamom extract as inhibitor of human platelet aggregation." *Phytother Res.* 19(5):437–40.

10. Kaunitz, H. 1986 (Mar-Apr). "Medium-chain triglycerides (MCT) in aging and arteriosclerosis." *J Environ Pathol Toxicol Oncol.* 6(3-4):115–21.

11. Cuban Ministry of Public Health, Havana. 1992. *Therapeutic Guide to Plant Pharmaceuticals and Honey Pharmaceuticals (Guia Terapeutica Dispensarial de Fitofarmacos y Apifarmacos).* Ministerio de Salud Publica, Ciudad de La Habana, Republica de Cuba.

12. Federal Republic of Germany. *Monographien der E-Kommission (Phyto-Therapie) (380 monographs). A therapeutic guide to herbal medicine evaluating the safety and efficacy of herbs for licensed medical prescribing in Germany.* Published between 1984 and 1994 in the Bundesanzeiger (official publication by the Federal Republic of Germany). Copies of the monographs are available at the Heilpflanzen-Welt Bibliothek: http://buecher.heilpflanzen-welt.de/BGA-Commission-E-Monographs/

13. Okada, Y., Tanaka, K., Sato, E., and Okajima, H. 2006 (Nov 21). "Kinetic and mechanistic studies of allicin as an antioxidant." *Org Biomol Chem.* 4(22):4113–17.

14. Fukao, H., Yoshida, H., Tazawa, Y., and Hada, T. 2007 (Jan). "Antithrombotic effects of odorless garlic powder both in vitro and in vivo." *Biosci Biotechnol Biochem.* 71(1):84–90.

15. Hsieh, C.L., Peng, C.H., Chyau, C.C., Lin, Y.C., Wang, H.E., and Peng, R.Y. 2007 (Apr 18). "Low-density lipoprotein, collagen, and thrombin models reveal that Rosmarinus officinalis L. exhibits potent antiglycative effects." *J Agric Food Chem.* 55(8):2884–91.

16. Goel, A., Kunnumakkara, A.B., and Aggarwal, B.B. 2008 (Feb 15). "Curcumin as 'Curecumin': From kitchen to clinic." *Biochem Pharmacol.* 75(4):787–809.

INTERSTITIAL CYSTITIS

1. Krenn, H., Daha, L.K., Oczenski, W., and Fitzgerald, R.D. 2003. "A case of cannabinoid rotation in a young woman with chronic cystitis." *J Pain Symptom Manage.* 25(1):3–4.

2. Twiss, Christian, Kilpatrick, Lisa, Craske, Michelle, Buffington, C.A. Tony, Ornitz, Edward, Rodríguez, Larissa V., Mayer, Emeran A., and Naliboff, Bruce D. 2009. "Increased acoustic startle responses in IBS patients during abdominal and non-abdominal threat." *The Journal of Urology* 181(5):2127–33.

3. Theoharides, T.C., Whitmore, K., Stanford, E., Moldwin, R., and O'Leary, M.P. 2008 (Dec). "Interstitial cystitis: Bladder pain and beyond." *Expert Opin Pharmacother.* 9(17):2979–94.

RHEUMATOID ARTHRITIS

1. Blake, D.R., Robson, P., Ho, M., Jubb, R.W., and McCabe, C.S. 2006. "Preliminary assessment of the efficacy, tolerability and safety of a cannabis-based medicine (Sativex) in the treatment of pain caused by rheumatoid arthritis." *Rheumatology* 45(1):50–52.

2. Lu, Dai, Kiran Vemuri, V., Duclos, Richard I., Jr., and Makriyannis, Alexandros. 2006 (Jul). "The cannabinergic system as a target for anti-inflammatory therapies." *Current Topics in Medicinal Chemistry* 6(13):1401–26(26). Bentham Science Publishers.

3. Burstein, Sumner H., and Zurier, Robert B. 2009 (Mar). "Cannabinoids, endocannabinoids, and related analogs in inflammation." *AAPS J.* 11(1):109–19.

4. Cobb, Sidney, MD, Stanislav V. Kasl, PhD., Edith Chen, MA, and Roger Christenfeld, MA. 1965 (Dec). "Some psychological and social characteristics of patients hospitalized for rheumatoid arthritis, hypertension, and duodenal ulcer." *Journal of Chronic Diseases* 18(12):1259–78.

5. Cheren, Stanley, MD, and Levitan, Harold, MD. 1989. "Chapter 4. Onset Situation in Three Psychosomatic Illnesses" in *Psychosomatic Medicine: Theory, Physiology and Practice* (Madison, Connecticut: International University Press, Inc., Vol. 1).

6. Johnson, Adelaide, MD, Shapiro, Louis B., MD, and Alexander, Franz, MD. "Preliminary Report on a Psychosomatic Study of Rheumatoid Arthritis." Paper presented at the Annual Meeting of the American Society for Research in Psychosomatic Problems, Atlantic City, New Jersey, May 3, 1947.

7. Cuban Ministry of Public Health, Havana. 1992. *Therapeutic Guide to Plant Pharmaceuticals and Honey Pharmaceuticals (Guia Terapeutica Dispensarial de Fitofarmacos y Apifarmacos)*. Ministerio de Salud Publica, Ciudad de La Habana, Republica de Cuba.

8. Khanna, D., Sethi, G., Ahn, K.S., Pandey, M.K., Kunnumakkara, A.B., Sung, B., Aggarwal, A., and Aggarwal, B.B. 2007 (Jun). "Natural products as a gold mine for arthritis treatment." *Curr Opin Pharmacol.* 7(3):344–51.

9. Tekeoglu, I., Dogan, A., Ediz, L., Budancamanak, M., and Demirel, A. 2007 (Sep). "Effects of thymoquinone (volatile oil of black cumin) on rheumatoid arthritis in rat models." *Phytother Res.* 21(9):895–97.

Gastro-Esophageal Reflux Disease (GERD)

1. Beaumont, H., Jensen, J., Carlsson, A., Ruth, M., Lehmann, A., and Boeckx-staens, G.E. 2009 (Jan). "Effect of Delta(9)-tetrahydrocannabinol, a cannabinoid receptor agonist, on the triggering of transient lower oesophageal sphincter relaxations in dogs and humans." *Br J Pharmacol.* 156(1):153–62.

2. Naliboff, Bruce D., PhD, Minou Mayer, MA, MFT, Ronnie Fass, MD, Leah Z. Fitzgerald, RN, MS, Lin Chang, MD, Roger Bolus, PhD, and Emeran A. Mayer, MD. 2004. "The effect of life stress on symptoms of heartburn." *Psychosomatic Medicine* 66:426–34.

3. Sharma, Abhishek, MD, PhD, Lukas Van Oudenhove, MD, PhD, Peter Paine, MD, PhD, Lloyd Gregory, PhD, and Qasim Aziz, MD, PhD. 2010 (Oct). "Anxiety increases acid-induced esophageal hyperalgesia." *Psychosomatic Medicine* 72(8):802–09.

Inflammatory Bowel Disease (IBS)

1. Ford, A.C., Talley, N.J., Spiegel, B.M., Foxx-Orenstein, A.E., Schiller, L., Quigley, E.M., and Moayyedi, P. "Effect of fibre, antispasmodics, and peppermint oil in the treatment of irritable bowel syndrome: Systematic review and meta-analysis." *BMJ* 337:a2313.

2. Izzo, A.A., and Sharkey, K.A. 2010 (Apr). "Cannabinoids and the gut: New developments and emerging concepts." *Pharmacol Ther.* 126(1):21–38.

3. Lu, Dai, Kiran Vemuri, V., Duclos, Richard I., Jr., and Makriyannis, Alexandros. 2006 (Jul). "The cannabinergic system as a target for anti-inflammatory therapies." *Current Topics in Medicinal Chemistry* 6(13):1401–26(26). Bentham Science Publishers.

4. Storr, M.A., Keenan, C.M., Emmerdinger, D., Zhang, H., Yüce, B., Sibaev, A., Massa, F., Buckley, N.E., Lutz, B., Göke, B., Brand, S., Patel, K.D., and Sharkey, K.A. 2008 (Aug). "Targeting endocannabinoid degradation protects against experimental colitis in mice: involvement of CB(1) and CB(2) receptors." *J Mol Med.* (Berl). 86(8):925–36.

5. Capasso, R., Borrelli, F., Aviello, G., Romano, B., Scalisi, C., Capasso, F., and Izzo, A. 2008 (Jul). "Cannabidiol, extracted from Cannabis sativa, selectively inhibits inflammatory hypermotility in mice." *Br J Pharmacol.* 154(5):1001–08.

6. Kaptchuk, Ted J., Elizabeth Friedlander, John M. Kelley, M. Norma Sanchez, Efi Kokkotou, Joyce P. Singer, Magda Kowalczykowski, Franklin G. Miller, Irving Kirsch, and Anthony J. Lembo. 2010 (Dec 22). "Placebos without deception: A randomized controlled trial in irritable bowel syndrome." *PLoS ONE* 5(12):e15591.

   Kaptchuk, Ted J., John M. Kelley, Lisa A. Conboy, Roger B. Davis, Catherine E. Kerr, Eric E. Jacobson, Irving Kirsch, Rosa N. Schyner, Bong Hyun Nam, Long T. Nguyen, Min Park, Andrea L. Rivers, Claire McManus, Efi Kokkotou, Douglas A. Drossman, Peter Goldman, and Anthony J. Lembo. 2008 (Apr). "Components of placebo effect: Randomized controlled trial in patients with irritable bowel syndrome." *BMJ* 336:999.

7. Whitehead, W.E., Palsson, O., and Jones, K.R. 2002 (Apr). "Systematic review of the comorbidity of irritable bowel syndrome with other disorders: What are the causes and implications?" *Gastroenterology* 122(4):1140–56.

8. Grace, William J., MD, and Graham, David T., MD. Dept. of Medicine of the New York Hospital–Cornell Medical Center. 1952 (July 1). "Relationship of specific attitudes and emotions to certain bodily diseases." *Psychosomatic Medicine* 14(4):243–51.

9. Ibid.

10. Ibid.

11. Bliss, D.Z., Jung, H.J., Savik, K., Lowry, A., LeMoine, M., Jensen, L., Werner, C., and Schaffer, K. 2001 (Jul-Aug). "Supplementation with dietary fiber improves fecal incontinence." *Nurs Res.* 50(4):203–13.

12. Goel, A., Kunnumakkara, A.B., and Aggarwal, B.B. 2008 (Feb 15). "Curcumin as 'Curecumin': From kitchen to clinic." *Biochem Pharmacol.* 75(4):787–809.

13. Hanai, H., Iida, T., Takeuchi, K., Watanabe, F., Maruyama, Y., Andoh, A., Tsujikawa, T., Fujiyama, Y., Mitsuyama, K., Sata, M., Yamada, M., Iwaoka, Y., Kanke, K., Hiraishi, H., Hirayama, K., Arai, H., Yoshii, S., Uchijima, M., Nagata, T., and Koide, Y. 2006 (Dec). "Curcumin maintenance therapy for ulcerative colitis: Randomized, multicenter, double-blind, placebo-controlled trial." *Clin Gastroenterol Hepatol.* 4(12):1502–06.

PANCREATITIS

1. Michalski, Christoph W., Milena Maier, Mert Erkan, Danguole Sauliunaite, Frank Bergmann, Pal Pacher, Sandor Batkai, Nathalia A. Giese, Thomas Giese, Helmut Friess, and Jörg Kleeff. 2008. "Cannabinoids reduce markers of inflammation and fibrosis in pancreatic stellate cells." *PLoS ONE* 3(2):e1701.

2. Dembiński, A., Warzecha, Z., Ceranowicz, P., Warzecha, A.M., Pawlik, W.W., Dembiński, M., Rembiasz, K., Sendur, P., Kuśnierz-Cabala, B., Tomaszewska, R., Chowaniec, E., and Konturek. P.C. 2008 (Sep 4). "Dual, time-dependent deleterious and protective effect of anandamide on the course of cerulein-induced acute pancreatitis. Role of sensory nerves." *Eur J Pharmacol.* 591(1-3):284–92.

3. Nakai, Y., Araki, T., Takahashi, S., Shimada, A., and Nakagawa, T. 1983. "Chronic pancreatitis as psychosomatic disorder." *Psychother Psychosom.* 39(4):201–12.

4. Goel, A., Kunnumakkara, A.B., and Aggarwal, B.B. 2008 (Feb 15). "Curcumin as 'Curecumin': From kitchen to clinic." *Biochem Pharmacol.* 75(4):787–809.

PERIDONTITIS

1. Napimoga, M.H., Benatti, B.B., Lima, F.O., Alves, P.M., Campos, A.C., Pena-Dos-Santos, D.R., Severino, F.P., Cunha, F.Q., and Guimarães, F.S. 2009 (Feb). "Cannabidiol decreases bone resorption by inhibiting RANK/RANKL expression and pro-inflammatory cytokines during experimental periodontitis in rats." *Int Immunopharmacol.* 9(2):216–22.

2. Vitaliano, Peter P., PhD, Rutger Persson, DDS, PhD, Asuman Kiyak, PhD, Hardeep Saini, BS, and Diana Echeverria, PhD. 2005. "Caregiving and gingival symptom reports: Psychophysiologic mediators." *Psychosomatic Medicine* 67:930–38.

3. Ibid.

4. Gazzani, G., Daglia, M., and Papetti, A. 2012 (Apr). "Food components with anticaries activity." *Curr Opin Biotechnol.* 23(2):153–59.

Insomnia

1. Fujimori, M., and Himwich, H.E. 1973. "Delta sup(9) Tetrahydrocannabinol and the sleep wakefulness cycle." *Physiology and Behavior* 11(3):291–95.

   Freemon, F.R. 1974. "The effect of Delta sup(9) tetrahydrocannabinol on sleep." *Psychopharmacologia* 35(1):39–44.

   Adams, P.M., and Barratt, E.S. 1975. "Effect of chronic marijuana administration on stages of primate sleep wakefulness. *Biological Psychiatry* 10(3):315–22.

   Feinberg, I., Jones, R., et al. 1975. "Effects of high-dosage delta-9-tetrahydrocannabinol on sleep patterns in man." *Clinical Pharmacology and Therapeutics* 17(4):458–66.

   Feinberg, I., Jones, R., et al. 1976. "Effects of marijuana extract and tetrahydrocannabinol on electroencephalographic sleep patterns." *Clinical Pharmacology and Therapeutics* 19(6):782–94.

   Freemon, F.R. 1982. "The effect of chronically administered delta-9-tetrahydrocannabinol upon the polygraphically monitored sleep of normal volunteers." *Drug and Alcohol Dependence* 10(4):345–53.

2. Nicholson, A.N., Turner, C., Stone, B.M., and Robson, P.J. 2004 (Jun). "Effect of Delta-9-tetrahydrocannabinol and cannabidiol on nocturnal sleep and early-morning behavior in young adults." *J Clin Psychopharmacol.* 24(3):305–13.

3. Fernández-Mendoza, Julio, MS, Antonio Vela-Bueno, MD, Alexandros N. Vgontzas, MD, María José Ramos-Platón, PhD, Sara Olavarrieta-Bernardino, MSc, Edward O. Bixler, PhD, and Juan José De la Cruz-Troca, MSc. 2010 (May). "Cognitive-emotional hyperarousal as a premorbid characteristic of individuals vulnerable to insomnia." *Psychosomatic Medicine* 72(4):397–403.

Libido

1. Parker, R.C., and Lux. 2008 (Jun). "Psychoactive plants in Tantric Buddhism; Cannabis and datura use in Indo-Tibetan Esoteric Buddhism." *Erowid Extracts* 14:6–11.

2. Sam'l O.L. Potter, MA, MD, MRCP (Lond.) 1892. *A Compend of Materia Medica and Therapeutics and Prescription Writing; with especial references to the physiological actions of drugs* (Philadelphia: P. Blakiston, Son & Co.), p. 40. Based on the last revision of the U.S. Pharmacopeia, 5th Edition.

3. Mahler, S.V., Smith, K.S., and Berridge, K.C. 2007 (Nov). "Endocannabinoid hedonic hotspot for sensory pleasure: Anandamide in nucleus accumbens shell enhances 'liking' of a sweet reward." *Neuropsychopharmacology* 32(11):2267–78.

4. Kassi, E., Papoutsi, Z., Fokialakis, N., Messari, I., Mitakou, S., and Moutsat-

sou, P. 2004 (Nov 17). "Greek plant extracts exhibit selective estrogen receptor modulator (SERM)-like properties." *J Agric Food Chem.* 52(23):6956–61.

5. Preuss, H.G., Echard, B., Polansky, M.M., and Anderson, R. 2006 (Apr). "Whole cinnamon and aqueous extracts ameliorate sucrose-induced blood pressure elevations in spontaneously hypertensive rats." *J Am Coll Nutr.* 25(2): 144–50.

6. Tajuddin Shamshad, Ahmad, Abdul Latif, and Iqbal A. Qasmi. 2003 (Oct 20). "Myristica fragrans Houtt. (nutmeg) and Syzygium aromaticum (L) Merr. & Perry (clove) in male mice: A comparative study." *BMC Complementary and Alternative Medicine* 3:6.

7. Qureshi, S., Shah, A.H., Tariq, M., and Ageel, A.M. 1989. "Studies on herbal aphrodisiacs used in Arab system of medicine." *Am J Chin Med.* 17(1-2):57–63.

8. Kamtchouing, P., Mbongue, G.Y., Dimo, T., Watcho, P., Jatsa, H.B., and Sokeng, S.D. 2002 (May). "Effects of Aframomum melegueta and Piper guineense on sexual behaviour of male rats." *Behav Pharmacol.* 13(3):243–47.

9. Dording, C.M., Fisher, L., Papakostas, G., Farabaugh, A., Sonawalla, S., Fava, M., and Mischoulon, D. 2008 (Fall). "A double-blind, randomized, pilot dose-finding study of maca root (L. meyenii) for the management of SSRI-induced sexual dysfunction." *CNS Neurosci Ther.* 14(3):182–91.

10. Tajuddin, Ahmad S. et al. 2003. "Aphrodisiac activity of 50% ethanolic extracts of Myristica fragrans. . ." (see note 6 above).

Lung Diseases

Asthma

1. Tashkin, D.P., Shapiro, B.J., and Frank, I.M. 1974 (Apr). "Acute effects of smoked marijuana and oral delta9-tetrahydrocannabinol on specific airway conductance in asthmatic subjects." *Am Rev Respir Dis.* 109(4):420–28.

2. Tashkin, D.P., Shapiro, B.J., Lee, Y.E., and Harper, C.E. 1975 (Sep). "Effects of smoked marijuana in experimentally induced asthma." *Am Rev Respir Dis.* 112(3):377–86.

3. Williams, S.J., Hartley, J.P., and Graham, J.D. 1976. "Bronchodilator effect of delta1-tetrahydrocannabinol administered by aerosol of asthmatic patients." *Thorax* 31(6):720–23.

4. Tashkin, D.P., Reiss, S., Shapiro, B.J., Calvarese, B., Olsen, J.L., and Lodge, J.W. 1977 (Jan). "Bronchial effects of aerosolized delta 9-tetrahydrocannabinol in healthy and asthmatic subjects." *Am Rev Respir Dis.* 115(1):57–65.

5. Hartley, J.P., Nogrady, S.G., and Seaton, A. 1978 (Jun). "Bronchodilator effect of delta1-tetrahydrocannabinol." *Br J Clin Pharmacol.* 5(6):523–25.

6. Gong, H., Jr., Tashkin, D.P., and Calvarese, B. 1983. "Comparison of bronchial effects of nabilone and terbutaline in healthy and asthmatic subjects." *Journal of Clinical Pharmacology* 23(4):127–33.

7. Lu, Dai, Kiran Vemuri, V., Duclos, Richard I., Jr., and Makriyannis, Alexandros. 2006 (Jul). "The cannabinergic system as a target for anti-inflammatory therapies." *Current Topics in Medicinal Chemistry* 6(13):1401–26(26). Bentham Science Publishers.

8. Grace, William J., MD, and Graham, David T., MD. Dept. of Medicine of the New York Hospital–Cornell Medical Center. 1952 (July 1). "Relationship of specific attitudes and emotions to certain bodily diseases." *Psychosomatic Medicine* 14(4):243–51.

9. Monday, J., Montplaisir, J., and Malo, J.L. 1987 (May). "Dream process in asthmatic subjects with nocturnal attacks." *Am J Psychiatry* 144(5):638–40.

10. Wood, James, M., Bootzin, Richard R., Quan, Stuart F., and Klink, Mary E. 1993 (Dec). "Prevalence of nightmares among patients with asthma and chronic obstructive airways disease." *Dreaming* 3(4):231–41.

11. William Ernest Henley (1849–1903). "Invictus."

12. Boskabady, M.H., and Ramazani-Assari, M. 2001 (Jan). "Relaxant effect of Pimpinella anisum on isolated guinea pig tracheal chains and its possible mechanism(s)." *J Ethnopharmacol.* 74(1):83–88.

13. Khan, A.U., and Gilani, A.H. 2006 (Dec). "Selective bronchodilatory effect of Rooibos tea (Aspalathus linearis) and its flavonoid, chrysoeriol." *Eur J Nutr.* 45(8):463–69.

14. Usmani, O.S., Belvisi, M.G., Patel, H.J., Crispino, N., Birrell, M.A., Korbonits, M., Korbonits, D., and Barnes, P.J. 2005 (Feb). "Theobromine inhibits sensory nerve activation and cough." *FASEB J.* 19(2):231–33.

15. Cuban Ministry of Public Health, Havana. 1992. *Therapeutic Guide to Plant Pharmaceuticals and Honey Pharmaceuticals (Guia Terapeutica Dispensarial de Fitofarmacos y Apifarmacos).* Ministerio de Salud Publica, Ciudad de La Habana, Republica de Cuba.

16. Boskabady, M.H., Javan, H., Sajady, M., and Rakhshandeh, H. 2007 Oct. "The possible prophylactic effect of Nigella sativa seed extract in asthmatic patients." *Fundam Clin Pharmacol.* 21(5):559–66.

17. Venkatesan, N., Punithavathi, D., and Babu, M. 2007. "Protection from acute and chronic lung diseases by curcumin." *Adv Exp Med Biol.* 595:379–405.

Chronic Obstructive Pulmonary Disease

1. Karl-Christian Bergmann. "Dronabinol—eine mögliche neue Therapieoption bei COPD-Patienten mit pulmonaler Kachexie." Paper presented

at the 2005 Conference of the German Society for Pneumology, Berlin, 17 March 2005.

2. Tan, W.C., Lo, C., Jong, A., Xing, L., Fitzgerald, M.J., Vollmer, W.M., Buist, S.A., and Sin, D.D. 2009 (Apr 14). "Marijuana and chronic obstructive lung disease: a population-based study." *CMAJ* 180(8):814–20.

Mental Disorders

Attention Deficit Hyperactivity Disorder

1. Bloom, B., Jones, L.I., and Freeman, G. 2013. "Summary health statistics for U.S. children: National Health Interview Survey, 2012." *Vital Health Stat* 10(258).

2. Kooij, S.J., Bejerot, S., Blackwell, A., Caci, H., Casas-Brugué, M., Carpentier, P.J., Edvinsson, D., Fayyad, J., Foeken, K., Fitzgerald, M., Gaillac, V., Ginsberg, Y., Henry, C., Krause, J., Lensing, M.B., Manor, I., Niederhofer, H., Nunes-Filipe, C., Ohlmeier, M.D., Oswald, P., Pallanti, S., Pehlivanidis, A., Ramos-Quiroga, J.A., Rastam, M., Ryffel-Rawak, D., Stes, S., and Asherson, P. 2010 (Sep 3). "European consensus statement on diagnosis and treatment of adult ADHD: The European Network Adult ADHD." *BMC Psychiatry* 10:67.

3. Drug Enforcement Administration. Office of Diversion Control. Drug & Chemical Evaluation Section. "Ritalin." May 2013. www.deadiversion.usdoj .gov/drug_chem_info/methylphenidate.pdf

4. Lafenêtre, P., Chaouloff, F., and Marsicano, G. 2009 (Dec). "Bidirectional regulation of novelty-induced behavioral inhibition by the endocannabinoid system." *Neuropharmacology* 57(7-8):715–21.

5. Castelli, M., Federici, M., Rossi, S., De Chiara, V., Napolitano, F., Studer, V., Motta, C., Sacchetti, L., Romano, R., Musella, A., Bernardi, G., Siracusano, A., Gu, H.H., Mercuri, N.B., Usiello, A., and Centonze, D. 2011 (Nov). "Loss of striatal cannabinoid CB1 receptor function in attention-deficit/hyperactivity disorder mice with point-mutation of the dopamine transporter." *Eur J Neurosci.* 34(9):1369–77.

6. Gururajan, A., Taylor, D.A., and Malone, DT. 2012 (Oct). "Cannabidiol and clozapine reverse MK-801-induced deficits in social interaction and hyperactivity in Sprague-Dawley rats." *J Psychopharmacol.* 26(10):1317–32.

7. Strohbeck-Kuehner, Peter, Skopp, Gisela, and Mattern, Rainer. 2008. "Case report: Cannabis improves symptoms of ADHD." *Cannabinoids* 3(1):1–3.

8. Loflin, M., Earleywine, M., De Leo, J., et al. 2013. Subtypes of attention deficit-hyperactivity disorder (ADHD) and cannabis use." *Subst Use Misuse.* 49(4):427–34.

9. Ly, C., and Gehricke, J.G. 2013 (Dec 30). "Marijuana use is associated with inattention in men and sleep quality in women with attention-deficit/hyperactivity disorder: A preliminary study." *Psychiatry Res.* 210(3):1310–12.

10. Posner, Michael I., and Rothbart, Mary K. 2009 (Jun 1). "Toward a physical basis of attention and self regulation." *Phys Life Rev.* 6(2):103–120.

   Klingberg, T., Forssberg, H., and Westerberg, H. 2002 (Sep). "Training of working memory in children with ADHD." *J Clin Exp Neuropsychol.* 24(6):781–91.

11. Sykes, D.H., Douglas, V.I., and Morgenstern, G. 1973 (Sep). "Sustained attention in hyperactive children." *J Child Psychol Psychiatry* 14(3):213–20.

12. Tang, Y.Y., Ma, Y., Wang, J., Fan, Y., Feng, S., Lu, Q., Yu, Q., Sui, D., Rothbart, M.K., Fan, M., and Posner, M.I. 2007 (Oct 23). "Short-term meditation training improves attention and self-regulation." *Proc Natl Acad Sci USA* 104(43):17152–56.

ANXIETY

1. Kessler, Ronald C., PhD, Wai Tat Chiu, AM, Olga Demler, MA, MS, and Ellen E. Walters, MS. 2005 (Jun). "Prevalence, severity, and comorbidity of 12-month *DSM-IV* disorders in the National Comorbidity Survey Replication." *Arch Gen Psychiatry* 62(6):617–27.

2. Witkin, J.M., Tzavara, E.T., and Nomikos, G.G. 2005 (Sep). "A role for cannabinoid CB1 receptors in mood and anxiety disorders." *Behav Pharmacol.* 16(5-6):315–31.

3. Wen Jiang, Yun Zhang, Lan Xiao, Jamie Van Cleemput, Shao-Ping Ji, Guang Bai, and Xia Zhang. 2005. "Cannabinoids promote embryonic and adult hippocampus neurogenesis and produce anxiolytic- and antidepressant-like effects." *J Clin Invest.* 115(11):3104–16.

4. Corless, I.B., Lindgren, T., Holzemer, W., Robinson, L., Moezzi, S., Kirksey, K., Coleman, C., Tsai, Y.F., Sanzero, Eller L., Hamilton, M.J., Sefcik, E.F., Canaval, G.E., Rivero Mendez, M., Kemppainen, J.K., Bunch, E.H., Nicholas, P.K., Nokes, K.M., Dole, P., and Reynolds, N. 2009 (May). "Marijuana effectiveness as an HIV self-care strategy." *Clin Nurs Res.* 18(2):172–93.

5. José Alexandre S. Crippa, Antonio Waldo Zuardi, and Jaime E.C. Hallak. 2010 (May). "Therapeutical use of the cannabinoids in psychiatry." *Revista Brasileira de Psiquiatria* 32(Suppl I).

AUTISM

1. "Graph by Autism Speaks." Accessed April 16, 2015. www.autismspeaks.org/docs/Prevalence_Graph_12_18_2009.pdf

2. Lovaas, O.I. 1987 (Feb). "Behavioral treatment and normal educational and intellectual functioning in young autistic children." *Consult Clin Psychol.* 55(1):3–9.

3. Cohen, Howard, Amerine-Dickens, Mila, and Smith, Tristram. 2006. "Early intensive behavioral treatment: Replication of the UCLA Model in a community setting." *Journal of Developmental & Behavioral Pediatrics* 27(2):145–55.

   Sallows, Glen O. & Graupner, and Tamlynn, D. 2005. "Intensive behavioral treatment for children with autism: Four-year outcome and predictors." *American Journal on Mental Retardation* 110(6):417–38.

   Myers, S.M., and Johnson, C.P. 2007 (Nov). "Management of children with autism spectrum disorders." *Pediatrics* 120(5):1162–82.

4. Ibid.

5. Ganz, M.L., MS, PhD. 2007. "The lifetime distribution of the incremental societal costs of autism." *Arch Pediatr Adolesc Med.* 161(4):343–49.

6. Autism Research Institute, 4182 Adams Ave., San Diego, CA 92116. "Medical Marijuana: A Valuable Treatment for Autism?" 2003. *Autism Research Review International* 17(1):3.

7. Treffert, Darold A. 2009 (May 27). "Extraordinary people: Understanding savant syndrome." *Philos Trans R Soc Lond B Biol Sci.* 364(1522):1351–57.

8. Derek Paravicini (born July 1979) can play any piece of music after hearing it but once.

9. Richard Wawro (born April 1952) creates phenomenal and extremely detailed and vivid land and seascape drawings, rendered from memory after seeing the landscapes but once.

10. Daniel Tammet (born January 1979) is well-known for his vivid and complex ability to see positive integers up to 10,000, each with its own unique shape, color, texture, and feeling.

11. Temple Grandin (born August 1947) is a U.S. doctor of animal science and Professor at Colorado State University.

12. Howlin, P., Goode, S., Hutton, J., and Rutter, M. 2009 (May 27). "Savant skills in autism: Psychometric approaches and parental reports." *Philos Trans R Soc Lond B Biol Sci.* 364(1522):1359–67.

Depression

1. World Health Organization (WHO). 2012. Mental Health. "Depression." Accessed April 16, 2015. www.who.int/mediacentre/factsheets/fs369/en/

2. Beal, J.E., Olson, R., Laubenstein, L., Morales, J.O., Bellman, P., Yangco, B., Lefkowitz, L., Plasse, T.F., and Shepard, K.V. 1995. "Dronabinol as a treatment for anorexia associated with weight loss in patients with AIDS." *Journal of Pain and Symptom Management* 10(2):89–97.

3. Neff, G.W., O'Brien, C.B., Reddy, K.R., Bergasa, N.V., Regev, A., Molina, E., Amaro, R., Rodriguez, M.J., Chase, V., Jeffers, L., and Schiff, E. 2002 (Aug). "Preliminary observation with dronabinol in patients with intractable pruritus secondary to cholestatic liver disease." *Am J Gastroenterol.* 97(8):2117–19.

4. Wen Jiang, Yun Zhang, Lan Xiao, Jamie Van Cleemput, Shao-Ping Ji, Guang Bai, and Xia Zhang. 2005. "Cannabinoids promote embryonic and adult hippocampus neurogenesis and produce anxiolytic- and antidepressant-like effects." *J Clin Invest.* 115(11):3104–16.

5. McLaughlin, R.J., Hill, M.N., Morrish, A.C., and Gorzalka, B.B. 2007 (Sep). "Local enhancement of cannabinoid CB1 receptor signalling in the dorsal hippocampus elicits an antidepressant-like effect." *Behav Pharmacol.* 18(5-6):431–38.

6. Bambico, F.R., Katz, N., Debonnel, G., and Gobbi, G. 2007. "Cannabinoids elicit antidepressant-like behavior and activate serotonergic neurons through the medial prefrontal cortex." *J Neurosci.* 27(43):11700–11.

7. Corless, I.B., Lindgren, T., Holzemer, W., Robinson, L., Moezzi, S., Kirksey, K., Coleman, C., Tsai, Y.F., Sanzero, Eller L., Hamilton, M.J., Sefcik, E.F., Canaval, G.E., Rivero Mendez, M., Kemppainen, J.K., Bunch, E.H., Nicholas, P.K., Nokes, K.M., Dole, P., and Reynolds, N. 2009 (May). "Marijuana effectiveness as an HIV self-care strategy." *Clin Nurs Res.* 18(2):172–93.

8. Crippa, J.A., Zuardi, A.W., and Hallak, J.E. 2010 (May). "Therapeutical use of the cannabinoids in psychiatry." *Rev Bras Psiquiatr.* 32 Suppl 1:S56–66.

9. El-Alfy, Abir T., Kelly Ivey, Keisha Robinson, Safwat Ahmed, Mohamed Radwan, Desmond Slade, Ikhlas Khan, Mahmoud ElSohly, and Samir Ross. 2010 (Jun). "Antidepressant-like effect of Δ9-tetrahydrocannabinol and other cannabinoids isolated from Cannabis sativa L." *Pharmacology Biochemistry and Behavior* 95(4):434–42.

10. Michalaka, Johannes, Rohdeb, Katharina, and Trojec, Nikolaus F. 2015 (Mar). "How we walk affects what we remember: Gait modifications through biofeedback change negative affective memory bias." *Journal of Behavior Therapy and Experimental Psychiatry* 46:121–25.

11. Bruinsma, K, and Taren, D.L. 1999 (Oct). "Chocolate: Food or drug?" *J Am Diet Assoc.* 99(10):1249–56.

12. Dhingra, D., and Sharma, A. 2006 (Spring). "Antidepressant-like activity of n-hexane extract of nutmeg (Myristica fragrans) seeds in mice." *J Med Food.* 9(1):84–89.

BIPOLAR AFFECTIVE DISORDER (BAD) OR MANIC-DEPRESSIVE DISORDER

1. Leverich, Gabriele S., and Post, Robert M. 2006 (Apr 1). "Course of bipolar illness after history of childhood trauma." *The Lancet* 367(9516):1040–42.

2. Baldessarini, R.J., Tondo, L., Davis, P., Pompili, M., Goodwin, F.K., and Hennen, J. 2006 (Oct). "Decreased risk of suicides and attempts during long-term lithium treatment: A meta-analytic review." *Bipolar Disord.* 8(5 Pt 2):625–39.

3. El-Alfy, Abir T., Kelly Ivey, Keisha Robinson, Safwat Ahmed, Mohamed Radwan, Desmond Slade, Ikhlas Khan, Mahmoud ElSohly, and Samir Ross. 2010 (Jun). "Antidepressant-like effect of Δ9-tetrahydrocannabinol and other cannabinoids isolated from Cannabis sativa L." *Pharmacology Biochemistry and Behavior* 95(4):434–42.

4. Zuardi, A., Crippa, J., Dursun, S., Morais, S., Vilela, J., Sanches, R., and Hallak, J. 2010 (Jan). "Cannabidiol was ineffective for manic episode of bipolar affective disorder." *J Psychopharmacol.* 24(1):135–37.

5. El-Mallakh, R.S., and Brown, C. 2007. "The effect of extreme marijuana use on the long-term course of bipolar I illness: A single case study." *J Psychoactive Drugs* 39(2):201–02.

6. Ashton, C.H., Moore, P.B., Gallagher, P., and Young, A.H. 2005 (May). "Cannabinoids in bipolar affective disorder: A review and discussion of their therapeutic potential." *J Psychopharmacol.* 19(3):293–300.

7. Grinspoon, L., and Bakalar, J.B. 1998 (Apr–Jun). "The use of cannabis as a mood stabilizer in bipolar disorder: Anecdotal evidence and the need for clinical research." *J Psychoactive Drugs* 30(2):171–77.

POST-TRAUMATIC STRESS DISORDER (PTSD)

1. Shin, L.M., Rauch, S.L., and Pitman, R.K. 2006 (Jul). "Amygdala, medial prefrontal cortex, and hippocampal function in PTSD." *Ann N Y Acad Sci.* 1071:67–79.

2. Ganon-Elazar, E., and Akirav, I. 2009 (Sep 9). "Cannabinoid receptor activation in the basolateral amygdala blocks the effects of stress on the conditioning and extinction of inhibitory avoidance." *J Neurosci.* 29(36):11078–88.

3. Ibid.

4. Fraser, G.A. 2009 (Winter). "The use of a synthetic cannabinoid in the management of treatment-resistant nightmares in posttraumatic stress disorder (PTSD)." *CNS Neurosci Ther.* 15(1):84–88.

5. Harloe, J.P., Thorpe, A.J., and Lichtman, A.H. 2008 (Oct 28). "Differential endocannabinoid regulation of extinction in appetitive and aversive Barnes maze tasks." *Learn Mem.* 15(11):806–09.

6. Wang, S., and Mason, J. 1999. "Elevations of serum T3 levels and their association with symptoms in World War II veterans with combat-related posttraumatic stress disorder: Replication of findings in Vietnam combat veterans." *Psychosom Med* 61:131–38.

7. Redondo, Roger L., Joshua Kim, Autumn L. Arons, Steve Ramirez, Xu Liu, and Susumu Tonegawa. 2014 (Sep 18). "Bidirectional switch of the valence associated with a hippocampal contextual memory engram." *Nature* 513(7518):426–30. doi:10.1038/nature13725.

SCHIZOPHRENIA

1. The extrapyramidal system is the part of the brain involved in reflexes, movements, and positional control. It is located outside the normal pyramidal pathways responsible for motion leading from the brain into the spinal cord.

2. Picchioni, Marco M., and Murray, Robin M. 2007 (July 14). "Schizophrenia." *BMJ* 335(7610):91–95.

3. Ibid.

4. Ibid

5. Ibid.

6. Ibid.

7. Read, J., van Os, J., Morrison, A.P., and Ross, C.A. 2005 (Nov). "Childhood trauma, psychosis and schizophrenia: A literature review with theoretical and clinical implications." *Acta Psychiatr Scand.* 112(5):330–50.

8. Giuffrida, A., Leweke, F.M., Gerth, C.W., Schreiber, D., Koethe, D., Faulhaber, J., Klosterkotter, J., and Piomelli, D. 2004 (Nov). "Cerebrospinal anandamide levels are elevated in acute schizophrenia and are inversely correlated with psychotic symptoms." *Neuropsychopharmacology* 29(11):2108–14.

9. Catechol-O-methyltransferase (COMT) valine (an amino acid) 158 allele

10. Caspi, A., Moffitt, T.E., Cannon, M., McClay, J. Murray, R., Harrington, H., Taylor, A., Arseneault, L., Williams, B., Braithwaite, A., Poulton, R., and Craig, I.W. 2005 (May 15). "Moderation of the effect of adolescent-onset cannabis use on adult psychosis by a functional polymorphism in the catechol-O-methyltransferase gene: Longitudinal evidence of a gene X environment interaction." *Biol Psychiatry.* 57(10):1117–27.

11. Henquet, Cécile, Robin Murray, Don Linszen, and Jim van Os. 2005 (Jul). "The environment and schizophrenia: The role of cannabis use." *Schizophr Bull.* 31(3):608–12.

12. Leweke, F.M., Koethe, D., Pahlisch, F., Schreiber, D., Gerth, C.W., Nolden, B.M., Klosterkötter, J., Hellmich, M., and Piomelli, D. 2009. "S39-02 Antipsychotic effects of cannabidiol." *European Psychiatry* 24, Supplement 1:S207.

13. Crippa, J.A., Zuardi, A.W., and Hallak, J.E. 2010 (May). "Therapeutical use of the cannabinoids in psychiatry." *Rev Bras Psiquiatr.* 32, Supplement 1:S56–66.

14. Parolaro, D., Realini, N., Vigano, D., Guidali, C., and Rubino, T. 2010

(Jul). "The endocannabinoid system and psychiatric disorders." *Exp Neurol.* 224(1):3–14.

Neurological Diseases

Cannabis and Neuroprotection in General

1. The United States of America as represented by the Department of Health and Human Services. (Aidan J. Hampson, Julius Axelrod, and Maurizio Grimaldi) Patent No. 09/674028 filed on 02/02/2001. Patent 6630507 issued on October 7, 2003. Estimated expiration date: 2021. Cannabinoids as antioxidants and neuroprotectants. www.patentstorm.us/patents/6630507.html

2. Hamelink, Carol, Hampson, Aidan, Wink, David A., Eiden, Lee E., and Eskay, Robert L. 2005 (Aug). "Comparison of cannabidiol, antioxidants, and diuretics in reversing binge ethanol-induced neurotoxicity." *JPET* 314(2):780–88.

3. Viscomi, M.T., Oddi, S., Latini, L., Pasquariello, N., Florenzano, F., Bernardi, G., Molinari, M., and Maccarrone, M. 2009 (Apr 8). "Selective CB2 receptor agonism protects central neurons from remote axotomy-induced apoptosis through the PI3K/Akt pathway." *J Neurosci.* 29(14):4564–70.

4. Touriño, C., Zimmer, A., and Valverde, O. 2010 (Feb 10). "THC prevents MDMA neurotoxicity in mice." *PLoS One* 5(2):e9143.

5. Chauhan, N.B., and Sandoval, J. 2007 (Jul). "Amelioration of early cognitive deficits by aged garlic extract in Alzheimer's transgenic mice." *Phytother Res.* 21(7):629–40.

6. Hsieh, C.L., Peng, C.H., Chyau, C.C., Lin, Y.C., Wang, H.E., and Peng, R.Y. 2007 (Apr 18). "Low-density lipoprotein, collagen, and thrombin models reveal that Rosmarinus officinalis L. exhibits potent antiglycative effects." *J Agric Food Chem.* 55(8):2884–91.

7. Goel, A., Kunnumakkara, A.B., and Aggarwal, B.B. 2008 (Feb 15). "Curcumin as 'Curecumin': From kitchen to clinic." *Biochem Pharmacol.* 75(4):787–809.

8. Natarajan, C., and Bright, J.J. 2002 (Jun 15). "Curcumin inhibits experimental allergic encephalomyelitis by blocking IL-12 signaling through Janus kinase-STAT pathway in T lymphocytes." *J Immunol.* 168(12):6506–13.

Alcohol Dependence/Abuse

1. Mikuriya, Tod H., MD. 1970. "Cannabis substitution. An adjunctive therapeutic tool in the treatment of alcoholism." *Medical Times* 98(4):187–91.

2. Mikuriya, Tod H., MD. 2004. "Cannabis as a substitute for alcohol: A harm-reduction approach." *Journal of Cannabis Therapeutics* 4(1).

3. Thanos, P.K., Dimitrakakis, E.S., Rice, O., Gifford, A., and Volkow, N.D. 2005 (Nov 7). "Ethanol self-administration and ethanol conditioned place

preference are reduced in mice lacking cannabinoid CB1 receptors." *Behav Brain Res.* 164(2):206–13.

4. Vinod, K.Y., Yalamanchili, R., Thanos, P.K., Vadasz, C., Cooper, T.B., Volkow, N.D., and Hungund, B.L. 2008 (Aug). "Genetic and pharmacological manipulations of the CB(1) receptor alter ethanol preference and dependence in ethanol preferring and nonpreferring mice." *Synapse* 62(8):574–81.

5. Hamelink, Carol, Hampson, Aidan, Wink, David A., Eiden, Lee E., and Eskay, Robert L. 2005 (Aug). "Comparison of cannabidiol, antioxidants, and diuretics in reversing binge ethanol-induced neurotoxicity." *JPET* 314(2):780–88.

6. Enoch, M.A. 2006 (Dec). "Genetic and environmental influences on the development of alcoholism: Resilience vs. risk." *Ann N Y Acad Sci.* 1094:193–201.

ALZHEIMER'S DISEASE

1. Jiaquan Xu, MD; Kenneth D. Kochanek, MA; Sherry L. Murphy, BS; and Betzaida Tejada-Vera, BS. May 20, 2010. "National Vital Statistics Reports. Deaths: Final Data for 2007." Volume 58, Number 19. U.S. Department of Health and Human Services. Centers for Disease Control and Prevention. National Center for Health Statistics. National Vital Statistics System.

2. Stern, Y. 2006 (Jul-Sep). "Cognitive reserve and Alzheimer disease." *Alzheimer Dis Assoc Disord.* 20(3 Suppl 2):S69–74.

3. Ramírez, B.G., Blázquez, C., Gómez del Pulgar, T., Guzmán, M., and de Ceballos, M.L. 2005 (Feb 23). "Prevention of Alzheimer's disease pathology by cannabinoids: Neuroprotection mediated by blockade of microglial activation." *J Neurosci.* 25(8):1904–13.

4. Tolón, R.M., Núñez, E., Pazos, M.R., Benito, C., Castillo, A.I., Martínez-Orgado, J.A., and Romero, J. 2009 (Jun). "The activation of cannabinoid CB2 receptors stimulates in situ and in vitro beta-amyloid removal by human macrophages." *Brain Res.* 5.

5. Bisogno, T., and Di Marzo, V. 2008. "The role of the endocannabinoid system in Alzheimer's disease: Facts and hypotheses." *Curr Pharm Des.* 14(23):2299–3305.

6. Passmore, M.J. 2008. "The cannabinoid receptor agonist nabilone for the treatment of dementia-related agitation." *Int J Geriatr Psychiatry* 23(1):116–17.

7. Tucker, Adrienne M., and Stern, Yaakov. 2011. "Cognitive reserve in aging." *Current Alzheimer Research*, 8.

8. Chauhan, N.B., and Sandoval, J. 2007 (Jul). "Amelioration of early cognitive deficits by aged garlic extract in Alzheimer's transgenic mice." *Phytother Res.* 21(7):629–40.

9. Goel, A., Kunnumakkara, A.B., and Aggarwal, B.B. 2008 (Feb 15). "Curcumin as 'Curecumin': From kitchen to clinic." *Biochem Pharmacol.* 75(4):787–809.

Aggarwal, B.B., Kumar, A., and Bharti, A.C. 2003 (Jan-Feb). "Anticancer potential of curcumin: Preclinical and clinical studies." *Anticancer Research* 23(1A):363–98.

10. Sommer, Andrei P., Jan Bieschke, Ralf P. Friedrich, Dan Zhu, Erich E. Wanker, Hans J. Fecht, Derliz Mereles, and Werner Hunstein. 2012 (Jan). "670 nm laser light and EGCG complementarily reduce amyloid-β aggregates in human neuroblastoma cells: Basis for treatment of Alzheimer's disease?" *Photomedicine and Laser Surgery* 30(1): 54–60.

Amyotrophic Lateral Sclerosis (ALS) or Lou Gehrig's Disease

1. Sejvar, J.J., Holman, R.C., Bresee, J.S., Kochanek, K.D., and Schonberger, L.B. 2005. "Amyotrophic lateral sclerosis mortality in the United States, 1979–2001." *Neuroepidemiology* 25(3):144–52.

2. Pablo, J., Banack, S.A., Cox, P.A., Johnson, T.E., Papapetropoulos, S., Bradley, W.G., Buck, A., and Mash, D.C. 2009 (Oct). "Cyanobacterial neurotoxin BMAA in ALS and Alzheimer's disease." *Acta Neurol Scand.* 120(4):216–25.

3. Horner, R.D., Kamins, K.G., Feussner, J.R., Grambow, S.C., Hoff-Lindquist, J., Harati, Y., Mitsumoto, H., Pascuzzi, R., Spencer, P.S., Tim, R., Howard, D., Smith, T.C., Ryan, M.A., Coffman, C.J., and Kasarskis. E.J. 2003 (Sep 23). "Occurrence of amyotrophic lateral sclerosis among Gulf War veterans." *Neurology* 61(6):742–49.

4. Haley, R.W. 2003 (Sep 23). "Excess incidence of ALS in young Gulf War veterans." *Neurology* 61(6):750–56.

5. Carter, G.T., Abood, M.E., Aggarwal, S.K., and Weiss, M.D. 2010 (Aug). "Cannabis and amyotrophic lateral sclerosis: Hypothetical and practical applications, and a call for clinical trials." *Am J Hosp Palliat Care* 27(5):347–56.

6. Weber, M., Goldman, B., and Truniger, S. 2010. "Tetrahydrocannabinol (THC) for cramps in amyotrophic lateral sclerosis: A randomized, double blind crossover trial." *J.Neurol.Neurosurg.Psychiatry* 81:1135–40.

7. Carter, G.T., et al. 2010. "Cannabis and amyotrophic lateral sclerosis" (see note 4 above).

8. Rossi, S., Bernardi, G., and Centonze, D. 2010 (Jul). "The endocannabinoid system in the inflammatory and neurodegenerative processes of multiple sclerosis and of amyotrophic lateral sclerosis." *Exp Neurol.* 224(1):92–102.

9. Centonze, D., Finazzi-Agrò, A., Bernardi, G., and Maccarrone, M. 2007 (Apr). "The endocannabinoid system in targeting inflammatory neurodegenerative diseases." *Trends Pharmacol Sci.* 28(4):180–87.

10. Weydt, P., Hong, S., Witting, A., Möller, T., Stella, N., and Kliot, M. 2005 (Sep). "Cannabinol delays symptom onset in SOD1 (G93A) transgenic mice

without affecting survival." *Amyotroph Lateral Scler Other Motor Neuron Disord.* 6(3):182–84.

11. Amtmann, D., Weydt, P., Johnson, K.L., Jensen, M.P., and Carter, G.T. 2004 (Mar-Apr). "Survey of cannabis use in patients with amyotrophic lateral sclerosis." *Am J Hosp Palliat Care* 21(2):95–104.

12. Carter, G.T., and Rosen, B.S. 2001 (Jul-Aug). "Marijuana in the management of amyotrophic lateral sclerosis." *Am J Hosp Palliat Care* 18(4):264–70.

13. Rabkin, Judith G., PhD, Glenn J. Wagner, PhD, and Maura Del Bene, RN, BSN. 2000. "Resilience and distress among amyotrophic lateral sclerosis patients and caregivers." *Psychosomatic Medicine* 62:271–79.

EPILEPTIC SEIZURE (STATUS EPILEPTICUS)

1. Jones, N.A., Hill, A.J., Smith, I., Bevan, S.A., Williams, C.M., Whalley, B.J., and Stephens, G.J. 2010 (Feb). "Cannabidiol displays anti-epileptiform and anti-seizure properties in vitro and in vivo." *J Pharmacol Exp Ther.* 332(2):569–77.

2. Romigi, A., Bari, M., Placidi, F., Marciani, M.G., Malaponti, M., Torelli, F., Izzi, F., Prosperetti, C., Zannino, S., Corte, F., Chiaramonte, C., and Maccarrone, M. 2010 (May). "Cerebrospinal fluid levels of the endocannabinoid anandamide are reduced in patients with untreated newly diagnosed temporal lobe epilepsy." *Epilepsia* 51(5):768–72.

3. Falenski, K.W., Carter, D.S., Harrison, A.J., Martin, B.R., Blair, R.E., and DeLorenzo, R.J. 2009. "Temporal characterization of changes in hippocampal cannabinoid CB(1) receptor expression following pilocarpine-induced status epilepticus." *Brain Res.* 1262:64–72.

4. Rüdiger, Lorenz. "Experiences with THC-treatment in children and adolescents." Paper presented at IACM 2nd Conference on Cannabinoids in Medicine, September 12-13, 2003, Cologne.

5. Pelliccia, A., Grassi, G., Romano, A., and Crocchialo, P. "Treatment with CBD in oily solution of drug-resistant paediatric epilepsies." Paper presented at the 2005 Congress on Cannabis and the Cannabinoids, Leiden, The Netherlands: International Association for Cannabis as Medicine.

6. Blumer, D. 1999. "Evidence supporting the temporal lobe epilepsy personality syndrome." *Neurology* 53(5 Suppl 2):S9–12.

7. Epstein, Arthur W., MD, and Ervin, Frank, MD. 1956. "Psychodynamic significance of seizure content in psychomotor epilepsy." *Psychosomatic Medicine* 18:43–55.

8. Barker, Wayne, MD. 1948. "Studies on epilepsy: The petit mal attack as a response within the central nervous system to distress in organism-environment integration." *Psychosomatic Medicine* 10:73–94.

9. Kemph, J.P., MD, Zegans, L.S., MD, Kooi, K.A., MD, and Waggoner, R.W., MD. 1963. "The emotionally disturbed child with a convulsive disorder." *Psychosomatic Medicine* 25:441–49.

10. Strauss, Hans, MD. 1944. "The effect of mental activity on the incidence of seizures and the electroencephalographic pattern in some epileptics." *Psychosomatic Medicine* 6:141–45.

11. Daly, David D., MD, and Barry, Maurice J., Jr., MD. 1957. "Musicogenic epilepsy: Report of three cases." *Psychosomatic Medicine* 19:399–408.

HUNTINGTON'S DISEASE

1. Lanska, D.J., Lavine, L., Lanska, M.J., and Schoenberg, B.S. 1988 (May). "Huntington's disease mortality in the United States." *Neurology* 38(5):769–72.

2. Sandyk, Reuven, Paul Consroe, Lawrence Z. Stern, and Stuart R. Snider, Tucson, AZ. 1986 (Apr). "Effects of cannabidiol in Huntington's disease." *Neurology* 36 (Suppl 1):342.

3. Consroe, P., Laguna, J., Allender, J., Snider, S., Stern, L., Sandyk, R., Kennedy, K., and Schram, K. 1991 (Nov). "Controlled clinical trial of cannabidiol in Huntington's disease." *Pharmacol Biochem Behav.* 40(3):701–08.

4. Sagredo, O., Ramos, J.A., Decio, A., Mechoulam, R., and Fernández-Ruiz, J. 2007 (Aug). "Cannabidiol reduced the striatal atrophy caused 3-nitropropionic acid in vivo by mechanisms independent of the activation of cannabinoid, vanilloid TRPV1 and adenosine A2A receptors." *Eur J Neurosci.* 26(4):843–51.

5. Sagredo, O., Pazos, M.R., Satta, V., Ramos, J.A., Pertwee, R.G., and Fernández-Ruiz, J. 2011 (Sep). "Neuroprotective effects of phytocannabinoid-based medicines in experimental models of Huntington's disease." *J Neurosci Res.* 89(9):1509–18.

6. Fernández-Ruiz, J., Moreno-Martet, M., Rodríguez-Cueto, C., Palomo-Garo, C., Gómez-Cañas, M., Valdeolivas, S., Guaza, C., Romero, J., Guzmán, M., Mechoulam, R., and Ramos, J.A. 2011 (Aug). "Prospects for cannabinoid therapies in basal ganglia disorders." *Br J Pharmacol.* 163(7):1365–78.

MULTIPLE SCLEROSIS (MS)

1. Elovaara, Irina, MD, PhD; Maritta Ukkonen, MD; Minna Leppakynnas, MD; Terho Lehtimaki, MD, PhD; Mari Luomala, MSc; Jukka Peltola, MD; and Prasun Dastidar, MD. 2000. "Adhesion molecules in multiple sclerosis—Relation to subtypes of disease and methylprednisolone therapy." *Arch Neurol.* 57:546–51.

2. Mestre, L., Docagne, F., Correa, F., Loría, F., Hernangómez, M., Borrell, J., and Guaza, C. 2009 (Feb). "A cannabinoid agonist interferes with the pro-

gression of a chronic model of multiple sclerosis by downregulating adhesion molecules." *Mol Cell Neurosci.* 40(2):258–66.

3. Aragona, M., Onesti, E., Tomassini, V., Conte, A., Gupta, S., Gilio, F., Pantano, P., Pozzilli, C., and Inghilleri, M. 2009 (Jan-Feb). "Psychopathological and cognitive effects of therapeutic cannabinoids in multiple sclerosis: A double-blind, placebo-controlled, crossover study." *Clin Neuropharmacol.* 32(1):41–47.

4. Conte, A., Bettolo, C.M., Onesti, E., Frasca, V., Iacovelli, E., Gilio, F., Giacomelli, E., Gabriele, M., Aragona, M., Tomassini, V., Pantano, P., Pozzilli, C., and Inghilleri, M. 2009 (May). "Cannabinoid-induced effects on the nociceptive system: A neurophysiological study in patients with secondary progressive multiple sclerosis." *Eur J Pain.* 13(5):472–77.

5. Di Filippo, M., Pini, L.A., Pelliccioli, G.P., Calabresi, P., and Sarchielli, P. 2008 (Nov). "Abnormalities in the cerebrospinal fluid levels of endocannabinoids in multiple sclerosis." *J Neurol Neurosurg Psychiatry* 79(11):1224–29.

6. Deutsch, S.I., Rosse, R.B., Connor, J.M., Burket, J.A., Murphy, M.E., and Fox, F.J. 2008 (May). "Current status of cannabis treatment of multiple sclerosis with an illustrative case presentation of a patient with MS, complex vocal tics, paroxysmal dystonia, and marijuana dependence treated with dronabinol." *Spectr.* 13(5):393–403.

7. Rog, D.J., Nurmikko, T.J., and Young, C.A. 2007 (Sep). "Oromucosal delta9-tetrahydrocannabinol/cannabidiol for neuropathic pain associated with multiple sclerosis: An uncontrolled, open-label, 2-year extension trial." *Clin Ther.* 29(9):2068–79.

8. Collin, C., Davies, P., Mutiboko, I.K., and Ratcliffe, S.: Sativex Spasticity in MS Study Group. 2007 (Mar). "Randomized controlled trial of cannabis-based medicine in spasticity caused by multiple sclerosis." *Eur J Neurol.* 14(3):290–96.

9. Centonze, D., Bari, M., Rossi, S., Prosperetti, C., Furlan, R., Fezza, F., De Chiara, V., Battistini, L., Bernardi, G., Bernardini, S., Martino, G., and Maccarrone, M. 2007 (Oct). "The endocannabinoid system is dysregulated in multiple sclerosis and in experimental autoimmune encephalomyelitis." *Brain* 130(Pt 10):2543–53.

10. Pryce, G., and Baker, D. 2007. "Control of spasticity in a multiple sclerosis model is mediated by CB1, not CB2, cannabinoid receptors." *British Journal of Pharmacology* 150:519–25.

11. Lu, Dai, Kiran Vemuri, V., Duclos, Richard I., Jr., and Makriyannis, Alexandros. 2006 (Jul). "The cannabinergic system as a target for anti-inflammatory therapies." *Current Topics in Medicinal Chemistry* 6(13):1401–26(26). Bentham Science Publishers.

12. Freeman, R.M., Adekanmi, O., Waterfield, M.R., Waterfield, A.E., Wright, D., and Zajicek, J. 2006 (Nov). "The effect of cannabis on urge incontinence in patients with multiple sclerosis: A multicentre, randomised placebo-controlled trial (CAMS-LUTS)." *Int Urogynecol J Pelvic Floor Dysfunct.* 17(6):636–41.

13. Barnes, M.P. 2006 (Apr). "Sativex: Clinical efficacy and tolerability in the treatment of symptoms of multiple sclerosis and neuropathic pain." *Expert Opin Pharmacother.* 7(5):607–15.

14. Yang, C., Hader, W., and Zhang, X. 2006 (Mar 3). "Therapeutic action of cannabinoid on axonal injury induced by peroxynitrite." *Brain Res.* 1076(1): 238–42.

15. Trebst, C., and Stangel, M. 2005 (Aug). "Cannabinoids in multiple sclerosis—therapeutically reasonable?" *Fortschr Neurol Psychiatr.* 73(8):463–69.

16. Rog, D.J., Nurmikko, T.J., Friede, T., and Young, C.A. 2005 (Sep 27). "Randomized, controlled trial of cannabis-based medicine in central pain in multiple sclerosis." *Neurology* 65(6):812–19.

17. Perras, C. 2005 (Sep). "Sativex for the management of multiple sclerosis symptoms." *Issues Emerg Health Technol.* 72:1–4.

18. Rog, D.J., et al. 2005. "Randomized, controlled trial. . ." See note 16.

19. Wade, D.T., Makela, P., Robson, P., House, H., and Bateman, C. 2004 (Aug). "Do cannabis-based medicinal extracts have general or specific effects on symptoms in multiple sclerosis? A double-blind, randomized, placebo-controlled study on 160 patients." *Mult Scler.* 10(4):434–41.

20. Brady, C.M., DasGupta, R., Dalton, C., Wiseman, O.J., Berkley, K.J., and Fowler, C.J. 2004. "An open-label pilot study of cannabis-based extracts for bladder dysfunction in advanced multiple sclerosis." *Multiple Sclerosis* 10(4):425–33.

21. Page, S.A., Verhoef, M.J., Stebbins, R.A., Metz, L.M., and Levy, J.C. 2003. "Cannabis use as described by people with multiple sclerosis." *Can J Neurol Sci* 30(3):201–05.

22. Consroe, P., Musty, R., Rein, J., Tillery, W., and Pertwee, R. 1997. "The perceived effects of smoked cannabis on patients with multiple sclerosis." *European Neurology* 38(1):44–48.

23. Martyn, C.N., Illis, L.S., and Thom, J. 1995. "Nabilone in the treatment of multiple sclerosis." *Lancet* 345(8949):579.

24. Greenberg, H.S., Werness, S.A.S., Pugh, J.E., Andrus, R.O., Anderson, D.J., and Domino, E.F. 1994. "Short-term effects of smoking marijuana on balance in patients with multiple sclerosis and normal volunteers." *Clinical Pharmacology and Therapeutics* 55:324–28.

25. Meinck, H.M., Schönle, P.W., and Conrad, B. 1989. "Effect of cannabinoids

on spasticity and ataxia in multiple sclerosis." *Journal of Neurology* 236(2): 120–22.

26. Ungerleider, J.T., Andyrsiak, T., Fairbanks, L., Ellison, G.W., and Myers, L.W. 1987. "Delta-9-THC in the treatment of spasticity associated with multiple sclerosis." *Advances in Alcohol and Substance Abuse* 7(1):39–50.

27. Petro, D.J., and Ellenberger, C., Jr. 1981. "Treatment of human spasticity with delta 9-tetrahydrocannabinol." *Journal of Clinical Pharmacology* 21(8-9 Suppl):413S–416S.

28. Varda Mei-Tal, MD, Sanford Meyerowitz, MD, and George L. Engel, MD. 1970. "The role of psychological process in a somatic disorder: Multiple sclerosis." *Psychosomatic Medicine* 32:67–86.

29. Kurt D. Ackerman, MD, PhD, Rock Heyman, MD, Bruce S. Rabin, MD, PhD, Barbara P. Anderson, PhD, Patricia R. Houck, MSH, Ellen Frank, PhD, and Andrew Baum, PhD. 2002. "Stressful life events precede exacerbations of multiple sclerosis." *Psychosomatic Medicine* 64:916–20.

    G. S. Philippopoulos, MD, E.D. Wittkower, MD, and A. Cousineaum, MA. 1958. "The etiologic significance of emotional factors in onset and exacerbations of multiple sclerosis." *Psychosomatic Medicine* 20:458–74.

30. Natarajan, C., and Bright, J.J. 2002 (Jun 15). "Curcumin inhibits experimental allergic encephalomyelitis by blocking IL-12 signaling through Janus kinase-STAT pathway in T lymphocytes." *J Immunol.* 168(12):6506–13.

31. Sundqvist, E., Bäärnhielm, M., Alfredsson, L., Hillert, J., Olsson, T., and Kockum, I. 2010 (Dec). "Confirmation of association between multiple sclerosis and CYP27B1." *Eur J Hum Genet.* 18(12):1349–52.

Parkinson's Disease

1. The United States of America as represented by the Department of Health and Human Services. (Aidan J. Hampson, Julius Axelrod, and Maurizio Grimaldi) Patent No. 09/674028 filed on 02/02/2001. Patent 6630507 issued on October 7, 2003. Estimated expiration date: 2021. Cannabinoids as antioxidants and neuroprotectants. http://www.patentstorm.us/patents/6630507.html

2. Venderova, K., Ruzicka, E., Vorisek, V., and Visnovsky, P. 2004. "Survey on cannabis use in Parkinson's disease: Subjective improvement of motor symptoms." *Movement Disorders* 19(9):1102–06.

3. Farooq, M.U., Ducommun, E., and Goudreau, J. 2009 (Mar). "Treatment of a hyperkinetic movement disorder during pregnancy with Dronabinol." *Parkinsonism Relat Disord.* 15(3):249–51.

4. Iuvone, T., Esposito, G., De Filippis, D., Scuderi, C., and Steardo, L. 2009

(Winter). "Cannabidiol: A promising drug for neurodegenerative disorders?" *CNS Neurosci Ther.* 15(1):65–75.

5. Aggarwal, B.B., Kumar, A., and Bharti, A.C. 2003 (Jan-Feb). "Anticancer potential of curcumin: Preclinical and clinical studies." *Anticancer Research* 23(1A):363–98.

TOURETTE SYNDROME

1. Moss, D.E., Manderscheid, P.Z, Montgomery, S.P., Norman, A.B., and Sanberg, P.R. 1989. "Nicotine and cannabinoids as adjuncts to neuroleptics in the treatment of Tourette syndrome and other motor disorders." *Life Sci.* 44(21):1521–25.

2. Müller-Vahl, K.R., Kolbe, H., Schneider, U., and Emrich, H.M. 1998 (Dec). "Cannabinoids: Possible role in patho-physiology and therapy of Gilles de la Tourette syndrome." *Acta Psychiatr Scand.* 98(6):502–06.

3. Müller-Vahl, K.R., Schneider, U., Koblenz, A., Jöbges, M., Kolbe, H., Daldrup, T., and Emrich, H.M. 2002 (Mar). "Treatment of Tourette's syndrome with Delta 9-tetrahydrocannabinol (THC): A randomized crossover trial." *Pharmacopsychiatry* 35(2):57–61.

Müller-Vahl, K.R., Koblenz, A., Jöbges, M., Kolbe, H., Emrich, H.M., and Schneider, U. 2001 (Jan). "Influence of treatment of Tourette syndrome with delta9-tetrahydrocannabinol (delta9-THC) on neuropsychological performance." *Pharmacopsychiatry* 34(1):19–24.

Müller-Vahl, K.R., Prevedel, H., Theloe, K., Kolbe, H., Emrich, H.M., and Schneider, U. 2003 (Feb). "Treatment of Tourette syndrome with delta-9-tetrahydrocannabinol (delta 9-THC): No influence on neuropsychological performance." *Neuropsychopharmacology* 28(2):384–88.

Curtis, A., Clarke, C.E., and Rickards, H.E. 2009 (Oct 7). "Cannabinoids for Tourette's Syndrome." *Cochrane Database Syst Rev.* (4):CD006565.

4. Hasan, A., Rothenberger, A., Münchau, A., Wobrock, T., Falkai, P., and Roessner, V. 2010 (Apr). "Oral delta 9-tetrahydrocannabinol improved refractory Gilles de la Tourette syndrome in an adolescent by increasing intracortical inhibition: A case report." *J Clin Psychopharmacol.* 30(2):190–92.

5. Curtis, A., Clarke, C.E., and Rickards, H.E. 2009 (Oct 7). "Cannabinoids for Tourette's Syndrome." *Cochrane Database Syst Rev.* (4):CD006565.

6. Müller-Vahl, K.R., Schneider, U., Prevedel, H., Theloe, K., Kolbe, H., Daldrup, T., and Emrich, H.M. 2003 (Apr). "Delta 9-tetrahydrocannabinol (THC) is effective in the treatment of tics in Tourette syndrome: A 6-week randomized trial." *J Clin Psychiatry* 64(4):459–65.

7. Müller-Vahl, K.R., Prevedel, H., Theloe, K., Kolbe, H., Emrich, H.M., and Schneider, U. 2003 (Feb). "Treatment of Tourette syndrome with

delta-9-tetrahydrocannabinol (delta 9-THC): No influence on neuropsychological performance." *Neuropsychopharmacology* 28(2):384–88.

8. Müller-Vahl, K.R., et al. 2002. "Treatment of Tourette's syndrome. . ." See note 3.

9. Müller-Vahl, K.R., et al. 2001. "Influence of treatment of Tourette syndrome . . ." (see note 3).

10. Schneider, U., Muller-Vahl, K.R., Stuhrmann, M., Gadzicki, D., Heller, D., Seifert, J., and Emrich, H.M. 2000 (Oct). "The importance of the endogenous cannabinoid system in various neuropsychiatric disorders." *Fortschr Neurol Psychiatr.* 68(10):433–38.

11. Müller-Vahl, K.R., Kolbe, H., Schneider, U., and Emrich, H.M. 1999 (Oct). "Cannabis in movement disorders." *Forsch Komplementarmed.* 6 Suppl 3:23–27.

12. Müller-Vahl, K.R., et al. 1998. "Cannabinoids: possible role. . ." See note 2.

13. Moss, D.E., Manderscheid, P.Z., Montgomery, S.P., Norman, A.B., and Sanberg, P.R. 1989. "Nicotine and cannabinoids as adjuncts to neuroleptics in the treatment of Tourette syndrome and other motor disorders." *Life Sci.* 44(21):1521–25.

OBGYN

1. Russo, Ethan, MD. 2002. "Cannabis treatments in obstetrics and gynecology: A historical review." *Journal of Cannabis Therapeutics* 2(3/4):5–35; and in *Women and Cannabis: Medicine, Science, and Sociology* (ed: Ethan Russo, Melanie Dreher, and Mary Lynn Mathre) (The Haworth Integrative Healing Press, an imprint of The Haworth Press, Inc., 2002, pp. 5–35).

2. Sam'l O.L. Potter, MA, MD, MRCP (Lond.) 1892. *A Compend of Materia Medica and Therapeutics and Prescription Writing; with especial references to the physiological actions of drugs* (Philadelphia: P. Blakiston, Son & Co.), p. 123. Based on the U.S. Pharmacopeia, 5th edition.

ABORTION, MISCARRIAGE, AND FERTILITY

1. Piomelli, Daniele. 2004. "THC: Moderation during implantation." *Nature Medicine* 10:19–20.

    Paria, B.C., H. Song, X. Wang, P.C. Schmid, R.J. Krebsbach, H.H. Schmid, T.I. Bonner, A. Zimmer, and S.K. Dey. 2001 (Jun 8). "Dysregulated cannabinoid signaling disrupts uterine receptivity for embryo implantation." *J Biol Chem.* 276(23):20523–28.

2. Paria, B.C., Wang, H., and Dey, S.K. 2002 (Dec 31). "Endocannabinoid signaling in synchronizing embryo development and uterine receptivity for implantation." *Chem Phys Lipids.* 121(1-2):201–10.

Childbirth Pains

1. L. Grinspoon, MD, and James Bakalar. 1997. *Marijuana, The Forbidden Medicine* (New Haven and London: Yale University Press. Revised and expanded edition).

Endometriosis

1. Dmitrieva, N., Nagabukuro, H., Resuehr, D., Zhang, G., McAllister, S.L., McGinty, K.A., Mackie, K., and Berkley, K.J. 2010 (Dec). "Endocannabinoid involvement in endometriosis." *Pain* 151(3):703–10.
2. Leconte, M., Nicco, C., Ngô, C., Arkwright, S., Chéreau, C., Guibourdenche, J., Weill, B., Chapron, C., Dousset, B., and Batteux, F. 2010 (Dec). "Antiproliferative effects of cannabinoid agonists on deep infiltrating endometriosis." *Am J Pathol.* 177(6):2963–70.
3. Heim, C., Ehlert, U., Hanker, J.P., and Hellhammer, H.H. 1998 (May 1). "Abuse-related posttraumatic stress disorder and alteration of the hypothalamic-pituitary-adrenal axis in women with chronic pelvic pain." *Psychosomatic Medicine* 60:302–18.

Menstrual Pain

1. Grotenhermen, F., and Schnelle, M. 2003. "Survey on the medical use of cannabis and THC in Germany." *J Cannabis Ther* 3(2):17–40.
2. Kassi, E., Papoutsi, Z., Fokialakis, N., Messari, I., Mitakou, S., and Moutsatsou, P. 2004 (Nov 17). "Greek plant extracts exhibit selective estrogen receptor modulator (SERM)-like properties." *J Agric Food Chem.* 52(23):6956–61.
3. Modaress Nejad, V., and Asadipour, M. 2006 (May-Jul). "Comparison of the effectiveness of fennel and mefenamic acid on pain intensity in dysmenorrhoea." *East Mediterr Health J.* 12(3-4):423–27.

Morning Sickness

1. Westfall, R.E., Janssen, P.A., Lucas, P., and Capler, R. 2006. "Survey of medicinal cannabis use among childbearing women: Patterns of its use in pregnancy and retroactive self-assessment of its efficacy against 'morning sickness'." *Complement Ther Clin Pract* 12(1):27–33.

Pregnancy

1, El-Talatini, M.R., Taylor, A.H., and Konje, J.C. 2010 (Apr). "The relationship between plasma levels of the endocannabinoid, anandamide, sex steroids, and gonadotrophins during the menstrual cycle." *Fertil Steril.* 93(6):1989–96.
2. Greenland, S., Richwald, G.A., and Honda, G.D. 1983 (Jun). "The effects of marijuana use during pregnancy. II. A study in a low-risk home-delivery population." *Drug Alcohol Depend.* 11(3-4):359–66.

Osteoporosis

1. Karsak, M., Cohen-Solal, M., Freudenberg, J., Ostertag, A., Morieux, C., Kornak, U., Essig, J., Erxlebe, E., Bab, I., Kubisch, C., de Vernejoul, M.C., and Zimmer, A. 2005 (Nov 15). "Cannabinoid receptor type 2 gene is associated with human osteoporosis." *Hum Mol Genet.* 14(22):3389–96.

2. Orr Ofek, Meliha Karsak, Nathalie Leclerc, Meirav Fogel, Baruch Frenkel, Karen Wright, Joseph Tam, Malka Attar-Namdar, Vardit Kram, Esther Shohami, Raphael Mechoulam, Andreas Zimmer, and Itai Bab. 2006 (Jan 17). "Peripheral cannabinoid receptor, CB2, regulates bone mass." *PNAS* 103(3):696–701.

3. Bab, I., Zimmer, A., and Melamed, E. 2009. "Cannabinoids and the skeleton: From marijuana to reversal of bone loss." *Ann Med.* 41(8):560–67.

4. Kassi, E., Papoutsi, Z., Fokialakis, N., Messari, I., Mitakou, S., and Moutsatsou, P. 2004 (Nov 17). "Greek plant extracts exhibit selective estrogen receptor modulator (SERM)-like properties." *J Agric Food Chem.* 52(23):6956–61.

Pain (in general)

1. Lee, W.M. 2004 (Jul). "Acetaminophen and the U.S. Acute Liver Failure Study Group: Lowering the risks of hepatic failure." *Hepatology* 40(1):6–9.

2. Green, G.A. 2001. "Understanding NSAIDs: From aspirin to COX-2." *Clin Cornerstone* 3(5):50–60.

3. Wolfe, Sidney M., MD, Larry D. Sasich, PharmD, MPH, Rose-Ellen Hope, RPh, and Public Citizen's Health Research Group. 1999. *Worst Pills, Best Pills—A Consumer's Guide to Avoiding Drug-Induced Death or Illness* (New York: Pocket Books).

4. Moore, T.J., Cohen, M.R., and Furberg, C.D. 2007 (Sep 10). "Serious adverse drug events reported to the Food and Drug Administration, 1998-2005." *Arch Intern Med.* 167(16):1752–59.

5. Weiner, Richard S., PhD (Editor). Chapter 31, written by Ethan B. Russo, MD, "The Role of Cannabis and Cannabinoids in Pain Management" in *Pain Management: A Practical Guide for Clinicians* (London, New York, Washington, DC: CRC Press, 2002).

6. Conte, A., Bettolo, C.M., Onesti, E., Frasca, V., Iacovelli, E., Gilio, F., Giacomelli, E., Gabriele, M., Aragona, M., Tomassini, V., Pantano, P., Pozzilli, C., and Inghilleri, M. 2009 (May). "Cannabinoid-induced effects on the nociceptive system: A neurophysiological study in patients with secondary progressive multiple sclerosis." *Eur J Pain* 13(5):472–77.

7. Welch, S.P., and Eads, M. 1999 (Nov 27). "Synergistic interactions of endogenous opioids and cannabinoid systems." *Brain Res.* 848(1-2):183–90.

8. Burstein, Sumner H., and Zurier, Robert B. 2009 (Mar). "Cannabinoids, endo-cannabinoids, and related analogs in inflammation." *AAPS J.* 11(1):109–19.

9. Wallace, M., Schulteis, G., Atkinson, J.H., Wolfson, T., Lazzaretto, D., Bentley, H., Gouaux, B., and Abramson, I. 2007 (Nov). "Dose-dependent effects of smoked cannabis on capsaicin-induced pain and hyperalgesia in healthy volunteers." *Anesthesiology* 107(5):785–96.

   Kraft, B., Frickey, N.A., Kaufmann, R.M., Reif, M., Frey, R., Gustorff, B., and Kress, H.G. 2008 (Jul). "Lack of analgesia by oral standardized cannabis extract on acute inflammatory pain and hyperalgesia in volunteers." *Anesthesiology* 109(1):101–10.

10. Weiner, Richard S., PhD (Editor). Chapter 31, *Pain Management.* See note 5 above.

11. Burstein and Zurier. 2009. "Cannabinoids. . ." See note 8 above.

12. Conte, A., et al. 2009. "Cannabinoid-induced effects. . ." See note 6 above.

13. Wallace, M., et al. 2007. "Dose-dependent effects of smoked cannabis. . ." See note 9 above.

14. Heinrich, U., Neukam, K., Tronnier, H., Sies, H., and Stahl, W. 2006 (Jun). "Long-term ingestion of high-flavanol cocoa provides photoprotection against UV-induced erythema and improves skin condition in women." *J Nutr.* 136(6):1565–69.

15. Gagnier, J.J., van Tulder, M.W., Berman, B., and Bombardier, C. 2007 (Jan 1). "Herbal medicine for low back pain: A Cochrane review." *Spine* 32(1):82–92.

16. Cuban Ministry of Public Health, Havana. 1992. *Therapeutic Guide to Plant Pharmaceuticals and Honey Pharmaceuticals (Guia Terapeutica Dispensarial de Fitofarmacos y Apifarmacos).* Ministerio de Salud Publica, Ciudad de La Habana, Republica de Cuba.

17. Federal Republic of Germany. *Monographien der E-Kommission (Phyto-Therapie) (380 monographs). A therapeutic guide to herbal medicine evaluating the safety and efficacy of herbs for licensed medical prescribing in Germany.* Published between 1984 and 1994 in the Bundesanzeiger (official publication by the Federal Republic of Germany). Copies of the monographs are available at the Heilpflanzen-Welt Bibliothek: http://buecher.heilpflanzen-welt.de/BGA-Commission-E-Monographs/

18. Beltran, J., Ghosh, A.K., and Basu, S. 2007 (Mar 1). "Immunotherapy of tumors with neuroimmune ligand capsaicin." *J Immunol.* 178(5):3260–64.

19. Elwakeel, H.A., Moneim, H.A., Farid, M., and Gohar, A.A. 2007 (Jul). "Clove oil cream: A new effective treatment for chronic anal fissure." *Colorectal Dis.* 9(6):549–52.

20. Chaieb, K., Hajlaoui, H., Zmantar, T., Kahla-Nakbi, A.B., Rouabhia, M., Mahdouani, K., and Bakhrouf, A. 2007 (Jun). "The chemical composition and biological activity of clove essential oil, Eugenia caryophyllata (Syzigium aromaticum L. Myrtaceae): A short review." *Phytother Res.* 21(6):501–06.

22. *Monographien der E-Kommission (Phyto-Therapie)* (380 monographs). See note 17.

23. Modaress, Nejad, V., and Asadipour, M. 2006 (May-Jul). "Comparison of the effectiveness of fennel and mefenamic acid on pain intensity in dysmenorrhoea." *East Mediterr Health J.* 12(3-4):423–27.

24. Cuban Ministry of Public Health, Havana. 1992. See note 16.

25. Ojewole, J.A. 2006 (Sep). "Analgesic, antiinflammatory and hypoglycaemic effects of ethanol extract of Zingiber officinale (Roscoe) rhizomes (Zingiberaceae) in mice and rats." *Phytother Res.* 20(9):764–72.

26. Umukoro, S., and Ashorobi, R.B. 2008 (Feb 12). "Further pharmacological studies on aqueous seed extract of Aframomum melegueta in rats." *J Ethnopharmacol.* 115(3):489–93.

27. Umukoro, S., and Ashorobi, R.B. 2007 (Feb 12). "Further studies on the antinociceptive action of aqueous seed extract of Aframomum melegueta." *J Ethnopharmacol.* 109(3):501–04.

28. *Monographien der E-Kommission (Phyto-Therapie)* (380 monographs). See note 17.

29. Nomicos, E.Y. 2007 (Nov-Dec). "Myrrh: medical marvel or myth of the magi?" *Holist Nurs Pract.* 21(6):308–23.

30. Cemek, M., Enginar, H., Karaca, T., and Unak, P. 2006 (Nov-Dec). "In vivo radioprotective effects of Nigella sativa L oil and reduced glutathione against irradiation-induced oxidative injury and number of peripheral blood lymphocytes in rats." *Photochem Photobiol.* 82(6):1691–96.

31. Cuban Ministry of Public Health, Havana. 1992. See note 16.

Chronic Non-Malignant Pains

1. Wolff, R., Clar, C., Lerch, C., and Kleijnen, J. 2011 (Feb). "Epidemiology of chronic non-malignant pain in Germany." *Schmerz.* 25(1):26–44.

2. Bujalska, M. 2008. "Effect of cannabinoid receptor agonists on Streptozotocin-induced hyperalgesia in diabetic neuropathy." *Pharmacology* 82(3):193–200.

3. Haroutiunian, S., Rosen, G., Shouval, R., and Davidson, E. 2008. "Open-label, add-on study of tetrahydrocannabinol for chronic nonmalignant pain." *J Pain Palliat Care Pharmacother.* 22(3):213–17.

Migraine

1. Zebenholzer, K., Rudel, E., Frantal, S., Brannath, W., Schmidt, K., Wöber-Bingöl, C., and Wöber, C. 2011 (Mar). "Migraine and weather: A prospective diary-based analysis." *Cephalalgia* 31(4):391–400.

2. Wöber, C., Brannath, W., Schmidt, K., Kapitan, M., Rudel, E., Wessely, P., Wöber-Bingöl, Ç. 2007. "Prospective analysis of factors related to migraine attacks: The PAMINA study." *Cephalalgia* 27(4):304–14.

3. Lay, C.L., and Broner, S.W. 2009 (May). "Migraine in women." *Neurologic Clinics* 27(2):503–11.

4. Etminan, M., Takkouche, B., Isorna, F.C., and Samii, A. 2005 (Jan 8). "Risk of ischaemic stroke in people with migraine: Systematic review and meta-analysis of observational studies." *BMJ* 330(7482):63.

5. Russo, Ethan B., MD. 2001. "Hemp for headache: An in-depth historical and scientific review of cannabis in migraine treatment." *Journal of Cannabis Therapeutics* 1(2).

   Russo, Ethan, MD. 1998. "Cannabis for migraine treatment: The once and future prescription? An historical and scientific review." *Pain* 76:3–8.

6. Russo, Ethan B., MD. 2004 (Feb-Apr). "Clinical Endocannabinoid Deficiency (CECD): Can this concept explain therapeutic benefits of cannabis in migraine, fibromyalgia, irritable bowel syndrome and other treatment-resistant conditions?" *Neuroendocrinology Letters* 25(1/2).

7. Raby, W.N., Modica, P.A., Wolintz, R.J., and Murtaugh, K. 2006 (Feb). "Dronabinol reduces signs and symptoms of idiopathic intracranial hypertension: A case report." *J Ocul Pharmacol Ther.* 22(1):68–75.

8. Volfe, Z., Dvilansky, A., and Nathan, I. 1985. "Cannabinoids block release of serotonin from platelets induced by plasma from migraine patients." *Int J Clin Pharm. Res* V(4):243–46.

9. Kozersky, S., Dewey, W.L., and Harris, L.S. 1973. "Antipyretic analgesic and anti-inflammatory effects of delta-9-THC in the rat." *Europ. J. Pharmacol.* 24:1.

10. Adams, M.D., Earnhardt, J.T., Dewey, W.L., and Harris, L.S. 1976. "Vasoconstrictor actions of delta-8 and delta-9-THC in the rat." *J. Pharmacol. Exp. Therap.* 196:649.

11. Mikuriya, T.H. 1969. "Marijuana in medicine: Past, present and future." *Calif. Med.* 110:34–40.

12. Grace, William J., MD, and Graham, David T., MD. Dept. of Medicine of the New York Hospital–Cornell Medical Center. 1952 (Jul 1). "Relationship of specific attitudes and emotions to certain bodily diseases." *Psychosomatic Medicine* 14(4):243–51.

13. Wöber, C., Brannath, W., Schmidt, K., Kapitan, M., Rudel, E., Wessely, P., and Wöber-Bingöl, Ç. 2007. "Prospective analysis of factors related to migraine attacks: The PAMINA study." *Cephalalgia* 27(4):304–14.

14. Evans, R.W., MD, and Couch, J.R., MD, PhD. 2001. "Orgasm and migraine." *Headache* 41:512–14.

15. Couch, J., and Bearss, C. 1990. "Relief of migraine with sexual intercourse." *Headache* 30:302.

Neuropathies (in general)

1. Burstein, Sumner H., and Zurier, Robert B. 2009 (Mar). "Cannabinoids, endo-cannabinoids, and related analogs in inflammation." *AAPS J.* 11(1):109–19.

2. Wilsey, B., Marcotte, T., Tsodikov, A., Millman, J., Bentley, H., Gouaux, B., and Fishman, S. 2008 (Jun). "A randomized, placebo-controlled, crossover trial of cannabis cigarettes in neuropathic pain." *J Pain* 9(6):506–21.

3. Attal, N., Brasseur, L., Guirimand, D., Clermond-Gnamien, S., Atlami, S., and Bouhassira, D. 2004 (Apr). "Are oral cannabinoids safe and effective in refractory neuropathic pain?" *Eur J Pain* 8(2):173–77.

4. Berman, J.S., Symonds, C., and Birch, R. 2004 (Dec). "Efficacy of two cannabis-based medicinal extracts for relief of central neuropathic pain from brachial plexus avulsion: Results of a randomised controlled trial." *Pain* 112(3):299–330.

5. Wade, D.T., Robson, P., House, H., Makela, P., and Aram, J. 2003 (Feb). "A preliminary controlled study to determine whether whole-plant cannabis extracts can improve intractable neurogenic symptoms." *Clin Rehabil.* 17(1): 21–29.

6. Karst, M., Salim, K., Burstein, S., Conrad, I., Hoy, L., and Schneider, U. 2003 (Oct 1). "Analgesic effect of the synthetic cannabinoid CT-3 on chronic neuropathic pain: A randomized controlled trial." *Journal of the American Medical Association* 290(13):1757–62.

Neuropathies—AIDS-Related

1. Abrams, D.I., Jay, C.A., Shade, S.B., Vizoso, H., Reda, H., Press, S., Kelly, M.E., Rowbotham, M.C., and Petersen, K.L. 2007 (Feb 13). "Cannabis in painful HIV-associated sensory neuropathy: A randomized placebo-controlled trial." *Neurology* 68(7):515–21.

2. Ellis, R.J., Toperoff, W., Vaida, F., van den Brande, G., Gonzales, J., Gouaux, B., Bentley, H., and Atkinson, J.H. 2009 (Feb). "Smoked medicinal cannabis for neuropathic pain in HIV: A randomized, crossover clinical trial." *Neuropsychopharmacology* 34(3):672–80.

PAIN DUE TO ADVANCED CANCER

1. Johnson, J.R., Burnell-Nugent, M., Lossignol, D., Ganae-Motan, E.D., Potts, R., and Fallon, M.T. 2010 (Feb). "Multicenter, double-blind, randomized, placebo-controlled, parallel-group study of the efficacy, safety, and tolerability of THC:CBD extract and THC extract in patients with intractable cancer-related pain." *J Pain Symptom Manage.* 39(2):167–79.

2. Ellis, R.J., Toperoff, W., Vaida, F., van den Brande, G., Gonzales, J., Gouaux, B., Bentley, H., and Atkinson, J.H. 2009 (Feb). "Smoked medicinal cannabis for neuropathic pain in HIV: A randomized, crossover clinical trial." *Neuropsychopharmacology* 34(3):672–80.

Prion Diseases

1. Mead, Simon, MRCP, Jerome Whitfield, MA, Mark Poulter, BSc, Paresh Shah, PhD, James Uphill, BSc, Tracy Campbell, BSc, Huda Al-Dujaily, BSc, Holger Hummerich, PhD, Jon Beck, BSc, Charles A. Mein, PhD, Claudio Verzilli, PhD, John Whittaker, PhD, Michael P. Alpers, FRS, and John Collinge, FRS. 2009. "A novel protective prion protein variant that colocalizes with kuru exposure." *N Engl J Med.* 361:2056–65.

2. Llewelyn, C.A., Hewitt, P.E., Knight, R.S., Amar, K., Cousens, S., Mackenzie, J., and Will, R.G. 2004. "Possible transmission of variant Creutzfeldt-Jakob disease by blood transfusion." *Lancet* 363:417–21.

3. Sevda Dirikoc, Suzette A. Priola, Mathieu Marella, Nicole Zsürger, and Joëlle Chabry. 2007 (Sep 5). "Nonpsychoactive cannabidiol prevents prion accumulation and protects neurons against prion toxicity." *J Neurosci.* 27(36):9537–44.

4. The United States of America as represented by the Department of Health and Human Services. (Aidan J. Hampson, Julius Axelrod and Maurizio Grimaldi) Patent No. 09/674028 filed on 02/02/2001. Patent 6630507 issued on October 7, 2003. Estimated expiration date: 2021. Cannabinoids as antioxidants and neuroprotectants. www.patentstorm.us/patents/6630507.html

5. Sevda Dirikoc, et al. 2007. "Nonpsychoactive cannabidiol. . ." See note 3 above.

6. Mice were treated intraperitoneally three times per week for the indicated period of time with 200 μl of 20 or 60 mg/kg CBD diluted 1:1:2 in an ethanol/cremophor/NaCl 0.9% mixture. CBD was from GW Pharmaceuticals (Wiltshire, UK), dissolved at 10–2 M in ethanol, and stored at −20°C until use.

Sickle Cell Disease

1. Howard, J., Anie, K.A., Holdcroft, A., Korn, S., and Davies, S.C. 2005. "Cannabis use in sickle cell disease: A questionnaire study." *Br J Haematol.* 131(1):123–28.

2. Kohli, D.R., Li, Y., Khasabov, S.G., Gupta, P., Kehl, L.J., Ericson, M.E., Nguyen, J., Gupta, V., Hebbel, R.P., Simone, D.A., and Gupta, K. 2010 (Jul 22). "Pain-related behaviors and neurochemical alterations in mice expressing sickle hemoglobin: Modulation by cannabinoids." *Blood* 116(3):456–65.

3. Shmist, Y.A., Goncharov, I., Eichler, M., Shneyvays, V., Isaac, A., Vogel, Z., and Shainberg, A. 2006 (Feb). "Delta-9-tetrahydrocannabinol protects cardiac cells from hypoxia via CB2 receptor activation and nitric oxide production." *Mol Cell Biochem* 283(1-2):75–83.

4. Levenson, James L., MD, Donna K. McClish, PhD, Bassam A. Dahman, BS, Viktor E. Bovbjerg, PhD, MPH, Vanessa de A. Citero, MD, Lynne T. Penberthy, MD, MPH, Imoigele P. Aisiku, MD, MSCR, John D. Roberts, MD, Susan D. Roseff, MD, and Wally R. Smith, MD. 2008. "Depression and anxiety in adults with sickle cell sisease: The PiSCES Project." *Psychosomatic Medicine* 70:192–96.

5. Zhang, C., Li, X., Lian, L., Chen, Q., Abdulmalik, O., Vassilev, V., Lai, C.S., and Asakura, T. 2004 (Jun). "Anti-sickling effect of MX-1520, a prodrug of vanillin: An in vivo study using rodents." *Br J Haematol.* 125(6):788–95.

Skin Diseases (in general)

1. Bíró, Tamás, Balázs I. Tóth, György Haskó, Ralf Paus, and Pál Pacher. 2009 (Aug). "The endocannabinoid system of the skin in health and disease: Novel perspectives and therapeutic opportunities." *Trends Pharmacol Sci.* 30(8):411–20.

2. Telek, A., Bíró, T., Bodó, E., Tóth, B.I., Borbíró, I., Kunos, G., and Paus, R. 2007 (Nov). "Inhibition of human hair follicle growth by endo- and exocannabinoids." *FASEB J.* 21(13):3534–41.

3. Stander, S., Reinhardt, H.W., and Luger, T.A. 2006 (Sep). "Topical cannabinoid agonists: An effective new possibility for treating chronic pruritus." *Hautarzt.* 57(9):801–07.

4. Neff, G.W., O'Brien, C.B., Reddy, K.R., Bergasa, N.V., Regev, A., Molina, E., Amaro, R., Rodriguez, M.J., Chase, V., Jeffers, L., and Schiff, E. 2002 (Aug). "Preliminary observation with dronabinol in patients with intractable pruritus secondary to cholestatic liver disease." *Am J Gastroenterol.* 97(8):2117–19.

5. Yosipovitch, G., Tang, M., Dawn, A.G., Chen, M., Goh, C.L., Huak, Y., and Seng, L.F. 2007. "Study of psychological stress, sebum production and acne vulgaris in adolescents." *Acta Derm Venereol.* 87(2):135–39.

6. Zorrilla, E.P., Luborsky, L., McKay, J.R., Rosenthal, R., Houldin, A., Tax, A., McCorkle, R., Seligman, D.A., and Schmidt, K. 2001 (Sep). "The relationship of

depression and stressors to immunological assays: A meta-analytic review." *Brain Behav Immun.* 15(3):199–26.

7. Marnewick, J., Joubert, E., Joseph, S., Swanevelder, S., Swart, P., and Gelderblom, W. 2005 (Jun 28). "Inhibition of tumour promotion in mouse skin by extracts of rooibos (Aspalathus linearis) and honeybush (Cyclopia intermedia), unique South African herbal teas." *Cancer Lett.* 224(2):193–202.

8. Heinrich, U., Neukam, K., Tronnier, H., Sies, H., and Stahl, W. 2006 (Jun). "Long-term ingestion of high-flavanol cocoa provides photoprotection against UV-induced erythema and improves skin condition in women." *J Nutr.* 136(6):1565–69.

9. Mitani, H., Ryu, A., Suzuki, T., Yamashita, M., Arakane, K., and Koide, C. 2007 (Apr-Jun). "Topical application of plant extracts containing xanthine derivatives can prevent UV-induced wrinkle formation in hairless mice." *Photodermatol Photoimmunol Photomed.* 23(2-3):86–94.

10. Mondello, F., De Bernardis, F., Girolamo, A., Cassone, A., and Salvatore, G. 2006 (Nov 3). "In vivo activity of terpinen-4-ol, the main bioactive component of Melaleuca alternifolia Cheel (tea tree) oil, against azole-susceptible and -resistant human pathogenic Candida species." *BMC Infect Dis.* 6:158.

11. Ferrini, A.M., Mannoni, V., Aureli, P., Salvatore, G., Piccirilli, E., Ceddia, T., Pontieri, E., Sessa, R., and Oliva, B. 2006 (Jul-Sep). "Melaleuca alternifolia essential oil possesses potent anti-staphylococcal activity extended to strains resistant to antibiotics." *Int J Immunopathol Pharmacol.* 19(3):539–44.

12. Vazquez, J.A., and Zawawi, A.A. 2002 (Sep-Oct). "Efficacy of alcohol-based and alcohol-free melaleuca oral solution for the treatment of fluconazole-refractory oropharyngeal candidiasis in patients with AIDS." *HIV Clin Trials* 3(5):379–85.

13. De Lucca, A.J., Bland, J.M., Vigo, C.B., Cushion, M., Selitrennikoff, C.P., Peter, J., and Walsh, T.J. 2002 (Apr). "CAY-I, a fungicidal saponin from Capsicum sp. fruit." *Med Mycol.* 40(2):131–37.

14. Bergsson, G., Steingrímsson, O., and Thormar, H. 1999 (Nov). "In vitro susceptibilities of Neisseria gonorrhoeae to fatty acids and monoglycerides." *Antimicrob Agents Chemother.* 43(11):2790–92.

15. Bergsson, G., Arnfinnsson, J., Steingrímsson, O., and Thormar, H. 2001 (Oct). "Killing of Gram-positive cocci by fatty acids and monoglycerides." *APMIS.* 109(10):670–78.

16. Bergsson, G., Arnfinnsson, J., Steingrímsson, O., and Thormar, H. 2001 (Nov). "In vitro killing of Candida albicans by fatty acids and monoglycerides." *Antimicrob Agents Chemother.* 45(11):3209–12.

17. Bergsson, G., Arnfinnsson, J., Karlsson, S.M., Steingrímsson, O., and Thormar, H. 1998 (Sep). "In vitro inactivation of Chlamydia trachomatis by fatty acids and monoglycerides." *Antimicrob Agents Chemother.* 42(9):2290–94.

18. Isaacs, C.E., Kim, K.S., and Thormar, H. 1994 (Jun 6). "Inactivation of enveloped viruses in human bodily fluids by purified lipids." *Ann N Y Acad Sci.* 724:457–64.

19. Tedeschi, P., Maietti, A,. Boggian, M., Vecchiati, G., and Brandolini, V. 2007 (Sep). "Fungitoxicity of lyophilized and spray-dried garlic extracts." *J Environ Sci Health B.* 42(7):795–99.

20. Umukoro, S., and Ashorobi, R.B. 2008 (Feb 12). "Further pharmacological studies on aqueous seed extract of Aframomum melegueta in rats." *J Ethnopharmacol.* 115(3):489–93.

21. Tampieri, M.P., Galuppi, R., Macchioni, F., Carelle, M.S., Falcioni, L., Cioni, P.L., and Morelli, I. 2005 (Apr). "The inhibition of Candida albicans by selected essential oils and their major components." *Mycopathologia.* 159(3):339–45.

22. Fu, Y., Zu, Y., Chen, L., Shi, X., Wang, Z., Sun, S., and Efferth, T. 2007 (Oct). "Antimicrobial activity of clove and rosemary essential oils alone and in combination." *Phytother Res.* 21(10):989–94.

23. Cuban Ministry of Public Health, Havana. 1992. *Therapeutic Guide to Plant Pharmaceuticals and Honey Pharmaceuticals (Guia Terapeutica Dispensarial de Fitofarmacos y Apifarmacos).* Ministerio de Salud Publica, Ciudad de La Habana, Republica de Cuba.

24. Goel, A., Kunnumakkara, A.B., and Aggarwal, B.B. 2008 (Feb 15). "Curcumin as 'Curecumin': From kitchen to clinic." *Biochem Pharmacol.* 75(4):787–809.

ACNE

1. Bíró, Tamás, Balázs I. Tóth, György Haskó, Ralf Paus, and Pál Pacher. 2009 (Aug). "The endocannabinoid system of the skin in health and disease: Novel perspectives and therapeutic opportunities." *Trends Pharmacol Sci.* 30(8):411–20.

2. Yosipovitch, Gil, Mark Tang, Aerlyn G. Dawn, Mark Chen, Chee Leok Goh, Yiong Huak Chan, and Lim Fong Seng. 2007 (Mar). "Study of psychological stress, sebum production and Acne vulgaris in adolescents." *Acta Dermato-Venereologica* 87(2):135–39.

DERMATITIS (ECZEMA)

1. Bíró, Tamás, Balázs I. Tóth, György Haskó, Ralf Paus, and Pál Pacher. 2009 (Aug). "The endocannabinoid system of the skin in health and disease: Novel perspectives and therapeutic opportunities." *Trends Pharmacol Sci.* 30(8):411–20.

2. Grace, William J., MD, and Graham, David T., MD. Dept. of Medicine of

the New York Hospital–Cornell Medical Center. 1952 (Jul 1). "Relationship of specific attitudes and emotions to certain bodily diseases." *Psychosomatic Medicine* 14(4):243–51.

Hair Growth—Unwanted (Hirsutism)

1. Bíró, Tamás, Balázs I. Tóth, György Haskó, Ralf Paus, and Pál Pacher. 2009 (Aug). "The endocannabinoid system of the skin in health and disease: Novel perspectives and therapeutic opportunities." *Trends Pharmacol Sci.* 30(8):411–20.
2. Fava, G.A., Grandi, S., Savron, G., Bartolucci, G., Santarsiero, G., Trombini, G., and Orlandi, C. 1989. "Psychosomatic assessment of hirsute women." *Psychother Psychosom.* 51(2):96–100.
3. Javidnia, K., Dastgheib, L., Mohammadi Samani, S., and Nasiri, A. 2003. "Antihirsutism activity of fennel (fruits of Foeniculum vulgare) extract. A double-blind placebo controlled study." *Phytomedicine* 10(6-7):455–58.

Hair Loss (Baldness)

1. Bíró, Tamás, Balázs I. Tóth, György Haskó, Ralf Paus, and Pál Pacher. 2009 (Aug). "The endocannabinoid system of the skin in health and disease: Novel perspectives and therapeutic opportunities." *Trends Pharmacol Sci.* 30(8):411–20.

Itching (Pruritis)

1. Bíró, Tamás, Balázs I. Tóth, György Haskó, Ralf Paus, and Pál Pacher. 2009 (Aug). "The endocannabinoid system of the skin in health and disease: Novel perspectives and therapeutic opportunities." *Trends Pharmacol Sci.* 30(8):411–20.
2. Grace, William J., MD, and Graham, David T., MD. Dept. of Medicine of the New York Hospital–Cornell Medical Center. 1952 (Jul 1). "Relationship of specific attitudes and emotions to certain bodily diseases." *Psychosomatic Medicine* 14(4):243–51.

Psoriasis

1. Bíró, Tamás, Balázs I. Tóth, György Haskó, Ralf Paus, and Pál Pacher. 2009 (Aug). "The endocannabinoid system of the skin in health and disease: Novel perspectives and therapeutic opportunities." *Trends Pharmacol Sci.* 30(8):411–20.
2. Aggarwal, B.B., Kumar, A., and Bharti, A.C. 2003 (Jan-Feb). "Anticancer potential of curcumin: Preclinical and clinical studies." *Anticancer Research* 23(1A):363–98.

Seborrhea

1. Schwartz, R.A., Janusz, C.A., and Janniger, C.K. 2006 (Jul 1). "Seborrheic dermatitis: An overview." *Am Fam Physician* 74(1):125–30.

2. Bíró, Tamás, Balázs I. Tóth, György Haskó, Ralf Paus, and Pál Pacher. 2009 (Aug). "The endocannabinoid system of the skin in health and disease: Novel perspectives and therapeutic opportunities." *Trends Pharmacol Sci.* 30(8):411–20.

SYSTEMIC SCLEROSIS

1. Bíró, Tamás, Balázs I. Tóth, György Haskó, Ralf Paus, and Pál Pacher. 2009 (Aug). "The endocannabinoid system of the skin in health and disease: Novel perspectives and therapeutic opportunities." *Trends Pharmacol Sci.* 30(8):411–20.

Vomiting

CHEMOTHERAPY-INDUCED NAUSEA AND VOMITING

1. Parker, L.A., Rock, E., and Limebeer, C. 2011 (Aug). "Regulation of nausea and vomiting by cannabinoids." *Br J Pharmacol.* 163(7):1411–22.
2. Pan, H., Mukhopadhyay, P., Rajesh, M., Patel, V., Mukhopadhyay, B., Gao, B., Haskó, G., and Pacher, P. 2009 (Mar). "Cannabidiol attenuates cisplatin-induced nephrotoxicity by decreasing oxidative/nitrosative stress, inflammation, and cell death." *J Pharmacol Exp Ther.* 328(3):708–14.
3. Meiri, E., Jhangiani, H., Vredenburgh, J.J., Barbato, L.M., Carter, F.J., Yang, H.M., and Baranowski, V. 2007. "Efficacy of dronabinol alone and in combination with ondansetron versus ondansetron alone for delayed chemotherapy-induced nausea and vomiting." *Curr Med Res Opin.* 23(3):533–43.
4. Walsh, D., Nelson, K.A., and Mahmoud, F.A. 2003 (Mar). "Established and potential therapeutic applications of cannabinoids in oncology." *Support Care Cancer.* 11(3):137–43.
5. Tramèr, Martin R., Dawn Carroll, Fiona A. Campbell, D. John, M. Reynolds, R. Andrew Moore, and Henry J. McQuay. 2001. "Cannabinoids for control of chemotherapy induced nausea and vomiting: Quantitative systematic review." *BMJ* 323:16–21.
6. Abrahamov, A., Abrahamov, A., and Mechoulam, R. 1995. "An efficient new cannabinoid antiemetic in pediatric oncology." *Life Sci.* 56(23-24):2097–2102.
7. Lane, M., Vogel, C.L., Ferguson, J., Krasnow, S., Saiers, J.L., Hamm, J., Salva, K., Wiernik, P.H., Holroyde, C.P., Hammill, S., et al. 1991 (Aug). "Dronabinol and prochlorperazine in combination for treatment of cancer chemotherapy-induced nausea and vomiting." *J Pain Symptom Manage.* 6(6):352–59.
8. Cunningham, D., Bradley, C.J., Forrest, G.J., et al. 1988. "A randomized trial of oral nabilone and prochlorperazine compared to intravenous metoclopramide and dexamethasone in the treatment of nausea and vomiting induced by chemotherapy regimens containing cisplatin or cisplatin analogues." *Eur J Cancer Clin Oncol* 24:685–689.

9. McCabe, M., Smith, F.P., Goldberg, D., Macdonald, J., Woolley, P.V., and Warren, R. Division of Medical Oncology, Vincent T. Lombardi Cancer Research Center, Georgetown University, Washington, DC. 1988. "Efficacy of tetrahydrocannabinol in patients refractory to standard anti-emetic therapy." *Investigational New Drugs* 6:243–46.

10. Vinciguerra, V., Moore, T., and Brennan. E. 1988. "Inhalation marijuana as an antiemetic for cancer chemotherapy." *New York State Journal of Medicine* 88: 525–27.

11. Chan, H.S., Correia, J.A., and MacLeod, S.M. 1987. "Nabilone versus pro-chlorperazine for control of cancer chemotherapy-induced emesis in children: A double-blind, crossover trial." *Pediatrics* 79:946–52.

12. Priestman, S.G., Priestman, T.J., and Canney, P.A. 1987. "A double-blind randomized cross-over comparison of nabilone and metoclopramide in the control of radiation-induced nausea." *Clin Radiol.* 38:543–44.

13. Crawford, S.M., and Buckman, R. 1986. "Nabilone and metoclopramide in the treatment of nausea and vomiting due to cisplatinum: A double-blind study." *Med Oncol Tumor Pharmacother.* 3(1):39–42.

14. Dalzell, A.M., Bartlett, H., and Lilleyman, J.S. 1986 (May). "Nabilone: An alternative antiemetic for cancer chemotherapy." *Arch Dis Child.* 61(5):502–05.

15. Pomeroy, M., Fennelly, J.J., and Towers, M. 1986. "Prospective random-ized double-blind trial of nabilone versus domperidone in the treatment of cytotoxic-induced emesis." *Cancer Chemother Pharmacol* 17(3):285–88.

16. Niiranen, A., and Mattson, K. 1985 (Aug). "A cross-over comparison of nabi-lone and prochlorperazine for emesis induced by cancer chemotherapy." *Ameri-can Journal of Clinical Oncology* 8(4):336–40.

17. Ahmedzai, S., Carlyle, D.L., Calder, I.T., and Moran, F. 1983 (Nov). "Anti-emetic efficacy and toxicity of nabilone, a synthetic cannabinoid, in lung can-cer chemotherapy." *Br J Cancer* 48(5):657–63.

18. George, M., Pejovic, M.H., Thuaire, M., Kramar, A., and Wolff, J.P. 1983. "Randomized comparative trial of a new anti-emetic, nabilone, in cancer patients treated with cisplatin." *Biomed Pharmacother.* 37(1):24–27.

19. Hutcheon, A.W., Palmer, J.B., Soukop, M., Cunningham, D., McArdle, C., Welsh, J., Stuart, F., Sangster, G., Kaye, S., Charlton, D., et al. 1983 (Aug). "A randomised multicentre single blind comparison of a cannabinoid anti-emetic (levonantradol) with chlorpromazine in patients receiving their first cytotoxic chemotherapy." *European Journal for Cancer and Clinical Oncology* 19(8):1087–90.

20. Ungerleider, J.T., Andrysiak, T., Fairbanks, L., Goodnight, J., Sarna, G., and

Jamison, K. 1982. "Cannabis and cancer chemotherapy: A comparison of oral delta-9-THC and prochlorperazine." *Cancer* 50:636–45.

21. Johansson, R., Kilkku, P., and Groenroos, M. 1982 (Dec). "A double-blind, controlled trial of nabilone vs. prochlorperazine for refractory emesis induced by cancer chemotherapy." *Cancer Treat Rev.* 9 Suppl B:25–33.

22. Jones, S.E., Durant, J.R., Greco, F.A., and Robertone, A. 1982 (Dec). "A multi-institutional Phase III study of nabilone vs. placebo in chemotherapy-induced nausea and vomiting." *Cancer Treat Rev.* 9 Suppl B:45–48.

23. Orr, L.E., and McKernan, J.F. 1981. "Antiemetic effect of delta9-tetrahydrocannabinol in chemotherapy-associated nausea and emesis as compared to placebo and compazine." *J Clin Pharmacol* 21:76S–80S.

24. Herman, T.S., Einhorn, L.H., Jones, S.E., Nagy, C., Chester, A.B., Dean, J.C., Furnas, B., Williams, S.D., Leigh, S.A., Dorr, R.T., and Moon, T.E. 1979 (Jun 7). "Superiority of nabilone over prochlorperazine as an antiemetic in patients receiving cancer chemotherapy." *N Engl J Med.* 300(23):1295–97.

25. Sallan, Stephen E., MD, Norman E. Zinberg, MD, and Emil Frei III, MD. 1975. "Antiemetic effect of Delta-9-Tetrahydrocannabinol in patients receiving cancer chemotherapy." *N Engl J Med* 293:795–97.

MOTION SICKNESS

1. Turner, M., and Griffin, M.J. 1999. "Motion sickness in public road transport: Passenger behavior and susceptibility." *Ergonomics* 42:444–61.

2. Cluny, N.L., Naylor, R.J., Whittle, B.A., and Javid, F.A. 2008 (Aug). "The effects of cannabidiol and tetrahydrocannabinol on motion-induced emesis in Suncus murinus." *Basic Clin Pharmacol Toxicol.* 103(2):150–56.

3. Chouker, Alexander, Ines Kaufmann, Simone Kreth, Daniela Hauer, Matthias Feuerecker, Detlef Thieme, Michael Vogeser, Manfred Thiel, and Gustav Schelling. 2010. "Motion sickness, stress and the endocannabinoid system." *PLoS One.* 5(5).

4. Grace, William J., MD, and Graham, David T., MD. Dept. of Medicine of the New York Hospital–Cornell Medical Center. 1952 (Jul 1). "Relationship of specific attitudes and emotions to certain bodily diseases." *Psychosomatic Medicine* 14(4):243–51.

5. Chouker, Alexander, et al. 2010. "Motion sickness, stress and the endocannabinoid system." See note 3.

6. Crockett, S.L., Schühly, W., and Bauer, R. 2007. "Pflanzliche antiemetika. Inhaltsstoffe, molekulare wirkmechanismen und klinische evidenz." *Pharm Unserer Zeit.* 36(5):381–88.

7. *Monographien der E-Kommission (Phyto-Therapie)* (380 monographs). *A ther-*

apeutic guide to herbal medicine evaluating the safety and efficacy of herbs for licensed medical prescribing in Germany. Published between 1984 and 1994 in the Bundesanzeiger (official publication by the Federal Republic of Germany). Copies of the monographs are available at the Heilpflanzen-Welt Bibliothek: http://buecher.heilpflanzen-welt.de/BGA-Commission-E-Monographs/

8. Schmid, R., Schick, T., Steffen, R., Tschopp, A., and Wilk, T. 1994 (Dec 1). "Comparison of seven commonly used agents for prophylaxis of seasickness." *J Travel Med.* 1(4):203–06.

9. Nanthakomon, T., and Pongrojpaw, D. 2006 (Oct). "The efficacy of ginger in prevention of postoperative nausea and vomiting after major gynecologic surgery." *J Med Assoc Thai.* 89 Suppl 4:S130–36.

10. Chittumma, P., Kaewkiattikun, K., and Wiriyasiriwach, B. 2007 (Jan). "Comparison of the effectiveness of ginger and vitamin B6 for treatment of nausea and vomiting in early pregnancy: A randomized double-blind controlled trial." *J Med Assoc Thai.* 90(1):15–20.

Wound Care (in general)

1. Radwan, S., El-Essawy, A., and Sarhan, M.M. 1984. "Experimental evidence for the occurrence in honey of specific substances active against microorganisms." *Zentral Microbiol.* 139:249–55.

   Ibrahim, A.S. 1985. "Antibacterial action of honey." *Bull Islam Med.* 1:363–65.

   Jeddar, A., Kharsany, A., Ramsaroop, U.G., Bhamjee, A., Hafejee, I.E., and Moosa, A. 1985. "The antibacterial action of honey." *South Afri Med J.* 67:257–58.

   Molan, P.C., Smith, I.M., and Reid, G.M. 1988. "A comparison of the antibacterial activities of some New Zealand honeys." *Journal of Agricultural Research* 27:252–56.

   Subramanyam, M. 1991. "Tropical application of honey in treatment of burns." *Br J Surg.* 78:497–98.

2. Cuban Ministry of Public Health, Havana. 1992. Therapeutic Guide to Plant Pharmaceuticals and Honey Pharmaceuticals (Guia Terapeutica Dispensarial de Fitofarmacos y Apifarmacos). Ministerio de Salud Publica, Ciudad de La Habana, Republica de Cuba.

3. Callaway, J., Schwab, U., Harvima, I., Halonen, P., Mykkanen, O., Hyvonen, P., and Jarvinen, T. 2005 (Apr). "Efficacy of dietary hempseed oil in patients with atopic dermatitis." *J Dermatolog Treat.* 16(2):87–94.

Fractured Bones

1. Joshua M. Abzug, MD, Aaron Johnson, MD, MS and Brandon S. Schwartz, MPH. Inappropriate Splint Application for Pediatric Fractures in the Emer-

gency Department and Urgent Care Environment. Presented at the National Conference of the American Academy of Pedeatrics. (San Diego, 2014).

2. Karsak M, Cohen-Solal M, Freudenberg J, Ostertag A, Morieux C, Kornak U, Essig J, Erxlebe E, Bab I, Kubisch C, de Vernejoul MC, Zimmer A. Cannabinoid receptor type 2 gene is associated with human osteoporosis. Department of Psychiatry, Life and Brain Center, University of Bonn, Germany. Hum Mol Genet. 2005 Nov 15;14(22):3389-96.

3. Orr Ofek, Meliha Karsak, Nathalie Leclerc, Meirav Fogel, Baruch Frenkel, Karen Wright, Joseph Tam, Malka Attar-Namdar, Vardit Kram, Esther Shohami, Raphael Mechoulam, Andreas Zimmer, and Itai Bab. Peripheral cannabinoid receptor, CB2, regulates bone mass. Bone Laboratory, Hebrew University of Jerusalem, P.O.B. 12272, Jerusalem 91120, Israel. PNAS January 17, 2006 vol. 103 no. 3 696-701.

4. Bab I, Zimmer A, Melamed E. Cannabinoids and the skeleton: from marijuana to reversal of bone loss. Bone Laboratory, the Hebrew University of Jerusalem, Jerusalem, Israel. Ann Med. 2009;41(8):560-7.

5. Kogan, N. M., Melamed, E., Wasserman, E., Raphael, B., Breuer, A., Stok, K. S., Sondergaard, R., Escudero, A. V., Baraghithy, S., Attar-Namdar, M., Friedlander-Barenboim, S., Mathavan, N., Isaksson, H., Mechoulam, R., Müller, R., Bajayo, A., Gabet, Y. and Bab, I. (2015). Cannabidiol, a Major Non-Psychotropic Cannabis Constituent Enhances Fracture Healing and Stimulates Lysyl Hydroxylase Activity in Osteoblasts. J Bone Miner Res.

Post-Surgery Wounds

1. Burstein, Sumner H., and Zurier, Robert B. 2009 (Mar). "Cannabinoids, endocannabinoids, and related analogs in inflammation." *AAPS J.* 11(1):109–19.

Spinal Cord Injuries

1. There are actually 33 spinal bones. The sacral spine consists of five vertebrae fused without discs in between. The coccyx part of the spine consists of four vertebrae fused without discs in between.

2. Dunn, M., and Davis, R. 1974 (Nov). "The perceived effects of marijuana on spinal cord injured males." *Paraplegia.* 12(3):175.

3. Hagenbach, U., Luz, S., Ghafoor, N., Berger, J.M., Grotenhermen, F., Brenneisen, R., and Mader, M. 2007 (Aug). "The treatment of spasticity with Delta(9)-tetrahydrocannabinol in persons with spinal cord injury." *Spinal Cord.* 45(8):551–62.

4. Kogel, R.W., Johnson, P.B., Chintam, R., Robinson, C.J., and Nemchausky,

B.A. 1995 (Oct). "Treatment of spasticity in spinal cord injury with dronab-inol, a tetrahydrocannabinol derivative." *Am J Ther.* 2(10):799–805.

5. Maurer, M., Henn, V., Dittrich, A., and Hofmann, A. 1990. "Delta-9-tetrahydrocannabinol shows antispastic and analgesic effects in a single case double-blind trial." *Eur Arch Psychiatry Clin Neurosci.* 240(1):1–4.

6. Malec, J., Harvey, R.F., and Cayner, J.J. 1982 (Mar). "Cannabis effect on spasticity in spinal cord injury." *Arch Phys Med Rehabil.* 63(3):116–18.

Chapter V: Integrating Mind-Body Medicine for Deeper Healing

1. Applying the Healing Balm of Deep Relaxation

1. Dusek, J.A., Hibberd, P.L., Buczynski, B., Chang, B.H., Dusek, K.C., John-ston, J.M., Wohlhueter, A.L., Benson, H., and Zusman, R.M. 2008 (Mar). "Stress management versus lifestyle modification on systolic hypertension and medication elimination: A randomized trial." *J Altern Complement Med.* 14(2):129–38.

2. Grainger, J., and Boachie-Ansah, G. 2001 (Nov). "Anandamide-induced relax-ation in sheep arteries: The role of the vascular endothelium, arachidonic acid metabolites and potassium channels." *Br. J. Pharmacol.* 134(5):1003–12.

3. Puente, N., Cui, Y., Lassalle, O., Lafourcade, M., Georges, F., Venance, L., Grandes, P., and Manzoni, O.J. 2011 (Nov 6). "Polymodal activation of the endo-cannabinoid system in the extended amygdala." *Nat Neurosci.* 14(12):1542–47.

4. Sudsuang, R., Chentanez, V., and Veluvan, K. 1991 (Sep). "Effect of Buddhist meditation on serum cortisol and total protein levels, blood pressure, pulse rate, lung volume and reaction time." *Physiol Behav.* 50(3):543–48.

Schneider, R.H., Alexander, C.N., Staggers, F., Orme-Johnson, D.W., Rainforth, M., Salerno, J.W., Sheppard, W., Castillo-Richmond, A., Barnes, V.A., and Nidich, S.I. 2005 (Jan). "A randomized controlled trial of stress reduction in African Americans treated for hypertension for over one year." *Am J Hypertens.* 18(1):88–98.

5. Rosenblatt, Lucy E., MA, Sasikanth Gorantla, MD, Jodi A. Torres, BA, Rubin S. Yarmush, BA, Surita Rao, MD, Elyse R. Park, PhD, MPH, John W. Den-ninger, MD, PhD, Herbert Benson, MD, Gregory L. Fricchione, MD, Bruce Bernstein, PhD, and John B. Levine, MD, PhD. 2011 (Nov). "Relaxation Response-based yoga improves functioning in children with autism: A pilot study." *J Altern Complement Med.* 17(11):1029–35.

2. Using Your Emotional Intelligence for Deeper Healing

1. Kiecolt-Glaser, J.K., McGuire, L., Robles, T.F., and Glaser, R. 2002. "Emotions,

morbidity, and mortality: New perspectives from psychoneuroimmunology." *Annu Rev Psychol.* 53:83–107.

Dickerson, Sally S., MA, Margaret E. Kemeny, PhD, Najib Aziz, MD, Kevin H. Kim, PhD, and John L. Fahey, MD. 2004. "Immunological effects of induced shame and guilt." *Psychosomatic Medicine* 66:124–31.

A. Taking Ownership of Where You are Right Now

1. Cunningham, Alastair J., OC, PhD, CPsych, and Watson, Kimberly, MA. 2004 (Sep). "How psychological therapy may prolong survival in cancer patients: New evidence and a simple theory." *Integr Cancer Ther.* 3(3):214–29.

2. Kubie, L.S., MD, and Margolin, S., MD. 1945 (May 1). "The therapeutic role of drugs in the process of repression, dissociation and synthesis." *Psychosomatic Medicine* 7(3):147–51.

3. Redondo, Roger L., Joshua Kim, Autumn L. Arons, Steve Ramirez, Xu Liu, and Susumu Tonegawa. 2014 (Sep 18). "Bidirectional switch of the valence associated with a hippocampal contextual memory engram." *Nature* 513(7518):426–30.

B. Releasing the Toxins of Suppressed/Repressed Emotions

1. Mann, S.J., and Delon, M. "Improved hypertension control after disclosure of decades-old trauma." *Psychosomatic Medicine* 57(5):501–05.

C. Identifying and Releasing Unhealthy Mental-Emotional Habits

1. Arnett, J.J. 2000 (Jul-Aug). "Optimistic bias in adolescent and adult smokers and nonsmokers." *Addict Behav.* 25(4):625–32.

2. Dickerson, S.S., Kemeny, M.E., Aziz, N., Kim, K.H., and Fahey, J.L. 2004 (Jan-Feb). "Immunological effects of induced shame and guilt." *Psychosom Med.* 66(1):124–31.

3. Boiten, Frans A., Nico H. Frijda, and Cornelis J.E. Wientjes. 1994 (Jul). "Emotions and respiratory patterns: Review and critical analysis." *International Journal of Psychophysiology* 17(2):103–28.

D. Exploring and Building Healthy Mental-Emotional Habits

Discernment, Curiosity and Tempered Positivity

1. Fredrickson, Barbara. 2003 (Jul-Aug). "The value of positive emotions: The emerging science of positive psychology is coming to understand why it's good to feel good." *American Scientist* 91(4):330.

2. Steptoe, A., Wardle, J., and Marmot, M. 2005. "Positive affect and health-related neuroendocrine, cardiovascular, and inflammatory processes." *Proc Natl Acad Sci USA* 102:6508–12.

3. Richman, L.S., Kubzansky, L., Maselko, J., Kawachi, I., Choo, P., and Bauer,

M. 2005 (Jul). "Positive emotion and health: going beyond the negative." *Health Psychol.* 24(4):422–29.

4. Danner, D.D., Snowdon, D.A., and Friesen, W.V. 2001 (May). "Positive emotions in early life and longevity: Findings from the nun study." *Pers Soc Psychol.* 80(5):804–13.

5. Ostir, G.V., Markides, K.S., Black, S.A., and Goodwin, J.S. 2000 (May). "Emotional well-being predicts subsequent functional independence and survival." *J Am Geriatr Soc.* 48(5):473–78.

6. Gibbons, H. 2009 (Jun). "Evaluative priming from subliminal emotional words: Insights from event-related potentials and individual differences related to anxiety." *Conscious Cogn.* 18(2):383–400.

7. Gottmann, John M., James Coan, Sybil Carrere, and Catherine Swanson. 1998 (Feb). "Predicting marital happiness and stability from newlywed interactions." *Journal of Marriage and the Family* 60:5–22.

8. Fredrickson, Barbara L., and. Losada, Marcial F. 2005 (Oct). "Positive affect and the complex dynamics of human flourishing." *Am Psychol.* 60(7): 678–86.

9. Heather Barry Kappesa, Gabriele Oettingena. 2011 (Jul). "Positive fantasies about idealized futures sap energy." *Journal of Experimental Social Psychology* 47(4):719–29.

10. Sevincer, A.T., Busatta, P.D., and Oettingen, G. 2014 (Feb). "Mental contrasting and transfer of energization." *Pers Soc Psychol Bull.* 40(2):139–52.

Oettingen, G., Mayer, D., Timur Sevincer, A., Stephens, E.J., Pak, H.J., and Hagenah, M. 2009 (May). "Mental contrasting and goal commitment: The mediating role of energization." *Pers Soc Psychol Bull.* 35(5):608–22.

Three Healing Habits: Gratitude, Compassion, and Forgiveness

1. McCraty, R., Barrios-Choplin, B., Rozman, D., Atkinson, M., and Watkins, A.D. 1998 (Apr-Jun). "The impact of a new emotional self-management program on stress, emotions, heart rate variability, DHEA and cortisol." *Integr Physiol Behav Sci.* 33(2):151–70.

2. Emmons, Robert A., and McCullough, Michael E. 2003. "Counting blessings versus burdens: An experimental investigation of gratitude and subjective well-being in daily life." *Journal of Personality and Social Psychology* 84(2):377–89.

3. Affleck, G., Tennen, H., Croog, S., and Levine, S. 1987. "Causal attributions, perceived benefits and morbidity after heart attack: An 8-year study." *Journal of Consulting and Clinical Psychology* 55:29–35.

4. Miller, T.Q., Smith, T.W., Turner, C.W., Guijarro, M.L., and Hallet, A.J. 1996. "A meta-analytic review of research on hostility and physical health." *Psychological Bulletin* 119:322–48.

5. Kok, B.E., Coffey, K.A., Cohn, M.A., Catalino, L.I., Vacharkulksemsuk, T., Algoe, S.B., Brantley, M., and Fredrickson, B.L. 2013 (Jul 1). "How positive emotions build physical health: Perceived positive social connections account for the upward spiral between positive emotions and vagal tone." *Psychol Sci.* 24(7):1123–32.

6. Hölzel, Britta K., James Carmody, Mark Vangel, Christina Congleton, Sita M. Yerramsetti, Tim Gard, and Sara W. Lazara. 2011 (Jan 30). "Mindfulness practice leads to increases in regional brain gray matter density." *Psychiatry Res.* 191(1): 36–43.

7. Tabak, Benjamin A., Michael E. McCullough, Angela Szeto, Armando J. Mendez, and Philip M. McCabe. 2011. "Oxytocin indexes relational distress following interpersonal harms in women." *Psychoneuroendocrinology* 36:115–22.

   Berry, J.W., and Worthington, E.L., Jr. 2001. "Forgivingness, relationship quality, stress while imagining relationship events, and physical and mental health." *Journal of Counseling Psychology* 48:447–55.

8. Witvliet, C.V., Ludwig, T.E., and Bauer, D.J. 2002. "Please forgive me: Transgressors' emotions and physiology during imagery of seeking forgiveness and victim responses." *Journal of Psychology and Christianity* 21:219–33.

9. Thoresen, C.E., Harris, A.H.S., and Luskin, F. 2000. *Forgiveness: Theory, Research, and Practice* (New York: Guilford Press), pp. 254–80.

   Greenwald, D.F., and Harder, D.W. 1994. "Sustaining fantasies and psychopathology in a normal sample." *Journal of Clinical Psychology* 50:707–10.

   Bono, Giacomo, and McCullough, Michael E. 2006. "Positive responses to benefit and harm: Bringing forgiveness and gratitude into cognitive psychotherapy." *University of Miami. Journal of Cognitive Psychotherapy: An International Quarterly* 20(2).

E. Transforming Unhealthy Emotional Habits Into Positive Ones

1. Hansen, E., and Bejenke, C. 2010 (Mar). "Negative and positive suggestions in anaesthesia: Improved communication with anxious surgical patients." *Anaesthesist.* 59(3):199–202, 204–06, 208–09.

2. Dusek, J.A., Out, H.H., Wohlhueter, A.L., Bhasin, M., Zerbini, L.F., Joseph, M.G., Benson, H., and Libermann, T.A. 2008 (Jul 2). "Genomic counterstress changes induced by the relaxation response." *PLoS One.* 3(7):e2576.

3. Using the Power of Choice for Ongoing Healing

1. Taylor, Jill Bolte, PhD. 2008. *My Stroke of Insight: A Brain Scientist's Personal Journey.* (New York: Viking Penguin).

2. Jill Bolte Taylor's "Stroke of Insight" speech at TED.com. To see the speech go to: www.ted.com/talks/jill_bolte_taylor_s_powerful_stroke_of_insight?language=en

3. Ibid.

4. Ibid.

5. Talarovicova, A., Krskova, L., and Kiss, A. 2007 (Nov). "Some assessments of the amygdala role in suprahypothalamic neuroendocrine regulation: A mini-review." *Endocr Regul.* 41(4):155–62.

6. Fredrickson, Barbara L., and Losada, Marcial F. 2005 (Oct). "Positive affect and the complex dynamics of human flourishing." *Am Psychol.* 60(7):678–86.

7. Gottmann, John M., James Coan, Sybil Carrere, and Catherine Swanson. 1998 (Feb). "Predicting marital happiness and stability from newlywed interactions." *Journal of Marriage and the Family* 60:5–22.

4. Reprogramming Unhealthy Beliefs and Building Beliefs that Heal

1. Blesching, U. 2001. *Emotional Authorship.* Master's Thesis, Western Institute for Social Research, Berkeley, CA.

2. For more information on Ayaan Hirsi Ali, go to her website at: http://theaha-foundation.org/

3. Lipton, Bruce, PhD. 2008. *Peak Vitality: Raising the Threshold of Abundance in Our Material, Spiritual and Emotional Lives* (Santa Rosa, CA: Elite Books).

4. Shin, L.M., Rauch, S.L., and Pitman, R.K. 2006 (Jul). "Amygdala, medial prefrontal cortex, and hippocampal function in PTSD." *Ann N Y Acad Sci.* 1071:67–79.

5. Kaptchuk, Ted J., Elizabeth Friedlander, John M. Kelley, M. Norma Sanchez, Efi Kokkotou, Joyce P. Singer, Magda Kowalczykowski, Franklin G. Miller, Irving Kirsch, and Anthony J. Lembo. 2010 (Dec 22). "Placebos without deception: A randomized controlled trial in irritable bowel syndrome." *PLoS ONE* 5(12):e15591. doi:10.1371/journal.pone.0015591

   Kaptchuk, Ted J., John M. Kelley, Lisa A. Conboy, Roger B. Davis, Catherine E. Kerr, Eric E. Jacobson, Irving Kirsch, Rosa N. Schyner, Bong Hyun Nam, Long T. Nguyen, Min Park, Andrea L. Rivers, Claire McManus, Efi Kokkotou, Douglas A. Drossman, Peter Goldman, and Anthony J. Lembo. 2008 (Apr 3). "Components of placebo effect: Randomized controlled trial in patients with irritable bowel syndrome." *BMJ* 336:999.

5. Finding the Silver Lining and Wisdom in Your Illness

1. LeShan, Lawrence, PhD. 1989. *Cancer as a Turning Point: A Handbook for People with Cancer, Their Families, and Health Professionals* (New York: A Plume Book).

2. Barefoot, J.C., Dahlstrom, W.G., and Williams, R.B., Jr. 1983 (Mar). "Hostility, CHD incidence, and total mortality: A 25-year follow-up study of 255 physicians." *Psychosomatic Medicine* 45(1):59–63.

3. McCraty, R., Barrios-Choplin, B., Rozman, D., Atkinson, M., and Watkins, A.D. 1998 (Apr-Jun). "The impact of a new emotional self-management program on stress, emotions, heart rate variability, DHEA and cortisol." *Integr Physiol Behav Sci.* 33(2):151–70.

4. Schneck, Jerome M. 1947. "The psychological component in a case of Herpes simplex." *Psychosomatic Medicine* 9:62–64.w

INDEX

Mad cow disease, 424

Maggot debridement therapy, 94

Manic-depressive disorder, 334–36

Marijuana. *See* Cannabis

Martyrdom, 37, 483, 484–86

Mechoulam, Raphael, 6

Meditation, 35, 41–43, 475, 491

Melanoma, 176–79

Menstrual pain, 396–98

Mental contrasting, 488–89

Mental disorders. *See also individual disorders*

diagnosing, 310–11

spiritual view of, 311

Methicillin-resistant *Staphylococcus aureus. See* MRSA

Mexican oregano *(Lippia graveolens)*, 10, 13

Migraine, 414–19

Mind-body medicine. *See also* Emotions; *individual diseases and symptoms*

benefits of, 31–32

choice and, 498–501

"disease as message" paradigm, 506–8

neuroprotection and, 351

overview of, 31–36

pain and, 408–10

questions for exploring, 65

relaxation response and, 473–75

resistance to healing and, 508–9

risk of adverse effects from, 35–36

Mindfulness, 42, 491

Miscarriage, 391

Morning sickness, 398–400

Motion sickness, 456–59

MRSA (methicillin-resistant *Staphylococcus aureus*), 91–94

Multiple sclerosis (MS), 375–82

Myrrh

cancer and, 132, 151, 170, 176, 179

inflammation and, 259, 264, 277, 412

respiratory ailments and, 104

N

Nausea. *See* Vomiting

Neisseria gonorrhea. See Gonorrhea

Nervous system, classification of, 348

Neurogenesis, 1, 2

Neurological diseases. *See also individual diseases*

cannabis and, 349–51

causes of, 349

classification of, 348

food and, 351–52

mind-body medicine and, 351

Neuropathies, 419–23

Nigella

asthma and, 307

cancer and, 132–33, 161, 181

cardiovascular disease and, 204

inflammation and, 259, 264, 277

radiation protection and, 134, 412

Night sweats, 153–55

Night vision, 241

Norepinephrine, 39, 53

NSAIDs (non-steroidal anti-inflammatory drugs), 405, 407

Nutmeg

depression and, 333

diabetes and, 231

libido enhancement and, 300–301

radiation protection and, 134

O

OBGYN (obstetrics and gynecology), 390–91. *See also individual conditions*

OCD (obsessive-compulsive disorder), 319

Ocimum. See Basil

Opioids, 39, 43, 405, 407

Oregano

cancer and, 133, 170

diabetes and, 231

fungi and, 437

oxidative stress reduction and, 235

Osteoarthritis, 259–64

Osteoporosis, 401–3

Oxidative stress reduction, 234, 235

Oxytocin, 39, 44–46, 147

ACKNOWLEDGMENTS

I would like to express my gratitude to the many people and plants who saw me through the creation of this new, revised, and expanded edition of *The Cannabis Health Index (CHI)*.

To the African bone setters from Aponchie Clinic in Accra, Ghana, who shared a secret that years later would be part of *CHI*. To my sister Bianca, my mom Christel, and Kirby Seid for their unwavering support. To my editor Leslie Larson for her combination of warmth of heart and cool, clear thinking that made the complexity of a new edition a breeze. Thanks to Tim McGee for his expert guidance in shaping the book, to the eagle eyes of my copyeditor Kathy Glass, whose attention to details made *CHI* more crisp, precise, and well organized. To designers Jasmine Hromjak and Brad Greene for their artful skills of making the book look clear and beautiful. To Howie Severson for his great cover ideas, which made it difficult to choose just one. To Joyce Thom for her support in clarifying the use of *CHI* and of *chi*. To Tim Sunderman, the sole force and creative artist behind the *CHI* app, *CHI* magazine and the CannabisHealthIndex .com website. And to the forces of synchronicity that directed Chris Keller and David Anderson to place *The Cannabis Health Index* into the hands of a friend, who passed it along to Steve DeAngelo of Harborside Health Center in Oakland, California, who in turn gave it to Richard Grossinger and Doug Reil of North Atlantic Books.

ABOUT THE AUTHOR

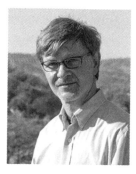

UWE BLESCHING is editor-in-chief of *CHI* magazine and author of *Spicy Healing: A Global Guide to Growing and Using Spices for Food and Medicine.* He is a medical journalist and regular contributor in the field of mind-body medicine. His current focus is on cannabinoid medicine and phytopharmacology as well as evidence-based illness prevention and treatment protocols. In addition to being informed by Blesching's lifelong passion for mind-body medicine, *The Cannabis Health Index* draws from rigorous in-depth research and Blesching's twenty years' experience in emergency medicine as a paramedic for the City of San Francisco. Blesching holds a BA in Humanities from the New College of California and an MA in Psychology and a PhD in Higher Education and Social Change from the Western Institute for Social Research.

Get the Free App and Monthly eMagazine to Support Your Copy of *The Cannabis Health Index*

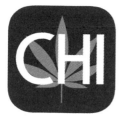

The CHI app puts evidence-based medicine for more than 100 diseases at your fingertips. It provides the same rating system as the book, making it easy to determine at a glance what the current scientific consensus says about how cannabis may work for a specific condition. The app offers practical ways that cannabis can improve your health, cutting-edge mind-body approaches that produce powerful healing, and suggestions for maintaining a positive approach to help you feel empowered and motivated as you heal.

CHI magazine keeps you up-to-date on the latest science and healing approaches. Monthly editions examine new research and offer innovative articles on topics such as mind-body medicine, cannabinoid-based medicine, and emotional intelligence. Published in Apple News.

For more information, visit CannabisHealthIndex.com.

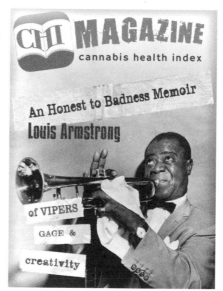